Carotid Disease

The Role of Imaging in Diagnosis and Management

Stroke is a major cause of morbidity and mortality, with carotid disease representing an important contributory risk factor. This book is a comprehensive review of the pathogenesis and management of carotid disease with specific focus on the role imaging has to play in the early recognition of symptomatic and asymptomatic disease as well as the treatment of the developed condition. Technological advances in imaging modalities now allow detailed analysis of the disease progression, the prediction of critical events leading to a stroke, as well as the identification of the most effective surgical or other interventional treatments. This book should be read by neurologists, cardiologists, vascular surgeons, neurosurgeons and radiologists involved in the care of patients with carotid disease, and also by researchers involved in the development of new diagnostic and therapeutic techniques and drugs.

Jonathan Gillard is a reader in neuroradiology at the University of Cambridge, and an honorary consultant radiologist at Cambridge University Hospital's NHS Foundation Trust.

Martin Graves is consultant clinical scientist in the Departments of Radiology and Medical Physics at Cambridge University Hospitals NHS Foundation Trust.

Thomas Hatsukami is a professor of vascular surgery at the University of Washington School of Medicine, Seattle, Washington.

Chun Yuan is a professor of radiology at the University of Washington, Seattle, Washington.

Carotid Disease

The Role of Imaging in Diagnosis and Management

Jonathan Gillard

University of Cambridge

Martin Graves

University of Cambridge

Thomas Hatsukami

University of Washington

Chun Yuan

University of Washington

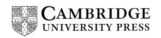

CAMBRIDGE UNIVERSITY PRESS

Cambridge, New York, Melbourne, Madrid, Cape Town, Singapore, São Paulo

Cambridge University Press
The Edinburgh Building, Cambridge CB2 2RU, UK
Published in the United States of America by Cambridge University Press, New York

www.cambridge.org
Information on this title: www.cambridge.org/9780521862264

First published 2007

Printed in the United Kingdom at the University Press, Cambridge

A catalogue record for this publication is available from the British Library

Library of Congress Cataloguing in Publication data

Carotid disease : the role of imaging in diagnosis and management / [edited by]
Jonathan Gillard ... [et al.].
   p. ; cm.
Includes bibliographical references and index.
ISBN-13:   978-0-521-86226-4 (hardback)
ISBN-10:   0-521-86226-4 (hardback)
1. Carotid artery—Imaging. 2. Carotid artery—Diseases—Diagnosis. I. Gillard,
Jonathan H., 1964-
[DNLM: 1. Carotid Artery Diseases—diagnosis. 2. Carotid Artery Diseases—therapy.
3. Diagnostic Imaging—methods. WL 355 C2933 2006] I. Title.
RC691.6.152C37 2006
616.1′36075—dc22

                                                                2006020517

ISBN-13   978-0-521-86226-4 hardback
ISBN-10   0-521-86226-4 hardback

Contents

Contributors

Pippa G. Al-Rawi, B.Sc.
University Department of Neurosurgery
Cambridge University Hospitals NHS Foundation
  Trust
Cambridge CB2 2QQ
UK

Donna K. Arnett, Ph.D.
Department of Epidemiology
University of Alabama at Birmingham School of
  Public Health
Birmingham, AL 35294
USA

Henry, J. M. Barnett, C.C., M.D., D.Sc., F.R.C.P.C.
Professor Emeritus, University of Western Ontario
Scientist Emeritus, Robarts Research Institute
London, Ontario N6A 5K8
Canada

Jonathan L. Brisman, M.D.
Department of Cerebrovascular and Endovascular
  Neurosurgery
New Jersey Neuroscience Institute
JFK Medical Center
65 James Street
Edison, NJ, 08818
USA

Allen Burke, M.D.
CVPath
The International Registry of Pathology
19 Firstfield Road
Gaithersburg MD 20878
USA

Andrew Carlson, M.D.
Department of Neurosurgery
University of New Mexico
Albuquerque New Mexico 87151
USA

Andrew G. Clifton
Department of Neuroradiology
2nd Floor, Atkinson Morley Wing
St George's Hospital
London SW17 0QT
UK

John Crouse
Department of Internal Medicine
Wake Forest University School of Medicine
Medical Center Boulevard
Winston-Salem NC 27175
USA

John R. Davies, B.Sc., M.B.B.S., M.R.C.P.
Department of Cardiovascular Medicine
University of Cambridge
Cambridge University Hospitals NHS Foundation
    Trust
Cambridge CB2 2QQ
UK

Zahi A. Fayad, Ph.D.
Mount Sinai School of Medicine
One Gustave L. Levy Place
Imaging Science Laboratories
Box 1234
New York, NY 10029
USA

Michael Gaunt, M.D., F.R.C.S.
Department of Surgery
Cambridge University Hospitals NHS Foundation
    Trust
Cambridge CB2 2QQ
UK

Matthew F. Giles, M.R.C.P.
Stroke Prevention Research Unit
University Department of Clinical Neurology
Radcliffe Infirmary
Woodstock Road
Oxford OX2 6HE
UK

Jonathan H. Gillard, M.D., F.R.C.R.
Department of Radiology
University of Cambridge
Cambridge CB2 2QQ
UK

Alison H. Goodall, Ph.D.
Department of Cardiovascular Sciences
University of Leicester
Glenfield Hospital
Leicester LE3 9QP
UK

Martin J. Graves, M.Sc.
Departments of Radiology & Medical Physics
Cambridge University Hospitals NHS Foundation
    Trust
Cambridge CB2 2QQ
UK

Jeroen van der Grond, M.D.
Department of Radiology
Leiden University Medical Center
Leiden 2300 RC
The Netherlands

Alison Halliday, M.S., F.R.C.S.
Department of Cardiological Sciences
St George's Hospital Medical School
London SW17 0RE
UK

Jamie Harle
Department of Medical Physics
Cambridge University Hospitals NHS Foundation
    Trust
Cambridge CB2 2QQ
UK

Thomas Hatsukami, M.D., F.A.C.S.
Department of Surgery
University of Washington School of Medicine
815 Mercer Street
Box 358050
Seattle WA 98109
USA

William Hollingworth, Ph.D.
Department of Radiology
University of Washington,
Seattle WA 98103
USA

Simon P. S. Howarth, M.R.C.S.
Department of Radiology
University of Cambridge
Cambridge CB2 2QQ
UK

Fabien Hyafil, M.D.
Mount Sinai School of Medicine
One Gustave L. Levy Place
Imaging Science Laboratories
Box 1234
New York, NY 10029
USA

William Kerwin, Ph.D.
Department of Radiology
University of Washington
Box 358050
815 Mercer Street
Seattle, WA 98109
USA

Peter J. Kirkpatrick, F.R.C.S. (S.N.)
University Department of Neurosurgery
Cambridge University Hospitals NHS Foundation
    Trust
Cambridge CB2 2QQ
UK

Frank D. Kolodgie, Ph.D.
CVPath
The International Registry of Pathology
19 Firstfield Road
Gaithersburg MD 20878
USA

Elena Ladich, M.D.
CVPath
The International Registry of Pathology
19 Firstfield Road
Gaithersburg MD 20878
USA

David Lester, Ph.D.
Pfizer Inc, Global Clinical Platforms
685 Third Avenue
Mailstop 685/19/7
New York, NY 10017
USA

Michael J. Lipinski, B.S.
Mount Sinai School of Medicine
One Gustave L. Levy Place
Imaging Science Laboratories
Box 1234
New York, NY 10029
USA

Fei Liu, Ph.D.
Department of Radiology
University of Washington
Seattle, WA 98195
USA

Aad van der Lugt, M.D., Ph.D.
Department of Radiology
Erasmus MC
University Medical Center
Rotterdam
The Netherlands

Charles B. L. M. Majoie, M.D., Ph.D.
Department of Neuroradiology
Academic Medical Center
PO Box 22700
1100 DE Amsterdam
The Netherlands

Greg McMahon, M.R.C.S.
Department of Cardiovascular Sciences
University of Leicester
Glenfield Hospital
Leicester LE3 9QP
UK

Stephen Meairs, M.D., Ph.D.
Faculty of Clinical Medicine Mannheim
University of Heidelberg
68167 Mannheim
Germany

Gregory Moneta, M.D.
Oregon Health and Science University
3181 SW Sam Jackson Park Road
Mail Code OP-11
Multnomah Pavilion 1600
Portland Oregon 97239-3098
USA

Marc R. Mayberg, M.D.
The Department of Neurosurgery
Seattle Neuroscience Institute
Seattle, WA 98122
USA

Alan Moody, F.R.C.P., F.R.C.R.
Department of Diagnostic Imaging
Sunnybrook Health Sciences Centre
H2075 Bayview
Toronto, Ontario M4N 3M5
Canada

Paul J. Nederkoorn, M.D., Ph.D.
Department of Neurology
Academic Medical Center
PO Box 22700
1100 DE Amsterdam
The Netherlands

Stephen Nicholls, M.B.B.S., Ph.D., F.R.A.C.P.
The Cleveland Clinic Foundation
Department of Cardiovascular Medicine/F15
9500 Euclid Avenue
Cleveland OH 44195
USA

Steven Nissen, M.D., F.A.C.C.
The Cleveland Clinic Foundation
Department of Cardiovascular Medicine/F15
9500 Euclid Avenue
Cleveland OH 44195
USA

Christopher O'Donnell, M.D., Ph.D.
Massachusetts General Hospital
Harvard Medical School
Framingham MA 01702
USA

Kuniaki Ogasawara, M.D.
Department of Neurosurgery
Iwate Medical University
Uchimaru 19-1
Morioka 020-8505
Japan

Mohamed Ouhlous, M.D.
Department of Radiology
Erasmus MC
University Medical Center
Rotterdam
The Netherlands

James Revkin, M.D.
Pfizer Inc, PGRD
50 Pequot Ave, MS-6025
A4115
New London, CT 06320
USA

Stephen S. Rich, Ph.D.
Department of Public Health Sciences
Wake Forest University School of Medicine
Winston-Salem NC 27157-1063
USA

Gaston A. Rodriguez-Granillo, M.D.
Interventional Cardiology, Room H922
Thoraxcenter Bd 406
Erasmus MC
Dr Molewaterplein 40
3015 GD Rotterdam
The Netherlands

John A. Ronald, M.Sc.
Imaging Research Laboratories
Robarts Research Institute
London, Ontario N6A 5KA
Canada

Peter M. Rothwell, M.D., Ph.D., F.R.C.P.
University Department of Clinical Neurology
Radcliffe Infirmary
Woodstock Road
Oxford OX2 6HE
UK

James H. F. Rudd, M.R.C.P., Ph.D.
Mount Sinai School of Medicine
One Gustave L. Levy Place
Imaging Science Laboratories
Box 1234
New York, NY 10029
USA

Brian K. Rutt, Ph.D.
Robarts Research Institute
London, Ontario N6A 5KA
Canada

Marc R. H. M. van Sambeek, M.D., Ph.D.
Department of Vascular Surgery
Erasmus MC
University Medical Center
Rotterdam
The Netherlands

Patrick Serruys, M.D., Ph.D.
Interventional Cardiology
Toraxcenter Bd 406
Erasmus MC
Dr Molewaterplein 40
3015 GD Rotterdam
The Netherlands

Jan Stam, M.D., Ph.D.
Department of Neurology
Academic Medical Center
PO Box 22700
1100 DE Amsterdam
The Netherlands

Dalin Tang, Ph.D.
Mathematical Sciences Department
Worcester Polytechnic Institute
Worcester, MA 01609
USA

Tjun Tang, M.R.C.S.
Department of Radiology
University of Cambridge
Cambridge CB2 2QQ
UK

Rikin Trivedi, M.R.C.P., M.R.C.S.
Department of Radiology
University of Cambridge
Cambridge CB2 2QQ
UK

E. Murat Tuzcu, M.D.
The Cleveland Clinic Foundation
Department of Cardiovascular Medicine/F15
9500 Euclid Avenue
Cleveland OH 44195
USA

Jean Marie U-King-Im, M.R.C.S.
Department of Radiology
University of Cambridge
Cambridge CB2 2QQ
UK

Stella Vig, M.Ch., F.R.C.S. (Gen. Surg.)
Department of Vascular Surgery
Mayday University Hospital
Croydon CR7 7YE
UK

Renu Virmani, M.D.
CVPath
The International Registry of Pathology,
19 Firstfield Road
Gaithersburg MD 20878
USA

Thomas de Weert, M.D.
Department of Radiology
Erasmus MC
University Medical Center
Rotterdam
The Netherlands

Peter L. Weissberg, M.D., F.R.C.P.
Department of Cardiovascular Medicine
University of Cambridge
Cambridge University Hospitals NHS Foundation
   Trust
Cambridge CB2 2QQ
UK

Nigel Wood, Ph.D.
Department of Chemical Engineering
Imperial College London
London SW7 2AZ
UK

Dongxiang Xu, Ph.D.
Department of Radiology
University of Washington
Seattle, WA 98195
USA

Yun Xu, Ph.D.
Department of Chemical Engineering
Imperial College London
London SW7 2AZ
UK

Chun Yang, Ph.D.
Mathematical Sciences Department
Worcester Polytechnic Institute
Worcester, MA 01609
USA

Howard Yonas, M.D.
Department of Neurosurgery
University of New Mexico
Albuquerque New Mexico 87151
USA

Chun Yuan, Ph.D.
Department of Radiology
University of Washington
Seattle, WA 98195
USA

Abbreviations

123I-IMP	N-isopropyl-p-[123I]-iodoamphetamine
[3H]DG	Tritiated deoxyglucose
18FDG PET	18Fluoro-deoxyglucose positron emission tomography
AAC	Abdominal aortic calcific (deposits)
ABP	Arterial blood pressure
ABC	Activity-based costing
ACA	Anterior cerebral artery
ACAPS	Asymptomatic carotid artery progression study
ACAS	Asymptomatic carotid atherosclerosis study
ACE	ASA and carotid endarterectomy trial
ACS	Acute coronary syndromes
ACST	Asymptomatic carotid surgery trial
ACST II	Asymptomatic carotid surgery trial II
ACT	Activated clotting time
AF	Atrial fibrillation
AHA	American Heart Association
AIF	Arterial input function
AP	Aortic plaque
ARIC	Arteriosclerosis risk in communities study
ARR	Absolute risk reduction
ASL	Arterial spin labeling
BC	Boundary conditions
BEACH	Boston scientific EPI-A carotid stenting trial for high risk surgical patients

BHI	Breath holding index	COSS	Carotid occlusion surgery study
BMI	Body mass index	COX-1	Cyclo-oxygenase-1
BOLD	Blood oxygen level-dependent	CPP	Cerebral perfusion pressure
BTO	Balloon test occlusion	CPR	Curved planar reformations
CABERNET	Carotid artery revascularization using the bostonscientific filter wire and the EndoTex nex stent	CPVI	Computational plaque vulnerability index
		CREST	Carotid revascularization endarterectomy versus stenting trial
CABG	Coronary artery bypass graft		
CAD	Coronary artery disease		
CAMELOT	Comparison of amlodipine vs. enalapril to limit occurrences of thrombosis	CRP	C-reactive protein
		CT	Computerized tomography
		CTA	Computerized tomography angiography
CAPRIE	Clopidogrel versus aspirin in patients at risk of ischemic events	CTP	Computerized tomography perfusion
CARESS	Clopidogrel and aspirin for reduction of emboli in symptomatic carotid stenosis	CURE	Effects of clopidogrel in addition to aspirin in patients with acute coronary syndromes without ST-segment elevation
CAS	Carotid artery stenting		
CASCADE	Computer-aided system for cardiovascular disease evaluation	CVD	Cardiovascular disease
		CVR	Cerebral vasodilatory response
CASL	Continuous arterial spin labeling	CW	Continuous wave
CASTIA	Clopidogrel in acute stroke and TIA	DCE	Dynamic contrast-enhanced
CAVATAS	Carotid and vertebral artery transluminal angioplasty study	DEP	Distal embolic protection
		DESPOT	Driven equilibrium single pulse observation of T1
CBF	Cerebral blood flow		
CBV	Cerebral blood volume	DESPOD	Driven equilibrium single pulse observation in three dimensions
CCA	Common carotid artery		
CCAIT	Canadian coronary atherosclerosis intervention trial	DIFF	Diffusion-based
		df	Degrees of freedom
CDFI	Color Doppler flow imaging	DIPLOMA	Double inversions with proximal labeling of both tag and control images
CEMRA	Contrast enhanced magnetic resonance angiography		
CE	Conformité Européene (European Conformity)	DIR	Double inversion recovery
		DNA	Deoxyribonucleic acid
CE MRI	Contrast-enhanced MRI	DOF	Degrees-of-freedom
CFD	Computational fluid dynamics	DSA	Digital subtraction angiography
CFR	Code of federal regulations	DSC-MRI	Dynamic susceptibility contrast magnetic resonance angiography
CHD	Coronary heart disease		
CHI	Contrast harmonic imaging	DTPA	Diethyltriaminepentaacetic acid
CHMP	Committee for medicinal products for human use	DUS	Duplex ultrasound
		DWI	Diffusion weighted imaging
CHS	Cardiovascular health study	DZ	Dyzygotic
CI	Confidence interval	EBCT	Electron beam CT
CLAS	Cholesterol lowering atherosclerosis study	ECA	External carotid artery

ECIC	Extracranial-intracranial	HMG-CoA	b-hydroxy-b-methylglutaryl-CoA
ECG	Electrocardiogram	HMPAO	Hexamethyl propylene amine oxime
ECST	European carotid surgery	HPS	Heart protection study
EDC	Ethyl cysteinate dimer	HPVI	Histopathological plaque vulnerability index
EEM	External elastic membrane		
EES	Extravascular extracellular space	HR	Hazard ratio
EMEA	European medicines agency	HU	Hounsfield units
EPI	Echo planar imaging	ICA	Internal carotid artery
EPISTAR	Echo-planar imaging and signal targeting with alternating RF	ICAM	Intercellular adhesion molecule
		ICC	Intraclass correlation coefficient
		ICER	Incremental cost effectiveness ratio
EPOM	Electromagnetic position and orientation measurement		
ER	Endoplasmic reticular	ICSS	International carotid stenting study
ERF	Erasmus rucphen family		
ESPS-2	European stroke prevention study 2	IDTCFA	Intravascular ultrasound derived thin cap fibroatheroma
EVA-3S	Endarterectomy versus angioplasty in patients with severe symptomatic carotid stenosis	IH	Internal hyperplasia
		IL	Interleukin
		ImQ	Image quality
F	Factor (clotting)	IMT	Intima media thickness
FAIR	Flow sensitive alternating inversion recovery	INR	International normalized ratio
		IPH	Intraplaque hemorrhage
FASTER	Fast assessment of stroke and transient ischemic attack to prevent early recurrence	IRON	Inversion recovery on-resonance water suppression
		IT	Intimal thickening
FATS	Familial Atherosclerosis Treatment Study	IVUS	Intravascular ultrasound
		IVUS-VH	Intravascular ultrasound-virtual histology
FC	Fibrous cap		
FDA	Food and Drug Administration	KAPS	Kupio atherosclerosis study
FE	Finite element	KFRS	Kalman filtering registration and smoothing
FSE	Fast-spin-echo		
FSI	Fluid-structure interaction	LCAS	Lipoprotein and coronary atherosclerosis study
FT	Fourier tranform		
FV	Flow velocity	LDF	Laser Doppler flowmetry
GP	Glycoprotein	LDL	Low-density lipoprotein
GPx	Glutathione peroxidase	LDL-C	Low-density lipoprotein cholesterol
GRAPPA	Generalized autocalibrating partially parallel acquisition		
		LMMSE	Linear minimum mean square error
GRASP	Gradient echo acquisition for superparamagnetic particles with positive contrast		
		LOD	Logarithmic of the odds
		LR	Lipid rich
Hb	Deoxyhemoglobin	LRNC	Lipid rich necrotic core
HbO2	Oxyhemoglobin	MAAS	Multicenter anti-atheroma study
HDL	High-density lipoprotein	MAP	Mean arterial pressure

MARS	Monitored atherosclerosis regression study	NS	Not significant
MATCH	Management of atherothrombosis with clopidogrel in high-risk patients	N-S	Navier-Stokes
		NWI	Normalized wall index
		OCT	Optical coherence tomography
		OEF	Oxygen extraction fraction
MAVERIC	Evaluation of the Medtronic AVE self-expanding carotid stent system with distal protection in the treatment of carotid stenosis	ORION	Outcome of rosuvastatin treatment on carotid artery atheroma
		OR	Odds ratio
		OSI	Oscillatory shear index
MBFV	Mean blood flow velocity	oxLDL	Oxidized LDL
MCA	Middle cerebral artery	PAI-1	Plasminogen inhibitor type-1
MCP-1	Monocyte chemotactic protein-1	PASL	Pulsed arterial spin labeling
M-CSF	Macrophage colony-stimulating factor	PC	Phase contrast
		PCA	Posterior cerebral artery
MDA-2	Radiolabeled malondialdehyde-2	PDI	Power Doppler imaging
MDT	Multidisciplinary team	PDW	Proton density weighted
MEPPS	Morphology-enhanced probabilistic plaque segmentation	PET	Positron emission tomography
		PH	Plaque hemorrhage
MES	Micro-embolic signals	PLAC	Pravastatin limitation of atherosclerosis in the coronary and carotid arteries
MIP	Maximum intensity projection		
MLD	Minimum lumen diameter		
MMBE	Matched mask bone elimination	POC	Proof of Concept
MMP	Matrix metalloproteinase	POM	Position and orientation measurement
MOTSA	Multiple overlapping thin slab acquisition		
		PON	Paraoxonase
MPO	Myeloperoxidase	PPV	Positive predictive value
MPR	Multi-planar reformations	PR	Plaque rupture
MR	Magnetic resonance	PROPELLER	Periodically overlapping parallel lines with enhanced reconstruction
MRA	Magnetic resonance angiography		
MRC	Medical research council		
MRI	Magnetic resonance imaging	PROVE-IT	Pravastatin or atorvastatin evaluation and infection therapy
MSCT	Multislice CT		
MSCTA	Multislice CTA	PS	Phosphatidyl serine
MSR	Macrophage scavenger receptor	PWV	Pulse wave velocity
MTT	mean transit time	QALY	Quality adjusted life years
MZ	Monozygotic	QCA	Quantitative coronary angiography
NAA	N-acetyl aspartate	QIR	Quadruple inversion recovery
NASCET	North American symptomatic carotid endarterectomy trial	QTL	Quantitative-trait loci
		QUIPPS	Quantitative imaging of perfusion using a single subtraction
NC	Necrotic core		
NI	New intimal		
NIRS	Near infrared spectroscopy	RARE	Rapid acquisition with relaxation enhancement
NNT	Number needed to treat		
NPV	Negative predictive value	RCT	Randomized clinical trial

rCVR	Regional cerebrovascular reactivity	SPIO	Superparamagnetic iron oxide
REGRESS	Regression growth evaluation statin study	SPIRIT	Stroke prevention in reversible ischemia trial
RES	Reticuloendothelial system	SSD	Shaded surface display
REVERSAL	Reversal of atherosclerosis with aggressive lipid lowering	SSFP	Steady-state free precession
		STA	Superficial temporal artery
REX	Rapid extended coverage	STARD	Standards for reporting of diagnostic accuracy
RF	Radiofrequency		
RFLP	Restriction fragment length polymorphisms	STLCOS	St. Louis carotid occlusion study
		TACIT	Transatlantic asymptomatic carotid interventional trial
RGB	Red-green-blue		
rHDL	Recombinant high-density lipoprotein	TCD	Transcranial Doppler
		TCFA	Thin cap fibroatheroma
ROC	Receiver operating curve	TE	Echo time
ROI	Region of interest	TF	Tissue factor
RRR	Relative risk reduction	TFPI	Tissue factor pathway inhibitor
rSO2	Regional oxygen saturation	TH	Thrombus
SAPPHIRE	Stent and angioplasty with protection for patients at high risk for endarterectomy	TxA2	Thromboxane A2
		TI	Inversion time
		TIA	Transient ischemic attack
SBA	Slab boundary artefact	TILT	Transfer insensitive labeling technique
SBP	Systolic blood pressure		
SE	Sensitivity	TNF	Tumour necrosis factor
SENSE	Sensitivity encoding	TNT	Treating to new targets
SEP	Sensory evoked potential	TOF	Time of flight
SHELTER	Stenting of high risk patients extracranial lesions trial with embolic removal	TOI	Tissue oxygen Index
		tPA	Tissue plasminogen activator
		TTP	Time to peak
SI	Signal intensity	TR	Repetition time
SjO2	Venous oxygen saturation	TRF	Telomeric repeat binding factor
SLINKY	Sliding interleaved kY	TRICKS	Time-resolved imaging of contrast kinetics
SMASH	Simultaneous acquisition of spatial harmonics		
		uPA	Urokinase-type plasminogen activator
SNP	Single nucleotide polymorphism		
SNR	Signal-to-noise ratio	US	Ultrasound
SP	Specificity	USPIO	Ultrasmall paramagnetic iron oxide
SPACE	Stent protected percutaneous angioplasty versus carotid endarterectomy trial		
		uTE	Ultrashort echo times
		VASST	Veterems administration symptomatic stenosis trial
SPARCL	Stroke prevention by aggressive reduction in cholesterol levels		
		VBA	Vertebrobasilar arteries
SPECT	Single positron emission computed tomography	VCAM	Vascular cell adhesion molecule
		VN	Vitronectin
SPGR	Spoiled gradient-recalled echo	VR	Volume rendering

VSMC	Vascular smooth muscle cells	WASID	Warfarin aspirin symptomatic intracranial disease
VWA	Vessel wall area		
VWF	von Willebrand factor	WHHL	Wantanabe heritable hyperlipidemic
WARSS	Warfarin aspirin recurrent stroke study	WSS	Wall shear stress

Introduction

Henry J. M. Barnett

Professor Emeritus, University of Western Ontario
Scientist Emeritus, Robarts Research Institute

The chronology of events that have led to the preparation of this book is fascinating and unique. When people of my generation went to medical school they heard very little about the importance of the main artery to the brain. Stroke was universally considered as a consequence of intra-cerebral hemorrhage or intracerebral arterial thrombosis particularly of the middle cerebral artery. Even the angiographic identification of internal carotid artery stenosis and occlusion in the late 1920s and early 1930s by Moniz failed to stimulate the worldwide medical community to adopt this diagnostic breakthrough, and to focus on the internal carotid artery. Legitimate concerns about the potential hazards of the use of radio-active thorotrast, the contrast medium used by the pioneers, with its biological half-life of hundreds of years, and the custom of cutting down on the carotid artery deterred enthusiasm for the use of the procedure. In the 1940s Hultquist and Fisher carried out postmortem studies of the previously neglected portion of the extracranial carotid artery independently in Sweden and Canada. They iden-tified this vessel as a common site of arteriosclero-tic disease causing stroke. Almost coincident with these illuminating publications came the introduc-tion of percutaneous angiography and the recogni-tion of transient ischemic attack as a harbinger of stroke. All this accumulated knowledge led to a 1954 *Lancet* case-report by Eastcott and Rob at St. Mary's Hospital, London, describing the surgical removal of the diseased portion of a symptomatic carotid artery. Within two decades, approximately one million carotid endarterectomies had been performed worldwide. Carotid surgery had arrived and so too had the rapid development of neuroradiology.

Concern about the unproven indications for carotid endarterectomy and the absence of any delineation of acceptable morbidity and mortality from the procedure led to the performance of two large randomized trials for symptomatic carotid artery disease (NASCET and ECST) and in time two trials examining the benefit for subjects with asymptomatic carotid disease (ACAS and ACST). Standards emerged from these large studies, determining who should and should not perform endarterectomy and on which patients. The symptomatic patients were all studied and the results analyzed based on conventional angiography. The asymptomatic studies were based on ultrasound evaluations of stenosis. Reasonable but not totally perfect correlations were effected converting ultrasound evaluations to what had come to be accepted as the NASCET method of measuring the severity of the disease. The single most important prognostic variable proved to be the degree of arterial stenosis.

The simplicity and safety of noninvasive methods of measurement made them desirable. Happily, innovative and ingenious imaging has begun to make these technological differences less consequential. As this book will describe, it is now possible with less invasive techniques to identify the role played by carotid disease, the need or not for surgical intervention, the extent of collateral circulation and the presence or absence of a cerebral perfusion defect.

We have come a long way in 50 years! It has been rewarding to have a front-row seat as all this has passed by. And there has been more than this coming from radiological progress. A rapidly spreading enthusiasm has developed for dilatation and/or stenting of diseased carotid, middle cerebral and even basilar arteries. The diagnostic radiologist has suddenly become a therapeutic radiologist. A word of caution: as with their surgical and neurological colleagues, the therapeutic radiologist is faced with the obligation of proving beyond equivocation that these excitingly promising procedures are as good as or better than the alternative and "standard" therapies that have evolved and whose risks and benefits have been carefully evaluated. The hope is that these therapeutic evaluations will be carried out as a collaborative effort involving bio-statisticians, stroke-oriented neurologists, and experts in vascular surgery. Popular acceptance and conventional wisdom based on clinical experience are not to be mistaken for proven fact. Perhaps it is wise for all who would study therapy to recall the words of Julius Caesar when he wrote: "Men willingly believe what they wish," or a similar thought expressed 1600 years later by Francis Bacon: "For what a man would like to be true, that he more readily believes."

What future problems remain in the realm of imaging related to the carotid circulation? While the randomized carotid trials demonstrated that the degree of luminal narrowing is an important prognostic factor, improvement in identification of the subset of patients at highest risk will aid in deciding appropriate therapy. Advancements in high-resolution imaging technology now permit detailed assessment of the characteristics of the extracranial carotid atheroma itself, and provide the opportunity to examine the role morphology, composition and functional/inflammatory status of the carotid plaque in the pathogenesis of stroke. Furthermore, these state-of-the-art imaging techniques show promise for directly assessing the effect of pharmacological intervention on the atherosclerotic lesion.

In conclusion it is not an exaggeration to state that radiologists have revolutionized and continue to rationalize the management of patients with cerebral ischemia. Stroke neurologists are deeply in their debt.

Pathology of carotid artery atherosclerotic disease

Renu Virmani, Allen Burke, Elena Ladich and Frank D. Kolodgie

The International Registry of Pathology, Gaithersburg MD, USA

Introduction

Stroke is the third leading cause of death in the United States, accounting for 600 000 cases each year, of which about 500 000 are first attacks (American Heart Association, 2001; Heart and Stroke Statistical Update. Dallas, TX, 2001). The pathologic events leading to stroke are complex, and involve atherosclerosis of the aorta and its branches, especially the carotid artery, obstruction of blood flow by increasing plaque burden, embolization of plaque components, especially of thrombotic material, and cerebrovascular factors. The importance of plaque components that predispose to plaque disruption, in addition to the degree of stenosis, has relatively recently been appreciated in relation to cerebral ischemic events. The purpose of this chapter is to characterize atherosclerotic carotid disease in light of our knowledge of coronary atherosclerosis and relate carotid plaque morphology to cerebral ischemic syndromes with special focus on features of plaque instability. A precise understanding of the histologic features of carotid atherosclerosis should help target specific treatments that are likely to be beneficial in the prevention of a subsequent event.

Pathologic features of atherosclerosis, lessons learned from aortic and coronary artery disease

The pathologic classification of atherosclerosis is in constant evolution, and should reflect in part variation based on the size of the artery involved. Two types of lesions were initially described based on gross examination of the aorta: the fatty streak and the atheromatous plaque. The fatty streak, as the less elevated and not prone to thrombosis, was considered a precursor lesion to the advanced atheromatous plaque. The fatty streak consists of smooth muscle cells, lipid-rich macrophages, and lymphocytes within a proteoglycan-collagenous matrix. The atheromatous or fibrofatty plaque is a raised lesion having a lipid-rich necrotic core containing cholesterol and cholesterol esters with an overlying fibrous cap. The atheromatous plaque, unlike the fatty streak, is prone to calcification, ulceration, thrombosis and hemorrhage.

The American Heart Association (Stary et al., 1994, 1995) proposed a numeric classification that was intended to approximate the stages of plaque progression, especially in the aorta. We recently published a modification of the AHA classification based on examination of over 200 cases of sudden coronary death, tailored more to the coronary artery (Virmani et al., 2000). A major modification includes the concept of thin-cap atheroma, which is thought to be a precursor lesion to plaque rupture, and hence a potentially more advanced lesion than the typical fibroatheroma (see Table 1.1). It is characterized by a necrotic core (~25% of plaque area), and a thin fibrous cap (<65 mm), heavily infiltrated by macrophages. A mechanistic term for the thin-cap atheroma is vulnerable plaque, based on the hypothetical

Carotid Disease: The Role of Imaging in Diagnosis and Management, ed. Jonathan Gillard, Martin Graves, Thomas Hatsukami and Chun Yuan. Published by Cambridge University Press. © Cambridge University Press 2007.

propensity of this lesion to rupture. Although the importance of developing imaging modalities for the identification of thin-cap atheroma is well recognized in the coronary arteries, the concept of thin-cap atheroma in the carotid circulation is less developed.

In the coronary circulation, a less common form of thrombosis than plaque rupture is the *plaque erosion*. The precursor lesion for plaque erosion is less clearly defined than for plaque rupture, and, based on underlying plaque morphology of acute lesions, includes plaques with a developed necrotic core (fibroatheroma) and those without, i.e. *pathologic intimal thickening*. The concept of eroded plaques in the carotid artery has only been recently described; approximately 10% of carotid thrombi in patients with strokes or transient ischemic attacks demonstrated plaque erosion on detailed histologic examination of plaque removed following endarterectomy (Spagnoli *et al.*, 2004).

The "calcified nodule" represents the least frequent cause of luminal thrombus accounting for 2–5% of coronary thrombi (Virmani *et al.*, 2000). This lesion is least well understood and is always accompanied by an underlying calcified plate with or without bone formation and shows multiple pieces of calcified nodules admixed with the thrombus adjacent to the lumen. Although calcification with nodule formation is common in carotid plaques, thrombosis as a result of exposure of calcified material to the luminal circulation has not been clearly described in the carotid circulation, but is likely not uncommon.

Percent stenosis and risk of stroke

It is generally accepted that the degree of luminal compromised, as assessed by imaging, is important in determining response to surgical treatment. In the North American Symptomatic Carotid Endarterectomy Trial (NASCET) endarterectomy was efficacious in reducing the risk of stroke and death up to 2 years in patients with 70–99% stenosis of the ipsilateral carotid artery (North American Symptomatic Carotid Endarterectomy Trial Collaborators, 1991). The benefit of carotid endarterectomy is reduced for those with 50–69% stenosis; however, for patients with less than 50% stenosis the failure rate was similar for endarterectomy or medical therapy (Barnett *et al.*, 1998, 2002). Subsequent studies in asymptomatic carotid stenosis of 60% or greater among patients who are good surgical candidates have demonstrated a reduced 5-year risk of ipsilateral stroke after carotid endarterectomy versus medical therapy (Endarterectomy for asymptomatic carotid artery stenosis, 1995).

The optimal approach for managing patients with lower degrees of stenosis than 69% remains uncertain. The asymptomatic carotid atherosclerosis study (ACAS) showed that a reduction in the aggregate risk for stroke and perioperative stroke or death over 50 years was 53% for patients with 60% or more carotid narrowing treated surgically compared with those treated medically (Endarterectomy for asymptomatic carotid artery stenosis, 1995). Identification of asymptomatic individuals with low-grade narrowing who would benefit from surgical management depends on methods of determining high-risk plaques and stratification of carotid atherosclerosis by plaque composition. Addressing the needs of this large population requires an understanding of the pathology of carotid atherosclerosis in relation to plaque instability and thrombosis.

The NASCET study focused on luminal narrowing as a primary measure for evaluating the benefits of endarterectomy in stroke patients and currently guides the management for patients with symptomatic stenosis above 69% (North American Symptomatic Carotid Endarterectomy Trial, 1991). However, the degree of stenosis does not always accurately predict those patients who will develop symptomatic lesions, as low-grade stenosis may also result in cerebrovascular events (Wasserman *et al.*, 2005). Pathologic studies suggest that other factors such as atherosclerotic plaque composition may represent an independent risk factor for ischemic stroke.

Plaque morphology in carotid atherosclerosis

It is difficult to correlate carotid, aortic and cerebrovascular plaque morphology at autopsy, for technical reasons. As a result, the mechanisms by which carotid atherosclerosis results in cerebrovascular symptoms are less understood than those linking coronary disease and myocardial symptoms. From studies of surgically excised carotid plaques, it is apparent that occlusive thrombus triggered by plaque rupture is relatively uncommon in the carotid circulation (Carr *et al.*, 1996; Golledge *et al.*, 2000; Chu *et al.*, 2004; Spagnoli *et al.*, 2004). The relatively low incidence of carotid plaque rupture is probably related to high blood flow and tendency for ulceration and embolization of plaque contents and mural thrombus. Unlike the myocardial circulation, it is likely that ischemic damage in the brain is more dependent on embolization than static occlusion of the artery.

In the carotid artery, as in the coronary circulation, plaque rupture is much more frequent in symptomatic vs. asymptomatic patients, as are fibrous cap thinning and infiltration of the fibrous cap by macrophages and T cells (Carr *et al.*, 1996; Golledge *et al.*, 2000; Chu *et al.*, 2004; Spagnoli *et al.*, 2004). Studies in our laboratory showed that symptomatic carotid artery disease is more frequently associated with plaque rupture (74%) than is asymptomatic disease (32%) (Carr *et al.*, 1996). Our observations suggest critical differences in plaque morphology between patients with symptomatic and asymptomatic disease (Table 1.2).

There have been other attempts correlating plaque morphology, degree of stenosis, and symptoms in patients with carotid atherosclerosis. In a study comparing carotid endarterectomy specimens from symptomatic high-grade stenosis lesions to asymptomatic autopsy specimens without high-grade carotid artery stenosis, Bassiouny *et al.* came to the conclusion that high-grade lesions were more likely ulcerated and thrombosed, reflecting luminal irregularity, than less stenotic asymptomatic plaques (Bassiouny *et al.*,

1989). They were unable to demonstrate that plaque composition, including collagen, DNA, and lipid content, were associated with symptomatic lesions (Bassiouny *et al.*, 1989). However, in a subsequent report, Bassiouny's group studied 99 endarterectomy specimens from symptomatic and asymptomatic patients. Plaques from symptomatic patients had certain morphologic characteristics more frequently than those from asymptomatic patients. The necrotic core was twice as close to the lumen in symptomatic plaques when compared with asymptomatic plaques; the number of macrophages infiltrating the region of the fibrous cap was three times greater in the symptomatic plaques compared with the asymptomatic plaques; and regions of fibrous cap disruption or ulceration were more commonly observed in the symptomatic plaques than in the asymptomatic plaques (32% vs. 20%). The percent area of necrotic core or calcification was similar for both groups (22% vs. 26% and 7% vs. 6%, respectively) (Bassiouny *et al.*, 1997). These observations confirm the importance of histologic parameters, especially inflammation and features of thin-cap atheroma, in the evolution of symptoms associated with carotid stenoses.

A recent study by Spagnoli *et al.* demonstrated that there are significant differences in the types of surface disruption in patients with major stroke, transient ischemic attack, and no symptoms (Spagnoli *et al.*, 2004). Thrombosis was defined by the presence of platelets or fibrin on the plaque surface with or without interspersed red and white blood cells. A thrombotically active plaque was observed more frequently in patients with ipsilateral major stroke, compared to patients with transient ischemic attack and those without symptoms (Table 1.3). In addition, the type of thrombus differed by patient symptoms. In patients with major stroke, 90.1% were associated with plaque rupture and 9.9% with luminal surface erosion. However, erosion was seen in approximately twice as many patients with transient ischemic attack than with stroke. Moreover, the study demonstrated that ruptured plaques of patients affected by stroke were characterized by the presence of

Table 1.1. Atherosclerotic plaque classifications

	Stary *et al.*	Virmani *et al.*	
		Initial	Progression
Early plaques	Type I: microscopic detection of lipid droplets in intima and small groups of macrophage foam cells	Intimal thickening	None
	Type II: fatty streaks visible on gross inspection, layers of foam cells, occasional lymphocytes and mast cells	Intimal xanthoma	None
	Type III (intermediate): extracellular lipid pools present among layers of smooth muscle cells	Pathologic intimal thickening	Thrombus (Erosion)
Intermediate plaque	Type IV: well defined lipid core; may develop surface disruption (fissure)	Fibrous-cap atheroma	Thrombus (Erosion)[c]
Late lesions		Thin fibrous-cap atheroma	Thrombus (Rupture) Hemorrhage/fibrin[d]
	Type Va: new fibrous tissue overlying lipid core (multilayered fibroatheroma)[a]	Healed plaque rupture, erosion	Repeated rupture or erosion with or without total occlusion
	Type Vb: calcification[b]	Fibrocalcific plaque (with or without necrotic core)	
	Type Vc: fibrotic lesion with minimal lipid (could be result of organized thrombi)		
Miscellaneous/ complicated features	Type VIa: surface disruption		
	Type VIb: intraplaque hemorrhage		
	Type VIc: thrombosis		
		Calcified nodule	Thrombus (usually nonocclusive)

[a]May overlap with healed plaque ruptures; [b]occasionally referred to as type VII lesion; [c]may further progress with healing (healed erosion); [d]may further progress with healing (healed rupture).

a more severe inflammatory infiltrate, constituted by monocytes, macrophages, and T lymphocyte cells compared with that observed in the transient ischemic attack and asymptomatic groups ($p = 0.001$). These findings support other data implicating the involvement of inflammatory cells, cytokines, adhesion molecules, and other inflammatory mediators in the pathogenesis of ischemic cerebrovascular injury (Frijns and Kappelle, 2002) and demonstrate a major role of carotid thrombosis and inflammation in ischemic stroke in patients affected by carotid atherosclerotic disease.

Effect of high flow and carotid plaque morphology

Atherosclerosis begins near branch ostia, bifurcations and bends, suggesting that flow dynamics play an important role in its induction. Laminar

Table 1.2. Gross and microscopic plaque characteristics in symptomatic and asymptomatic patients undergoing carotid endarterectomy

Gross morphology	Symptomatic, % ($n=25$)	Asymptomatic, % ($n=17$)	p-value
% Stenosis(Duplex)	74±17	77±15	ns
Ulceration	94	64	0.02
Plaque hemorrhage	47	52	ns
Microscopic characteristics			
Plaque rupture	74	32	0.004
Thin fibrous cap	95	48	0.003
Cap foam cells	84	44	0.006
Intraplaque fibrin	100	68	0.008
Intraplaque hemo.	84	56	0.06
Necrotic core	84	72	ns
Ulceration	11	8	ns
Calcified nodule	7	7	ns
Thrombus	63	80	ns
SMC rich area	5	0	ns
Eccentric shape	68	64	ns

Abbreviations: hemo = hemorrhage; ns = non significant.
Modified from Carr *et al.*, 1996

Table 1.3. Thrombotically active plaques, cap rupture, and cap erosion by study groups

	No. of plaques %			p-value		
	Patients with major ipsilateral stroke ($n=96$) (%)	Patients with TIA ($n=91$) (%)	Asymptomatic patients ($n=82$) (%)	Stroke vs. TIA	Stroke vs. asymptomatic	TIA vs. asymptomatic
Thrombotically active plaque	71 (74)	32 (35.2)	12 (14.6)	<0.001	<0.001	0.002
Cap rupture	64 (66.7)	21 23.1)	11 (13.4)	<0.001	<0.001	0.004
Cap erosion	7 (7.3)	11 (12.1)	1 (1.2)	0.51	0.09	0.03

Abbreviation: TIA = transient ischemic attack.
Reproduced with permission from Spagnoli, L. G., *et al.* (2004). *Journal of the American Medical Association*, **292**:1845–52.

flow is disturbed at carotid bifurcation regions, resulting in decreased shear stress and atherosclerotic plaque accumulation on the outer wall of the proximal segment of the sinus of the internal carotid artery (Zarins *et al.*, 1983; Anayiotos *et al.*, 1994; Masawa *et al.*, 1994). The intimal thickness is the least on the flow divider side at the junction of the internal and external carotid arteries where wall stress is the highest (Figure 1.1) (Glagov *et al.*, 1988).

High flow rates and the shear forces caused by the bifurcation of the common carotid artery into the internal and external carotids result in unique features of carotid plaque morphology as compared to the coronary circulation. Most importantly, the ulcerated plaque, which is uncommon in the coronary artery circulation, is relatively common in the carotid and other elastic arteries. Ulcerated plaque is a term used when the thrombus and a portion of the plaque have embolized, leaving an excavation in the remaining lesion (Figure 1.2). Another feature of carotid atherosclerosis is the infrequency of total occlusion relative to the coronary circulation. Occlusive carotid disease is reported in 3% of patients with posterior circulation infarcts, 14% in those with partial anterior circulation infarcts and 29% in patients with total anterior circulation infarcts; however, in coronary circulation the incidence of chronic total occlusion in patients dying suddenly is 40% (Golledge *et al.*, 2000; Burke *et al.*, 2001). The explanation for the low rate of total occlusions in carotid plaques is most likely related to high-flow rates that limit thrombotic occlusions unless there is severe luminal narrowing caused by repeated plaque ruptures.

Role of embolism and symptomatic carotid disease

The high rate of ulcerated plaques in the carotid circulation suggests that high-flow states result in relatively large amounts of embolized lipid material in cases of carotid plaque rupture. The reduction of stroke risk after carotid endarterectomy is attributed to removal of the cerebral embolic source in most patients. Transcranial Doppler-detected microembolic signals emanating from the ipsilateral middle cerebral artery have been associated with high-grade stenosis and recent stroke, and decrease after endarterectomy (Stork *et al.*, 2002). They have been associated with ulcerated plaques

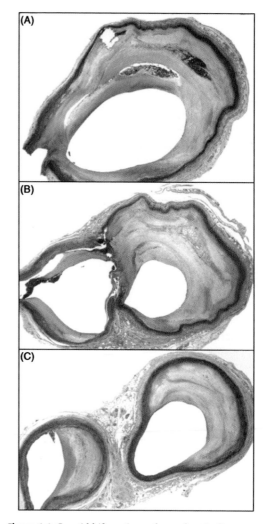

Figure 1.1 Carotid bifurcation, atherosclerotic disease. Panel A demonstrates the common carotid artery. There is moderate narrowing by atherosclerotic plaque, with two hemorrhagic necrotic cores. This layering indicates repeated surface disruption (rupture) and healing with smooth muscle cells. Panel B demonstrates the bifurcation, with the flow divider illustrated in the center. Note that the flow dividers on either side are relatively devoid of plaque, indicating the high shear stress in this site is relatively protective of accumulation of atherosclerotic material. Panel C shows the internal carotid artery (right), with the external carotid (left). Note the positive remodeling of the internal carotid artery at the site of atherosclerotic plaque.

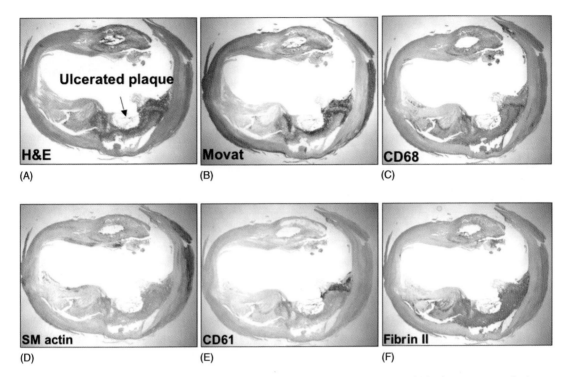

Figure 1.2 Plaque rupture with thrombosis and ulceration. Unlike coronary arteries, in which ulcers are unusual, plaque disruption in the carotid artery frequently results in embolization and crater formation. (A) demonstrates a routine hematoxylin eosin section of a carotid artery with thrombus and ulcer. (B) shows the corresponding Movat pentachrome stain, which highlights collagen (yellow) and elastic tissue (black). (C–F) are immunohistochemical stains for macrophages (Kp-1), smooth muscle cells (alpha actin), platelets (CD61) and fibrin (fibrin II). Note that at the ulcer crater, there are abundant macrophages (C) with few smooth muscle cells (D). The thrombus itself has largely embolized; there are residual platelets (E) and fibrin (E) at one edge of the crater.

as assessed by ultrasound (Valton *et al.*, 1998) and histologically disrupted plaques (Sitzer *et al.*, 1995). An association with plaque characteristics has not been uniformly demonstrated, however (Droste *et al.*, 1999; Stork *et al.*, 2002; Verhoeven *et al.*, 2005).

Comparison of coronary and carotid atherosclerosis

In our laboratory, we have compared the histomorphometric features of unstable coronary and carotid atherosclerotic plaques. The mean fibrous cap thickness in carotid plaque rupture was nearly three times greater than coronary plaque rupture (72 ± 15 microns vs. 23 ± 17 microns), respectively (Figure 1.3). We measured carotid vulnerable plaques (necrotic core with overlying thin cap and infiltration by macrophages, Figure 1.4) and found a mean cap thickness of 72 ± 24 microns, which is greater than the 65-micron upper limit of a thin-cap fibroatheroma in the coronary artery. In addition, there are fewer macrophages in the fibrous cap of carotid plaque ruptures than coronary plaque ruptures ($13.5 \pm 10.9\%$ vs. $26 \pm 20\%$). Similarly, in carotid-vulnerable plaques the number of macrophages

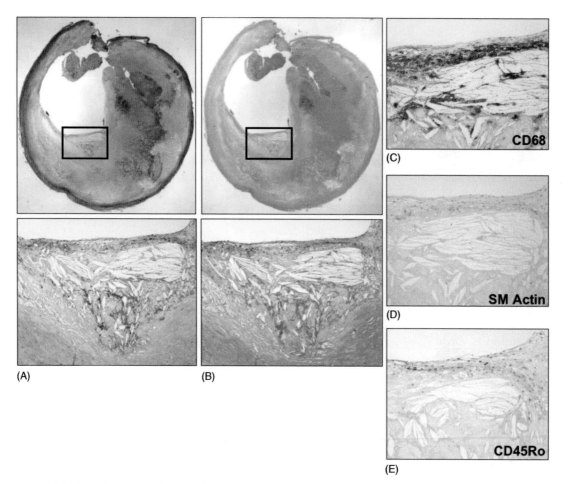

Figure 1.3 Vulnerable plaque with hemorrhage. Panel A (Movat stain) and panel B (hematoxylin-eosin stain) show carotid endarterectomy specimens with a thin fibrous cap (boxed areas, and insets below). Panels C (CD 68 for macrophages), D (alpha actin for smooth muscle cells) and E (CD45Ro for T-cells) demonstrate that, in the area of thinning of the cap, there are numerous macrophages, no smooth muscle cells, and a sprinkling of T lymphocytes.

is fewer than coronary-vulnerable plaques ($10\pm 1.8\%$ vs. $14\pm 10\%$). (Virmani *et al.*, 2000)

The role of angiogenesis in plaque progression has been studied in the coronary arteries (Kolodgie *et al.*, 2003). The role of vasa vasorum in precipitation of acute coronary syndromes and aortic plaque disruption is the focus of ongoing research. Plaque vascularity has, in addition, been shown to correlate with intraplaque hemorrhage and the presence of symptomatic carotid disease (Mofidi *et al.*, 2001). Imaging techniques for detection of vasa vasorum in carotid plaques may be important in future evaluation of carotid stenosis.

Plaque hemorrhage in the carotid artery (Figure 1.5) is far more frequent than in the coronary arteries and may be related to high-flow

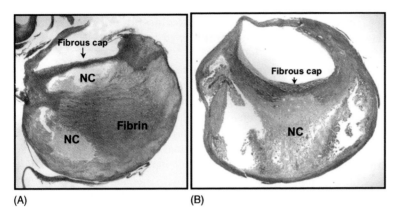

Figure 1.4 Fibrous cap, carotid atherosclerosis. These photographs of carotid plaques (Masson trichrome stain) demonstrate multiple necrotic cores (NC), with a fibrin-rich central area, and a thin fibrous cap (arrow) with collagen staining blue (A). Panel B shows a single large necrotic core, with a thicker fibrous cap than shown in panel A (arrow).

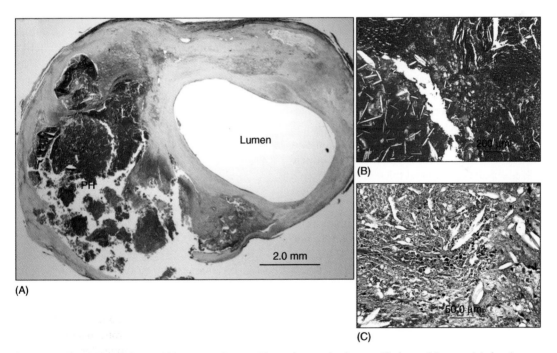

Figure 1.5 Plaque hemorrhage within a necrotic core. Photomicrograph of a carotid plaque (Movat stain) showing intraplaque hemorrhage with the necrotic core (nc), note the fibrous cap is thick (symptomatic patient). (B) shows a high power of the hemorrhage, which shows areas of well-formed red cells with interspersed free cholesterol crystals, and similar crystals are seen in areas where the red cells cannot be recognized and no foam cells are identified, suggestive that the free cholesterol may be derived from the red cell membranes that are rich in free cholesterol. (C) is high power showing hemosiderin (brown pigment) lying free as well as within macrophages.

rates and pressures in the lumen and the vasa vasorum. The maximum frequency of hemorrhage is observed in arteries with 50–75% cross-sectional area luminal narrowing. We have reported in coronary plaques that intraplaque hemorrhage is responsible for necrotic core enlargement and excessive foamy macrophages in the fibrous caps (Kolodgie *et al.*, 2003). Red blood cell membranes are the richest source of cholesterol as compared to any other cell in the body. The free cholesterol in the necrotic core is believed to arise from apoptotic cell death of foamy macrophages. However, we have shown that free cholesterol in fibroatheromas, thin-cap fibroatheromas and plaque ruptures is also derived from erythrocytes that become trapped in the necrotic core when intraplaque hemorrhages occur (Kolodgie *et al.*, 2003). Takaya *et al.* recently reported that patients with carotid intraplaque hemorrhage at 18 months follow-up had larger necrotic cores as well as accelerated plaque progression as compared to patients without intraplaque hemorrhage (Takaya *et al.*, 2005).

The frequency of calcification is similar in coronary and carotid arteries, with maximum calcification seen in carotid arteries narrowed greater than 70% cross-sectional area. Calcification in the carotid artery similar to coronary artery is at first speckled and occurs in areas rich in smooth muscle cells like pathologic intimal thickening and occurs at sites of smooth muscle cell loss. The next most frequent site is the base of the necrotic core, close to the media (Figure 1.6). Calcium in the carotid plaque is often fragmented and may be located deep in the plaque or close to the surface. However, the frequency of calcified nodules (with surface thrombus) (Figure 1.7), a form of calcification that results in irregular nodules of calcium, is higher in carotid disease (approximately 6–7%), as compared to coronary artery disease (1–2%). In contrast, plaque erosion, while common in the coronary circulation, is somewhat less frequent in the carotid artery. In carotid arteries, percent stenosis was highest in healed plaque ruptures and was greater than thin-cap atheromas and acute plaque ruptures.

Is luminal narrowing the only determinant of vulnerability of a plaque?

Vulnerable plaque is a concept well accepted in the coronary circulation but not so well established in the carotid plaque. In studies carried out in the coronary circulation it has been shown that plaque ruptures often occur at low degrees of luminal narrowing and that percent stenosis is a poor predictor of plaque rupture. Ambrose *et al.* showed in retrospective analysis of angiograms of patients with acute myocardial infarction, that the median stenosis of the initial angiogram in the artery that caused the infarction was 48% (Ambrose *et al.*, 1988). This concept subsequently has been now repeatedly proven to be correct; we have shown in sudden coronary death that at least 40% of patients dying suddenly with a luminal thrombus have underlying plaques <75% narrowed in the cross-sectional area (Farb *et al.*, 1995). Wasserman *et al.* have suggested that in the carotid artery it is time to look beyond stenosis (Figure 1.8). They state that "although retrospective angiographic studies of extracranial carotid atherosclerosis and stroke have not been reported, the mechanism of plaque rupture may be similar to that seen in the coronary artery" (Wasserman *et al.*, 2005).

Plaque progression through repeated silent ruptures (Figure 1.9)

Morphologic studies of coronary plaques have suggested that plaques beyond 50% cross-sectional area narrowing occur through repeated ruptures, which are most often clinically silent (Burke *et al.*, 2001). The sites of healed plaque ruptures can be recognized by the presence of a necrotic core with a discontinuous fibrous cap which is made up of type I collagen identified by either Movat and/or Sirius red-stained sections of the artery with an overlying neointimal tissue that is rich in smooth muscle cells in a proteoglycan-rich matrix and type III collagen (Figure 1.9). In the coronary circulation

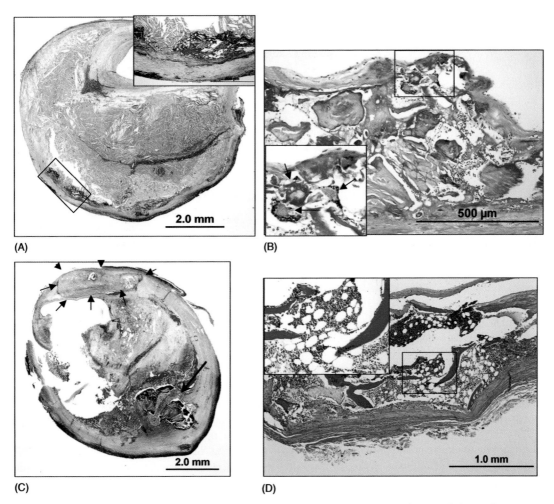

Figure 1.6 Calcification and bone formation in atherosclerotic plaques. (A) is a section of a carotid plaque showing plaque hemorrhage within a necrotic core, note presence of calcification at the periphery of the necrotic core close to the outer wall, which is highlighted in the insert. (B) is a another section of the carotid artery showing both a calcified sheet (small arrows) and two nodules of calcification (large arrow) that have likely resulted from a break in calcified sheet close and within the necrotic core that shows presence of hemorrhage. (C) shows a high power of multiple calcified nodules close to the lumen with interspersed osteoclasts (highlighted in the insert). (D) shows low and high power of an area of bone formation with surrounding marrow, which may be seen in at least 10% of carotid plaques.

Mann and Davies showed that the frequency of healed-plaque ruptures increased as the luminal narrowing increased (Mann and Davies, 1999). Burke *et al.* reported that healed-plaque ruptures were found in 61% of patients dying suddenly from coronary artery disease (Burke *et al.*, 2001). The sites of acute plaque rupture showed presence of underlying healed ruptures and the *de novo* acute plaque rupture was an infrequent phenomenon (11%).

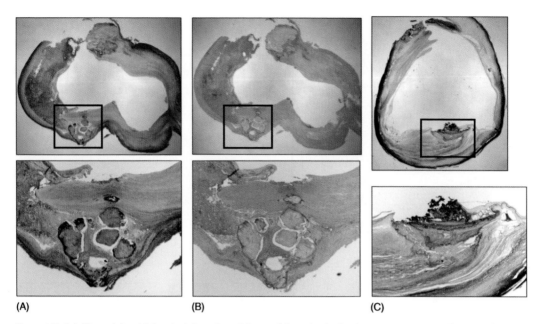

(A)   (B)   (C)

Figure 1.7 Calcific nodule with luminal thrombus. A form of thrombosis that is more common in the carotid artery than in the coronary is the nodular calcified plaque. Panel A shows a Movat pentachrome and panel B a hematoxylin-eosin stain of a carotid endarterectomy specimen with a nodular calcified area (boxes, and insets below). Panel C demonstrates an area of surface thrombus (boxed area, and inset below) overlying the nodular calcification.

Extensive calcification and bone formation in carotid plaques (Figure 1.6)

The degree of calcification and presence of lamellar bone has been studied in a series of carotid endarterectomies and correlated with symptoms and risk factors (Hunt *et al.*, 2002). Extensive calcification was found to be inversely correlated with ulceration and plaque hemorrhage. Bone formation was present in 13% of plaques, and was associated with a history of diabetes mellitus and coronary artery disease. An association between bone formation and cerebrovascular symptoms was not demonstrated, however (Hunt *et al.*, 2002).

Magnetic resonance imaging and components of carotid atherosclerosis

The development of high-resolution MRI holds promise for the evaluation of carotid atherosclerosis in vivo. Ultrasound is valuable for plaque characterization and assessment of stroke risk, but lipid core and intraplaque hemorrhage cannot be distinguished, and calcification can obscure plaque visualization. The advent of MRI has allowed for delineation of the outer wall, fibrous cap and lipid core. Carotid plaque components, including fibrous tissue, calcium and lipid, can be identified using signal intensity variation from four different weightings (Zhao *et al.*, 2001). High-resolution MRI has been utilized to assess the effect of lipid-lowering treatment on carotid plaque composition (Zhao *et al.*, 2001) and has been verified in ex vivo models (Shinnar *et al.*, 1999). Furthermore, determination of plaque components of low-grade carotid stenosis using MRI techniques holds great promise in risk assessment of individuals without severe degrees of luminal narrowing (Wasserman *et al.*, 2005). High-resolution MRI has been utilized for the detection of intraplaque hemorrhage, which predicts subsequent

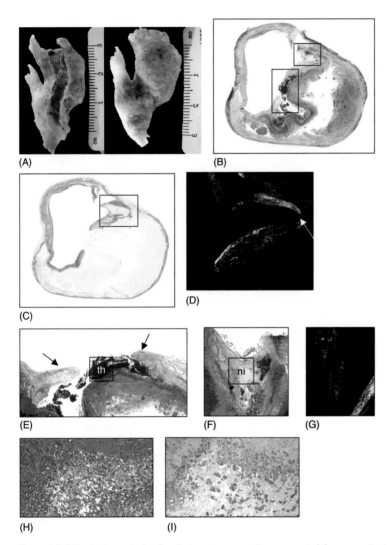

Figure 1.8 Histologic analysis of endarterectomy specimen resected from a patient who presented with hyperlipidemia and left vertebral ischemic events that had occurred in the last 3 months. Imaging techniques showed insignificant narrowing of the carotid artery. (A) is a Gross bisected specimen. (B) and (C) show low-power photomicrographs of the carotid plaque at the rupture site stained by Movat and by Sirius red stains, respectively. (D) is a boxed area in (C) showing the site of previous rupture under polarized light. This highlights the rupture site (arrow) in the type I collagen-rich fibrous cap (yellow−pink) and the newly formed neointima, which is rich in type II collagen (green). (E) is a high-power view of the rupture site (large boxed area in (B)). Black arrows highlight the ruptured fibrous cap and the thrombus (th) is seen in red at the site of discontinuous cap. (F) is a high-power view of the small boxed area in (B) showing the previous rupture site with hemorrhage in the necrotic core and a small area of new intimal (ni) growth representing the healed thrombus, which is seen in Sirius red stain under polarized light as green in (G). (H) and (I) are regions close to the fibrous cap showing macrophage infiltration by hematoxylin and eosin and CD68 stains, respectively. Red staining in (H) corresponds with hemorrhage, also seen as areas of red staining in (B) beneath the fibrous cap. (Reproduced with permission from Wasserman *et al.* (2005). *Stroke*, **36**, 2504−13.)

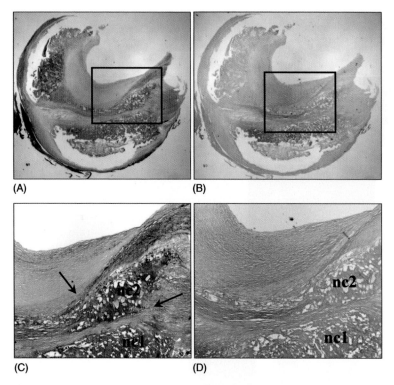

Figure 1.9 Healed plaque rupture. Atherosclerotic plaque from a patient with symptomatic carotid disease who underwent carotid endarterectomy. The internal carotid artery is severely narrow and there are two necrotic cores (nc1 and 2). The deeper necrotic core (nc1) is separated by a fibrous cap and the cap is disrupted (arrow). There is a second necrotic core (nc2) overlying the cap which is also disrupted (arrow) and the overlying neointimal tissue is rich in proteoglycans and type III collagen. (A) and (B) (Movat stains) and (C) and (D) (hematoxylin and eosin stains) are low- and high-power views highlighting the sites of previous ruptures that resulted in severe narrowing.

progression (Takaya *et al.*, 2005). MRI has been utilized to demonstrate ethnically-based differences in carotid plaque morphology, with Chinese patients demonstrating larger necrotic cores and lesser degrees of calcification than USA counterparts (Saam *et al.*, 2005).

Risk factors contributing to symptomatic carotid disease and correlation with plaque morphology

The correlation of risk factors with stroke is complicated by the multiple etiologic categories of stroke, including carotid atherothrombosis, aortic arch plaque embolization, thromboembolism for ischemic strokes, and hypertensive hemorrhagic strokes. Overall, the major independent risk factor is elevated blood pressure. In general, however, carotid risk factors show a spectrum similar to coronary disease, and include hypertension, and atherogenic and thrombotic factors.

Although hypertension is by far the most important risk factor for the development of all strokes, other risks include hypertension, impaired cardiac function, diabetes, nonvalvular atrial fibrillation, migraine, family history, and others. Modifiable risk factors are listed as cigarette smoking, low level of physical activity, and obesity (Wolf, 1998; Wolf and Grotta, 2000). The incidence of stroke increases in proportion to both systolic and diastolic blood pressure, and is elevated in Blacks, who have a high rate of hypertension (Goldstein *et al.*, 2001).

Serum lipids have long been associated with coronary artery disease, but not with cerebro-vascular disease. However, clinical trials using β-hydroxy-β-methylglutaryl-CoA (HMG-CoA) reductase inhibitors (statins) have shown a reduction of stroke risk in patients with coronary artery disease and elevated cholesterol levels. The relative risk of ischemic stroke in diabetic patients ranges from 1.8- to 6-fold greater in case-control studies. More recently attention has focused on inflammatory markers of atherosclerosis. High C-reactive protein (CRP) levels have been shown to be a predictor of risk of future cardiovascular events. Similarly, independent of other cardiovascular risk factors, elevated plasma CRP levels significantly predict the risk of future ischemic stroke and TIA in the asymptomatic elderly population (Rost *et al.*, 2001). High CRP at hospital discharge is a predictor of future cardiovascular events and death in patients admitted with ischemic stroke.

Smoking, another independent risk factor for stroke, is associated with an increased arterial wall stiffness, increase in fibrinogen levels, increased platelet aggregation and hematocrit, and decreased HDL-cholesterol (Goldstein *et al.*, 2001). Hypercoagulable states associated with the development of stroke include antiphospholipid syndrome, factor V Leiden, prothrombin 20210 mutation, protein C and S deficiency and high fibrinogen levels. Nonfasting total homocysteine levels are an independent risk factor for incidence of stroke in elderly persons (Bostom *et al.*, 1999).

Several studies have correlated plaque morphology to risk factors in the carotid and coronary circulation. Spagnoli *et al.* have shown that the fibrous carotid plaque correlated with aging and diabetes, the granulomatous plaque with hypertensive females, and the foam-cell rich

xanthomatous plaque exhibiting extensive alciano-philia with hypercholesterolemia. In smokers, plaques were frequently complicated by mural thrombosis (Spagnoli *et al.*, 1994). Mauriello *et al.* studying carotid endarterectomy specimens showed that patients with the highest tertile of fibrinogen (>407 mg/dl) had a high incidence of thrombosis (67%) compared with plaques of subjects with the lower and middle tertile (22% and 29%, $p=0.002$ and $p=0.009$, respectively) (Mauriello *et al.*, 2000). Plaque rupture was significantly associated with high fibrinogen level (54%, $p=0.003$). Multivariate analysis revealed that hyperfibrinogenemia was an independent predictor of fibrous cap thickness (inverse correlation), macrophage foam cell infiltration of the cap, and thrombosis. When accounting for the other risk factors, hyperfibrinogenemia remained an independent predictor of carotid thrombosis (Mauriello *et al.*, 2000). It is becoming increasingly evident that more studies correlating plaque morphology with risk factors are needed to further improve our understanding of carotid disease and target risk factor modification as more detailed assessment of plaque composition is possible with improved imaging techniques.

It has been shown that lipid-lowering therapy selectively depletes the lipid cores in carotid plaques. Zhao *et al.* analyzed carotid endarterectomy specimens from patients treated for 10 years with lipid-lowering agents in the Familial Atherosclerosis Treatment Study (FATS). This study demonstrated that the lipid core was significantly smaller in treated patients, although the extent of calcification was greater than non-treated controls, and the fibrous tissue content was the same (Zhao *et al.*, 2001).

In the coronary circulation, we have shown in patients dying suddenly that hypercholesterolemia correlates with plaque rupture and that smoking is more frequent in men and women dying with acute thrombus, whether due to plaque erosion or rupture (Burke *et al.*, 1997). Hypercholesterolemia also correlates with the number of thin-cap atheromas. Burke *et al.* also demonstrated that CRP is significantly elevated in patients dying suddenly with severe coronary disease, both with and without coronary thrombosis, and correlates with plaque burden. Mean staining intensity for CRP of plaques (necrotic core and macrophage) was significantly higher with high serum CRP than those with low CRP, as was mean number of thin-cap atheromas (Burke *et al.*, 2002).

Restenosis of carotid endarterectomy

The rate of recurrent carotid stenosis after carotid endarterectomy varies from 4 to 10% and usually occurs >3 months following surgery (Hunter *et al.*, 1997; Das *et al.*, 2000). In a series of 1726 endarterectomies performed at the Cleveland Clinic from 1983 to 1997, 65 (3.8%) patients were reoperated on for recurrent carotid stenosis occurring 3 to 194 months (mean 42 months) after the initial procedure. Of these patients, approximately half were symptomatic with neurologic symptoms and half were asymptomatic. The recurrence interval was 57 months in specimens with atherosclerotic disease ($n = 37$) whereas in specimens with myointimal hyperplasia ($n = 28$), the recurrence interval was 21 months ($p = 0.0007$). In recurrent disease, the myointimal hyperplasia consisted of smooth muscle cells in a proteoglycan matrix interspersed with fibrin; the collagen and elastin representing organization of the thrombus is sparse. Neovascularity may be present but is usually not extensive and surface thrombi tend to be platelet rich. Evidence of surface thrombosis was found in 77% of cases but intraplaque thrombi are uncommon; only 15% are found in specimens collected <36 months post the initial endarterectomy. A recent review of the literature by Ecker *et al.* representing a collection of >500 carotid endarterectomies that reported restenosis with follow-up varying from 18 to 82 months, show a recurrence rate ranging from 0.7 to 7.9% over an average of 3.5 years. Their own 7.1-year follow-up

of 975 patients however, yielded a restenosis rate (defined as $\geq 70\%$ stenosis) of only 0.1% (Ecker *et al.*, 2003).

In our experience, recurrent endarterectomy specimens collected up to 36 months post procedure typically contain myointimal hyperplasia and beyond this interval, atherosclerotic lesions are more common (Clagett *et al.*, 1986). Seventy-four percent of specimens with atherosclerotic lesions usually contain fibrin-rich surface thrombi, which are in continuity with an intraplaque thrombus (Figure 1.10). Extensive neovascularity in lesions with atherosclerosis is common. The plaque components include foam cells, cholesterol clefts, abundant collagen with focal areas of necrosis and calcification. Some cases may show myointimal hyperplasia in the deep intima, but it is usually interspersed with atherosclerotic plaque. Although all the components of atherosclerosis are present in primary and recurrent lesions, the atherosclerotic elements are arranged in a less orderly manner in the latter. Primary plaques demonstrate a central necrotic core with cholesterol clefts beneath a fibrous cap, whereas in recurrent lesions, the necrotic core is superficial and often unsupported by a dense layer of collagen. In recurrent lesions, the thrombus is contained within the plaque whereas in primary lesions it is usually associated with intraplaque hemorrhage, which is rarely observed in recurrent lesions (Clagett *et al.*, 1986; Hunter and Edgar, 1997).

In a recent paper Pauletto *et al.* report that examination of primary endarterectomy lesions may be predictive of maximum intimal-medial thickness (M-IMT) of revascularized vessels. Plaques with an abundance of smooth muscle cells, mostly of the fetal type (antismooth muscle cell [SM]-myosin heavy chain [MyHC positive]) were more likely to develop greater neointimal growth after surgery compared with lesions rich in macrophages and lymphocytes (Pauletto *et al.*, 2000).

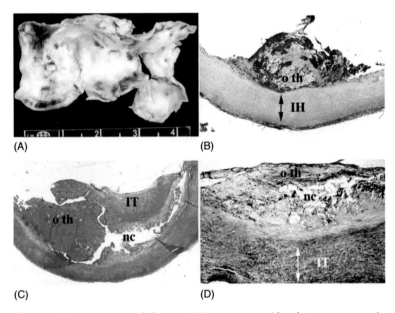

Figure 1.10 Recurrent carotid disease. (A) Recurrent carotid endarterectomy specimen showing a mostly pearly white appearance from fibrointimal hyperplasia with focal thrombi. (B) Histologic section of the same specimen showing organizing thrombus on the luminal surface with underlying fibrointimal hyperplasia (IH). (C) Low-power view of another specimen of a later recurrent lesion showing atherosclerotic change with necrotic core (nc) with fibrointimal thickening (IT) towards the lumen and organizing thrombus (o th) on the left. (D) High-power view of another atherosclerotic plaque: note, fibrointimal thickening (IT) underneath the necrotic core (nc) and surface organizing fibrin thrombus (o th). Note the presence of cholesterol clefts with interspersed macrophages. ([B, D]: Movat stain; [C]: hematoxylin and eosin stain.) Reproduced with permission from Virmani *et al.* (2001). *Pathology Case Reviews*, **6**, 242, Figure 1.5.

Atherosclerosis of the aortic arch and ischemic stroke

Recent evidence shows that atherosclerotic disease of the aortic arch may be a source of cerebral emboli (Davila-Roman *et al.*, 1994). Plaques located proximal to the ostium of the subclavian artery are reported in 60% of patients ≥60 years of age with ischemic stroke and the association was strongest when the plaques were ≥4 mm in thickness (Amarenco *et al.*, 1994). In 1996, "The French Study of Aortic Plaques in Stroke Group" collected data on patients >60 years old who had been admitted for brain infarction and followed with transesophageal echocardiography to determine the presence of aortic atherosclerotic disease.

The incidence of recurrent brain infarction was 11.9/100 person-years in patients with aortic wall thickness of ≥4 mm, as compared with 2.8/100 person-years in patients with a wall thickness <1 mm ($p < 0.001$) (The French Study of Aortic Plaques in Stroke Group F, 1996). It is not unusual to see plaque calcification in the aortic arch of sudden coronary death victims. Plaque ulceration and thrombosis is not an unusual finding at autopsy in patients >60 years of age (Figure 1.11).

Conclusions

Atherosclerosis, regardless of the arterial location, shares common features of intimal smooth

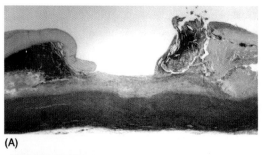

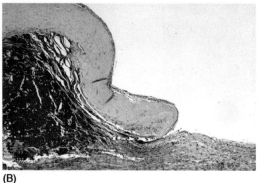

Figure 1.11 Aortic ulcer. Not all cerebrovascular ischemia is the result of carotid disease. Aortic plaques in the area of the arch and great vessels may undergo rupture and ulceration, with embolization of the plaque and thrombus to the brain. (A) demonstrates a low magnification of a healed rupture site in the aorta near the innominate artery ostium. (B) is a higher magnification of the lip of the ulcer crater.

muscle cells, inflammation, thrombosis, and extracellular accumulation of matrix, lipid, and calcification. However, the histopathology of carotid atherosclerotic disease shows distinct differences from that of the coronary circulation. Whereas small mural thrombi are common, occlusive luminal thrombosis is typically not a major feature of carotid disease. Plaque ulceration, with embolization of large amounts of necrotic core, is a common feature of carotid atherosclerosis and is infrequent in the coronary circulation. Similar to coronary disease, symptomatic carotid disease is predominantly associated with plaque rupture, and plaque erosion is relatively uncommon (10%). Calcified nodule, another cause of thrombosis, is

perhaps more frequent in the carotid artery compared to the coronary circulation, but its role in carotid thrombosis remains to be established. Although there is a higher incidence of plaque rupture in symptomatic carotid disease compared to asymptomatic patients, the extent of lipid area, necrotic core size, and calcification may not be different. Instead, the location of the lipid core and presence of thin-cap atheroma may be more important determinants of symptomatic disease. Not all cerebrovascular ischemia originates from the carotid atherosclerotic plaque and may frequently arise from atherosclerotic aortic arch disease. Therefore, in patients presenting with ischemic stroke, assessment of both the carotid artery and aortic arch is indicated. Ongoing research defining histopathologic parameters of symptomatic plaques are needed in order that imaging may predict future ischemic events, and novel therapeutic interventions be devised.

REFERENCES

Ambrose, J. A., Tannenbaum, M. A., Alexopoulos, D., *et al.* (1988). Angiographic progression of coronary artery disease and the development of myocardial infarction. *Journal of American College of Cardiology*, **12**, 56–62.

Amarenco, P., Cohen, A., Tzourio, C., *et al.* (1994). Atherosclerotic disease of the aortic arch and the risk of ischemic stroke. *New England Journal of Medicine*, **331**, 1474–9.

Anayiotos, A. S., Jones, S. A., Giddens, D. P., Glagov, S. and Zarins, C. K. (1994). Shear stress at a compliant model of the human carotid bifurcation. *Journal of Biomechanical Engineering*, **116**, 98–106.

Barnett, H. J., Taylor, D. W., Eliasziw, M., *et al.* (1998). Benefit of carotid endarterectomy in patients with symptomatic moderate or severe stenosis. North American Symptomatic Carotid Endarterectomy Trial Collaborators. *New England Journal of Medicine*, **339**, 1415–25.

Barnett, H. J., Meldrum, H. E. and Eliasziw, M. (2002). The appropriate use of carotid endarterectomy. *Canadian Medical Association Journal*, **166**, 1169–79.

Bassiouny, H. S., Davis, H., Massawa, N., *et al.* (1989). Critical carotid stenoses: morphologic and chemical similarity between symptomatic and asymptomatic plaques. *Journal of Vascular Surgery*, **9**, 202–12.

Bassiouny, H. S., Sakaguchi, Y., Mikucki, S. A., *et al.* (1997). Juxtalumenal location of plaque necrosis and neoformation in symptomatic carotid stenosis. *Journal of Vascular Surgery*, **26**, 585–94.

Bostom, A. G., Rosenberg, I. H., Silbershatz, H., *et al.* (1999). Nonfasting plasma total homocysteine levels and stroke incidence in elderly persons: the Framingham Study. *Annals of Internal Medicine*, **131**, 352–5.

Burke, A. P., Farb, A., Malcom, G. T., *et al.* (1997). Coronary risk factors and plaque morphology in men with coronary disease who died suddenly. *New England Journal of Medicine*, **336**, 1276–82.

Burke, A. P., Kolodgie, F. D., Farb, A., *et al.* (2001). Healed plaque ruptures and sudden coronary death: evidence that subclinical rupture has a role in plaque progression. *Circulation*, **103**, 934–40.

Burke, A. P., Tracy, R. P., Kolodgie, F., *et al.* (2002). Elevated C-reactive protein values and atherosclerosis in sudden coronary death: association with different pathologies. *Circulation*, **105**, 2019–23.

Carr, S., Farb, A., Pearce, W. H., Virmani, R. and Yao, J. S. (1996). Atherosclerotic plaque rupture in symptomatic carotid artery stenosis. *Journal of Vascular Surgery*, **23**, 755–65; discussion 765–756.

Chu, B., Kampschulte, A., Ferguson, M. S., *et al.* (2004). Hemorrhage in the atherosclerotic carotid plaque: a high-resolution MRI study. *Stroke*, **35**, 1079–84. Epub 2004 Apr 1071.

Clagett, G. P., Robinowitz, M., Youkey, J. R., *et al.* (1986). Morphogenesis and clinicopathologic characteristics of recurrent carotid disease. *Journal of Vascular Surgery*, **3**, 10–23.

Das, S. K., Brow, T. D. and Pepper, J. (2000). Continuing controversy in the management of concomitant coronary and carotid disease: an overview. *International Journal of Cardiology*, **74**, 47–65.

Davila-Roman, V. G., Barzilai, B., Wareing, T. H., *et al.* (1994). Atherosclerosis of the ascending aorta. Prevalence and role as an independent predictor of cerebrovascular events in cardiac patients. *Stroke*, **25**, 2010–16.

Droste, D. W., Dittrich, R., Kemeny, V., Schulte-Altedorneburg, G. and Ringelstein, E. B. (1999). Prevalence and frequency of microembolic signals in 105 patients with extracranial carotid artery occlusive disease. *Journal of Neurology, Neurosurgery and Psychiatry*, **67**, 525–8.

Ecker, R. D., Pichelmann, M. A., Meissner, I. and Meyer, F. B. (2003). Durability of carotid endarterectomy. *Stroke*, **34**, 2941–4.

Endarterectomy for asymptomatic carotid artery stenosis. (1995). Executive Committee for the Asymptomatic Carotid Atherosclerosis Study. *Journal of the American Medical Association*, **273**, 1421–8.

Farb, A., Tang, A. L., Burke, A. P., *et al.* (1995). Sudden coronary death. Frequency of active coronary lesions, inactive coronary lesions, and myocardial infarction. *Circulation*, **92**, 1701–9.

Frijns, C. J. and Kappelle, L. J. (2002). Inflammatory cell adhesion molecules in ischemic cerebrovascular disease. *Stroke*, **33**, 2115–22.

Glagov, S., Zarins, C., Giddens, D. P. and Ku, D. N. (1988). Hemodynamics and atherosclerosis. Insights and perspectives gained from studies of human arteries. *Archives of Pathology and Laboratory Medicine*, **112**, 1018–31.

Goldstein, L. B., Adams, R., Becker, K., *et al.* (2001). Primary prevention of ischemic stroke: A statement for healthcare professionals from the Stroke Council of the American Heart Association. *Circulation*, **103**, 163–82.

Golledge, J., Greenhalgh, R. M. and Davies, A. H. (2000). The symptomatic carotid plaque. *Stroke*, **31**, 774–81.

Hunt, J. L., Fairman, R., Mitchell, M. E., *et al.* (2002). Bone formation in carotid plaques: a clinicopathological study. *Stroke*, **33**, 1214–19.

Hunter, G. C. and Edgar, J. (1997). Poth Memorial/W. L. Gore and Associates, Inc. Lectureship. The clinical and pathological spectrum of recurrent carotid stenosis. *American Journal of Surgery*, **174**, 583–8.

Kolodgie, F. D., Gold, H. K., Burke, A. P., *et al.* (2003). Intraplaque hemorrhage and progression of coronary atheroma. *New England Journal of Medicine*, **349**, 2316–25.

Mann, J. and Davies, M. J. (1999). Mechanisms of progression in native coronary artery disease: role of healed plaque disruption. *Heart*, **82**, 265–8.

Masawa, N., Glagov, S. and Zarins, C. K. (1994). Quantitative morphologic study of intimal thickening at the human carotid bifurcation: I. Axial and circumferential distribution of maximum intimal thickening in asymptomatic, uncomplicated plaques. *Atherosclerosis*, **107**, 137–46.

Mauriello, A., Sangiorgi, G., Palmieri, G., *et al.* (2000). Hyperfibrinogenemia is associated with specific histocytological composition and complications of atherosclerotic carotid plaques in patients affected by transient ischemic attacks. *Circulation*, **101**, 744–50.

Mofidi, R., Crotty, T. B., McCarthy, P., *et al.* (2001). Association between plaque instability, angiogenesis and symptomatic carotid occlusive disease. *British Journal of Surgery*, **88**, 945–50.

North American Symptomatic Carotid Endarterectomy Trial Collaborators. (1991). Beneficial effect of carotid endarterectomy in symptomatic patients with high-grade carotid stenosis. *New England Journal of Medicine*, **325**, 445–53.

North American Symptomatic Carotid Endarterectomy Trial. (1991). Methods, patient characteristics, and progress. *Stroke*, **22**, 711–20.

Pauletto, P., Puato, M., Faggin, E., *et al.* (2000). Specific cellular features of atheroma associated with development of neointima after carotid endarterectomy: the carotid atherosclerosis and restenosis study. *Circulation*, **102**, 771–8.

Rost, N. S., Wolf, P. A., Kase, C. S., *et al.* (2001). Plasma concentration of C-reactive protein and risk of ischemic stroke and transient ischemic attack: the Framingham study. *Stroke*, **32**, 2575–9.

Saam, T., Cai, J. M., Cai, Y. Q., *et al.* (2005). Carotid plaque composition differs between ethno-racial groups: an MRI pilot study comparing mainland Chinese and American Caucasian patients. *Arteriosclerosis, Thrombosis and Vascular Biology*, **25**, 611–16. Epub 2005 Jan 2013.

Shinnar, M., Fallon, J. T., Wehrli, S., *et al.* (1999). The diagnostic accuracy of ex vivo MRI for human atherosclerotic plaque characterization. *Arteriosclerosis, Thrombosis and Vascular Biology*, **19**, 2756–61.

Sitzer, M., Muller, W., Siebler, M., *et al.* (1995). Plaque ulceration and lumen thrombus are the main sources of cerebral microemboli in high-grade internal carotid artery stenosis. *Stroke*, **26**, 1231–3.

Spagnoli, L. G., Mauriello, A., Palmieri, G., *et al.* (1994). Relationships between risk factors and morphological patterns of human carotid atherosclerotic plaques. A multivariate discriminant analysis. *Atherosclerosis*, **108**, 39–60.

Spagnoli, L. G., Mauriello, A., Sangiorgi, G., *et al.* (2004). Extracranial thrombotically active carotid plaque as a risk factor for ischemic stroke. *Journal of the American Medical Association*, **292**, 1845–52.

Stary, H. C., Chandler, A. B., Dinsmore, R. E., *et al.* (1995). A definition of advanced types of atherosclerotic lesions and a histological classification of atherosclerosis. A report from the Committee on Vascular Lesions of the Council on Arteriosclerosis, American Heart Association. *Circulation*, **92**, 1355–74.

Stary, H. C., Chandler, A. B., Glagov, S., *et al.* (1994). A definition of initial, fatty streak, and intermediate lesions of atherosclerosis. A report from the Committee on Vascular Lesions of the Council on Arteriosclerosis, American Heart Association. *Circulation*, **89**, 2462–78.

Stork, J. L., Kimura, K., Levi, C. R., *et al.* (2002). Source of microembolic signals in patients with high-grade carotid stenosis. *Stroke*, **33**, 2014–18.

Takaya, N., Yuan, C., Chu, B., *et al.* (2005). Presence of intraplaque hemorrhage stimulates progression of carotid atherosclerotic plaques: a high-resolution magnetic resonance imaging study. *Circulation*, **111**, 2768–75.

The French Study of Aortic Plaques in Stroke Group F. (1996). Atherosclerotic disease of the aortic arch as a risk factor for recurrent ischemic stroke. *New England Journal of Medicine*, **334**, 1216–21.

Valton, L., Larrue, V., le Traon, A. P., Massabuau, P. and Geraud, G. (1998). Microembolic signals and risk of early recurrence in patients with stroke or transient ischemic attack. *Stroke*, **29**, 2125–8.

Verhoeven, B. A., de Vries, J. P., Pasterkamp, G., *et al.* (2005). Carotid atherosclerotic plaque characteristics are associated with microembolization during carotid endarterectomy and procedural outcome. *Stroke*, **36**, 1735–40. Epub 2005 Jul 1737.

Virmani, R., Kolodgie, F. D., Burke, A. P., *et al.* (2000). Lessons from sudden coronary death: a comprehensive morphological classification scheme for atherosclerotic lesions. *Arteriosclerosis, Thrombosis and Vascular Biology*, **20**, 1262–75.

Wasserman, B. A., Wityk, R. J., Trout H. H. 3rd and Virmani, R. (2005). Low-grade carotid stenosis: looking beyond the lumen with MRI. *Stroke*, **36**, 2504–13. Epub 2005 Oct 2520.

Wolf, P. A. (1998). Prevention of stroke. *Lancet*, **352** (Suppl. 3), SIII15–18.

Wolf, P. A. and Grotta, J. C. (2000). Cerebrovascular disease. *Circulation*, **102** (Suppl. 4), IV75–80.

Zarins, C. K., Giddens, D. P., Bharadvaj, B. K., *et al.* (1983). Carotid bifurcation atherosclerosis. Quantitative correlation of plaque localization with flow velocity profiles and wall shear stress. *Circulation Research,* **53**, 502–14.

Zhao, X. Q., Yuan, C., Hatsukami, T. S., *et al.* (2001). Effects of prolonged intensive lipid-lowering therapy on the characteristics of carotid atherosclerotic plaques in vivo by MRI: a case-control study. *Arteriosclerosis,- Thrombosis and Vascular Biology,* **21**, 1623–9.

2

Epidemiology of carotid artery atherosclerosis

Christopher J. O'Donnell

National Heart, Lung and Blood Institute and its Framingham Heart Study, Bethesda, MD, and Department of Medicine, Massachusetts General Hospital, Harvard Medical School, Boston, MA, USA

Introduction

Cardiovascular disease, including stroke and myocardial infarction, is the leading cause of death and disability in the Western world (Thom *et al.*, 2006). When considered separately from other cardiovascular diseases, stroke is a leading cause of mortality, ranked third behind diseases of the heart and cancer (Thom *et al.*, 2006). There are estimated to be 500 000 newly diagnosed cases of stroke in the USA annually, the majority of which are ischemic in nature (Thom *et al.*, 2006). The age-adjusted incidence rate of stroke is substantially greater in Blacks than Whites (White *et al.*, 2005).

Atherosclerotic cardiovascular disease in general, and ischemic stroke in particular, is usually preceded by the presence of subclinical atherosclerosis that develops in the carotid arteries and other vessels. The pathological characteristics of carotid artery atherosclerosis are described in elegant detail by Virmani *et al.* in Chapter 1. Here, we review the epidemiology of carotid artery atherosclerosis, including its distribution, determinants and risks conferred by its presence. The available evidence demonstrates that carotid artery atherosclerosis is common and high risk, and the identification and treatment of carotid artery atherosclerosis may substantially reduce the burden of cardiovascular disease.

Subclinical atherosclerosis precedes clinically apparent disease

From the current pathological evidence, subclinical atherosclerosis appears to be common and to precede most cases of clinically apparent disease. Atherosclerotic lesions of the human aorta, both fatty streaks and fibrous plaques, are commonly noted in autopsy studies of combatant soldiers and other teenage and young adult victims of premature noncoronary death (Solberg and Strong, 1983; Strong, 1995). Abdominal aortic calcific deposits (AAC) occur early in the progression of atherosclerosis (Strong, 1995). These seminal studies contributed to a large body of pathological evidence, described in this book by Virmani *et al.* (Chapter 1), suggesting that atherosclerosis in the large arteries begins with the gross appearance of a fatty streak that subsequently progresses to an atheromatous plaque.

The spectrum of plaque progression is described by the most recent classification of atherosclerosis by the American Heart Association (Stary *et al.*, 1994, 1995). More recently, there has been focus on the concept of vulnerability of atherosclerotic plaques to rupture and lead to atherothrombotic sequellae, such as stroke for plaque rupture in the carotid arteries or myocardial infarction for plaque rupture in the coronary arteries

Carotid Disease: The Role of Imaging in Diagnosis and Management, ed. Jonathan Gillard, Martin Graves, Thomas Hatsukami and Chun Yuan. Published by Cambridge University Press. © Cambridge University Press 2007.

(Naghavi *et al.*, 2003a,b). In particular, it has been noted that plaques with thin-cap atheroma, characterized by a necrotic core and a thin fibrous cap, with heavy macrophage infiltration, are predisposed to plaque rupture (Virmani *et al.*, 2000). Elegant clinical-pathological studies have been performed on humans with carotid artery segments that were first imaged by magnetic resonance and subsequently removed by carotid endarterectomy (Yuan *et al.*, 2002). These studies demonstrate that subjects with stroke or transient ischemic attack were more likely to have had a thin fibrous cap both by imaging and pathology (Yuan *et al.*, 2002).

Physical examination of the carotid artery

In the Framingham study, the incidence of carotid bruit is 7.0% in individuals aged 65−79 (Wolf *et al.*, 1981; Brand *et al.*, 1989). Women aged 50−84 years with carotid bruits experience a significantly increased risk of stroke and myocardial infarction. Both men and women with carotid bruits have a higher total mortality in an 8-year follow-up period (Wolf *et al.*, 1981). Interestingly, presence of carotid bruit is poorly predictive of an ipsilateral cerebral infarction (Wolf *et al.*, 1981). The predictive value of carotid bruit for ipsilateral angiographic carotid atherosclerosis is 77%, compared to 85% for extracranial carotid atherosclerosis at any site (Ingall *et al.*, 1989). Thus, carotid bruits serve as markers for generalized atherosclerosis. While inexpensive and clinically useful, carotid bruits are generally considered to be neither sensitive nor specific for detection of clinically significant carotid artery disease. In persons who are preoperative candidates for coronary artery bypass grafting, the prevailing practice in many institutions is to unselectively order an imaging test, such as carotid ultrasonography, rather than rely on physical examination alone, to screen for individuals with hemodynamically significant (e.g. >70%) carotid artery stenosis who may be candidates for carotid endarterectomy concomitant with bypass surgery (Fukuda *et al.*, 2000; Archbold *et al.*, 2001). Nevertheless, a retrospective study suggested that a clinical strategy that limits imaging to those with a carotid bruit, older age or prior cerebrovascular disease would reduce imaging test burden by 40% with negligible impact on surgical management or postoperative neurological outcomes (Durand *et al.*, 2004).

Imaging of subclinical carotid artery disease for epidemiological assessment

High-resolution imaging modalities are now available to provide reproducible, quantitative assessment of the degree of luminal obstruction or wall disease of the carotid artery. The reliance on available data from subjects undergoing invasive imaging, such as carotid artery angiography, while accurate, may lead to substantial bias in assessment of the distribution of carotid artery disease (Sharrett, 1993). To be useful for epidemiological assessments, an imaging modality must be noninvasive or minimally invasive, reproducible, widely available, and able to be conducted during an examination of brief duration. Imaging with computed tomography (Chapters 12 and 15) or magnetic resonance (Chapters 11 and 14) offers substantially greater degrees of resolution, including delineation of plaque components, particularly when imaging is enhanced by use of noninvasive contrast. However, the imaging modality that fits these criteria and is widely used for epidemiological assessment is Doppler ultrasound imaging of the carotid arteries. The ultrasound technique is described in detail in Chapter 9 of this book. The vast majority of epidemiological information to date has been provided by studies using Doppler ultrasonography.

Since continuous wave Doppler was first employed for evaluation of cerebrovascular disease, continuous development of new ultrasound techniques led to introduction of cerebrovascular ultrasound modalities that are still in use today.

These modalities include B-mode imaging, duplex systems that combine B-mode and pulse wave measurements, and color-flow Doppler imaging. In particular, high-resolution B-mode imaging ultrasonography is useful for detection of the degree of luminal stenosis or of intimal medial thickness (IMT) of the common carotid artery, carotid bulb, and the internal carotid artery. These findings may occur in subjects who are asymptomatic or in those who are symptomatic, having experienced a prior transient ischemic attack or stroke. Continuous wave and pulse wave Doppler techniques are used for detection of stenosis or occlusion in the extracranial arteries.

Ultrasound measures of carotid stenosis and IMT have been the mainstay of epidemiological investigations of carotid atherosclerosis. Therefore, much of this chapter will focus on the extensive literature on these measures. Other measures of atherosclerosis that have been reported to be feasible using ultrasound imaging, such as focal calcifications or plaque area, may provide more quantitative assessments of the burden of atherosclerosis in the carotid artery (Spence and Hegele, 2004). However, to date these measures have not been widely collected or reported in population-based studies.

Distribution and prevalence of carotid stenosis and carotid IMT

Data regarding hemodynamically nonsignificant degrees of carotid stenosis provide a strong indicator of the high prevalence of carotid atherosclerosis. Such nonsignificant degrees of carotid stenosis are typically asymptomatic. For example, in the Cardiovascular Health Study, which consisted of men and women aged 65 years or older, detectable carotid stenosis was present in 75% of men and 62% of women (O'Leary et al., 1992). However, there was a low prevalence of moderate or greater (>50%) stenosis – 7% in men and 5% in women (O'Leary et al., 1992). The maximum stenosis and maximum wall thickness increases with age and was consistently and significantly greater in men compared with women at all ages (O'Leary et al., 1992).

In addition to the clear increases in carotid artery disease with increasing age, carotid artery stenosis and carotid IMT are both significantly associated with cardiovascular risk factors in cross-sectional and longitudinal studies. In studies of carotid artery stenosis in elderly men and women in the Cardiovascular Health Study, moderate to severe degrees of carotid stenosis are associated with hypertension, smoking, and reduced high-density lipoprotein (HDL) cholesterol levels (O'Leary et al., 1992). Similar cross-sectional associations of carotid stenosis with hypertension, smoking and reduced HDL cholesterol levels were noted in another elderly cohort, the Rotterdam Heart Study (Bots et al., 1992), as well as in a smaller cohort that included elderly persons but spanned a younger age range (Fabris et al., 1994). Similar studies have been conducted to relate risk factors to measures of carotid IMT, with similar results. In the Cardiovascular Health Study, significant relations were noted of carotid IMT with hypertension, smoking, and reduced HDL cholesterol levels (O'Leary et al., 1992).

It is possible that single measurements of cardiovascular risk factors in cross-sectional studies may not reflect a person's past exposure to risk factors. In the Framingham Heart Study, longitudinal ("time-integrated") measurements of risk factors measured serially over 34 years were related to carotid artery stenosis detected in elderly men and women (Wilson et al., 1997). In men, there were statistically significant increased odds for moderate carotid stenosis with increases in systolic blood pressure, cigarette smoking and total cholesterol, with similar nonsignificant increases in women (Wilson et al., 1997).

Other measures of focal carotid plaque have been reported. These measures are correlated with the more commonly conducted IMT and stenosis measures, and there is evidence for relations of these measures to risk factors.

Carotid IMT and stenosis have been related to a number of novel risk factors. Measures of carotid IMT and stenosis are related to markers of inflammation, consistent with the notion that inflammatory markers detected in the blood are markers of the presence and burden of atherosclerosis. Increasing C-reactive protein (CRP) levels are modestly associated with carotid stenosis and increases in internal but not common carotid artery IMT, even after adjustment for risk factors, in 3173 men and women of the Framingham Heart Study (Wang et al., 2002). Similarly, in the Rotterdam Study, CRP levels are associated with presence of carotid plaques (Van et al., 2006) and with progression of carotid IMT (Van et al., 2002). Circulating white blood cell counts have also been associated with carotid IMT in several studies (Elkind et al., 2001; Chapman et al., 2004), however, in one of these studies, consisting of 1111 Australian persons randomly selected from the population, circulating levels of CRP were not associated with carotid IMT (Chapman et al., 2004). In a number of other studies, there are strong associations between CRP and carotid IMT in unadjusted or age-adjusted analyses, but these associations are attenuated or eliminated after adjustment for other traditional risk factors (Folsom et al., 2001; Kivimaki et al., 2005; Makita et al., 2005). Thus, there are generally consistent associations of CRP with measures of carotid atherosclerosis but associations are not always noted to be independent of other risk factors. Since CRP is a nonspecific marker, other markers of inflammation, such as interleukin (IL)-6, may prove to be more sensitive markers of carotid IMT.

A number of other novel risk markers have also been examined in relation with measures of carotid atherosclerosis. Levels of circulating homocysteine have been reported to be associated with carotid stenosis and IMT. In a meta-analysis of many such studies, there is a clear association of homocysteine with carotid IMT across studies, although the magnitude of association was noted to be weak (Durga et al., 2004). Measures of glucose intolerance, such as elevations in hemoglobin A1C, have also been linked to increases in carotid IMT (Jorgensen et al., 2004). Relations of numerous other novel risk factors with carotid measures have been reported — including fibrinogen and other hemostatic factors, other inflammatory factors, and metabolic markers. However, in general none of these factors have shown strong, graded associations with increases in carotid stenosis or IMT that are similar in magnitude as associations with other established risk factors or are independent of established risk factors.

In addition to associations with established and novel risk factors, carotid atherosclerosis is clearly heritable, by several lines of evidence. First, a strong familial predisposition to clinically apparent disease is a strong indicator of future risk. Measures of carotid IMT and/or stenosis are increased in persons with evidence of parental premature coronary heart disease (Wang et al., 2003), earlier age of parental death (Baldassarre et al., 2005), and in Mexican Americans with a family history of adult onset diabetes mellitus (Kao et al., 2005). These findings suggest that one pathway for familial cardiovascular disease is via the occurrence and burden of subclinical atherosclerosis. Further, several traditional family-based heritability analyses have been conducted to assess for a heritable component to the interindividual variability in carotid measures (Manolio et al., 2004). Heritability has been reported in family studies ranging in size from several dozen to several hundred, with heritability estimates suggesting a statistically significant moderate magnitude of heritability ~0.40, with a range from 0.21 to 0.86, for carotid IMT even after adjustment for potential confounding risk factors (Manolio et al., 2004). For example, in a heritability study of 906 men and 980 women from 586 extended families (1630 sibpairs) from the Offspring cohort of the Framingham Heart Study, the multivariable-adjusted heritability of both internal carotid IMT was 0.35 and for common carotid IMT, 0.38, indicating that 38% of the variability in IMT is attributed to the role of genetics (Fox et al., 2003).

Other published heritability studies include studies of Caucasian twins (Jartti *et al.*, 2002; Swan *et al.*, 2003), African American and Caucasian families ascertained for diabetes (Lange *et al.*, 2005), Hispanic families with hypertension (Xiang *et al.*, 2002), and Mexican American families with coronary heart disease (CHD) (Wang *et al.*, 2005). Additionally, significant heritability has been demonstrated in several family studies ascertained for otherwise healthy Mexicans (Duggirala *et al.*, 1996), Caribbean Hispanics (Hank Juo *et al.*, 2004), Native Americans (North *et al.*, 2002), and Caucasians (Zannad *et al.*, 1998). Finally, evidence for familial aggregability has been reported in 4737 family members from multiple ethnicities (the NHLBI Family Heart Study, which includes Caucasian, Hispanic and African American families, including 2514 high CHD-risk families) (Pankow *et al.*, 2004), and in 733 Mexican American family members (Hunt *et al.*, 2002).

In Chapter 3, there is a detailed summary of the results of population genetic studies conducted using the methods of either genetic linkage or genetic association. In brief, the results of three family studies in which genetic linkage was conducted suggest that there are chromosomal segments harboring genetic variant(s) that predispose to susceptibility to increased carotid IMT (Fox *et al.*, 2004; Pankow *et al.*, 2004; Wang *et al.*, 2005). In the Framingham Heart Study, there is evidence for genomewide significant linkage of internal carotid IMT to chromosome 12, a region harboring the gene for macrophage scavenger receptor, type 1 (SCARB1), variation which is highly associated with internal carotid IMT (Fox *et al.*, 2004). Results of association studies have been recently summarized (Manolio *et al.*, 2004), and to date there have been very few replication studies conducted of sufficiently large sample size in high quality cohort studies. Only a very limited number of replicated associations of carotid measures have been observed, including associations with variants in the gene matrix metalloproteinase (MMP) 3 as well as possibly PON1 (Manolio *et al.*, 2004), and a meta-analysis of the association of the −174G/C

polymorphism of the IL-6 gene with carotid IMT also suggests a modest but consistent association for this variant (Mayosi *et al.*, 2005).

Prediction of prevalent cardiovascular disease and future risk for cardiovascular disease

Carotid stenosis as well as internal carotid IMT and common carotid IMT are each associated with prevalent cardiovascular disease (O'Leary *et al.*, 1992). Of these three ultrasound measures, maximum internal carotid artery IMT was the best correlate for a history of coronary disease, and common carotid artery IMT the best correlate for stroke. In age- and sex-adjusted multiple regression models that included all three ultrasound findings, both maximum internal carotid and common carotid IMT were significant correlates of both prevalent coronary heart disease and prevalent stroke (O'Leary *et al.*, 1992). Similarly, in the atherosclerosis risk in communities (ARIC) study of 13 870 black and white men and women, the prevalence of cardiovascular disease was consistently greater with increasing carotid IMT in women more so than in men, and particularly in persons with coexisting peripheral vascular disease (Burke *et al.*, 1995).

In prospective studies, carotid IMT also predicts both incident CHD and stroke in the elderly even after adjustment for traditional risk factors (Bots *et al.*, 1997; O'Leary *et al.*, 1999; del Sol *et al.*, 2001; Lorenz *et al.*, 2006). In a nested case-control study drawn from participants in the Rotterdam Study 55 years and older and including 98 myocardial infarctions and 95 strokes, there was a significant 34% increased risk for stroke and a marginal 25% increased risk for myocardial infarction after adjustment for risk factors in approximately 3 years of follow-up (Bots *et al.*, 1997). In a follow-up study of longer duration in the Rotterdam Study that included 374 incident cases of myocardial infarction or stroke, the addition of carotid IMT to the risk-factor-adjusted model resulted in only a modest increase in discrimination of risk using a receiver operating curve (ROC) analysis (del Sol et al., 2001). In a separate prospective study conducted in 1289 Japanese men free of cardiovascular disease followed for 4.5 years, the incidence of stroke was associated with increased common carotid artery IMT and more so with the combination of common carotid artery and internal carotid artery IMT, even after multivariable adjustment. Focal plaque was also a significant multivariable predictor (Kitamura et al., 2004).

In 4476 subjects free of prevalent cardiovascular disease in the Cardiovascular Health Study, the relative risk of both stroke and myocardial infarction increased with increasing carotid IMT (O'Leary et al., 1999). In models adjusting for risk factors, there were statistically significant increasing risks across the second through fifth quintiles of carotid IMT for the incidence of either stroke or myocardial infarction, and similar results were noted for the individual outcomes of stroke and myocardial infarction. Multivariable-adjusted increases in risks were statistically significant across the second through fifth quintiles and were 54%, 84%, 101%, and 215%, respectively. Of note, maximal internal carotid artery IMT was a similar predictor for stroke and a better predictor for myocardial infarction compared with maximal common carotid artery IMT (O'Leary et al., 1999). The IMT thicknesses (in mm) for each quintile were <0.90, 0.91–1.10, 1.11–1.39, 1.40–1.80, and ≥1.81, respectively, for internal carotid artery IMT, and <0.90, 0.87–0.96, 0.97–1.05, 1.06–1.17, and ≥1.18, respectively, for common carotid artery IMT (O'Leary et al., 1999). In a related study of the roles of CRP and carotid IMT in prediction of stroke in the Cardiovascular Health Study, the association of CRP with stroke was stronger in persons with increased carotid IMT (Cao et al., 2003).

Prospective data are also available from several cohorts which include younger persons and large numbers of black as well as white subjects (Chambless et al., 2004; Rosvall et al., 2005a,b; Lorenz et al., 2006). In a study of 5163 Swedish middle-aged men and women followed for 7 years, common carotid IMT, carotid plaque and carotid stenosis were each associated with increased risk for coronary events even after adjustment for risk factors (Rosvall et al., 2005a). In the same cohort, carotid IMT predicted incidence of stroke more so than carotid plaque, even after adjustment for risk factors (Rosvall et al., 2005b). In the ARIC study, the inclusion of carotid IMT in models that also include other nontraditional as well as traditional risk factors resulted in a very modest incremental increase in the area under the ROC curve for prediction of ischemic stroke (Chambless et al., 2004). More recently, results reported for the Carotid Atherosclerosis Progression study, consisting of 5056 men and women ranging in age from 19 to 90 years (mean age 50.1 years), provided information regarding prediction of carotid IMT in younger persons (Lorenz et al., 2006). As expected, the measurement range of IMT was substantially lower than in the older cohorts such as the Cardiovascular Health Study, underscoring the profound age dependence of carotid IMT. In unadjusted analyses, IMT in the internal and common carotid arteries as well as the bifurcation was highly predictive of stroke, myocardial infarction and death, but after adjustment for age, sex and risk factors, IMT in the common carotid artery and bulb were significant predictors for myocardial infarction and the combined endpoint, with higher relative risks noted for younger compared with older persons (Lorenz et al., 2006).

In their totality, the results from prospective, population-based data provide data that both internal and common carotid artery IMT are significant predictors of incrementally increased risks for stroke and myocardial infarction in asymptomatic elderly subjects and possibly also in younger persons. In recent years, there has been increasing focus on the potential use of high-resolution atherosclerosis imaging modalities such as carotid ultrasonography, computed tomography and magnetic resonance imaging for clinical risk prediction and screening (Smith et al., 2000; Greenland et al., 2001; Redberg et al., 2003). Risk prediction algorithms are now well established based upon traditional risk factors, such as those reported from the Framingham Heart Study for the prediction of risks for stroke (Wolf *et al.*, 1991), and coronary heart disease (Wilson *et al.*, 1998), the latter serving as the basis for cholesterol-lowering treatment guidelines from the National Cholesterol Education Program Expert Panel on Detection, Evaluation, and Treatment of High Blood Cholesterol in Adults (Third Report of the NCEP, 2002). Several consensus panels have suggested that use of carotid IMT and other measures should be examined closely for risk stratification in men and women who are at intermediate risk by established risk factors (Greenland *et al.*, 2000; Taylor *et al.*, 2003). However, at present, data are insufficient for clinical or population benefit from use of such tests, and there are not yet consensus guidelines that strongly advocate for screening of subclinical carotid disease in otherwise asymptomatic persons. Further data from prospective epidemiologic observational and treatment studies of carotid imaging by ultrasonography and magnetic resonance imaging are awaited. If carotid ultrasound or magnetic resonance imaging for IMT is to one day be considered for use in screening, a number of technical issues will need to be addressed, including the high degree of additional training required for the conduct of this testing, the need for careful attention to reproducibility, and the lack of uniform imaging standards, as well as high cost for magnetic resonance imaging.

Carotid disease in different arterial segments may lead to differences in disease risk

A number of lines of evidence suggest that wall disease in the common versus the internal carotid arterial segments may reflect somewhat different pathophysiologies. In many of the earlier studies of carotid ultrasound imaging, carotid IMT was defined by either IMT in the common carotid artery alone or the common carotid artery plus the bulb. In a limited number of population studies, both measures have been conducted. Common carotid artery IMT may represent diffuse wall thickening resulting from smooth muscle accumulation and matrix deposition. Internal carotid artery IMT may represent the cumulation of focal atherosclerotic plaques (O'Leary *et al.*, 1996), possibly related to endothelial dysfunction and hemodynamic shear forces (Crouse *et al.*, 1987; Malek *et al.*, 1999). The observation that ICA IMT is somewhat more strongly associated with increased risks of incident cardiovascular disease (O'Leary *et al.*, 1999), or that addition of internal carotid IMT to the common carotid IMT confers greater risk (Kitamura *et al.*, 2004) supports this contention. The arterial bulb, or bifurcation, is also a lesion-prone area, and with an increased activity of atherosclerosis and its risk factors (Grabowski and Lam, 1995), including lipid deposition and thrombosis, possibly related to hemodynamic factors (Topper *et al.*, 1996). In vitro models support the contention of the relations of shear forces to formation of plaques at the bifurcation and internal carotid artery (Zarins *et al.*, 1983; Asakura and Karino, 1990). By contrast, blood flow in the common carotid artery is laminar and nonturbulent, and common carotid artery IMT appears to be inversely related to shear stress, independent of age, body mass index and other risk factors (Gnasso *et al.*, 1996; Carallo *et al.*, 1999; Irace *et al.*, 1999; Jiang *et al.*, 2000). Lower shear stresses may increase the time of exposure of the common carotid artery IMT to atherogenic processes such as exposure to oxidized low-density lipoprotein (LDL). Indeed, risk factor associations appear to differ according to each of the three carotid segments, internal carotid IMT versus common carotid IMT versus the bulb IMT, with blood pressure and weight more related to common carotid artery IMT and levels of apolipoprotein B related to internal carotid artery IMT (Schott *et al.*, 2004). These considerations indicate that it may well be useful in future studies to independently examine the environmental and genetic risk factors for common versus internal carotid artery IMT, the differential predictive abilities of these beds, and the response of these beds to treatment in progression studies. Other ultrasound-based plaque measures should also be considered, if they prove reproducible and feasible in large-scale population-based research (Spence and Hegele, 2004). However, one of the more exciting directions for future research is the more exquisite characterization offered by magnetic resonance imaging. Epidemiological studies of carotid atherosclerosis using magnetic resonance imaging are currently underway and will provide further important evidence regarding the epidemiology of plaque components.

Carotid IMT progression

A growing and now large body of evidence has focused on the epidemiology of carotid artery disease progression. The annual rate of progression of carotid IMT is slow, in the range of 0.01–0.03 mm/year. There is substantial variability in carotid IMT measurements to be able to identify carotid IMT change over short time spans; optimal progression studies contain thousands of individuals with follow-up of multiple years using accurate, semiautomated, unbiased measurements conducted by a highly trained sonographer. Risk factors for carotid IMT progression have been identified in a follow-up study conducted in 15 792 middle-aged subjects in the ARIC. Increases in IMT using different model adjustments were associated with a number of risk factors, including baseline diabetes mellitus, current smoking, HDL cholesterol, pulse pressure, white blood cell count, and fibrinogen (Chambless et al., 2002), as well as with lower socioeconomic status (Ranjit et al., 2006).

Repeat measurements of carotid IMT have been conducted in a number of longitudinal studies that have examined the impact of lipid-lowering therapies on progression of carotid IMT (Blankenhorn et al., 1993; Furberg et al., 1994; Smilde et al., 2001; Taylor et al., 2002, 2004). In general, these studies have demonstrated a slowing of the progression of

carotid IMT in those treated with active therapy. Similarly, other randomized trials have demonstrated efficacy on carotid IMT progression with intensive versus conventional diabetes treatment (Nathan et al., 2003), calcium antagonists versus placebo (Pitt et al., 2000), and beta-blocking drugs (metoprolol) versus placebo (Hedblad et al., 2001; Wiklund et al., 2002). While there is consistency in some of these findings, comparison of results between studies is made somewhat difficult by use of different measurement protocols. Despite these overall favorable results, there is still no published evidence that slowing of carotid IMT progression is associated with reduction in clinically apparent cardiovascular disease. There is currently no consensus on which measure of carotid IMT progression (e.g. internal vs. common carotid IMT) should be used as a primary endpoint, and the adoption of standardized protocols for imaging and determination of progression will be essential to aid the interpretation and synthesis of these data for use in clinical prevention and treatment (O'Leary and Polak, 2002). Ongoing studies in cohort studies including the Framingham Heart Study and the Multiethnic Study of Atherosclerosis will provide these data.

Conclusion

The totality of epidemiologic evidence demonstrates a high burden of subclinical carotid disease in middle-aged and elderly men and women. While carotid disease can be imaged with a number of high-resolution imaging modalities, the vast majority of evidence is available from studies using carotid ultrasonography for stenosis and IMT imaging. From these studies, it is clear that both carotid stenosis and IMT are heritable measures that are related to many established and emerging risk factors and are associated with increased risks for stroke and myocardial infarction. Studies of carotid progression demonstrate clear associations of increased carotid IMT progression with established risk factors and slowing of progression by treatment with drugs that treat risk factors, such as intensive diabetic treatment, blood-pressure-lowering drugs such as calcium antagonists or beta-blockers, and lipid-lowering drugs. A number of important questions are under intensive investigation at present, including the utility of carotid IMT measurements over and above risk factors for risk prediction and treatment decisions, the utility of carotid IMT progression for prediction of cardiovascular disease, and the genetic architecture of carotid IMT and stenosis. Among the important objectives for future research and clinical use will be the development of standardized carotid ultrasound protocols and the introduction of newer modalities, such as carotid magnetic resonance imaging.

REFERENCES

Archbold, R. A., Barakat, K., Magee, P. and Curzen, N. (2001). Screening for carotid artery disease before cardiac surgery: is current clinical practice evidence based? *Clinical Cardiology*, **24**, 26–32.

Asakura, T. and Karino, T. (1990). Flow patterns and spatial distribution of atherosclerotic lesions in human coronary arteries. *Circulation Research*, **66**, 1045–66.

Baldassarre, D., Amato, M., Veglia, F., *et al.* (2005). Correlation of parents' longevity with carotid intima-media thickness in patients attending a Lipid Clinic. *Atherosclerosis*, **179**, 111–17.

Blankenhorn, D. H., Selzer, R. H., Crawford, D. W., *et al.* (1993). Beneficial effects of colestipol-niacin therapy on the common carotid artery. Two- and four-year reduction of intima-media thickness measured by ultrasound. *Circulation*, **88**, 20–8.

Bots, M. L., Breslau, P. J., Briet, E., *et al.* (1992). Cardiovascular determinants of carotid artery disease. The Rotterdam Elderly Study. *Hypertension*, **19**, 717–20.

Bots, M. L., Hoes, A. W., Koudstaal, P. J., Hofman, A. and Grobbee, D. E. (1997). Common carotid intima-media thickness and risk of stroke and myocardial infarction: the Rotterdam Study. *Circulation*, **96**, 1432–7.

Brand, F. N., Abbott, R. D. and Kannel, W. B. (1989). Diabetes, intermittent claudication, and risk of cardio-vascular events. The Framingham Study. *Diabetes*, **38**, 504–9.

Burke, G. L., Evans, G. W., Riley, W. A., *et al.* (1995). Arterial wall thickness is associated with prevalent cardiovascular disease in middle-aged adults. The Atherosclerosis Risk in Communities (ARIC) Study. *Stroke*, **26**, 386–91.

Cao, J. J., Thach, C., Manolio, T. A., *et al.* (2003). C-reactive protein, carotid intima-media thickness, and incidence of ischemic stroke in the elderly: the Cardiovascular Health Study. *Circulation*, **108**, 166–70.

Carallo, C., Irace, C., Pujia, A., *et al.* (1999). Evaluation of common carotid hemodynamic forces. Relations with wall thickening. *Hypertension*, **34**, 217–21.

Chambless, L. E., Heiss, G., Shahar, E., Earp, M. J. and Toole, J. (2004). Prediction of ischemic stroke risk in the Atherosclerosis Risk in Communities Study. *American Journal of Epidemiology*, **160**, 259–69.

Chambless, L. E., Folsom, A. R., Davis, V., *et al.* (2002). Risk factors for progression of common carotid athero-sclerosis: the Atherosclerosis Risk in Communities Study, 1987–1998. *American Journal of Epidemiology*, **155**, 38–47.

Chapman, C. M., Beilby, J. P., McQuillan, B. M., Thompson, P. L. and Hung, J. (2004). Monocyte count, but not C-reactive protein or interleukin-6, is an independent risk marker for subclinical carotid athero-sclerosis. *Stroke*, **35**, 1619–24.

Crouse, J. R., Toole, J. F., McKinney, W. M., *et al.* (1987). Risk factors for extracranial carotid artery atherosclerosis. *Stroke*, **18**, 990–6.

del Sol, A. I., Moons, K. G., Hollander, M., *et al.* (2001). Is carotid intima-media thickness useful in cardiovascular disease risk assessment? The Rotterdam Study. *Stroke*, **32**, 1532–8.

Duggirala, R., Gonzalez, V. C., O'Leary, D. H., Stern, M. P. and Blangero, J. (1996). Genetic basis of variation in carotid artery wall thickness. *Stroke*, **27**, 833–7.

Durand, D. J., Perler, B. A., Roseborough, G. S., *et al.* (2004). Mandatory versus selective preoperative carotid screening: a retrospective analysis. *Annals of Thoracic Surgery*, **78**, 159–66.

Durga, J., Verhoef, P., Bots, M. L. and Schouten, E. (2004). Homocysteine and carotid intima-media thickness: a critical appraisal of the evidence. *Atherosclerosis*, **176**, 1–19.

Elkind, M. S., Cheng, J., Boden-Albala, B., Paik, M. C. and Sacco, R. L. (2001). Elevated white blood cell count and carotid plaque thickness: the Northern Manhattan stroke study. *Stroke*, **32**, 842–9.

Fabris, F., Zanocchi, M., Bo, M., *et al.* (1994). Carotid plaque, aging, and risk factors. A study of 457 subjects. *Stroke*, **25**, 1133–40.

Folsom, A. R., Pankow, J. S., Tracy, R. P., *et al.* (2001). Association of C-reactive protein with markers of prevalent atherosclerotic disease. *American Journal of Cardiology*, **88**, 112–17.

Fox, C. S., Polak, J. F., Chazaro, I., *et al.* (2003). Genetic and environmental contributions to atherosclerosis phenotypes in men and women: heritability of carotid intima-media thickness in the Framingham Heart Study. *Stroke*, **34**, 397–401.

Fox, C. S., Cupples, L. A., Chazaro, I., *et al.* (2004). Genomewide linkage analysis for internal carotid artery intimal medial thickness: evidence for linkage to chromosome 12. *American Journal of Human Genetics*, **74**, 253–61.

Fukuda, I., Gomi, S., Watanabe, K. and Seita, J. (2000). Carotid and aortic screening for coronary artery bypass grafting. *Annals of Thoracic Surgery*, **70**, 2034–9.

Furberg, C. D., Adams, H. P. Jr, Applegate, W. B., *et al.* (1994). Effect of lovastatin on early carotid atherosclerosis and cardiovascular events. Asymptomatic Carotid Artery Progression Study (ACAPS) Research Group. *Circulation*, **90**, 1679–87.

Gnasso, A., Carallo, C., Irace, C., *et al.* (1996). Association between intima-media thickness and wall shear stress in common carotid arteries in healthy male subjects. *Circulation*, **94**, 3257–62.

Grabowski, E. F. and Lam, F. P. (1995). Endothelial cell function, including tissue factor expression, under flow conditions. *Thrombosis and Haemostasis*, **74**, 123–8.

Greenland, P., Smith, S. C. Jr and Grundy, S. M. (2001). Improving coronary heart disease risk assessment in asymptomatic people: role of traditional risk factors and noninvasive cardiovascular tests. *Circulation*, **104**, 1863–7.

Greenland, P., Abrams, J., Aurigemma, G. P., *et al.* (2000). Prevention Conference V: Beyond secondary prevention: identifying the high-risk patient for primary prevention: noninvasive tests of atherosclerotic burden: Writing Group III. *Circulation*, **101**, E16–E22.

Hank Juo, S. H., Lin, H. F., Rundek, T., *et al.* (2004). Genetic and Environmental Contributions to Carotid Intima-Media Thickness and Obesity Phenotypes in the Northern Manhattan Family Study. *Stroke*, **35**, 2243–7.

Hedblad, B., Wikstrand, J., Janzon, L., Wedel, H. and Berglund, G. (2001). Low-dose metoprolol CR/XL and fluvastatin slow progression of carotid intima-media thickness: Main results from the Beta-Blocker Cholesterol-Lowering Asymptomatic Plaque Study (BCAPS). *Circulation*, **103**, 1721–6.

Hunt, K. J., Duggirala, R., Goring, H. H., *et al.* (2002). Genetic basis of variation in carotid artery plaque in the San Antonio Family Heart Study. *Stroke*, **33**, 2775–80.

Ingall, T. J., Homer, D., Whisnant, J. P., Baker, H. L. Jr and O'Fallon, W. M. (1989). Predictive value of carotid bruit for carotid atherosclerosis. *Archives of Neurology*, **46**, 418–22.

Irace, C., Carallo, C., Crescenzo, A., *et al.* (1999). NIDDM is associated with lower wall shear stress of the common carotid artery. *Diabetes*, **48**, 193–7.

Jartti, L., Ronnemaa, T., Kaprio, J., *et al.* (2002). Population-based twin study of the effects of migration from Finland to Sweden on endothelial function and intima-media thickness. *Arteriosclerosis, Thrombosis and Vascular Biology*, **22**, 832–7.

Jiang, Y., Kohara, K. and Hiwada, K. (2000). Association between risk factors for atherosclerosis and mechanical forces in carotid artery. *Stroke*, **31**, 2319–24.

Jorgensen, L., Jenssen, T. and Joakimsen, O. (2004). Glycated hemoglobin level is strongly related to the prevalence of carotid artery plaques with high echogenicity in nondiabetic individuals: the Tromso study. *Circulation*, **110**, 466–70.

Kao, W. H., Hsueh, W. C., Rainwater, D. L., *et al.* (2005). Family history of type 2 diabetes is associated with increased carotid artery intimal-medial thickness in Mexican Americans. *Diabetes Care*, **28**, 1882–9.

Kitamura, A., Iso, H., Imano, H., *et al.* (2004). Carotid intima-media thickness and plaque characteristics as a risk factor for stroke in Japanese elderly men. *Stroke*, **35**, 2788–94.

Kivimaki, M., Lawlor, D. A., Juonala, M., *et al.* (2005). Lifecourse socioeconomic position, C-reactive protein, and carotid intima-media thickness in young adults: the cardiovascular risk in Young Finns Study. *Arteriosclerosis, Thrombosis and Vascular Biology*, **25**, 2197–202.

Lange, L. A., Bowden, D. W., Langefeld, C. D., *et al.* (2002). Heritability of carotid artery intima-medial thickness in type 2 diabetes. *Stroke*, **33**, 1876–81.

Lorenz, M. W., von, K. S., Steinmetz, H., Markus, H. S. and Sitzer, M. (2006). Carotid intima-media thickening indicates a higher vascular risk across a wide age range: prospective data from the Carotid Atherosclerosis Progression Study (CAPS). *Stroke*, **37**, 87–92.

Makita, S., Nakamura, M. and Hiramori, K. (2005). The association of C-reactive protein levels with carotid intima-media complex thickness and plaque formation in the general population. *Stroke*, **36**, 2138–42.

Malek, A. M., Alper, S. L. and Izumo, S. (1999). Hemodynamic shear stress and its role in atherosclerosis. *Journal of the American Medical Association*, **282**, 2035–42.

Manolio, T. A., Boerwinkle, E., O'Donnell, C. J. and Wilson, A. F. (2004). Genetics of ultrasonographic carotid atherosclerosis. *Arteriosclerosis, Thrombosis and Vascular Biology*, **24**, 1567–77.

Mayosi, B. M., Avery, P. J., Baker, M., *et al.* (2005). Genotype at the −174G/C polymorphism of the interleukin-6 gene is associated with common carotid artery intimal-medial thickness: family study and meta-analysis. *Stroke*, **36**, 2215–19.

Naghavi, M., Libby, P., Falk, E., *et al.* (2003a). From vulnerable plaque to vulnerable patient: a call for new definitions and risk assessment strategies: Part I. *Circulation*, **108**, 1664–72.

Naghavi, M., Libby, P., Falk, E., *et al.* (2003b). From vulnerable plaque to vulnerable patient: a call for new definitions and risk assessment strategies: Part II. *Circulation*, **108**, 1772–8.

Nathan, D. M., Lachin, J., Cleary, P., *et al.* (2003). Intensive diabetes therapy and carotid intima-media thickness in type 1 diabetes mellitus. *New England Journal of Medicine*, **348**, 2294–303.

North, K. E., MacCluer, J. W., Devereux, R. B., *et al.* (2002). Heritability of carotid artery structure and function: the Strong Heart Family Study. *Arteriosclerosis, Thrombosis and Vascular Biology*, **22**, 1698–703.

O'Leary, D. H. and Polak, J. F. (2002). Intima-media thickness: a tool for atherosclerosis imaging and event prediction. *American Journal of Cardiology*, **90**, 18L–21L.

O'Leary, D. H., Polak, J. F., Kronmal, R. A., *et al.* (1992). Distribution and correlates of sonographically detected carotid artery disease in the Cardiovascular Health Study. The CHS Collaborative Research Group. *Stroke*, **23**, 1752–60.

O'Leary, D. H., Polak, J. F., Kronmal, R. A., *et al.* (1996). Thickening of the carotid wall. A marker for atherosclerosis in the elderly? Cardiovascular Health Study Collaborative Research Group. *Stroke*, **27**, 224–31.

O'Leary, D. H., Polak, J. F., Kronmal, R. A., *et al.* (1999). Carotid-artery intima and media thickness as a risk factor for myocardial infarction and stroke in older adults. Cardiovascular Health Study Collaborative Research Group, see comments. *New England Journal of Medicine*, **340**, 14–22.

Pankow, J. S., Heiss, G., Evans, G. W., *et al.* (2004). Familial aggregation and genome-wide linkage analysis of carotid artery plaque: the NHLBI family heart study. *Human Heredity*, **57**, 80–9.

Pitt, B., Byington, R. P., Furberg, C. D., *et al.* (2000). Effect of amlodipine on the progression of atherosclerosis and the occurrence of clinical events. PREVENT Investigators. *Circulation*, **102**, 1503–10.

Ranjit, N., Diez-Roux, A. V., Chambless, L., *et al.* (2006). Socioeconomic differences in progression of carotid intima-media thickness in the Atherosclerosis Risk in Communities study. *Arteriosclerosis, Thrombosis and Vascular Biology*, **26**, 411–16.

Redberg, R. F., Vogel, R. A., Criqui, M. H., *et al.* (2003). 34th Bethesda Conference: Task force 3 – What is the spectrum of current and emerging techniques for the noninvasive measurement of atherosclerosis? *Journal of the American College of Cardiology*, **41**, 1886–98.

Rosvall, M., Janzon, L., Berglund, G., Engstrom, G. and Hedblad, B. (2005a). Incident coronary events and case fatality in relation to common carotid intima-media thickness. *Journal of Internal Medicine*, **257**, 430–7.

Rosvall, M., Janzon, L., Berglund, G., Engstrom, G. and Hedblad, B. (2005b). Incidence of stroke is related to carotid IMT even in the absence of plaque. *Atherosclerosis*, **179**, 325–31.

Schott, L. L., Wildman, R. P., Brockwell, S., *et al.* (2004). Segment-specific effects of cardiovascular risk factors on carotid artery intima-medial thickness in women at midlife. *Arteriosclerosis, Thrombosis and Vascular Biology*, **24**, 1951–6.

Smilde, T. J., van, W. S., Wollersheim, H., *et al.* (2001). Effect of aggressive versus conventional lipid lowering on atherosclerosis progression in familial hypercholesterolaemia (ASAP): a prospective, randomised, double-blind trial. *Lancet*, **357**, 577–81.

Smith, S. C. Jr, Greenland, P. and Grundy, S. M. (2000). AHA Conference Proceedings. Prevention conference V: Beyond secondary prevention: Identifying the high-risk patient for primary prevention: executive summary. American Heart Association. *Circulation*, **101**, 111–16.

Solberg, L. A. and Strong, J. P. (1983). Risk factors and atherosclerotic lesions: a review of autopsy studies. *Atherosclerosis*, **3**, 187–98.

Spence, J. D. and Hegele, R. A. (2004). Noninvasive phenotypes of atherosclerosis: similar windows but different views. *Stroke*, **35**, 649–53.

Stary, H. C., Chandler, A. B., Dinsmore, R. E., *et al.* (1995). A definition of advanced types of athero-sclerotic lesions and a histological classification of atherosclerosis. A report from the Committee on Vascular Lesions of the Council on Arteriosclerosis, American Heart Association. *Circulation*, **92**, 1355–74.

Stary, H. C., Chandler, A. B., Glagov, S., *et al.* (1994). A definition of initial, fatty streak, and interme-diate lesions of atherosclerosis. A report from the Committee on Vascular Lesions of the Council on Arteriosclerosis, American Heart Association. *Circulation*, **89**, 2462–78.

Strong, J. P. (1995). Natural history and risk factors for early human atherogenesis. Pathobiological Determi-nants of Atherosclerosis in Youth (PDAY) Research Group. *Clinical Chemistry*, **41**, 134–8.

Swan, L., Birnie, D. H., Inglis, G., Connell, J. M. and Hillis, W. S. (2003). The determination of carotid intima medial thickness in adults – a population-based twin study. *Atherosclerosis*, **166**, 137–41.

Taylor, A. J., Kent, S. M., Flaherty, P. J., *et al.* (2002) ARBITER: Arterial Biology for the Investigation of the Treatment Effects of Reducing Cholesterol: a randomized trial comparing the effects of atorvastatin and pravastatin on carotid intima medial thickness. *Circulation*, **106**, 2055–60.

Taylor, A. J., Merz, C. N. and Udelson, J. E. (2003). 34th Bethesda Conference: Executive summary–can atherosclerosis imaging techniques improve the detection of patients at risk for ischemic heart disease? *Journal of the American College of Cardiology*, **41**, 1860–2.

Taylor, A. J., Sullenberger, L. E., Lee, H. J., Lee, J. K. and Graee, K. A. (2004). Arterial Biology for the Investigation of the Treatment Effects of Reducing Cholesterol (ARBITER) 2: a double-blind, placebo-controlled study of extended-release niacin on atherosclerosis progres-sion in secondary prevention patients treated with statins. *Circulation*, **110**, 3512–17.

Third Report of the National Cholesterol Education Program (NCEP) Expert Panel on Detection, Evaluation, and Treatment of High Blood Cholesterol in Adults (Adult Treatment Panel III) final report. (2002). *Circulation*, **106**, 3143–421.

Thom, T., Haase, N., Rosamond, W., *et al.* (2006). Heart Disease and Stroke Statistics–2006 Update. A Report From the American Heart Association Statistics Committee and Stroke Statistics Subcommittee. *Circulation*, 2006 January 11.

Topper, J. N., Cai, J., Falb, D. and Gimbrone, M. A. Jr. (1996). Identification of vascular endothelial genes differentially responsive to fluid mechanical stimuli: cyclooxygenase-2, manganese superoxide dismutase, and endothelial cell nitric oxide synthase are selectively up-regulated by steady laminar shear stress. *Procceed-ings of the National Academy of Science USA*, **93**, 10417–22.

Van der Meer, I. M., Oei, H. H., Hofman, A., *et al.* (2006). Soluble Fas, a mediator of apoptosis, C-reactive protein, and coronary and extracoronary atherosclero-sis. The Rotterdam Coronary Calcification Study. *Atherosclerosis*.

Van der Meer, I. M., De Maat, M. P., Hak, A. E., *et al.* (2002). C-reactive protein predicts progression of atherosclero-sis measured at various sites in the arterial tree: the Rotterdam Study. *Stroke*, **33**, 2750–5.

Virmani, R., Kolodgie, F. D., Burke, A. P., Farb, A. and Schwartz, S. M. (2000). Lessons from sudden coronary death: a comprehensive morphological classification scheme for atherosclerotic lesions. *Arteriosclerosis, Thrombosis and Vascular Biology*, **20**, 1262–75.

Wang, T. J., Nam, B. H., Wilson, P. W., *et al.* (2002). Association of C-reactive protein with carotid athero-sclerosis in men and women: the Framingham Heart Study. *Arteriosclerosis, Thrombosis and Vascular Biology*, **22**, 1662–7.

Wang, T. J., Nam, B. H., D'Agostino, R. B., *et al.* (2003). Carotid intima-media thickness is associated with premature parental coronary heart disease: the Framingham Heart Study. *Circulation*, **108**, 572–6.

Wang, D., Yang, H., Quinones, M. J., *et al.* (2005). A genome-wide scan for carotid artery intima-media thickness: the Mexican-American Coronary Artery Disease family study. *Stroke*, **36**, 540–5.

White, H., Boden-Albala, B., Wang, C., *et al.* (2005). Ischemic stroke subtype incidence among whites, blacks, and Hispanics: the Northern Manhattan Study. *Circulation*, **111**, 1327–31.

Wiklund, O., Hulthe, J., Wikstrand, J., *et al.* (2002). Effect of controlled release/extended release metoprolol on carotid intima-media thickness in patients with hypercholesterolemia: a 3-year randomized study. *Stroke*, **33**, 572−7.

Wilson, P. W., Hoeg, J. M., D'Agostino, R. B., *et al.* (1997). Cumulative effects of high cholesterol levels, high blood pressure, and cigarette smoking on carotid stenosis. *New England Journal of Medicine*, **337**, 516−22.

Wilson, P. W., D'Agostino, R. B., Levy, D., *et al.* (1998). Prediction of coronary heart disease using risk factor categories. *Circulation*, **97**, 1837−47.

Wolf, P. A., Kannel, W. B., Sorlie, P. and McNamara, P. (1981). Asymptomatic carotid bruit and risk of stroke. The Framingham Study. *Journal of the American Medical Association*, **245**, 1442−5.

Wolf, P. A., D'Agostino, R. B., Belanger, A. J. and Kannel, W. B. (1991). Probability of stroke: a risk profile from the Framingham Study. *Stroke*, **22**, 312−18.

Xiang, A. H., Azen, S. P., Buchanan, T. A., *et al.* (2002). Heritability of subclinical atherosclerosis in Latino families ascertained through a hypertensive parent. *Arteriosclerosis, Thrombosis and Vascular Biology*, **22**, 843−8.

Yuan, C., Zhang, S. X., Polissar, N. L., *et al.* (2002). Identification of fibrous cap rupture with magnetic resonance imaging is highly associated with recent transient ischemic attack or stroke. *Circulation*, **105**, 181−5.

Zannad, F., Visvikis, S., Gueguen, R., *et al.* (1998). Genetics strongly determines the wall thickness of the left and right carotid arteries. *Human Genetics*, **103**, 183−8.

Zarins, C. K., Giddens, D. P., Bharadvaj, B. K., *et al.* (1983). Carotid bifurcation atherosclerosis. Quantitative correlation of plaque localization with flow velocity profiles and wall shear stress. *Circulation Research*, **53**, 502−14.

3

Genetics of carotid atherosclerosis

Stephen S. Rich[1] and Donna K. Arnett[2]

[1]Wake Forest University School of Medicine, Winston-Salem, NC, USA
[2]University of Alabama at Birmingham School of Public Health, Birmingham, AL, USA

Introduction

Carotid atherosclerosis is a multifactorial pheno-type that is the end product of an array of genetic and environmental causes. The number of cell types and factors that influence the interaction of inflammatory, metabolic and hemodynamic mechanisms is likely to be large. Each of these processes may have both "public" and "private" genetic determinants. Increasing knowledge of genes, their sequence variation, and their expression has provided novel insights regarding the contribution of individual genetic factors to atherosclerosis risk and potential biological pathways that mediate that risk.

Human genetic research has a recent history, starting from Mendel's reading of his paper, "Experiments on Plant Hybridization," in 1865 and publication in 1866. Mapping and identification of genes for human traits require three essential ingredients – a heritable trait, biological material (DNA), and DNA polymorphisms. DNA polymorphisms are heritable markers that can be scored in human populations. Many of the early investigations in human genetics were restricted to Mendelian (single gene) disorders in families that exhibited either dominant or recessive inheritance patterns. The DNA polymorphisms were restricted to blood group or serological markers, and were relatively infrequent in the human genome. Human genetic studies were revolutionized by the development of a new class of markers (restriction fragment length polymorphisms, RFLPs) and an analytic framework to enhance gene discovery (Botstein et al., 1980). Over the past 25 years, rapid progress in genomic technologies (Wolfsberg et al., 2003; Altshuler et al., 2005) has provided increasingly effective means to provide highly informative and remarkably dense sets of genetic markers. These events have led to the identification of many single gene disorders; however, the great challenge for human genetics is the identification of genes that influence the risk of common disease, such as carotid atherosclerosis.

Studies of the genetic basis of any complex human disease, and particularly carotid athero-sclerosis, require that the phenotype must be heritable. Requirements of careful clinical evaluation of phenotype are mandatory, as measurement error can have highly detrimental effects on heritability, the ability to map, and subsequently identify genes. For carotid atherosclerosis assessment in free-living human populations, the primary phenotype is intima media thickness (IMT), determined by B-mode ultrasound using standardized protocols that have been developed in major epidemiologic studies (Howard et al., 1994). A typical protocol would involve imaging performed on both the right and left extracranial carotid arteries by trained ultrasound technicians. A preliminary exploratory transverse study would be performed to assess the participant's anatomy and to detect the presence of significant athero-sclerotic disease. Standardized longitudinal images would be obtained of the near and far walls of the distal 10-mm portion of the common carotid artery at five predefined interrogation angles spaced 30° apart on each side. The "measured phenotype" for IMT would represent the mean value of 20 arterial segments, often of the common carotid IMT. This estimate of carotid atherosclerosis would have potentially different characteristics than other measures using fewer readings, or readings at different angles or locations. Thus, the phenotype, including the measurement and errors of measurement, are critical to finding (and replicating) genes. Once a phenotype has been appropriately determined, the extent of familial aggregation or genetic variation of the phenotype (heritability) is an important parameter for determining the likelihood of successful gene identification.

Familial aggregation and heritability of carotid atherosclerosis (IMT)

Extensive research with many study designs and diverse populations over more than 30 years has revealed a consistent pattern of familial influence on atherosclerosis (Hopkins and Williams, 1986). A positive family history of early cardiovascular disease (CVD) and myocardial infarction (MI) are significant independent risk factors for atherosclerosis. Between 20% and 50% of subjects with atherosclerosis have a positive family history of CVD or MI, even when including such risks as total cholesterol, LDL, HDL, blood pressure, diabetes, and cigarette smoking (Hopkins et al., 1988; Schildkraut et al., 1989; Williams et al., 2001).

Although there is ample evidence that genes play an important role in atherosclerosis, relatively few studies have estimated the extent of genetic contribution to measures of subclinical disease risk. Based upon an epidemiologic survey of households in Mexico City, the IMT measured at the common carotid artery (CCA) and the internal carotid artery (ICA) were obtained using ultrasonography (Duggirala et al., 1996). Genetic analyses of CCA IMT and ICA IMT measurements with models

incorporating cardiovascular risk factors (lipids, diabetes, blood pressure and smoking) resulted in significant estimates of heritability for CCA IMT ($h^2 = 0.92 \pm 0.05$) and ICA IMT ($h^2 = 0.86 \pm 0.13$). Of the observed variance in CCA IMT, genetic factors accounted for 66.0% of the total variation; for ICA IMT, genetic factors explained a similarly high proportion (74.9%) of total variation. These results suggested that substantial proportions of variance in CCA IMT and ICA IMT were attributable to shared genetic factors.

Other studies also observed significant evidence for familial aggregation of IMT in a variety of populations and ascertainment schemes. Familial aggregation of carotid IMT in the presence of type 2 diabetes was studied in 252 individuals with type 2 diabetes identified from 122 families (Lange et al., 2002). The age-, sex- and race-adjusted heritability estimate for carotid IMT was significantly elevated ($h^2 = 0.32 \pm 0.17$). Further adjustment for total cholesterol, hypertension status, and current smoking status increased the estimate ($h^2 = 0.41 \pm 0.16$). IMT heritability estimates in Latino families ascertained through a hypertensive proband (Xiang et al., 2002) were measured in 204 adult offspring of 69 hypertensive probands, along with 82 parents (54 probands and 28 spouses). In the offspring, heritability of IMT was significantly elevated ($h^2 = 0.64$) after adjustment for significant cardiovascular risk factors. In this population, genetic factors accounted for 50% of the total variation in IMT, compared to 22% of variation explained by "recognized" cardiovascular risk factors.

In the Framingham Offspring cohort, longitudinal measurements of carotid IMT were made from 1996 to 1998 in 906 men and 980 women from 586 extended families (Fox et al., 2003). B-mode ultrasonography was used to define mean and maximum IMT of the CCA and ICA. Multivariable-adjusted estimates of heritability were $h^2 = 0.38$ for the mean CCA IMT and $h^2 = 0.35$ for the mean ICA IMT. In the Northern Manhattan Family Study (Juo et al., 2004), 440 subjects from 77 Caribbean Hispanic families were examined for both mean

IMT and maximum IMT at the ICA, CCA, and carotid bifurcation, and the total IMT was determined as the mean value of IMT at all segments. The heritability estimates for IMT ranged from $h^2 = 0.09$ to $h^2 = 0.40$, with the highest for total maximum IMT and lowest for ICA maximum IMT. Using a bivariate genetic analysis method, there were significant genetic (but not environmental) correlations between IMT and measures of obesity (body mass index [BMI], waist circumference, and skin-fold thickness), a strong risk factor for atherosclerosis in Hispanic populations These results suggest that obesity and IMT may share common genetic factors.

A special study design often used in human genetics is the twin study. The comparison of monozygotic (MZ) twins (who share all their genes and their early environment) with dizygotic (DZ) twins (who share one-half their genes and their early environment) can provide an estimate of the effect of genetic factors on a phenotype that is highly age-dependent. Since carotid atherosclerosis is likely to have important age effects, comparisons made with twins (rather than parent-offspring or even siblings) can provide a "control" for effects on carotid atherosclerosis that differ by age. In a recent study (Swan et al., 2003) B-mode carotid artery ultrasound images were acquired on 264 twins (142 MZ and 122 DZ). An increased carotid IMT was significantly associated with known cardiovascular risk factors (total cholesterol and systolic blood pressure) and with a history of coronary events. Carotid IMT exhibited significant familial aggregation (intraclass correlation of 0.54 for MZ vs. 0.39 for DZ). Although the estimated heritability was similar to that observed in other studies ($h^2 = 0.31$), the small sample size did not permit the estimate to reach statistical significance.

Familial aggregation and heritability of other measures of carotid atherosclerosis

In contrast to IMT, the presence (or absence) of carotid artery plaque was examined for evidence of genetic contribution to carotid atherosclerosis (Hunt et al., 2002). Extracranial focal carotid artery plaque was identified by B-mode ultrasound bilaterally in the internal carotid artery or the carotid bulb. In this population (same as that of Durrigrala et al., 1996), 51 of 461 women and 57 of 289 men had evidence of a plaque in the right and/or left carotid artery. The age- and sex-adjusted heritability for carotid artery plaque was significant ($h^2 = 0.28 \pm 0.15$) and, after adjustment for other risk factors (diabetes, hypertension, BMI, waist circumference, and smoking status), the heritability remained significant ($h^2 = 0.23 + 0.15$). These data indicate that after established cardiovascular risk factors are included, the variation of carotid artery plaque (just as IMT) is under significant genetic influence.

In addition to IMT, the Erasmus Rucphen Family (ERF) study investigated the heritability of carotid-femoral pulse wave velocity (PWV) and carotid plaque score in 930 individuals connected in a single pedigree from an isolated population (Sayed-Tabatabaei et al., 2005). PWV was measured between the carotid and femoral arteries as an indicator of aortic stiffness. CCA IMT and plaque score, quantifying alterations in arterial wall structure, were measured by ultrasonography. After adjustment for risk factors, the heritability estimates were $h^2 = 0.26$ for PWV, $h^2 = 0.35$ for CCA IMT, and $h^2 = 0.21$ for plaque score. Genetic factors explained ~12% of the total variability for each of the phenotypes. Reduced arterial distensibility, or increased arterial stiffness, is a common correlate of carotid atherosclerosis. In the Northern Manhattan Family Study (Juo et al., 2005), measures of distensibility (strain, stiffness, distensibility, and elastic modulus) were obtained from the right CCA. From 88 families (605 relatives), the heritability estimates (age- and sex-adjusted) were $h^2 = 0.25$ for strain, $h^2 = 0.17$ for distensibility, $h^2 = 0.20$ for stiffness, and $h^2 = 0.20$ for elastic modulus. These results suggested that genetic factors explained a moderate proportion of the variability of carotid distensibility. The observed correlations between distensibility and IMT, however, were mainly attributable to age and sex effects, suggesting different underlying genetic mechanisms that generate the observed correlations and risk for carotid atherosclerosis.

An important feature of these reports is that, despite differing populations and study designs, there were consistently moderate to high heritability estimates of carotid IMT (or associated phenotypes) that could not be explained by traditional risk factors. The magnitude of heritability for carotid IMT across multiple ethnic groups appears relatively consistent. This is particularly important information, as there are clear ethnic differences in other risk factors for atherosclerosis (diabetes, obesity, hypertension) that do not appear to be absorbing the genetic effects on carotid atherosclerosis.

Gene discovery – candidate genes

The search for genes related to the cause of common complex disorders such as carotid atherosclerosis and CVD has been frustrating, partly because of the many factors known to contribute to disease and the potential "distance" of disease as a phenotype from genes and gene products. Linkage and association studies for phenotypes more proximal in the pathway from DNA sequence variation to overt clinical disease, such as ultrasound-defined carotid atherosclerosis, may potentially be more enlightening. A large and ever-growing list of candidate genes has been investigated, typically in a case-control design of association. Although early work using candidate genes has been equivocal, several candidate genes appear to have consistent associations with carotid atherosclerosis. One of these, stromelysin (or matrix metalloproteinases [MMP]-3), is discussed in detail below. Other candidate genes are mentioned for historical perspective, recognizing that the list is increasing in length and depth.

Gene discovery – MMP3 (stromelysin, transin)

Human fibroblast stromelysin (MMP3, or transin) is a secreted metalloprotease produced predominantly by connective tissue cells that can degrade the major components of the extracellular matrix, including fibronectin, laminin and type IV collagen (Sellers and Murphy, 1981). As with many candidate genes, the role of MMPs and atherosclerosis has been determined on the basis of gene function, rather than gene discovery. Expression of MMPs interstitial collagenase (MMP-1) gelatinases (MMP-2 and MMP-9) and stromelysin (MMP-3) and their endogenous inhibitors (TIMPs 1 and 2) were studied in human atherosclerotic plaques and in uninvolved arterial specimens (Galis et al., 1994). It was suggested that focal over-expression of activated MMP could promote destabilization and complications of atherosclerotic plaques.

The location of stromelysin I (MMP3) is on chromosome 11 in humans. In fact, this region of human chromosome 11 contains a cluster of metalloproteinase genes, including MMP3 (stromelysin I), MMP1 (fibroblast collagenase), and MMP10 (stromelysin II [MMP10], within a 135-kb region. The family of MMP genes have been mapped to multiple chromosomal sites, including chromosomes 11, 14 (MMP14), 16 (MMP2), 20 (MMP9), and 22 (MMP11). Several MMP genes are clustered on the long arm of chromosome 11q22 (MMP8, MMP10), (MMP1, MMP3, MMP12), (MMP7, MMP13). A common variant in the promoter of MMP3 causing reduced enzyme expression has been evaluated with respect to the progression of coronary atherosclerosis (Gnasso et al., 2000). Although serum matrix MMP-3 levels did not differ significantly among genotypes for the promoter polymorphism, CCA diameter and IMT were significantly larger in those homozygous (6A/6A) for the promoter polymorphism. Further, wall shear stress was lower in 6A/6A subjects, suggesting that the stromelysin promoter was associated with structural and functional characteristics of the CCA. In this study, individuals with the

6A/6A genotype (associated with lower enzyme activity) had increased wall thickness, enlarged arterial lumen, and local reduction of wall shear stress, predisposing them to atherosclerotic plaque localization.

It is unlikely that any single functional polymorphism will fully account for the observed variation in carotid atherosclerosis risk. An example of the genetic complexity is the potential interaction of genes on risk. The functional 5A/6A polymorphism of the MMP3 promoter has been implicated as a potential genetic marker for the progression of angiographically determined atherosclerosis in patients with coronary artery disease. In particular, it has been noted that there is a complex interaction between smoking, MMP3 genotype and risk of coronary heart disease (CHD) in healthy middle-aged men (Humphries *et al.*, 2002). Current smoking nearly doubled the risk for CHD, and suggested that in nonsmoking men (compared with the 5A/5A group) the risk was significantly increased in those with the 6A/6A genotype. Smoking differentially increased risk in all genotype groups. The data indicated a key role for variants in the MMP3 gene in the atherosclerotic process.

A functional interleukin-6 (IL-6) promoter polymorphism (−174G/C) was analyzed with the MMP3 in an effort to determine whether interaction of matrix and inflammation genes could increase risk for carotid atherosclerosis (Rauramaa *et al.*, 2000). The MMP3 genotype was significantly associated with IMT, and this relationship remained significant after adjustments for known risk factors (age, cardiorespiratory fitness, BMI, smoking, LDL cholesterol, and systolic blood pressure). The 5A/6A polymorphism independently explained 7% of the variance in carotid bifurcation IMT. The IL-6 polymorphism was also significantly associated with increased IMT, with men homozygous for the G allele having IMT that was 11% greater than men homozygous for the C allele. Men who were homozygous for both the 6A and G alleles had a covariate-adjusted IMT that was 36% greater than men who were homozygous for

neither allele. These data suggest that genetic factors that predispose to reduced matrix remodeling (MMP3 6A-allele) and to increased inflammation (IL-6 G-allele) combine to increase IMT in the carotid bifurcation. In a similar approach, MMP3 5A/6A homozygotes were found to have significantly higher aortic input and arterial stiffness than heterozygotes (Medley *et al.*, 2003). Differences in gene expression for 5A homozygotes (higher levels) and 6A homozygotes (lower levels) versus 5A/6A heterozygotes suggested that the MMP3 genotype may be an important determinant of vascular remodeling and atherosclerosis.

It should be noted that the polymorphisms investigated for MMP3 (and other candidate genes) are focused on "functional" polymorphisms; i.e. sites whose genotypes have a difference in level of enzymatic activity or a structural protein. While these "functional" sites are obvious candidates within a recognized candidate gene, it is not necessarily the case that only the functional sites are important in variation in activity or disease risk. Recent evidence of genetic risk factors for Crohn's disease (Hugot *et al.*, 2001), asthma (Van Eerdewegh *et al.*, 2002) and schizophrenia (Chumakov *et al.*, 2002) suggest that polymorphisms in noncoding (nonfunctional) regions may be important in disease susceptibility through gene regulation or alternative splicing. Thus, the careful examination of MMP3 (Figure 3.1) suggests that many polymorphic sites require consideration for association with carotid atherosclerosis. As shown in Figure 3.1, numerous polymorphic sites are present throughout the MMP3 gene, few of which are coding or reside in exons, but many of which are intronic.

Gene discovery − other genes

There are numerous candidate genes that could feasibly contribute to carotid atherosclerosis. The most consistent is MMP3, yet others have been proposed at different times. A series of candidate genes that lie in a narrow genomic region on

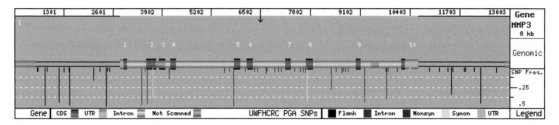

Figure 3.1 Structure and polymorphic sites/frequency of SNPs in the MMP3 gene. MMP3 has 10 exons and four coding SNPs (two in exon 2, exon 6 and exon 8); the nonsynonymous SNP located in exon 2 is of high frequency. Figure obtained from *SeattleSNPs, the NHLBI Program for Genomic Applications, SeattleSNPs, Seattle, WA (URL: http://pga.gs. washington.edu) [December, 2005]*. View of MMP3 obtained using Vh2 software (Nickerson *et al.* [1988]. *Nature Genetics*, **19**, 233–40).

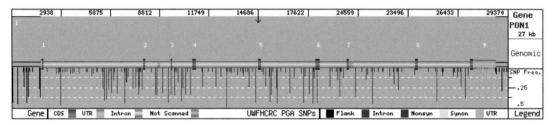

Figure 3.2A Structure and polymorphic sites/frequency of SNPs in the PON1 gene. PON1 has nine exons and only two coding SNPs (one in exon 3, the other in exon 6). Figure obtained from *SeattleSNPs, the NHLBI Program for Genomic Applications, SeattleSNPs, Seattle, WA (URL: http://pga.gs.washington.edu) [December, 2005]*. View of PON1 obtained using Vh2 software (Nickerson *et al.* [1988]. *Nature Genetics*, **19**, 233–40).

human chromosome 7 is paraoxonase system (PON1, PON2, PON3). A polymorphism in PON1 (L55M) has been weakly associated with carotid atherosclerosis. Another common polymorphism at codon 192 in PON1 has been shown to be associated with increased risk for CHD in Caucasian populations. However, these findings have not been reported consistently in all Caucasian and non-Caucasian populations, suggesting that this site may not represent a functional mutation; however, it may be in linkage disequilibrium with a functional site in either PON1 or a nearby gene (possibly PON2 or PON3). Identification of additional polymorphisms in the PON-gene cluster may help to locate the functional polymorphism. The extent of polymorphisms in the PON cluster is seen in Figure 3.2 (Figure 3.2A, PON1; Figure 3.2B, PON2; Figure 3.2C, PON3). As can be seen, there are numerous polymorphic

sites in each of the PON genes and, despite the genes having the appearance of duplications, there are numerous differences in structure and diversity that could lead to differences in function. Thus, failure to replicate a single polymorphism association with carotid atherosclerosis could be due to lack of information at that site (but an adjacent site in linkage disequilibrium could be informative).

Examination of all polymorphic sites (or those that account for the observed pattern of linkage disequilibrium in the candidate gene) better accounts for genetic association than examination of a single (albeit functional) candidate polymorphism. In addition, methods of genetic analysis have been evolving, so that methods of genomic control or individual admixture mapping can be used when family-based association is not feasible. Admixture methods may reduce the effects of population stratification. A recent example of this approach is

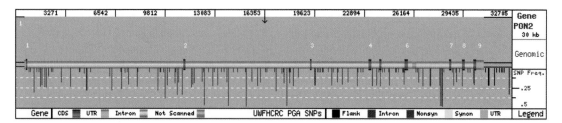

Figure 3.2B Structure and polymorphic sites/frequency of SNPs in the PON2 gene. PON2 has nine exons (same as PON1) although they are placed differently in the gene and are of different size. PON2 has three coding SNPs (exon 5, exon 6 and exon 9). Figure obtained from *SeattleSNPs, the NHLBI Program for Genomic Applications, SeattleSNPs, Seattle, WA (URL: http://pga.gs.washington.edu) [December, 2005]*. View of PON2 obtained using Vh2 software (Nickerson *et al.* [1988]. *Nature Genetics*, **19**, 233–40).

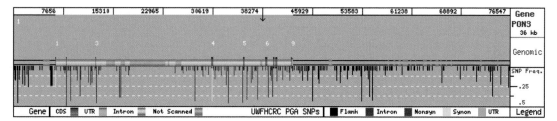

Figure 3.2C Structure and polymorphic sites/frequency of SNPs in the PON3 gene. PON3 has 9 exons (same as PON1 and PON2) although they are placed differently in the gene and are of different size. PON3 remains incompletely scanned for polymorphic sites, and has two relatively infrequent coding SNPs (exon 5 and exon 6). Figure obtained from *SeattleSNPs, the NHLBI Program for Genomic Applications, SeattleSNPs, Seattle, WA (URL: http://pga.gs.washington.edu) [December, 2005]*. View of PON2 obtained using Vh2 software (Nickerson *et al.* [1998]. *Nature Genetics*, **19**, 233–40).

the examination of risk of carotid atherosclerosis in subjects with type 2 diabetes. As atherosclerosis in type 2 diabetic patients has been linked to increased oxidative stress, genes that contribute to the anti-oxidant defense of the vascular wall, such as glutathione peroxidase-1 (GPx-1), would be an appropriate target. The GPx-1 gene was screened in Japanese type 2 diabetic patients, and four polymorphisms (−602A/G, +2C/T, Ala(5)/Ala(6), and Pro198Leu) were identified (Hamanishi *et al.*, 2004). Among these polymorphisms, all were in strong linkage disequilibrium with one another. The mean IMT of CCA and the prevalence of cardiovascular and peripheral vascular disease were significantly higher in the Pro/Leu group than in the Pro/Pro group. Follow-up with in vitro functional studies suggested

that the combination of Ala(6)/198Leu of GPx-1 had a 40% decrease in enzyme activity, while the −602G/+2T combination had a 25% decrease in activity.

Genomewide linkage scans for carotid atherosclerosis

In contrast to candidate gene studies, in which the investigator expresses knowledge about the proposed candidate as a component of a biological pathway important in the etiology of carotid atherosclerosis, the genomewide linkage scan professes no prior knowledge. The purpose of the genomewide linkage scan is to conduct a systematic evaluation of the entire human genome using families to examine the similarity of phenotype (IMT) with sharing of alleles at polymorphic genetic markers. As carotid IMT has been shown to be a heritable quantitative measure of atherosclerosis, a genomewide linkage scan could identify previously unrecognized genomic regions that could harbor genes contributing to variation in IMT. Because the genomewide linkage scan requires family material (families or sibships), relatively few scans have been performed for IMT or other measures of carotid atherosclerosis.

In the Framingham Offspring study (Fox et al., 2004), a genomewide linkage scan was conducted to localize quantitative-trait loci (QTLs) that contribute to variation in carotid IMT in 596 men and 629 women from 311 extended families (1242 sib pairs). In this set of families, significant evidence for linkage to ICA IMT (LOD = 4.1) was found at a region 161 cM from the tip of the short arm of chromosome 12. No region in the genome had suggestive evidence for linkage for CCA IMT. For ICA IMT, a strong candidate gene (a "positional candidate") was identified (SCARB1). Family-based association analysis of a SCARB1 SNP in exon 1 suggested a protective association with decreased ICA IMT compared with subjects homozygous for the common allele. This particular polymorphism contributed only a minor amount (2%) to the total variation in ICA IMT. Further, the polymorphism did not account for the evidence of linkage for IMT. Thus, there is strong evidence for a gene (or genes) in the region of chromosome 12 contributing to variation in ICA IMT. The variant of SCARB1 is not likely to be the sole contributing factor.

A genomewide linkage scan was recently performed using data from 91 two-generation Mexican American families, in which the criteria for ascertainment was that the family had a parent with coronary artery disease (Wang et al., 2005). In this set of families, the strongest evidence of linkage was found on chromosome 2 (LOD = 3.08). Other regions in the genome that supported evidence of linkage with carotid IMT were on chromosome 6 (LOD = 2.21) and chromosome 13 (LOD = 1.34).

In the NHLBI Family Heart Study (Pankow et al., 2004), a cross-sectional analysis of 2223 members of 525 randomly-ascertained families and 2514 members of 589 high CHD-risk families was performed. In contrast to other studies, the genome scan revealed no regions of significant or suggestive linkage for carotid plaque, although suggestive linkage (LOD = 2.43) was found on chromosome 2p11.2. Numerous other markers with nominal evidence ($p < 0.05$) for linkage were found, including those on chromosomes 2p25, 2q24–q32, and 6q21–q23. Thus, although there is little significant evidence for direct overlap of regions in the three genomewide linkage scans, there are suggestions that overlap in regions may occur.

Future of genetic studies of carotid atherosclerosis

When considering the future of identification of genetic determinants of carotid atherosclerosis, there are a number of issues to be considered. The first is the phenotype. There are numerous advantages in studying anatomically-defined atherosclerosis noninvasively as opposed to clinical events. First, atherosclerotic lesions are the necessary and specific prerequisite for most clinical cardiovascular events. Their presence is highly predictive of future clinical events (Hodis et al., 1998; O'Leary et al., 1999). In absence of direct evaluation of anatomically-defined lesions, the measurement of highly correlated phenotypes (such as IMT) provides a wealth of information that is amenable to genetic studies. In this respect, the clinical cardiovascular event is a more remote, complex, multifactorial and imprecise phenotype for genetic studies than the phenotype defined by anatomical means or imaging. Thus, continued exploration and examination of noninvasive measurement of carotid atherosclerosis is warranted to permit a closer relationship with the anticipated genetic variants. The second aspect is the development and implementation of novel statistical methods that will allow for simultaneous assessment of multiple genes, interacting with one another and with the environment to alter the phenotype. Such models will provide insight into small, meaningful, but relevant contributions of DNA variation contributing to carotid athero-sclerosis. Third, the characterization of the DNA sequence should allow correlation of variation in DNA with variation in phenotype. The current "gold standard" for polymorphic characterization of DNA in large studies is the dense SNP map (500 K or 1 M) across the human genome. However, in the next 5 years, it is anticipated that a complete $(1\times)$ sequencing coverage of the human genome may become affordable. Thus, the information available from every individual will exponentially increase. With appropriate informatics and analysis capability, it is not beyond the realm of imagination to obtain the DNA sequence of cases with carotid atherosclerosis and controls in a defined population for elegantly measured phenotypes. Once these technologies become available, the future of molecular medicine and individually tailored interventions and therapies for carotid atherosclerosis becomes possible.

REFERENCES

Altshuler, D., Brooks, L. D., Chakravarti, A., *et al.* (2005). A haplotype map of the human genome. *Nature*, **437**, 1299–320.

Botstein, D., White, R. L., Skolnick, M. and Davis, R. W. (1980). Construction of a genetic linkage map in man using restriction fragment length polymorphisms. *American Journal of Human Genetics*, **32**, 314–31.

Chumakov, I., Blumenfeld, M., Guerassimenko, O., *et al.* (2002). Genetic and physiological data implicating the new human gene G72 and the gene for D-amino acid oxidase in schizophrenia. *Proceedings of the National Academy of Science USA*, **99**, 13675–80.

Duggirala, R., Gonzalez Villalpando, C., O'Leary, D. H., Stern, M. P. and Blangero, J. (1996). Genetic basis of variation in carotid artery wall thickness. *Stroke*, **27**, 833–77.

Fox, C. S., Polak, J. F., Chazaro, I., *et al.* (2003). Genetic and environmental contributions to atherosclerosis pheno-types in men and women: heritability of carotid intima-media thickness in the Framingham Heart Study. *Stroke*, **34**, 397–401.

Fox, C. S., Cupples, L. A., Chazaro, I., *et al.* (2004). Genomewide linkage analysis for internal carotid artery intimal medial thickness: evidence for linkage to chromosome 12. *American Journal of Human Genetics*, **74**, 253–61.

Galis, Z. S., Sukhova, G. K., Lark, M. W. and Libby, P. (1994). Increased expression of matrix metalloprotein-ases and matrix degrading activity in vulnerable regions of human atherosclerotic plaques. *Journal of Clinical Investigation*, **94**, 2493–503.

Gnasso, A., Motti, C., Irace, C., *et al.* (2000). Genetic variation in human stromelysin gene promoter and common carotid geometry in healthy male subjects. *Arteriosclerosis, Thrombosis and Vascular Biology*, **20**, 1600–5.

Hamanishi, T., Furuta, H., Kato, H., *et al.* (2004). Functional variants in the glutathione peroxidase-1 (GPx-1) gene are associated with increased intima-media thickness of carotid arteries and risk of macro-vascular diseases in Japanese type 2 diabetic patients. *Diabetes*, **53**, 2455–60.

Hodis, H. N., Mack, W. J., LaBree, L., *et al.* (1998). The role of carotid arterial intima-media thickness in predicting clinical coronary events. *Annals of Internal Medicine*, **128**, 262–9.

Hopkins, P. N. and Williams, R. R. (1986). Identification and relative weight of cardiovascular risk factors. *Cardiology Clinic*, **4**, 3–31.

Hopkins, P. N., Williams, R. R., Kuida, H., *et al.* (1988). Family history as an independent risk factor for incident coronary artery disease in a high-risk cohort in Utah. *American Journal of Cardiology*, **62**, 703–7.

Howard, G., Burke, G. L., Evans, G. W., *et al.* (1994). Relations of intimal-medial thickness among sites within the carotid artery as evaluated by B-mode ultrasound. Atherosclerosis Risk in Communities. *Stroke*, **25**, 1581–7.

Hugot, J. P., Chamaillard, M., Zouali, H., *et al.* (2001). Association of NOD2 leucine-rich repeat variants with susceptibility to Crohn's disease. *Nature*, **411**, 599–603.

Humphries, S. E., Martin, S., Cooper, J. and Miller, G. (2002). Interaction between smoking and the stromely-sin-1 (MMP3) gene 5A/6A promoter polymorphism and risk of coronary heart disease in healthy men. *Annals of Human Genetics*, **66**, 343–52.

Hunt, K. J., Duggirala, R., Goring, H. H., *et al.* (2002). Genetic basis of variation in carotid artery plaque in the San Antonio Family Heart Study. *Stroke*, **33**, 2775–80.

Juo, S. H., Lin, H. F., Rundek, T., *et al.* (2004). Genetic and environmental contributions to carotid intima-media thickness and obesity phenotypes in the Northern Manhattan Family Study. *Stroke*, **35**, 2243–7.

Juo, S. H., Rundek, T., Lin, H. F., *et al.* (2005). Heritability of carotid artery distensibility in Hispanics: the Northern Manhattan Family Study. *Stroke*, **36**, 2357–61.

Lange, L. A., Bowden, D. W., Langefeld, C. D., *et al.* (2002). Heritability of carotid artery intima-medial thickness in type 2 diabetes. *Stroke*, **33**, 1876–81.

Medley, T. L., Kingwell, B. A., Gatzka, C. D., Pillay, P. and Cole, T. J. (2003). Matrix metalloproteinase-3 genotype contributes to age-related aortic stiffening through modulation of gene and protein expression. *Circulation Research*, **92**, 1254–61.

Nickerson, D. A., Taylor, S. L., Weiss, K. M., *et al.* (1998). DNA sequence diversity in a 9.7-kb region of the human lipoprotein lipase gene. *Nature Genetics*, **19**, 233–40.

O'Leary, D. H., Polak, J. F., Kronmal, R. A., *et al.* (1999). Carotid-artery intima and media thickness as a risk factor for myocardial infarction and stroke in older adults. Cardiovascular Health Study Collaborative Research Group. *New England Journal of Medicine*, **340**, 14–22.

Pankow, J. S., Heiss, G., Evans, G. W., *et al.* (2004). Familial aggregation and genome-wide linkage analysis of carotid artery plaque: the NHLBI family heart study. *Human Heredity*, **57**, 80–9.

Rauramaa, R., Vaisanen, S. B., Luong, L. A., *et al.* (2000). Stromelysin-1 and interleukin-6 gene promoter polymorphisms are determinants of asymptomatic carotid artery atherosclerosis. *Arteriosclerosis, Thrombosis and Vascular Biology*, **20**, 2657–62.

Sayed-Tabatabaei, F. A., van Rijn, M. J., Schut, A. F., *et al.* (2005). Heritability of the function and structure of the arterial wall: findings of the Erasmus Rucphen Family (ERF) study. *Stroke*, **36**, 2351–6.

Schildkraut, J. M., Myers, R. H., Cupples, L. A., Kiely, D. K. and Kannel, W. B. (1989). Coronary risk associated with age and sex of parental heart disease in the Framingham Study. *American Journal of Cardiology*, **64**, 555–9.

Sellers, A. and Murphy, G. (1981). Collagenolytic enzymes and their naturally occurring inhibitors. *International Review of Connective Tissue Research*, **9**, 151–90.

Swan, L., Birnie, D. H., Inglis, G., Connell, J. M. and Hillis, W. S. (2003). The determination of carotid intima medial thickness in adults – population-based twin study. *Atherosclerosis*, **166**, 137–41.

Van Eerdewegh, P., Little, R. D., Dupuis, J., *et al.* (2002). Association of the ADAM33 gene with asthma and bronchial hyperresponsiveness. *Nature*, **418**, 426–30.

Wang, D., Yang, H., Quinones, M. J., *et al.* (2005). A genome-wide scan for carotid artery intima-media thickness: the Mexican-American Coronary Artery Disease family study. *Stroke*, **36**, 540–5.

Williams, R. R., Hunt, S. C., Heiss, G., *et al.* (2001). Usefulness of cardiovascular family history data for population-based preventive medicine and medical research (the Health Family Tree Study and the NHLBI Family Heart Study). *American Journal of Cardiology*, **87**, 129–35.

Wolfsberg, T. G., Wetterstrand, K. A., Guyer, M. S., Collins, F. S. and Baxevanis, A. D. (2003). A user's guide to the human genome. *Nature Genetics*, **35** (Suppl. 1), 4.

Xiang, A. H., Azen, S. P., Buchanan, T. A., *et al.* (2002). Heritability of subclinical atherosclerosis in Latino families ascertained through a hypertensive parent. *Arteriosclerosis, Thrombosis and Vascular Biology*, **22**, 843–8.

4

Hematological processes in emboli formation

Alison H. Goodall and Greg McMahon

University of Leicester, Leicester, UK

Introduction

Spontaneous plaque rupture, or damage to the vessel wall during therapeutic interventions will lead to the formation of a thrombus at the site of vascular damage. Emboli can be released either as a result of shearing of the thrombus from the vessel wall, or as smaller emboli propagated at the surface of the growing thrombus. In either case the released emboli can lead to downstream vascular occlusion and subsequent ischemia.

Cerebrovascular events related to carotid artery disease are caused in the majority of cases by atherothrombotic emboli dislodging from the carotid plaque (Foulkes *et al.*, 1988; Sitzer *et al.*, 1995; Lammie *et al.*, 1999; Jander *et al.*, 2001). Embolization of platelet thrombus into the circulation is also a well recognized complication of surgical intervention (carotid endarterectomy) or carotid stenting (Riles *et al.*, 1994; Jordan *et al.*, 1999) and is the main cause of postoperative stroke and transient ischemic attack (TIA) (Spencer, 1997). It can generally be considered that embolization that occurs during the dissection phase of carotid endarterectomy is associated with carotid plaque instability, whereas embolic events observed after endarterectomy, following restoration of flow and in the early postoperative period, are related to excessive thrombus formation at the endarterectomy and clamping sites. The risk of developing embolization during carotid endarterectomy has been shown to be independent of surgical artefacts (Gaunt *et al.*, 1996), and may be linked to endogenous, patient-specific factors since the rate of embolization seen in patients who undergo a second procedure is correlated with that seen during their first operation (Hayes *et al.*, 2001). In this chapter we outline the hemostatic response to vascular damage in the carotid artery and consider the endogenous hemostatic factors that may determine the likelihood of embolization in patients.

A thrombus is formed through the interaction of platelets, coagulation and fibrinolytic factors. It is the balance between these components, and their inhibitors that determines the size and nature of the thrombus and the risk of embolization. Thrombus formed in the arterial system is predominantly platelet-rich (white thrombus) and many strands of evidence including investigation of pathological material, studies in flow-based laboratory systems and in animal models have demonstrated the importance of platelets in the regulation of thrombus formation. It is becoming clear that platelets are also key players in regulating the risk of embolization.

Mechanisms involved in thrombus formation and stabilization

Platelets adhere to the damaged vessel wall where they become activated and recruit further platelets into an aggregate. Adherent platelets expose a procoagulant surface that promotes the generation of thrombin, resulting in the cleavage of fibrinogen to fibrin, which stabilizes the aggregate. If the resultant thrombus is unstable it can be sheared from the vessel wall and travel downstream. Alternatively if the thrombus continues to be thrombogenic it can generate emboli at the surface, which may be shed and then cause downstream vascular occlusion (Figure 4.1). Thus the formation of emboli is a balance between thrombus size, stability and composition. Antiplatelet agents such as aspirin, abciximab and clopidogrel have proven efficacy as antithrombotic agents (Antithrombotic Trialists Collaboration, 2002) but understanding how they affect the dynamic process of thrombus formation and subsequent embolization is important in optimizing the treatment for patients with carotid artery disease.

Our understanding of hemostasis has advanced significantly over the past few decades. Concepts developed in the 1970s and 1980s saw the coagulation cascade and the platelets as relatively separate entities. This has subsequently been modified by work from many laboratories, but most notably from Harold Robert's group at Chapel Hill, that has given rise to the concept of a "cell-based" model of hemostasis in which the platelet plays a central role in the formation of a mature thrombus (Hoffman and Monroe, 2001; Hoffman, 2003).

Thrombus formation is initiated when vascular damage or plaque rupture allows tissue factor (TF) to become exposed to the plasma (Day et al., 2005). TF is found in abundance in the vascular intima and is often present in large amounts in atherosclerotic plaques (Wilcox et al., 1989; Fernandez-Ortiz et al., 1994). Once in contact with the plasma, TF rapidly binds trace amounts of activated Factor VII (FVIIa) that are present in the blood (Morissey et al., 1993). This activates Factor X (FX) to FXa, which can then generate thrombin from prothrombin. This reaction is rapidly shut down by tissue factor pathway inhibitor (TFPI), which binds to the TF-FVIIa-FXa complex. However the small amount of thrombin generated, together with collagen released from the intima/plaque, is sufficient to allow some platelets to become activated at the site of damage, which can promote further platelet activation and thrombin generation (Hoffman and Monroe, 2001).

Platelets initially adhere to von Willebrand factor (VWF) in the vessel wall. This interaction occurs under high wall shear rates, when the VWF undergoes a shear-induced conformational change, allowing it to bind to the glycoprotein (GP)Ibα receptor on the platelet (Ruggeri, 1997); a process that does not require the platelets to be activated. Consequent platelet activation by collagen and thrombin, and adenosine diphosphate (ADP) released from activated platelets and damaged cells, causes a conformational change in the GPIIb–IIIa receptor complex (Savage et al., 2001). This "final common pathway" of platelet activation allows the receptor to bind to fibrinogen, resulting in platelet-platelet aggregation, and so recruiting further platelets to the growing thrombus. Activated platelets also generate thromboxane A_2 (TxA$_2$) through metabolism of arachidonic acid by cyclo-oxygenase-1 (COX-1), which acts as a secondary agonist, augmenting the effects of the primary agonists by promoting degranulation and stabilizing the binding of fibrinogen to GPIIb–IIIa.

Activated platelets also play an important role in the generation and maintenance of a thrombus by propagating and amplifying thrombin generation through mechanisms that are not inhibited by TFPI. Platelet activation, in particular by collagen, can induce plasma membrane phospholipids to "flip" to the outer surface of the phospholipid bilayer, producing a negatively charged surface (Zwaal and Schroit, 1997). This allows the formation of the tenase and prothrombinase complexes on their surface, leading to a local increase in thrombin generation (Lentz, 2003). Locally

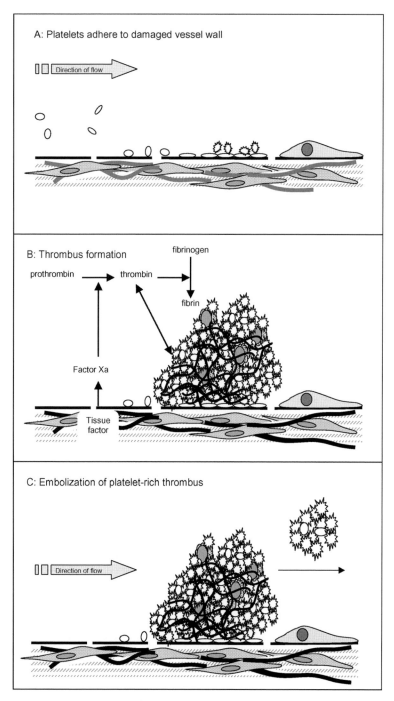

Figure 4.1 Pathways to embolization of a thrombus. (A) Platelets adhere to damaged blood vessel wall at high sheer rates through the interaction of platelet membrane glycoprotein Ibα with von Willebrand factor in the vessel wall. Platelet agonists released locally activate platelets. (B) Tissue factor in the vessel wall initiates coagulation, leading to thrombin generation. This activates platelets allowing aggregates to form, and cleaves fibrinogen to form fibrin. (C) As the thrombus forms, a section of platelet-rich thrombus can break away and travel downstream as emboli.

generated thrombin activates more platelets and cleaves fibrinogen to fibrin, which cross-links to produce a stable meshwork of fibers. Platelets therefore provide a reinforced loop in the generation of a thrombus, providing a source of thrombin to recruit new platelets and propagate clot formation.

Activated platelets also degranulate, releasing factors that potentiate the thrombotic response. These include hemostatic factors such as fibrinogen and Factor XIII (FXIII), released from the platelet α-granules, and platelet agonists such as ADP, released from the dense granules. Degranulation causes platelets to express P-selectin (CD62P) on their surface; a glycoprotein found in the membrane of platelet α-granules that is translocated to the platelet surface where it can bind to leucocytes via the PSGL-1 receptor, and recruit them to the growing thrombus (Larsen *et al.*, 1989; McEver *et al.*, 1989; Furie *et al.*, 2001). Here the leucocytes can release inflammatory factors, proteases and fibrinolytic inhibitors that variously aid the formation and stabilization of the thrombus.

The structure of fibrin is an important factor in clot structure and strength, and therefore in determining thrombus stability. Two key players in controlling the architecture of the fibrin fibers are thrombin and FXIII. Higher levels of thrombin lead to thinner fibers, which form more branches and cross-links, and therefore lead to a more stable clot (Collet *et al.*, 2003; Wolberg *et al.*, 2003; Scott *et al.*, 2004; Weisel, 2005). Factor XIII, which is present both in plasma, and released from the platelet α-granules, is activated by thrombin to FXIIIa, which cross-links the fibrin, so stabilizing the clot (Ariens *et al.*, 2002; Kobbervig and Williams, 2004).

Once a stable thrombus has been formed the process of fibrinolysis begins to eventually remove the clot. The two main fibrinolytic agents are tissue plasminogen activator (tPA) and urokinase-type plasminogen activator (uPA), both derived principally from endothelial cells (Lijnen and Collen, 1997). Both cleave plasminogen to release plasmin, which breaks down the fibrin clot. The principle inhibitor of these factors is plasminogen inhibitor Type-1 (PAI-1) found in significant amounts in the plasma but also in the platelet α-granules (Vaughan, 2005).

Many key factors in the hemostatic process have an influence on embolization (Table 4.1). Much of our understanding of hemostasis has come from the study of platelets and coagulation in relatively static systems. However, thrombi form under conditions of flow which may range from $\sim$200 sec^{-1} in a normal carotid artery to >3500 sec^{-1} in a stenotic vessel (Goldsmith and Turitto, 1986). To understand the regulation of thrombus formation and embolization it is therefore important to study the process under conditions of dynamic flow.

Evidence from in vitro models and animal studies

Several in vitro models of flow have been developed, most based on a flow chamber principle originally described by Hans Baumgartner in which blood, or blood components are flowed at controlled shear rates over a thrombogenic surface such as collagen, VWF, or subendothelial matrix (Tschopp *et al.*, 1979; Sakariassen *et al.*, 1989; Sakariassen *et al.*, 2004). Platelet deposition can be visualized microscopically and quantified either using radiolabeled platelets or by quantitative image analysis. An alternative, simple flow model is also provided by the Chandler loop, in which recalcified blood is placed in a closed loop and rotated to produce a thrombus (Chandler, 1958; Robbie *et al.*, 1997). The thrombi produced in this system are remarkably similar to arterial thrombi, with a platelet-rich head and a fibrin-rich tail (Robbie *et al.*, 1997). However, in many in vitro models the blood is anticoagulated and most models lack key features of a blood vessel, in particular the endothelium; drawbacks that can be overcome by studying thrombus formation in vivo in animal models.

Table 4.1. Key hemostatic factors that regulate thrombus formation and embolization

Platelet adhesion receptors (and their ligands)	Consequence of inhibition/deficiency
GPIbα (von Willebrand factor)	Platelets fail to adhere to the vessel. Thrombus does not form
GPIIb–IIIa (fibrinogen)	Platelets adhere but do not form a stable thrombus
P-selectin (leucocyte PSGL-1/ GPIbα on platelets)	Affects thrombus stability
CD40L (CD40)	Affects thrombus stability
Platelet agonists	
Thrombin	Platelet activation significantly reduced or prevented
Collagen	Platelet deposition significantly reduced
	Affects rate of thrombin generation within thrombus
Thromboxane A$_2$	Platelet aggregation reduced
	Affects thrombus stability
ADP	Reduces thrombus growth
	Specifically affects production of emboli
Hemostatic factors	
Fibrinogen	Thrombus can form but fibrinogen level affects thrombus stability
Thrombin	The level of thrombin generated within the thrombus regulates fibrin structure.
	Affects thrombus stability and resistance to lysis
FXIII	Cross-links fibrin and so affects thrombus stability and resistance to lysis
PAI-1	Affects resistance to lysis

Animal models of thrombosis

The model developed by Folts, Willerson and colleagues, which used endothelial damage to produce an occlusive thrombus (Folts *et al.*, 1976; Yao *et al.*, 1992), highlighted the importance of platelets in embolization. In this model the damage to the vessel wall results in the formation of an occlusive, platelet-rich thrombus which then embolizes and reforms so that cyclic variation in flow is recorded. Originally developed as a canine model of coronary artery disease, this model has been adapted to other species including the pig, rabbit and baboon, and to study carotid artery stenosis (Samana *et al.*, 1992; Golino *et al.*, 1995; Harker *et al.*, 1998).

In recent years, intravital microscopy has been used in whole animals to visualize thrombus formation and embolization at a site of damage, induced either by mechanical or laser injury, or by applying ferric chloride to the outside of an exposed vessel, in particular to explore the hemostatic system in knock-out or genetically modified mice (Day *et al.*, 2004; Mackman, 2004). A number of different vessels have been studied in this way, including the carotid artery. In an elegant series of studies, examining thrombus formation in mouse cremaster vessels, Bruce Furies' laboratory has demonstrated in vivo the sequence of events that occur when a thrombus forms (Sim *et al.*, 2005). These experiments have confirmed that the first element to appear at the site of vessel damage is TF, followed by platelets, which rapidly accumulate to form a large aggregate. Fibrin appears later, and predominantly in the "tail" of the thrombus, nearest the site of damage, so that the platelet-rich "head" of the thrombus extends downstream into the flow of blood (Falati *et al.*, 2002, 2003), and it is this platelet-rich region that can break off into emboli. Once this structure has formed, clot retraction can be seen as the links between the platelets and fibrin are stabilized and strengthened.

Factors affecting the formation of emboli

Platelet adhesion receptors

The GPIb-IX-V and GPIIb–IIIa complexes play synergistic roles, the former serving to initiate platelet deposition and thrombus formation and the latter stabilizing the thrombus (Ruggeri *et al.*, 1999). If adhesion of platelet GPIbα to VWF is blocked (for example, with antibodies), or absent (as in blood from patients with either Bernard-Soulier syndrome; a deficiency in the platelet GPIb complex, or severe, type III von Willebrand's disease; a deficiency in VWF), platelet adhesion is prevented at flow shear rates above 350 s^{-1} and no thrombus can form (Ruggeri, 1997; Tsuji *et al.*, 1999). There appears to also be a specific role for the GPV component of the GPIb-IX-V complex in thrombus formation. In an arteriolar model, mice lacking GPV (GPV$^{-/-}$) developed thrombus at a faster rate and produced more emboli than wild-type mice (Ni *et al.*, 2001). This is thought to reflect the binding of thrombin by GPV, which serves to enhance thrombin-induced platelet activation, rather than an effect on the adhesion of the GPIb-V-IX complex to VWF.

Many animal studies have demonstrated that blockade of fibrinogen binding to platelet GPIIb–IIIa with antibodies, or pharmacological agents, inhibits thrombus formation. The initial demonstration of the efficacy of the 7E3 antibody, which was subsequently developed into the clinically effective antiplatelet drug abciximab, was in the Folts model (Coller *et al.*, 1989). This observation has been replicated in numerous in vitro and animal studies using antibody-based and synthetic GPIIb–IIIa receptor antagonists (Topol *et al.*, 1999;

Quinn *et al.*, 2003), and using platelets from patients with Glanzmann's thrombasthenia (a deficiency in the GPIIb–IIIa complex) (Baumgartner *et al.*, 1994; Tsuji *et al.*, 1999). In general the effect of blocking fibrinogen binding to GPIIb–IIIa is to limit the growth of the thrombus, thus reducing the risk of embolization by preventing the accumulation of platelets at the site of damage.

Once the initial interaction of platelets with fibrinogen has occurred there is a phase of stabilization of the platelet aggregate. This involves a number of receptor ligand systems, most notably the interaction of fibrinogen with GPIIb–IIIa, which generates outside-in signaling, leading to clustering of the fibrinogen receptors and reinforcement of the binding of the ligand with its receptor (Parise, 1999). Interactions between other accessory molecules are also involved. These include the interaction of CD40 with its ligand on platelets (Anand *et al.*, 2003; Prasad *et al.*, 2004), the interaction between ephrins and Eph kinases (Prevost *et al.*, 2005) and the binding of Gas6 to its receptors (Angelillo-Scherrer *et al.*, 2001, 2005), all of which have been shown to influence thrombus stability.

P-selectin also helps to stabilize the thrombus. Using a blocking antibody to P-selectin in the canine Folts model, platelet-mediated thrombus formation was reduced (Ueyama *et al.*, 1997). P-selectin knock-out mice also show reduced thrombus formation in response to carotid injury (Ikeda *et al.*, 1999; Yokoyama *et al.*, 2005), with longer time to occlusion and spontaneous reflow, indicative of thrombus embolization. The mechanism of stabilization of a thrombus by P-selectin appears to be partly stabilization of platelet-platelet aggregates (Merten and Thiagarajan, 2000) but mostly through recruitment of leucocytes via interaction of P-selectin with PSGL-1 (Geng *et al.*, 2004; Yokoyama *et al.*, 2005).

Platelet ligands and soluble factors

It is both logical to assume, and experimentally demonstrated, that the interaction of platelets with fibrinogen/fibrin plays a critical role in the regulation of thrombus size and stability. Elevated plasma fibrinogen is a well-recognized risk factor for thrombosis (Koenig, 2003; Danesh *et al.*, 2005). Fibrinogen is an acute phase protein that is elevated in a wide range of clinical conditions, in smokers and in older subjects (Koenig, 2003); all factors that are associated with increased risk of thrombosis. There is a large body of experimental evidence that fibrinogen concentration has a marked effect on clot structure (Carr and Hermans, 1978; Blomback, 1994; Collet *et al.*, 2003; Scott *et al.*, 2004; Weisel, 2005). The level of fibrinogen may also affect the risk of embolization. For example, increasing the level of fibrinogen in the plasma of rats increased the number of emboli arising from an in vivo thrombus in a dose-related manner (Doutremepuich *et al.*, 1998). Conversely in an in vitro model, blood from patients with severe afibrinogenemia failed to form stable thrombi at shear rates >1500 sec^{-1} (Tsjui *et al.*, 1999). Similar findings come from studies in fibrinogen-deficient knock-out mice (Fgn$^{-/-}$) which formated large, platelet-rich thrombi in mesenteric arterioles that were rapidly released downstream as large emboli, due to shearing at the vessel wall (Ni *et al.*, 2000).

The stabilizing role of fibrinogen is dependent on both its interaction with the platelets, and its ability to form an effective fibrin network. In Fgn$^{-/-}$ mice the role of fibrinogen was replaced by fibronectin, which allowed platelet-platelet aggregation, but not stabilization of the clot. In FgnγΔ5 mice, in which the fibrinogen had been modified to lack the terminal five amino acids of the fibrinogen γ-chain (QADVG) that binds to GPIIb–IIIa, thrombi formed more rapidly and were smaller than in the wild-type animals, but produced larger numbers of small emboli that were released from the outer surface of the thrombus (Ni *et al.*, 2003). The FgnγΔ5 molecule retains clotting function and the ability to cross-link fibrin to FXIIIa but does not bind to platelet GPIIb–IIIa. These observations have been replicated using an antibody to the fibrinogen γ-chain (7E6) and in a model of carotid stenosis (Jirouskova *et al.*, 2004).

Although it is well established that VWF and fibrinogen are essential for platelet adhesion and aggregation, respectively, thrombi can still form in mice lacking both molecules (Ni *et al.*, 2000). In these animals other ligands such as fibronectin, thrombospondin and vitronectin (Vn) seem to be able to replace VWF and fibrinogen (Reheman *et al.*, 2005). The role of vitronectin is particularly interesting. In Vn$^{-/-}$ mice, thrombi that were formed in two different arteriolar models were small and unstable compared to those in wild-type mice (Konstantinides *et al.*, 2001; Reheman *et al.*, 2005). Vitronectin is a protein with multiple roles, including binding to platelet GPIIIa. It also forms a complex with PAI-1 in which the PAI-1 is stabilized into its active form (Preissner, 1991). PAI-1- deficient mice also produce small, unstable thrombi. But mice deficient in both Vn and PAI-1 showed no increase in the rate or number of emboli produced compared to the mice with the single deficiency (Koschnick *et al.*, 2005), indicating that these two molecules act in concert.

Platelets play a role in regulating the activity of PAI-1 in a thrombus. They contain a significant pool of PAI-1 in their α-granules, although <5% of this is active (DeClerck *et al.*, 1988; Simpson *et al.*, 1990). Recent data suggest that platelets regulate the interaction of PAI-1 and Vn via protein kinase A (PKA) bound to their surface (Morgenstern *et al.*, 2001). Upon activation, platelet PKA phosphorylates vitronectin causing it to dissociate from PAI-1. This would have the overall effect of stabilizing a thrombus by inhibiting fibrinolysis.

Platelet agonists and emboli

Platelets respond to a wide range of physiological agonists. These can be considered as primary agonists (thrombin and collagen) that initiate the platelet response, and secondary agonists (including ADP and TxA$_2$), released from, or generated by platelets following their initial activation by thrombin and collagen (Cattaneo *et al.*, 1990; Gachet, 2001; Woulfe *et al.*, 2001).

Blocking the response to thrombin or collagen has a marked effect on reducing all emboli, largely because thrombus formation is significantly impaired. The resulting effect is therefore to prevent deposition of platelets at the site of vascular damage, thus limiting the growth of the thrombus.

Agonists that have a secondary or augmenting role seem to play a particularly important role in the generation of the smaller emboli. The importance of the role of TxA$_2$ in thrombus formation has long been established in animal models (Folts *et al.*, 1976) and aspirin is an effective antiplatelet agent for the prevention of cardiovascular events including stroke (Antithrombotics Trialists Collaboration, 2002). Inhibition of platelet thromboxane production may specifically reduce embolization. For example, in a rabbit arteriolar model, blocking the TxA$_2$-mediated platelet response reduced the extent (but not the rate) of embolization (oude Egbrink *et al.*, 1993).

The role of ADP in regulating thrombus formation and embolization may be even more important. ADP has two receptors on the platelet surface, P2Y$_1$ and P2Y$_{12}$; both members of the purinergic receptor family of G-protein coupled receptors (Jin and Kunapuli, 1998; Gachet and Hechler, 2005). Both receptors are required for a full response of the platelet to ADP. Stimulation of the P2Y$_1$ receptor mobilizes Ca^{2+} ions in the cytosol, leading to initiation of aggregation. Stimulation of the P2Y$_{12}$ receptor causes inhibition of adenylate cyclase, leading to PI3-kinase-mediated activation of the GPIIb–IIIa complex, allowing fibrinogen to bind, and thus promoting platelet aggregation (Storey, 2001; Gachet and Hechler, 2005). Antiplatelet drugs that target the P2Y$_{12}$ receptor include the theinopyridine derivatives ticlopidine and clodiogrel and newer synthetic agents such as the AR-C series of compounds (Ingall *et al.*, 1999; Gachet, 2001; Storey, 2001). Antagonism of P2Y$_{12}$ has been found to have a significant antithrombotic effect in both cardiovascular disease and stroke

(Hass *et al.*, 1989; CAPRIE Steering Committee, 1996; Geiger *et al.*, 1999; CURE Investigators, 2001; Storey *et al.*, 2001). This efficacy may, at least in part, be linked to a reduction of thromboembolism as has been elegantly demonstrated in a rabbit model of thrombosis and embolization (van Gestel *et al.*, 2002). In this study, calcium mobilization (a primary event in platelet activation) was measured within single, fluo-3-labeled platelets that were being incorporated into a thrombus formed at a site of damage in mesenteric arterioles. Calcium mobilization in single platelets within the growing thrombus was prolonged and accompanied by other markers of platelet activation such as shape change and degranulation. However, platelets that were incorporated into a developing embolus exhibited only a transient rise in intracellular calcium with little evidence of significant levels of platelet activation, indicative of a weaker, ADP-mediated response (van Gestel *et al.*, 2002). It was subsequently shown that blockade of P2Y$_{12}$, in addition to inhibiting thrombus formation per se, specifically reduced the rate of downstream embolization (van Gestel *et al.*, 2003). Similar evidence has come from studies in P2Y$_{12}$$^{-/-}$ mice which produce smaller and less stable thrombi both in vitro and in vivo (Leon *et al.*, 2001; Andre *et al.*, 2003; Gachet and Hechler, 2005), implying that ADP plays a key role in the generation of emboli.

Evidence from clinical studies

Many of these studies in vitro or in animal models point to a range of potential factors involved in regulating the risk of embolization in patients with carotid artery disease; specifically highlighting the importance of platelets (Table 4.1). However, demonstration of significant effects on embolization in model systems and in animals, whilst informative, does not demonstrate clinical effect.

GPIIb–IIIa antagonists initially promised to be the antiplatelet drug of choice (Lefkovits *et al.*, 1995; Topol *et al.*, 1999; Vorcheimer *et al.*, 1999) as these block the final common pathway of platelet activation and prevent aggregation. However, concerns about the risk of bleeding have limited their use in stroke prevention. There is some limited evidence that tirofiban, a selective, nonpeptide GPIIb–IIIa antagonist, that has a relatively short-lived effect, can prevent circulating cerebral microemboli (Junghans and Siebler, 2003).

Although aspirin therapy has been shown to reduce the relative risk of thromboembolic stroke in patients undergoing carotid endarterectomy by 20–25%, a significant number of patients will still suffer an ischemic stroke in the perioperative period (Barnett et al., 1995; Goertler et al., 1999). This was confirmed in a prospective trial in this center, in patients undergoing carotid endarterectomy on standardized aspirin treatment (150 mg), which found no correlation between the magnitude of embolization and the ability of aspirin to inhibit platelet aggregation induced by arachidonic acid (Hayes et al., 2003). However, a link was found between the level of the platelet response to ADP and postoperative embolization. The platelet response to ADP varies considerably between individuals but remains remarkably consistent within an individual (O'Donnell et al., 2001; Fontana et al., 2003; Hetherington et al., 2005). In patients with enhanced preoperative sensitivity to ADP, there were significantly greater numbers of postoperative emboli when compared to the group of low ADP responders (Hayes et al., 2003). A subsequent trial in 100 patients, randomized to aspirin alone or to aspirin combined with a low dose of clopidogrel (75 mg), given the night before surgery, showed that the combined therapy reduced the rate of embolization in all subjects to below a clinically-significant level (Naylor et al., 2000), without an increase in bleeding (Payne et al., 2004). This finding has been supported by recent results from the CARESS (clopidogrel and aspirin for reduction of emboli in symptomatic carotid stenosis) trial, which found a reduction in both the appearance and rate of emboli in patients on a combination of aspirin compared to those on aspirin alone (Markus et al., 2005).

Conclusion

Many factors are involved in forming a stable thrombus and consequently there are many candidates for regulating the risk of embolization. Embolization can occur when a thrombus shears from the vessel wall and travels downstream; an event that is normally related to plaque instability, with or without intervention therapy. Antiplatelet and antithrombotic therapies are of benefit in limiting the growth of thrombus within the carotid vessel. However other targets, such as limiting plaque progression with statin therapy may prove effective in prevention of these events.

A thrombus that forms in the carotid artery can remain attached to the vessel wall but be thrombogenic, generating emboli at the surface that are shed into the circulation. Such events can be seen in the immediate postoperative period in patients undergoing carotid endarterectomy. Evidence from in vitro models and animal studies point to these emboli being predominantly platelet-rich. It is therefore unsurprising that this embolization can be affected by factors that stabilize platelets within the thrombus, such as secondary adhesion molecules, or secondary agonists. In particular ADP seems to have a very specific role in regulating embolization. Promising early results in randomized trials of clopidogrel therapy suggest this may be the therapeutic target of choice.

REFERENCES

Anand, S. X., Viles-Gonzalez, J. F., Badimon, J. J., Cavusoglu, E. and Marmur, J. D. (2003). Membrane-associated CD40L and sCD40L in atherothrombotic disease. *Thrombosis & Haemostasis*, **90**, 377–84.

Andre, P., Delaney, S. M., LaRocca, T., *et al.* (2003). P2Y12 regulates platelet adhesion/activation, thrombus growth, and thrombus stability in injured arteries. *Journal of Clinical Investigation*, **112**, 398–406.

Angelillo-Scherrer, A., de Frutos, P., Aparicio, C., *et al.* (2001). Deficiency or inhibition of Gas6 causes platelet dysfunction and protects mice against thrombosis. *Nature Medicine*, **7**, 215–21.

Angelillo-Scherrer, A., Burnier, L., Flores, N., *et al.* (2005). Role of Gas6 receptors in platelet signalling during thrombus stabilization and implications for antithrombotic therapy. *Journal of Clinical Investigation*, **115**, 237–56.

Antithrombotic Trialists' Collaboration. (2002). Collaborative meta-analysis of randomised trials of antiplatelet therapy for prevention of death, myocardial infarction and stroke in high risk patients. *British Medical Journal*, **321**, 71–86.

Ariens, R. A., Lai, T. S., Weisel, J. W., Greenberg, C. S. and Grant, P. J. (2002). Role of factor XIII in fibrin clot formation and effects of genetic polymorphisms. *Blood*, **100**, 743–54.

Barnett, H. J., Eliasiw, M. and Meldrum, H. E. (1995). Drugs and surgery in the prevention of ischaemic stroke. *New England Journal of Medicine*, **332**, 238–48.

Baumgartner, H. R., Mannucci, P. M. and Meyer, D. (1994). The role of platelet von Willebrand factor in platelet adhesion and thrombus formation: a study of 34 patients with various subtypes of type I von Willebrand disease. *British Journal of Haematology*, **86**, 327–32.

Blomback, B. (1994). Fibrinogen structure, activation, polymerization and fibrin gel structure. *Thrombosis Research*, **75**, 327–8.

CAPRIE steering committee. (1996). A randomized, blinded, trial of clopidogrel versus aspirin in patients at risk of ischemic events. *Lancet*, **348**, 1329–39.

Carr, M. E. Jr and Hermans, J. (1978). Size and density of fibrin fibers from turbidity. *Macromolecules*, **11**, 46–50.

Cattaneo, M., Canciani, M. T., Lecchi, A., *et al.* (1990). Released adenosine diphosphate stabilizes thrombin-induced human platelet aggregates. *Blood*, **75**, 1081–6.

Chandler, A. B. (1958). *In vitro* thrombotic coagulation of the blood. *Laboratory Investigations*, **7**, 110–14.

Coller, B. S., Folts, J. D., Smith, S. R., Scudder, L. E. and Jordan, R. (1989). Abolition of in vivo platelet thrombus formation in primates with monoclonal antibodies to the platelet GPIIb/IIIa receptor. Correlation with bleeding time, platelet aggregation, and blockade of GPIIb/IIIa receptors. *Circulation*, **80**, 1766–74.

Collet, J. P., Lesty, C., Montalescot, G. and Weisel, J. W. (2003). Dynamic changes of fibrin architecture during fibrin formation and intrinsic fibrinolysis of fibrin-rich clots. *Journal of Biological Chemistry*, **278**, 21331–5.

CURE investigators. (2001). Effects of clopidogrel in addition to aspirin in patients with acute coronary syndromes without ST-segment elevation. *New England Journal of Medicine*, **345**, 494–502.

Danesh, J., Lewington, S., Thompson, S. G., *et al.* (2005). Fibrinogen Studies Collaboration. Plasma fibrinogen level and the risk of major cardiovascular diseases and nonvascular mortality: an individual participant meta-analysis. *Journal of the American Medical Association*, **294**, 1799–809.

Day, S. M., Reeve, J. L., Myers, D. D. and Fay, W. P. (2004). Murine thrombosis models. *Thrombosis & Haemostasis*, **92**, 486–94.

Day, S. M., Reeve, J. L., Pedersen, B., *et al.* (2005). Macrovascular thrombosis is driven by tissue factor derived primarily from the blood vessel wall. *Blood*, **105**, 192–8.

DeClerck, P. J., Alessi, M. C., Verstreken, M., *et al.* (1988). Measurement of plasminogen activator inhibitor 1 in biologic fluids with a murine monoclonal antibody-based enzyme-linked immunosorbent assay. *Blood*, **71**, 220–5.

Doutremepuich, F., Aguejouf, O., Belougne-Malfatti, E. and Doutremepuich, C. (1998). Fibrinogen as a factor of thrombosis: experimental study. *Thrombosis Research*, **90**, 57–64.

Falati, S., Gross, P., Merrill-Skoloff, G., *et al.* (2002). Real-time in vivo imaging of platelets, tissue factor and fibrin during arterial thrombus formation in the mouse. *Nature Medicine*, **8**, 1175–81.

Falati, S., Liu, Q., Gross, P., *et al.* (2003). Accumulation of tissue factor into developing thrombi in vivo is dependent upon microparticle P-selectin glycoprotein ligand 1 and platelet P-selectin. *Journal of Experimental Medicine*, **197**, 1585–98.

Fernandez-Ortiz, A., Badimon, J. J., Falk, E., *et al.* (1994). Characterization of the relative thrombogenicity of atherosclerotic plaque components: implications for consequences of plaque rupture. *Journal of the American College of Cardiology*, **23**, 1562–9.

Folts, J. D., Crowell, E. B. Jr and Rowe, G. G. (1976). Platelet aggregation in partially obstructed vessels and its elimination with aspirin. *Circulation*, **54**, 365–70.

Fontana, P., Dupont, A., Gandrille, S., *et al.* (2003). Adenosine diphosphate-induced platelet aggregation is associated with P2Y12 gene sequence variations in healthy subjects. *Circulation*, **108**, 989–95.

Foulkes, M. A., Wolf, P. A., Price, T. R., Mohr, J. P. and Hier, D. B. (1988). The Stroke Data Bank: design, methods, and baseline characteristics. *Stroke*, **19**, 547–54.

Furie, B., Furie, B. C. and Flaumenhaft, R. (2001). A journey with platelet P-selectin: the molecular basis of granule secretion, signalling and cell adhesion. *Thrombosis & Haemostasis*, **86**, 214–21.

Gachet, C. (2001). ADP receptors of platelets and their inhibition. *Thrombosis & Haemostasis*, **86**, 222–32.

Gachet, C. and Hechler, B. (2005). The platelet P2 receptors in thrombosis. *Seminars in Thrombosis & Hemostasis*, **31**, 162–7.

Gaunt, M. E., Smith, J. L., Ratliff, D. A., Bell, P. R. and Naylor, A. R. (1996). A comparison of quality control methods applied to carotid endarterectomy. *European Journal of Vascular & Endovascular Surgery*, **11**, 4–11.

Geiger, J., Brich, J., Honig-Liedl, P., *et al.* (1999). Specific impairment of human platelet P2Y$_{AC}$ ADP receptor-mediated signaling by the antiplatelet drug clopidogrel. *Arteriosclerosis, Thrombosis and Vascular Biology*, **19**, 2007–11.

Geng, J. G., Chen, M., Chou, K. C. (2004). P-selectin cell adhesion molecule in inflammation, thrombosis, cancer growth and metastasis. *Current Medicinal Chemistry*, **11**, 2153–60.

Goertler, M., Baeumer, M., Kross, R., *et al.* (1999). Rapid decline of cerebral microemboli of arterial origin after intravenous acetylsalicylic acid. *Stroke*, **30**, 66–9.

Goldsmith, H. L. and Turitto, V. T. (1986). Rheological aspects of thrombosis and haemostasis: basic principles and applications. ICTH-Report–Subcommittee on Rheology of the International Committee on Thrombosis and Haemostasis. *Thrombosis & Haemostasis*, **55**, 415–35.

Golino, P., Ragni, M., and Cirillo, P., *et al.* (1995). Aurintricarboxylic acid reduces platelet deposition in stenosed and endothelially injured rabbit carotid arteries more effectively than other antiplatelet interventions. *Thrombosis & Haemostasis*, **74**, 974–9.

Harker, L. A., Marzec, U. M., Kelly, A. B., *et al.* (1998). Clopidogrel inhibition of stent, graft, and vascular thrombogenesis with antithrombotic enhancement by aspirin in nonhuman primates. *Circulation*, **98**, 2461–9.

Hass, W. K., Easton, J. D., Adams, H. P. J., *et al.* (1989). A randomized trial comparing ticlopidine hydrochloride with aspirin for the prevention of stroke in high-risk patients. *New England Journal of Medicine*, **321**, 501–7.

Hayes, P. D., Payne, D., Lloyd, A. J., Bell, P. R. and Naylor, A. R. (2001). Patients' thromboembolic potential between bilateral carotid endarterectomies remains stable over time. *European Journal of Vascular & Endovascular Surgery*, **22**, 496–8.

Hayes, P. D., Box, H., Tull, S., *et al.* (2003). Patients' thromboembolic potential after carotid endarterectomy is related to the platelets' sensitivity to adenosine diphosphate. *Journal of Vascular Surgery*, **38**, 1226–31.

Hetherington, S. L., Singh, R. K., Lodwick, D., *et al.* (2005). Dimorphism in the P2RY1 ADP receptor gene is associated with increased platelet activation response to ADP. *Arteriosclerosis, Thrombosis and Vascular Biology*, **25**, 252–7.

Hoffman, M. (2003). Remodelling the blood coagulation cascade. *Journal of Thrombosis and Thrombolysis*, **16**, 17–20.

Hoffman, M. and Monroe, D. M. 3rd. (2001). A cell-based model of hemostasis. *Thrombosis & Haemostasis*, **85**, 958–65.

Ikeda, H., Ueyama, T., Murohara, T., *et al.* (1999). Adhesive interaction between P-selectin and sialyl Lewis(x) plays an important role in recurrent coronary arterial thrombosis in dogs. *Arteriosclerosis, Thrombosis and Vascular Biology*, **19**, 1083–90.

Ingall, A. H., Dixon, J., Bailey, A., *et al.* (1999). Antagonists of the platelet P$_{2T}$ receptor: a novel approach to antithrombotic therapy. *Journal of Medicinal Chemistry*, **42**, 213–20.

Jander, S., Sitzer, M., Wendt, A., *et al.* (2001). Expression of tissue factor in high-grade carotid artery stenosis: association with plaque destabilization. *Stroke*, **32**, 850–4.

Jin, J. and Kunapuli, S. P. (1998). Coactivation of two different G protein-coupled receptors is essential for ADP-induced platelet aggregation. *Proceedings of the New York Academy of Sciences USA*, **95**, 8070–4.

Jirouskova, M., Chereshnev, I., Vaananen, H., Degen, J. L. and Coller, B. S. (2004). Antibody blockade or mutation of the fibrinogen gamma-chain C-terminus is more effective in inhibiting murine arterial thrombus formation than complete absence of fibrinogen. *Blood*, **103**, 1995–2002.

Jordan, W. D., Voellinger, D. C., Doblar, D. D., *et al.* (1999). Microemboli detected by transcranial Doppler monitoring in patients during carotid angioplasty versus carotid endarterectomy. *Cardiovascular Surgery*, **7**, 33–8.

Junghans, U. and Siebler, M. (2003). Cerebral microembolism is blocked by tirofiban, a selective nonpeptide platelet glycoprotein IIb/IIIa receptor antagonist. *Circulation*, **107**, 2717–21.

Kobbervig, C. and Williams, E. (2004). FXIII polymorphisms, fibrin clot structure and thrombotic risk. *Biophysical Chemistry*, **112**, 223–8.

Koenig, W. (2003). Fibrin(ogen) in cardiovascular disease: an update. *Thrombosis & Haemostasis*, **89**, 601–9.

Konstanitinides, S., Scafer, K., Thinnes, T. and Loskutoff, D. J. (2001). Plasminogen activator inhibitor-1 and its cofactor vitronectin stabilize arterial thrombi after vascular injury in mice. *Circulation*, **103**, 576–83.

Koschnick, S., Konstanitinides, S., Scafer, K., Crain, K. and Loskutoff, D. J. (2005). Thrombotic phenotype of mice with a combined deficiency in plasminogen activator inhibitor 1 and vitronectin. *Journal of Thrombosis & Haemostasis*, **3**, 2290–5.

Lammie, G. A., Sandercock, P. A. and Dennis, M. S. (1999). Recently occluded intracranial and extracranial carotid arteries: relevance of the unstable atherosclerotic plaque. *Stroke*, **30**, 1319–25.

Larsen, E. A., Celi, G. E., Gilbert, B. C., *et al.* (1989). PADGEM protein: a receptor that mediates the interaction of activated platelets with neutrophils and monocytes. *Cell*, **59**, 305–12.

Lefkovits, J., Plow, E. F. and Topol, E. J. (1995). Platelet glycoprotein IIb/IIIa receptors in cardiovascular medicine. *New England Journal of Medicine*, **332**, 1553–9.

Lentz, B. R. (2003). Exposure of platelet membrane phosphatidylserine regulates blood coagulation. *Progress in Lipid Research*, **42**, 423–38.

Leon, C., Freund, M., Ravanat, C., *et al.* (2001). Key role of the P2Y1 receptor in tissue factor induced thrombin dependent acute thromboembolism. Studies in P2Y1 knockout mice and mice treated with a P2Y1 antagonist. *Circulation*, **103**, 718–23.

Lijnen, H. R. and Collen, D. (1997). Endothelium in hemostasis and thrombosis. *Progress in Cardiovascular Diseases*, **39**, 343–50.

Mackman, N. (2004). Mouse models in haemostasis and thrombosis. *Thrombosis & Haemostasis*, **92**, 440–3.

McEver, R. P., Beckstead, J. H., Moore, K. L., Marshall-Carlson, L. and Bainton, D. F. (1989). GMP-140, a platelet alpha-granule membrane protein, is also synthesized by vascular endothelial cells and is localized in Weibel-Palade bodies. *Journal of Clinical Investigation*, **84**, 92–9.

Markus, H. S., Droste, D. W., Kaps, M., *et al.* (2005). Dual antiplatelet therapy with clopidogrel and aspirin in symptomatic carotid stenosis evaluated using Doppler embolic signal detection: the Clopidogrel and Aspirin for Reduction of Emboli in Symptomatic Carotid Stenosis (CARESS) trial. *Circulation*, **111**, 2233–40.

Merten, M. and Thiagarajan, P. (2000). P-selectin expression on platelets determines size and stability of platelet aggregates. *Circulation*, **102**, 1931–6.

Morgenstern, E., Gnad, U., Preissner, K. T., *et al.* (2001). Localization of protein kinase A and vitronectin in resting platelets and their translocation onto fibrin fibers during clot formation. *European Journal of Cell Biology*, **80**, 87–98.

Morrissey, J. H., Macik, B. G., Neuenschwander, P. F. and Comp, P. C. (1993). Quantitation of activated factor VII levels in plasma using a tissue factor mutant selectively deficient in promoting factor VII activation. *Blood*, **81**, 734–44.

Naylor, A. R., Hayes, P. D., Allroggen, H., *et al.* (2000). Reducing the risk of carotid surgery: A seven-year audit of the role of monitoring and quality control assessment. *Journal of Vascular Surgery*, **32**, 750–9.

Ni, H., Denis, C. V., Subbarao, S., *et al.* (2000). Persistence of platelet thrombus formation in arterioles of mice lacking both von Willebrand factor and fibrinogen. *Journal of Clinical Investigation*, **106**, 385–92.

Ni, H., Ramakrishnan, V., Ruggeri, Z. M., *et al.* (2001). Increased thrombogenesis and embolus formation in mice lacking glycoprotein V. *Blood*, **98**, 368–73.

Ni, H., Papalia, J. M., Degen, J. L. and Wagner, D. D. (2003). Control of thrombus embolization and fibronectin internalization by integrin alpha IIb beta 3 engagement of the fibrinogen gamma chain. *Blood*, **102**, 3609–14.

O'Donnell, C. J., Larson, M. G., Feng, D., *et al.* (2001). Framingham Heart Study. Genetic and environmental contributions to platelet aggregation: the Framingham heart study. *Circulation*, **103**, 3051–6.

oude Egbrink, M. G., Tangelder, G. J., Slaaf, D. W. and Reneman, R. S. (1993). Different roles of prostaglandins in thromboembolic processes in arterioles and venules in vivo. *Thrombosis & Haemostasis*, **70**, 826–33.

Parise, L. V. (1999). Integrin alpha(IIb)beta(3) signalling in platelet adhesion and aggregation. *Current Opinion in Cell Biology*, **11**, 597–601.

Payne, D. A., Jones, C. I., Hayes, P. D., *et al.* (2004). Beneficial effects of clopidogrel combined with aspirin in reducing cerebral emboli in patients undergoing carotid endarterectomy. *Circulation*, **109**, 1476–81.

Prasad, K. S., Andre, P., He, M., *et al.* (2004). Soluble CD40 ligand induces beta3 integrin tyrosine phosphorylation and triggers platelet activation by outside-in signaling.

Proceedings of the National Academy of Sciences of the United States of America, **100**, 12367–71.

Preissner, K. T. (1991). Structure and biological role of vitronectin. *Annual Review of Cell Biology*, **7**, 275–310.

Prevost, N., Woulfe, D. S., Jiang, H., *et al.* (2005). Eph kinases and ephrins support thrombus growth and stability by regulating integrin outside-in signaling in platelets. *Proceedings of the National Academy of Sciences of the United States of America*, **102**, 9820–5.

Quinn, M. J., Byzova, T. V., Qin, J., Topol, E. J. and Plow, E. F. (2003). Integrin alphaIIbbeta3 and its antagonism. *Arteriosclerosis, Thrombosis and Vascular Biology*, **23**, 945–52.

Reheman, A., Gross, P., Yang, H., *et al.* (2005). Vitronectin stabilizes thrombi and vessel occlusion but plays a dual role in platelet aggregation. *Journal of Thrombosis & Haemostasis*, **3**, 875–83.

Riles, T. S., Imparato, A. M., Jacobowitz, G. R., *et al.* (1994). The cause of perioperative stroke after carotid endarterectomy. *Journal of Vascular Surgery*, **19**, 206–14.

Robbie, L. A., Young, S. P., Bennett, B. and Booth, N. A. (1997). Thrombi formed in a Chandler loop mimic human arterial thrombi in structure and PAI-1 content and distribution. *Thrombosis & Haemostasis*, **77**, 510–15.

Ruggeri, Z. M. (1997). Mechanisms initiating platelet thrombus formation. *Thrombosis & Haemostasis*, **78**, 611–16.

Ruggeri, Z. M., Dent, J. A. and Saldivar, E. (1999). Contribution of distinct adhesive interactions to platelet aggregation in flowing blood. *Blood*, **94**, 172–8.

Sakariassen, K. S., Muggli, R. and Baumgartner, H. R. (1989). Measurements of platelet interaction with components of the vessel wall in flowing blood. *Methods in Enzymology*, **169**, 37–70.

Sakariassen, K. S., Turitto, V. T. and Baumgartner, H. R. (2004). Recollections of the development of flow devices for studying mechanisms of hemostasis and thrombosis in flowing whole blood. *Journal of Thrombosis & Haemostasis*, **2**, 1681–90.

Samama, C. M., Bonnin, P., Bonneau, M., *et al.* (1992). Comparative arterial antithrombotic activity of clopidogrel and acetyl salicylic acid in the pig. *Thrombosis & Haemostasis*, **68**, 500–5.

Savage, B., Cattaneo, M. and Ruggeri, Z. M. (2001). Mechanisms of platelet aggregation. *Current Opinions in Hematology*, **8**, 270–6.

Scott, E. M., Ariens, R. A. and Grant, P. J. (2004). Genetic and environmental determinants of fibrin structure and function: relevance to clinical disease. *Arteriosclerosis, Thrombosis and Vascular Biology*, **24**, 1558–66.

Sim, D., Flaumenhaft, R. and Furie, B. (2005). Interactions of platelets, blood-borne tissue factor, and fibrin during arteriolar thrombus formation in vivo. *Microcirculation*, **12**, 301–11.

Simpson, A. J., Booth, N. A., Moore, N. R. and Bennett, B. (1990). The platelet and plasma pools of plasminogen activator inhibitor (PAI-1) vary independently in disease. *British Journal of Haematology*, **75**, 543–8.

Sitzer, M., Muller, W., Siebler, M., *et al.* (1995). Plaque ulceration and lumen thrombus are the main sources of cerebral microemboli in high-grade internal carotid artery stenosis. *Stroke*, **26**, 1231–3.

Spencer, M. P. (1997). Transcranial Doppler monitoring and causes of stroke from carotid endarterectomy. *Stroke*, **28**, 685–91.

Storey, R. F. (2001). The P2Y12 receptor as a therapeutic target in cardiovascular disease. *Platelets*, **12**, 197–209.

Storey, R. F., Oldroyd, K. G. and Wilcox, R. G. (2001). Open multicentre study of the P_{2T} receptor antagonist AR-C69931 MX assessing safety, tolerability and activity in patients with acute coronary syndromes. *Thrombosis & Haemostasis*, **85**, 401–7.

Topol, E. J., Byzova, T. V. and Plow, E. F. (1999). Platelet GP IIb/IIIa blockers. *Lancet*, **353**, 227–31.

Tschopp, T. B., Baumgartner, H. R., Silberbauer, K. and Sinzinger, H. (1979). Platelet adhesion and platelet thrombus formation on subendothelium of human arteries and veins exposed to flowing blood in vitro. A comparison with rabbit aorta. *Haemostasis*, **8**, 19–29.

Tsuji, S., Sugimoto, M., Miyata, S., *et al.* (1999). Real-time analysis of mural thrombus formation in various platelet aggregation disorders: distinct shear-dependent roles of platelet receptors and adhesive proteins under flow. *Blood*, **94**, 968–75.

Ueyama, T., Ikeda, H., Haramaki, N., Kuwano, K. and Imaizumi, T. (1997). Effects of monoclonal antibody to P-selectin and analogue of sialyl Lewis X on cyclic flow variations in stenosed and endothelium-injured canine coronary arteries. *Circulation*, **95**, 1554–9.

van Gestel, M. A., Heemskerk, J. W., Slaaf, D. W., *et al.* (2002). Real-time detection of activation patterns in individual platelets during thromboembolism in vivo: differences between thrombus growth and embolus formation. *Journal of Vascular Research*, **39**, 534–43.

van Gestel, M.A., Heemskerk, J.W., Slaaf, D.W., *et al.* (2003). In vivo blockade of platelet ADP receptor P2Y12 reduces embolus and thrombus formation but not thrombus stability. *Arteriosclerosis, Thrombosis and Vascular Biology*, **23**, 518–23.

Vaughan, D.E. (2005). PAI-1 and atherothrombosis. *Journal of Thrombosis & Haemostasis*, **3**, 1879–83.

Vorchheimer, D.A., Badimon, J.J. and Fuster, V. (1999). Platelet glycoprotein IIb/IIIa receptor antagonists in cardiovascular disease. *Journal of the American Medical Association*, **281**, 1407–14.

Weisel, J.W. (2005). Fibrinogen and fibrin. *Advances in Protein Chemistry*, **70**, 247–99.

Wilcox, J.N., Smith, K.M., Schwartz, S.M., *et al.* (1989). Localization of tissue factor in the normal vessel wall and in the atherosclerotic plaque. *Proceedings of the National Academy of Sciences USA*, **86**, 2839–43.

Wolberg, A.S., Monroe, D.M., Roberts, H.R. and Hoffman, M. (2003). Elevated prothrombin results in clots with an altered fiber structure: a possible mechanism of the increased thrombotic risk. *Blood*, **101**, 3008–13.

Woulfe, D., Yang, J. and Brass, L. (2001). ADP and platelets: the end of the beginning. *Journal of Clinical Investigation*, **107**, 1503–5.

Yao, S.K., Ober, J.C., Krishnaswami, A., *et al.* (2002). Endogenous nitric oxide protects against platelet aggregation and cyclic flow variations in stenosed and endothelium-injured arteries. *Circulation*, **86**, 1302–9.

Yokoyama, S., Ikeda, H., Haramaki, N., *et al.* (2005). Platelet P-selectin plays an important role in arterial thrombogenesis by forming large stable platelet-leukocyte aggregates. *Journal of the American College of Cardiology*, **45**, 1280–6.

Zwaal, R.F. and Schroit, A.J. (1997). Pathophysiologic implications of membrane phospholipid asymmetry in blood cells. *Blood*, **89**, 1121–32.

5

Medical treatment for carotid stenosis

Matthew F. Giles and Peter M. Rothwell

University Department of Clinical Neurology, Radcliffe Infirmary, Oxford, OX2 6HE, UK

Introduction

Reviews of the surgical or interventional management of patients with symptomatic or asymptomatic carotid stenosis are commonplace but consideration of what constitutes best medical treatment in these particular patients has generally been less detailed, and there have been few randomized trials of pharmacological interventions specifically in these patient groups. This paucity of research is due partly to the effectiveness of carotid endarterectomy and stenting in preventing stroke and the tendency for trials of medical treatments in prevention of stroke not to distinguish between patients with different underlying pathologies. Recommendations for particular medical treatments in patients with carotid disease are therefore often made on the basis of extrapolation from trials and observational studies in broader populations of patients with cerebrovascular disease.

However, although carotid endarterectomy and stenting can substantially reduce the risk of stroke in patients with symptomatic carotid stenosis, optimal medical treatment is still essential. First, a significant group of patients with symptomatic carotid stenosis (and a larger group with asymptomatic disease) decide against intervention or are not appropriate for various reasons. Second, given the particularly high risk of recurrent stroke in patients with symptomatic carotid stenosis following minor stroke or transient ischemic attack (TIA) (Lovett *et al.*, 2004) and the frequent delays to

carotid endarterectomy in such patients (Fairhead *et al.*, 2005), medical treatment plays a very important role in this high-risk window between event and surgery. Third, atherothrombosis in vascular territories other than the carotid artery of interest commonly causes stroke or nonstroke vascular events, irrespective of any carotid intervention. This chapter will therefore review the evidence for specific medical treatments in patients with carotid stenosis. Management of symptomatic carotid stenosis will be considered primarily, but many of the issues are common to management of asymptomatic patients.

Antiplatelet agents

Antiplatelet therapy reduces the risk of recurrent stroke and vascular death in patients with TIA or ischemic stroke and it is unlikely that these agents will be ineffective in patients with carotid disease. However, as mentioned above, few randomized clinical trials (RCT) have distinguished between subtypes of stroke, and those which have, were small and used surrogate outcomes such as microembolic signals detected with transcranial Doppler ultrasound imaging.

In the North American symptomatic carotid endarterectomy trial (NASCET) (North American Symptomatic Carotid Endarterectomy Trial Collaborators, 1991), it was recommended that patients receive 1300 mg of aspirin per day for

Carotid Disease: The Role of Imaging in Diagnosis and Management, ed. Jonathan Gillard, Martin Graves, Thomas Hatsukami and Chun Yuan. Published by Cambridge University Press. © Cambridge University Press 2007.

stroke prevention. The treatment was not mandated by the protocol and therefore, individual physicians in the study could prescribe lower-dose aspirin, other antiplatelet agents, or warfarin if they desired. Nevertheless, 1300 mg of aspirin was considered an element of "best medical therapy" when NASCET began in 1987 and 60% of patients were on an antiplatelet agent at randomization and the vast majority went onto antiplatelet agents during follow-up. There was no protocol-mandated dose of aspirin in the European carotid surgery trial (ECST) although 84% of patients were on an antiplatelet agent at randomization (European Carotid Surgery Trialists' Collaborative Group, 1991).

In the absence of large-scale studies in patients with carotid stenosis, conclusions must be drawn from those including patients with noncardioembolic stroke or TIA in general. The Antithrombotic Trialists Collaboration showed a 25% relative risk reduction in the composite outcome of stroke, myocardial infarction, or vascular death conferred by aspirin compared to placebo (Antithrombotic Trialists Collaboration, 2002). Since the majority of patients with symptomatic carotid stenosis will have artery-to-artery emboli of platelet-fibrin material as the mechanism for their symptoms, it is reasonable to assume that antiplatelet therapy will be at least as effective in this group. Indeed, a meta-analysis of six trials of aspirin versus placebo after carotid endarterectomy, although involving only 907 patients, identified a significant reduction in the risk of stroke during follow-up (OR = 0.58, $p = 0.04$) (Engelter and Lyrer, 2003).

For some patients, aspirin is not tolerated or is contra-indicated and alternative antiplatelet agents must be used. Clopidogrel is a thienopyridine derivative, the efficacy of which was established in the clopidogrel versus aspirin in patients at risk of ischemic events (CAPRIE) study (CAPRIE Steering Committee, 1996). This was a randomized, blinded, multicenter trial of clopidogrel 75 mg per day versus aspirin 325 mg per day in patients with either recent ischemic stroke or MI or symptomatic peripheral vascular disease. In 19 185 patients,

it was found that there was a 8.7% relative risk reduction in the composite outcome of ischemic stroke, myocardial infarction, or vascular death in favor of clopidogrel (95% CI, 0.3–16.5; $p = 0.043$), with an absolute risk reduction of 0.5%. *Post hoc* analysis identified those with either previous coronary artery grafting, diabetes or vascular disease in more than one vascular bed, all of whom might be expected to have greater prevalence of carotid stenosis, as subgroups in whom clopidogrel had greater benefit. However, no data are available on the comparative efficacy of clopidogrel versus aspirin specifically in patients with extracranial carotid stenosis.

The use of drug combinations has the theoretical advantage of inhibiting platelet activity through more than one pharmacological mechanism, hence potentially conferring a greater antiplatelet effect. However, there have been no large-scale trials of combination antiplatelet agents specifically in patients with carotid stenosis. The combination of aspirin and dipyridamole, a cyclic nucleotide phosphodiesterase inhibitor, in ischemic stroke and TIA has been studied in a number of trials, including the European stroke prevention study 2 (ESPS-2) (Diener *et al.*, 1996). Although there are no data specifically in patients with carotid stenosis, a recent meta-analysis of these trials showed recurrent stroke was reduced by combined aspirin and dipyridamole compared to aspirin alone (odds ratio [OR], 0.78; 95% CI, 0.65–0.93) as was the composite outcome of nonfatal stroke, nonfatal myocardial infarction and vascular death (OR, 0.84; 95% CI, 0.72–0.97) (Leonardi-Bee *et al.*, 2005).

The combination of aspirin and clopidogrel was studied in the management of atherothrombosis with clopidogrel in high-risk patients (MATCH) trial (Diener *et al.*, 2004). Patients with recent ischemic stroke or TIA and at least one additional vascular risk factor were randomized between clopidogrel (75 mg once a day) and the combination of aspirin and clopidogrel (both 75 mg once a day). Over 18 months follow-up, there was a nonsignificant reduction in the primary endpoint (a composite of ischemic stroke, myocardial infarction, vascular death or hospitalization for acute ischemia) from 16.7% to 15.7% (absolute risk reduction [ARR] 1% [95% CI, 0.6−2.7]) in favor of combination treatment. However this was at the expense of a significant increase in life-threatening bleedings (2.6% vs. 1.3%; absolute risk increase 1.3% [95% CI, 0.6−1.9]).

What studies there are of combination antiplatelet agents specifically in patients with carotid stenosis have been small and have used microembolic signals (MES) detected on transcranial Doppler (TCD) as a surrogate endpoint. Asymptomatic MES are more common in high-risk patients including those with recent symptoms, plaque ulceration and tight or symptomatic stenosis and are thought to be independently predictive of TIA and recurrent stroke. In a group of nine patients with recent TIA or minor stroke due to medium or high-grade carotid stenosis of the ICA, intravenous aspirin (500 mg) caused a rapid and significant drop in MES rate in the middle cerebral artery (MCA) on the symptomatic side (Goertler et al., 1999). In the clopidogrel and aspirin for reduction of emboli in symptomatic carotid stenosis (CARESS) trial, 107 patients with recently symptomatic ≥50% carotid stenosis and MES detected on TCD were randomized to either aspirin alone (75 mg once a day) or the combination of aspirin and clopidogrel (300 mg loading then 75 mg once a day) (Markus et al., 2005). The primary endpoint (MES positivity at 7 days after randomization) was significantly reduced in the dual-therapy patients as compared to monotherapy patients (43.8% vs. 72.7%, relative risk reduction [RRR] 39.8%; 95% CI, 13.8−58.0; $p = 0.0046$) and there were fewer recurrent strokes or TIAs in the dual-therapy group although this was not statistically significant.

Given the favorable findings of the CARESS trial and the observation from the MATCH trial suggesting a trend toward benefit in the combination therapy arm when randomization was within the first week after the qualifying ischemic event, studies of aggressive antiplatelet therapy are ongoing in the acute phase after minor stroke or TIA. The FASTER trial (fast assessment of stroke and transient ischemic attack to prevent early recurrence) (Kennedy et al., 2003) is a 2×2 factorial design trial comparing aspirin plus clopidogrel (300 mg load followed by 75 mg/day) versus aspirin alone and simvastatin 40 mg versus placebo in patients who have had a TIA or minor ischemic stroke within the previous 24 hours. Treatment is for 1 month and the main outcome is recurrent stroke; the initial pilot phase aims to recruit 500 patients and should report findings in 2007. The CASTIA (clopidogrel in acute stroke and TIA) trial will randomize over 2400 patients with acute TIA or minor ischemic stroke within 24 hours of symptom onset to clopidogrel (300 mg load followed by 75 mg/day) or placebo. All patients will be treated with aspirin 75 mg/day. The composite outcome will include clinical stroke, new magnetic resonance imaging (MRI) findings of stroke, myocardial infarction, and vascular death at 90 days.

Anticoagulants

Although no trial has looked at anticoagulation versus antiplatelet agents specifically in patients with carotid disease, there is no evidence to support the use of anticoagulation in patients with recently symptomatic carotid stenosis who are in sinus rhythm. Warfarin with a target international normalized ratio (INR) of 3−4.5 was harmful in the SPIRIT trial (The Stroke Prevention in Reversible Ischemia Trial [SPIRIT] study group, 1997), and there was no additional benefit from warfarin over aspirin at a mean INR of 1.8 (target INR 1.4−2.8) in the WARSS trial (Warfarin Aspirin Recurrent Stroke Study Group, 2001). Although this trial excluded patients with stroke attributable to high-grade carotid stenosis for which surgery was planned, the authors commented that aspirin "was slightly but not significantly superior to warfarin in patients with large-vessel infarcts". Another related indication for which anticoagulation has been studied recently is intracranial stenosis. A previous small, retrospective, nonrandomized study found that the recurrent stroke rate was lower in patients with symptomatic 50–99% intracranial stenosis treated with warfarin, compared to aspirin (Chimowitz *et al.*, 1995). Eighty-eight patients treated with warfarin were followed for a median of 14.7 months and 63 patients on aspirin therapy were followed for a median duration of 19.3 months. Vascular risk factors and mean percent stenosis of the symptomatic artery were similar in the two groups. The rate of major vascular event per 100 patient years of follow-up was 18.1 in the aspirin group compared to 8.4 in the warfarin group ($p = 0.01$) and the corresponding rate of stroke was 10.4 versus 3.6 ($p = 0.02$). However, the hypothesis that warfarin is superior to aspirin for stroke prevention in intracranial stenosis was not supported in the warfarin aspirin symptomatic intracranial disease (WASID) trial (Chimowitz *et al.*, 2005). Patients with TIA or stroke caused by angiographically verified ≥50% stenosis of a major intracranial artery were randomized to receive either warfarin (target INR 2–3) or aspirin (1300 mg per day). The trial was stopped early due to a significant excess of deaths from any cause, major hemorrhage and sudden death or myocardial infarction in the warfarin group, although there was no significant difference in the primary endpoint of ischemic stroke, brain hemorrhage or death from vascular causes other than stroke between the groups.

Problems arise in clinical practice, however, in patients with TIA or ischemic stroke who have both an apparently symptomatic carotid stenosis and atrial fibrillation (AF). Warfarin is usually indicated in patients with TIA or ischemic stroke in AF, but the need for anticoagulation and/or endarterectomy in this situation depends to some extent on whether the recent TIA or stroke was cardioembolic or due to carotid thromboembolism. Echocardiography may reveal apical thrombus or atrial enlargement, in which case anticoagulation will probably be necessary. Alternatively, echocardiography may be normal and the pattern of ischemic lesions on brain imaging may be suggestive of carotid thromboembolism, in which case endarterectomy alone may be required. Occasionally, brain imaging also shows asymptomatic recent infarction in other arterial territories, suggesting that cardioembolism is the underlying cause. Diffusion-weighted MR imaging is the most useful modality in this situation (Figure 5.1).

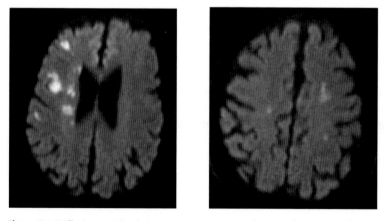

Figure 5.1 Diffusion-weighted imaging (DWI) in two patients with recent right-carotid transient ischemic attack (TIA) or minor ischemic stroke, atrial fibrillation and 70–80% right sided internal carotid artery stenosis. (left) shows multifocal ischemic lesions in the right hemisphere, typical of symptomatic carotid stenosis; (right) shows bilateral lesions typical of cardiac embolic source.

Cholesterol lowering

Although epidemiological studies do not suggest a strong association between cholesterol and ischemic stroke (Prospective Studies Collaboration, 1995), trials of statins have shown reductions in the risk of stroke in patients with coronary heart disease (Waters *et al.*, 2002; Amarenco *et al.*, 2004) although not clearly in patients with previous TIA or stroke (Heart Protection Study Collaborative Group, 2002, 2004). However, no RCT has yet addressed cholesterol-lowering treatment and stroke reduction specifically in patients with carotid artery stenosis. Cholesterol lowering is the one current medical treatment that was not used in the majority of patients in the RCTs of endarterectomy: 34% of the patients in the NASCET (North American Symptomatic Carotid Endarterectomy Trial Collaborators, 1991) and only 9% of those in the ECST (European Carotid Surgery Trialists' Collaborative Group, 1991) were on a lipid-lowering drug at randomization, although use will have increased during follow-up.

The heart protection study (HPS) is the largest trial of statins in cerebrovascular disease, having included 3280 patients with previous stroke or TIA, in addition to 17 256 with other occlusive arterial disease or diabetes (Heart Protection Study Collaborative Group, 2002, 2004). All patients were randomized to either simvastatin 40 mg daily or placebo, initiated at a mean 4.3 years after the qualifying event. Although there was no subgroup analysis according to prior stroke etiology among all patients with preexisting cerebrovascular disease, there was no apparent reduction in the stroke rate in the simvastatin group compared to placebo (169 [10.3%] vs. 170 [10.4%], relative risk 0.98 [0.79–1.22], NS), but there was a highly significant 20% (95% CI, 8–29%) reduction in the rate of any major vascular event (406 [24.7%] vs. 488 [29.8%], $p = 0.001$). There was no significant difference in hemorrhagic stroke rates either in those with or without preexisting cerebrovascular disease. Interestingly, in all the 20 536 participants in the study, there was a significant decrease in the rate of carotid endarterectomy or angioplasty in the statin arm compared to placebo (42 [0.4%] vs. 82 [0.8%], RRR 0.54 [0.38–0.77]; $p = 0.0003$).

A recent meta-analysis of all RCTs of statins in which stroke events were reported included data from over 90 000 patients. In 26 trials studying statins in seven different populations (coronary artery disease, hypercholesterolemia, normocholesterolemia, the elderly, hypertensives, diabetics and those with previous stroke) the relative risk reduction for any stroke was 21% (odds ratio [OR] 0.79, 95% CI, 0.73–0.85, $p < 0.0001$) and for fatal stroke was 9% (OR 0.91 95% CI, 0.65–1.22, $p = 0.37$) with no heterogeneity between trials. The implications of HPS along with the many trials of lipid lowering in coronary heart disease showing a reduction in stroke rate with statins, are for all patients with ischemic stroke or TIA to receive a statin; there is no reason to exclude those with carotid stenosis from this recommendation. More direct evidence will come from the publication of the stroke prevention by aggressive reduction cholesterol levels (SPARCL) trial in 2007 (Amarenco *et al.*, 2003). The study compared atorvastatin 80 mg versus placebo in stroke and TIA patients and the provisionally reported results show a significant reduction in fatal and ischaemic strokes, with a trend to fewer nonfatal strokes with atorvastatin at the expense of a small but significant increase in the risk of haemorrhagic stroke. The results will be reported in the near future, probably according to etiological subtype as the presence of carotid stenosis has been recorded.

Although evidence suggests that statins stabilize and/or cause regression of atherosclerotic plaque, thereby reducing the risk of thrombotic rupture, clear associations are lacking first between cholesterol level and ischemic stroke in the general population and second between the rates of cholesterol lowering by statin therapy and onset of beneficial action. Debate has therefore arisen over the precise mode of action of statins and mechanisms in addition to cholesterol lowering have been proposed (Vaughan *et al.*, 1996; Takemoto and Liao, 2001). Statins may act on

Table 5.1. Hazard ratios (95% CI) for the risk of stroke in patients categorized according to the severity of carotid disease within the pre-specified blood pressure groups. The hazard ratios are derived from a Cox proportional hazards model, stratified by trial, and adjusted for age, sex and previous coronary heart disease. Patients with bilateral <70% stenosis are allocated a hazard of 1

Stenosis group	Systolic blood pressure (mm Hg)			
	<130	130–149	150–169	≥170
Bilateral <70%	1	1	1	1
Unilateral ≥70%	1.90 (1.24–2.89)	1.18 (0.92–1.51)	1.27 (0.99–1.64)	1.64 (1.15–2.33)
	$p = 0.02$	$p = 0.30$	$p = 0.13$	$p = 0.03$
Bilateral ≥70%	5.97 (2.43–14.68)	2.54 (1.47–4.39)	0.97 (0.4–2.35)	1.13 (0.50–2.54)
	$p < 0.001$	$p = 0.001$	$p = 0.95$	$p = 0.77$

promoters of plaque stability through so-called pleiotropic effects. For example, in animal models of atherosclerosis, statins have been shown to increase collagen formation, reduce the size of the plaque lipid core and have antiinflammatory properties, by decreasing macrophage numbers and metalloproteinase production (Aikawa *et al.*, 2001). Similarly, in a trial of 24 patients scheduled for carotid endarterectomy, 11 were randomized to pravastatin and 13 to placebo and surgery was performed after 3 months of treatment (Crisby *et al.*, 2001). On analysis of tissue removed at operation, a positive effect of pravastatin was found on all biological parameters studied, including macrophage count, oxidized low-density lipoprotein (LDL), apoptotic cell count, metalloproteinases and smooth muscle cell proliferation. In addition, statins may modulate cerebral vasoreactivity and endothelial function through paracrine effects on nitric oxide synthase (Amin-Hanjani *et al.*, 2001; Laufs *et al.*, 2002). Lastly, statins may confer neuroprotection through antioxidant effects; by inhibiting leucocyte adhesion and migration, statins may protect the ischemic penumbra against injury by free radicals (Rosenson, 2004).

Blood-pressure-lowering drugs

Blood pressure lowering has been shown to be effective for secondary prevention of stroke (Progress Collaborative Group, 2001), although the effect in different etiological subtypes of ischemic stroke is unknown. However, it is likely that most patients with large-artery atherosclerosis will benefit. Many physicians are, however, cautious about lowering blood pressure, particularly in patients with bilateral severe carotid stenosis. These patients often also have disease of the vertebral arteries, the carotid siphon, and the cerebral arteries (Thiele *et al.*, 1980; Gorelick, 1993) and have a particularly high risk of recurrent stroke. Loss of the normal autoregulatory capacity of the cerebral circulation, such that cerebral blood flow is directly dependent on perfusion pressure, is common and there has been concern that blood pressure lowering may reduce cerebral perfusion and increase the risk of stroke (Vander Grond *et al.*, 1995; Grubb *et al.*, 1998).

Surprisingly, there is no mention of carotid disease in hypertension treatment guidelines, and no data on carotid disease were recorded in the trials of blood pressure lowering after stroke or TIA. However, some conclusions can be drawn from an analysis of the risk of stroke in prespecified categories of systolic blood pressure (SBP) stratified according to the presence or absence of flow-limiting (≥70%) carotid stenosis in patients randomized to medical treatment in ECST and NASCET (Table 5.1) (Rothwell *et al.*, 2003). Major increases in stroke risk were seen in association with bilateral flow-limiting stenosis in patients with SBP < 130 and SBP = 130–149, but not in patients with higher SBP. The 5-year risk of stroke in patients with bilateral ≥70% stenosis was 64.3% in those with SBP < 150 mmHg (median value) versus 24.2% at higher blood pressures ($p = 0.002$). This difference in risk was not present in the group who had been randomized to endarterectomy (13.4% vs. 18.3%, $p = 0.6$) suggesting a causal effect and indicating that aggressive blood pressure lowering without endarterectomy would probably be harmful in patients with bilateral severe carotid stenosis or severe symptomatic stenosis with contralateral occlusion. However, the relationship between blood pressure and stroke risk is positive in patients with only unilateral ≥70% stenosis (Rothwell et al., 2003), suggesting that blood pressure lowering is likely to be safe and beneficial in this group and following endarterectomy on one side in patients with bilateral severe carotid stenosis or severe symptomatic stenosis with contralateral occlusion.

Lifestyle modification

Lifestyle modification is frequently overlooked by busy hospital clinicians and although evidence for such interventions based on RCTs specifically in patients with carotid stenosis is lacking, it is important not to overlook simple measures which may well provide effective vascular prevention. The adverse effects of smoking on vascular and cancer risk are clearly established. However, the best methods of assisting smoking cessation are less clear although advice from physicians on quitting (including to a smoking partner), nicotine replacement therapy and bupropion in conjunction with behavioral support are all of some value (Molyneux, 2004).

Although dietary modification has mainly been studied in primary prevention and coronary artery disease, it may provide benefit for patients with carotid stenosis. A "Mediterranean diet", with a high intake of vegetables, fruits, cereals and fish and low in saturated (animal) fats has been shown to reduce cardiac death and myocardial infarction compared to a "Western diet" in patients with established ischemic heart disease, probably through its effects on lipid metabolism as opposed to reduction in total calorific intake (de Lorgeril et al., 1999). Salt restriction through dietary modification has been shown to reduce blood pressure slightly in hypertensive individuals, both on and off treatment, and in normotensives (Hooper et al., 2002). However, there are no clear data on the effects of salt restriction on "harder" endpoints such as mortality or vascular morbidity. The role of dietary antioxidants in vascular prevention has been much debated. A clear association between elevated plasma homocysteine levels and vascular disease was first demonstrated in individuals with homozygous homocystinuria and has since been shown in the general population although it is complicated by the interaction with age, lipid profile, diabetes and smoking (Kaplan, 2003). However, a recent RCT of multivitamin supplementation with folic acid, vitamin B6 and B12 compared to placebo in patients with recent ischemic stroke also on best medical therapy showed no benefit on vascular outcome over a 2-year period despite a significant but moderate reduction in plasma homocysteine levels (Toole et al., 2004). Other RCTs studying vitamin supplementation and vascular risk over longer follow-up periods are ongoing (VITATOPS Trials Study Group, 2002).

Medical treatment and intima-media thickness

Pignoli et al. were the first to demonstrate that common carotid intima-media thickness (IMT) measured by B-mode ultrasound in vitro corresponded with measurements made directly in autopsy specimens (Pignoli et al., 1986). IMT is correlated with the presence of cardiovascular risk factors and possibly with the future risk of vascular events including stroke and myocardial infarction (Mancini et al., 2004). In addition, sequential IMT measurement with ultrasound is safe, fast, reliable and reproducible, and this has led to its frequent use in clinical trials as a surrogate outcome marker for atherosclerosis. Statins in particular have been shown to cause a slowing in progression, or even a reduction, in IMT (Mercuri *et al.*, 1996; Amarenco *et al.*, 2004) as have ACE inhibitors (Lonn *et al.*, 2001), beta-blockers (Hedblad *et al.*, 2001), weight loss in obese subjects and various interventions in patients with diabetes (Kodama *et al.*, 2000; Hosomi *et al.*, 2001; Langenfeld *et al.*, 2005). However, the use of surrogate markers to predict clinical benefit is complex and treatment recommendations should not be made on the basis of the above studies alone.

Selection of patients for endarterectomy

Effect of treatment in clinical subgroups

Analysis of pooled data from both NASCET (North American Symptomatic Carotid Endarterectomy Trial Collaborators, 1991) and ECST (European Carotid Surgery Trialists' Collaborative Group, 1991) has provided statistical power to determine subgroup treatment interactions and has identified several clinically important observations (Rothwell *et al.*, 2004). Sex ($p = 0.003$), age ($p = 0.03$), and time from the last symptomatic event to randomization ($p = 0.009$) modified the effectiveness of surgery. Benefit from surgery was greatest in men, patients aged ≥75 years, and patients randomized within 2 weeks after their last ischemic event and fell rapidly with increasing delay. For patients with ≥50% stenosis, the number of patients needed to undergo surgery (number needed to treat, NNT) to prevent one ipsilateral stroke in 5 years was 9 for men versus 36 for women, 5 for age ≥75 versus 18 for age <65 years, and 5 for patients randomized within 2 weeks after their last ischemic event versus 125 for patients randomized >12 weeks. These observations were consistent across the 50–69% and ≥70% stenosis groups and similar trends were present in both ECST and NASCET.

Women had a lower risk of ipsilateral ischemic stroke on medical treatment and a higher operative risk in comparison to men. For recently symptomatic carotid stenosis, surgery is very clearly beneficial in women with ≥70% stenosis, but not in women with 50–69% stenosis. In contrast, surgery reduced the 5-year absolute risk of stroke by 8.0% (3.4–12.5) in men with 50–69% stenosis. This sex difference was statistically significant even when the analysis of the interaction was confined to the 50–69% stenosis group.

Benefit from carotid endarterectomy increased with age in the pooled analysis, and was particularly marked in patients aged over 75 years. However, this observation might not be generalizable to routine clinical practice because trial patients generally have a better prognosis (Stiller, 1994) and elderly patients might have a greater operative risk in clinical practice. There is some evidence of a higher operative risk in administrative database studies, particularly in patients aged over 85 years (Wennberg *et al.*, 1998), but a recent systematic review of published surgical case-series reported pooled odds of stroke and death of 1.2 (95% CI, 1.0–1.4; $p = 0.08$, 19 studies) for patients aged over 75 versus under 75 years and 1.2 (0.9–1.5; $p = 0.19$, 11 studies) for patients aged over 80 versus under 80 years (Bond *et al.*, 2005). There is, therefore, no justification for withholding carotid endarterectomy in patients aged over 75 who are deemed to be medically fit to undergo surgery. The evidence suggests that benefit is likely to be greatest in this group because of their high risk of stroke on medical treatment, although it should be noted that the trials included very few patients over the age of 80 years.

In the pooled analysis, benefit from surgery tended to be greatest in patients with stroke and to progressively decline in patients with cerebral TIA and retinal events in both the 50–69% and ≥70% stenosis groups. There was also a trend towards greater benefit in patients with irregular plaque than a smooth plaque in both stenosis groups. However, these treatment effects by subgroup interactions failed to reach statistical

Table 5.2. Independent predictors of ipsilateral ischemic stroke within 5 years in patients with recently symptomatic carotid stenosis randomized to medical treatment only in the European carotid surgery trial (Rothwell *et al.*, 2005)

Risk factor	Hazard ratio (95% CI)	*p*-value
Stenosis (per 10%)	1.18 (1.10, 1.25)	<0.0001
Near occlusion	0.49 (0.19, 1.24)	0.1309
Male sex	1.19 (0.81, 1.75)	0.3687
Age (per 10 years)	1.12 (0.89, 1.39)	0.3343
Time since last event (per 7 days)	0.96 (0.93, 0.99)	0.0039
Presenting event		
Ocular	1.00	
Single TIA	1.41 (0.75, 2.66)	
Multiple TIAs	2.05 (1.16, 3.60)	0.0067
Minor stroke	1.82 (0.99, 3.34)	
Major stroke	2.54 (1.48, 4.35)	
Diabetes	1.35 (0.86, 2.11)	0.1881
Previous MI	1.57 (1.01, 2.45)	0.0471
PVD	1.18 (0.78, 1.77)	0.4368
Treated hypertension	1.24 (0.88, 1.75)	0.2137
Irregular/ulcerated plaque	2.03 (1.31, 3.14)	0.0015

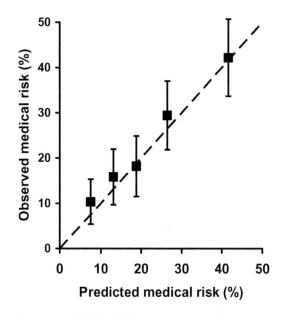

Figure 5.2 Reliability of the European Carotid Surgery Trial prognostic model (Table 5.2) for the 5-year risk of stroke on medical treatment in patients with 50–99% stenosis in the North American Symptomatic Carotid Endarterectomy Trial (NASCET). Observed medical risk in NASCET is plotted against predicted medical risk in quintile groups of predicted risk. Error bars represent 95% confidence intervals. (Rothwell *et al.*, 2005.)

significance either overall (*p* = 0.10 for irregular plaque and *p* = 0.16 for primary symptomatic event) or when the analysis was restricted to patients with ≥50% stenosis (*p* = 0.06 for irregular plaque and *p* = 0.1 for primary symptomatic event).

Effect of treatment in risk groups

Although carotid endarterectomy reduces the relative risk of stroke by about 30% over the next 3 years in patients with a recently symptomatic severe stenosis, only 20% of such patients have a stroke on medical treatment alone. The operation is therefore of no value in the other 80% of patients who, despite having a symptomatic stenosis, are destined to remain stroke free without surgery and

can only be harmed with surgery. Although the univariate subgroup analyses are of some help in selecting patients for surgery, it would be more useful to be able to identify and operate on, only those patients with a high risk of stroke on medical treatment alone, but a relatively low operative risk. One such model was derived from the patients randomized in the ECST (Table 5.2) (European Carotid Surgery Trialists' Collaborative Group, 1991; Rothwell *et al.*, 1999, 2005).

The potential usefulness of the ECST model is illustrated in Figure 5.2, which shows the risk of stroke on medical treatment in patients with 50–99% symptomatic carotid stenosis who were randomized to medical treatment in NASCET stratified into quintiles of predicted risk according

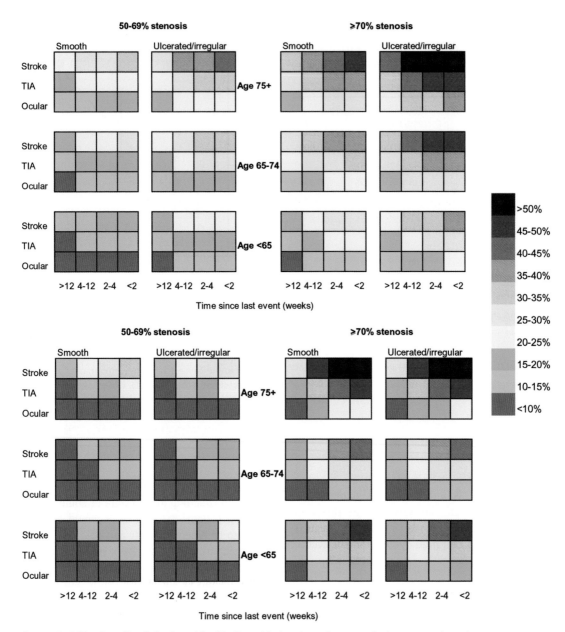

Figure 5.3 Table of predicted absolute risk of ipsilateral ischemic stroke on medical treatment in patients with recently symptomatic carotid stenosis. Stroke/transient ischemic attack (TIA)/ocular refers to the most severe symptomatic ipsilateral ischemic event in the past 6 months: stroke > cerebral TIA > ocular events only. (Rothwell *et al.*, 2005.)

to the ECST model. There was close agreement between predicted and observed medical risk ($x^2_{Heterogeneity} = 43.1$, df = 4, $p < 0.0001$; Mantel-Haenszel $x^2_{Trend} = 41.2$, df = 1, $p < 0.0001$). The likelihood of benefit from endarterectomy, which has a 5–7% operative risk of stroke and death followed by a residual stroke risk of about 1% per year, will clearly vary between these groups. Figure 5.3 shows a risk table derived from the ECST model indicating the 5-year risk of ipsilateral ischemic stroke in patients with recently symptomatic carotid stenosis on medical treatment based on the five variables that were both significant predictors of risk in the ECST model (Table 5.2) and yielded clinically important univariate subgroup treatment effect interactions in the analysis of pooled data from the relevant trials.

Conclusion

Patients with carotid stenosis are at high risk of stroke and acute ischemic events in other vascular territories and require intensive medical treatment. Medical treatment is particularly important in the high-risk period between the presenting event and carotid endarterectomy or stenting, and in patients who decline intervention or for whom intervention is not possible. Antiplatelet agents, cholesterol-lowering drugs and blood-pressure-lowering drugs should be considered in all patients with carotid stenosis.

REFERENCES

Aikawa, M., Rabkin, E., Sugiyama, S., et al. (2001). An HMG-CoA reductase inhibitor, cerivastatin, suppresses growth of macrophages expressing matrix metalloproteinases, and tissue factor in vivo, and in vitro. Circulation, **103**, 276–83.

Amarenco, P., Bogousslavsky, J., Callahan, A. S., et al. (2003). Design and baseline characteristics of the stroke prevention by aggressive reduction in cholesterol levels (SPARCL) study. Cerebrovascular Disease, **16**, 389–95.

Amarenco, P., Labreuche, J., Lavallee, P. and Touboul, P. J. (2004). Statins in stroke prevention and carotid atherosclerosis: systematic review and up-to-date meta-analysis. Stroke, **35**, 2902–9.

Amin-Hanjani, S., Stagliano, N. E., Yamada, M., et al. (2001). Mevastatin, an HMG-CoA reductase inhibitor, reduces stroke damage and upregulated endothelial nitric oxide synthase in mice. Stroke, **32**, 980–6.

Antithrombotic Trialists Collaboration. (2002). Collaborative meta-analysis of randomised trials of antiplatelet therapy for prevention of death, myocardial infarction, and stroke in high-risk patients. British Medical Journal, **324**, 71–86.

Bond, R., Rerkasem, K., Cuffe, R. and Rothwell, P. M. (2005). A systematic review of the associations between age and sex and the operative risks of carotid endarterectomy. Cerebrovascular Disease, **20**, 69–77.

CAPRIE Steering Committee. (1996). A randomised, blinded, trial of clopidogrel versus aspirin in patients at risk of ischaemic events (CAPRIE). Lancet, **348**, 1329–39.

Chimowitz, M. I., Kokkinos, P., Strong, J., et al. (1995). For the Warfarin-Aspirin Symptomatic Intracranial Disease Study Group. The warfarin-aspirin symptomatic intracranial disease study. Neurology, **45**, 1488–93.

Chimowitz, M. I., Lynn, M. J., Howlett-Smith, H., et al. (2005). Comparison of warfarin and aspirin for symptomatic intracranial arterial stenosis. New England Journal of Medicine, **352**, 1305–16.

Crisby, M., Nordin-Fredricksson, G., Shah, P. K., et al. (2001). Pravastatin treatment increases collagen content and decreases lipid content, inflammation, metalloproteinases, and cell death in human carotid plaques. Implications for plaque stabilization. Circulation, **103**, 926–33.

de Lorgeril, M., Salen, P., Martin, J.-L., et al. (1999). Mediterranean diet, traditional risk factors, and the rate of cardiovascular complications after myocardial infarction: final report of the Lyon Diet Heart Study. Circulation, **99**, 779–85.

Diener, H. C., Bogousslavsky, J., Brass, I. M., et al. (2004). Aspirin and clopidogrel compared with clopidogrel alone after recent ischemic stroke or transient ischemic attack in high-risk patients (MATCH): randomised double-blind, placebo-controlled trial. Lancet, **364**, 331–7.

Diener, H. C., Cunha, L., Forbes, C., *et al.* (1996). European Stroke Prevention Study. 2. Dipyridamole and acetyl-salicylic acid in the secondary prevention of stroke. *Journal of the Neurological Sciences*, **143**, 1–13.

Engelter, S. and Lyrer, P. (2003). Antiplatelet therapy for preventing stroke and other vascular events after carotid endarterectomy. *Cochrane Database System Review*, CD001458.

European Carotid Surgery Trialists' Collaborative Group. (1991). MRC European Carotid Surgery Trial. Interim results for symptomatic patients with severe (70–99%) or with mild (0–29%) carotid stenosis. *Lancet*, **337**, 1235–43.

Fairhead, J. F., Mehta, Z. and Rothwell, P. M. (2005). Population-based study of delays in carotid imaging and surgery and the risk of recurrent stroke. *Neurology*, **65**, 371–5.

Goertler, M., Baeumer, M., Kross, R., *et al.* (1999). Rapid decline of cerebral microemboli of arterial origin after intravenous acetylsalicylic acid. *Stroke*, **30**, 66–9.

Gorelick, P. B. (1993). Distribution of atherosclerotic cerebrovascular lesions. Effects of age, race, and sex. *Stroke*, **24**, 116–19.

Grubb, R. L. Jr, Derdeyn, C. P., Fritsch, S. M., *et al.* (1998). Importance of hemodynamic factors in the prognosis of symptomatic carotid occlusion. *Journal of the American Medical Association*, **280**, 1055–60.

Heart Protection Study Collaborative Group. (2002). MRC/BHF Heart Protection Study of cholesterol lowering with simvastatin in 20 536 high-risk patients: a randomised placebo-controlled trial. *Lancet*, **360**, 7–22.

Heart Protection Study Collaborative Group. (2004). Effects of cholesterol lowering with simvastatin on stroke and other major vascular events in 20 536 people with cerebrovascular disease or other high risk conditions. *Lancet*, **363**, 757–7.

Hedblad, B., Wikstrand, J., Janzon, L., Wedel, H. and Berglund, G. (2001). Low-dose metoprolol CR/XL and fluvastatin slow progression of carotid intima-media thickness: main results from the Beta-Blocker Cholesterol-Lowering Asymptomatic Plaque Study (BCAPS). *Circulation*, **103**, 1721–26.

Hooper, L., Bartlett, C., Davey Smith, G. and Ebrahim, S. (2002). Systematic review of long term effects of advice to reduce dietary salt in adults. *British Medical Journal*, **325**, 628–32.

Hosomi, N., Mizushige, K., Ohyama, H., *et al.* (2001). Angiotensin-converting enzyme inhibition with enalapril slows progressive intima-media thickening of the common carotid artery in patients with non-insulin-dependent diabetes mellitus. *Stroke*, **32**, 1539–45.

Kaplan, E. D. (2003). Association between homocysteine levels and risk of vascular events. *Drugs Today (Barc)*, **39**, 175–92.

Kennedy, J., Eliasziw, M., Hill, M. D. and Buchan, A. M. (2003). The Fast Assessment of Stroke and Transient Ischemic Attack to prevent Early Recurrence (FASTER) Trial. *Seminars in Cerebrovascular Diseases and Stroke*, **3**, 25–30.

Kodama, M., Yamasaki, Y., Sakamoto, K., *et al.* (2000). Antiplatelet drugs attenuate progression of carotid intima-media thickness in subjects with type 2 diabetes. *Thrombosis Research*, **97**, 239–45.

Langenfeld, M. R., Forst, T., Hohberg, C., *et al.* (2005). Pioglitazone decreases carotid intima-media thickness independently of glycemic control in patients with type 2 diabetes mellitus: results from a controlled randomized study. *Circulation*, **111**, 2525–31.

Laufs, U., Gertz, K., Dirnagl, U., *et al.* (2002). Rosuvastatin, a new HMG-CoA reductase inhibitor, upregulates endothelial nitric oxide synthase and protects from ischemic stroke in mice. *Brain Research*, **28**, 23–30.

Leonardi-Bee, J., Bath, P. M., Bousser, M. G., *et al.* (2005). Dipyridamole in Stroke Collaboration (DISC). Dipyridamole for preventing recurrent ischemic stroke and other vascular events: a meta-analysis of individual patient data from randomized controlled trials. *Stroke*, **36**, 162–8.

Lonn, E., Yusuf, S., Dzavik, V., *et al.* (2001). Effects of ramipril and vitamin E on atherosclerosis: the Study to Evaluate Carotid Ultrasound Changes in Patients Treated With Ramipril and Vitamin E (SECURE). *Circulation*, **103**, 919–25.

Lovett, J. K., Coull, A., Rothwell, P. M., on behalf of the Oxford Vascular Study. (2004). Early risk of recurrent stroke by aetiological subtype: implications for stroke prevention. *Neurology*, **62**, 569–74.

Mancini, G. B., Dahlof, B. and Diez, J. (2004). Surrogate markers for cardiovascular disease: structural markers. *Circulation*, **109** (Suppl. 1), 22–30.

Markus, H. S., Droste, D. W., Kaps, M., *et al.* (2005). Dual antiplatelet therapy with clopidogrel and aspirin in symptomatic carotid stenosis evaluated using Doppler embolic signal detection: the Clopidogrel and Aspirin for Reduction of Emboli in Symptomatic Carotid Stenosis (CARESS) trial. *Circulation*, **111**, 2233–40.

Mercuri, M., Bond, M. G., Sirtori, C. R., *et al.* (1996). Pravastatin reduces carotid intima-media thickness progression in an asymptomatic hypercholesterolemic Mediterranean population: The Carotid Atherosclerosis Italian Ultrasound Study. *American Journal of Medicine*, **101**, 627–34.

Molyneux, A. (2004). Nicotine replacement therapy. *British Medical Journal*, **328**, 454–6.

North American Symptomatic Carotid Endarterectomy Trial Collaborators (1991). Beneficial effect of carotid endarterectomy in symptomatic patients with high-grade carotid stenosis. *New England Journal of Medicine*, **325**, 445–53.

Pignoli, P., Tremoli, E., Poli, A., Oreste, P. and Paoletti, R. (1986). Intimal plus medial thickness of the arterial wall: a direct measurement with ultrasound imaging. *Circulation*, **74**, 1399–406.

Progress Collaborative Group. (2001). Randomised trial of a perindopril-based blood-pressure-lowering regimen among 6,105 individuals with previous stroke or transient ischaemic attack. *Lancet*, **358**, 1033–41.

Prospective Studies Collaboration (1995). Cholesterol, diastolic blood pressure, and stroke: 13,000 strokes in 450,000 people in 45 prospective cohorts. *Lancet*, **346**, 1647–53.

Rosenson, R. S. (2004). Statins in atherosclerosis: lipid-lowering agents with antioxidant capabilities. *Atherosclerosis*, **173**, 1–12.

Rothwell, P. M., Eliasziw, M., Gutnikov, S. A., Warlow, C. P. and Barnett, H. J. (2004). Carotid Endarterectomy Trialists Collaboration Endarterectomy for symptomatic carotid stenosis in relation to clinical subgroups and timing of surgery. *Lancet*, **363**, 915–24.

Rothwell, P M., Howard, S. C. and Spence, D. (2003). Relationship between blood pressure and stroke risk in patients with symptomatic carotid occlusive disease. *Stroke*, **34**, 2583–90.

Rothwell, P. M., Mehta, Z., Howard, S. C., Gutnikov, S. A. and Warlow, C. P. (2005). From subgroups to individuals: general principles and the example of carotid endartectomy. *Lancet*, **365**, 256–65.

Rothwell, P. M., Warlow, C. P. on behalf of the ECST Collaborators. (1999). Prediction of benefit from carotid endarterectomy in individual patients: A risk-modelling study. *Lancet*, **353**, 2105–10.

Stiller, C. A. (1994). Centralised treatment, entry to trials and survival. *British Journal of Cancer*, **70**, 352–62.

Stroke Prevention in Reversible Ischemia Trial (SPIRIT) Study Group. (1997). A randomized trial of anticoagulants versus aspirin after cerebral ischemia of presumed arterial origin. *Annals of Neurology*, **42**, 857–65.

Takemoto, M. and Liao, J. K. (2001). Pleiotropic effects of 3-hydroxy-3-methylglutaryl coenzyme A reductase inhibitors. *Arteriosclerosis, Thrombosis and Vascular Biology*, **21**, 1712–19.

Thiele, B. L., Young, J. V., Chikos, P. M., Hirsch, J. H. and Strandness, D. E. (1980). Correlation of arteriographic findings and symptoms in cerebrovascular disease. *Neurology*, **30**, 1041–6.

Toole, J. F., Malinow, M. R., Chambless, L. E., *et al.* (2004). Lowering homocysteine in patients with ischemic stroke to prevent recurrent stroke, myocardial infarction, and death: the Vitamin Intervention for Stroke Prevention (VISP) randomized controlled trial. *Journal of the American Medical Association*, **291**, 565–75.

Van der Grond, J., Balm, R., Kappelle, J., Eikelboom, B. C. and Mali, W. P. (1995). Cerebral metabolism of patients with stenosis or occlusion of the internal carotid artery. *Stroke*, **26**, 822–8.

Vaughan, C. J., Murphy, M. B. and Buckley, B. M. (1996). Statins do more than just lower cholesterol. *Lancet*, **348**, 1079–82.

VITATOPS Trial Study Group. (2002). The VITATOPS (Vitamins to Prevent Stroke) Trial: rationale and design of an international, large, simple, randomised trial of homocysteine-lowering multivitamin therapy in patients with recent transient ischaemic attack or stroke. *Cerebrovascular Disease*, **13**, 120–6.

Warfarin Aspirin Recurrent Stroke Study Group. (2001). A comparison of warfarin and aspirin for the prevention of recurrent ischemic stroke. *New England Journal of Medicine*, **345**, 1444–51.

Waters, D. D., Schwartz, G. G., Olsson, A. G., *et al.* (2002). Effects of atorvastatin on stroke in patients with unstable angina or non-Q-wave myocardial infarction. A Myocardial Ischemia Reduction with Aggressive Cholesterol Lowering (MIRACL) substudy. *Circulation*, **106**, 1690–5.

Wennberg, D. E., Lucas, F. L., Birkmeyer, J. D., Bredenberg, C. E. and Fisher, E. S. (1998). Variation in carotid endarterectomy mortality in the Medicare population: trial hospitals, volume, and patient characteristics. *Journal of the American Medical Association*, **279**, 1278–81.

6

Surgical management of symptomatic carotid disease: carotid endarterectomy and extracranial-intracranial bypass

Jonathan L. Brisman[1] and Marc R. Mayberg[2]

[1]New Jersey Neuroscience Institute, Edison, NJ, USA
[2]Seattle Neuroscience Institute, Seattle, WA, USA

Introduction

Stroke is a major health care problem in the United States, representing the third leading cause of death and the primary cause of disability (Mayberg, 1996). It is estimated that 700 000 people suffer a stroke in the United States annually resulting in approximately 53.6 billion dollars in direct and indirect costs (Hanel *et al.*, 2005). These numbers are expected to increase with an aging population.

Symptomatic carotid stenosis or occlusion is, by some estimates, responsible for 25% of all ischemic stroke (Hanel *et al.*, 2005) with an estimated 6–7% estimated annual stroke rate for patients with both symptomatic carotid stenosis or completed occlusion (Mayberg, 1996; Grubb and Powers, 2001). Sufficient evidence is now available from several clinical trials (MRC European Carotid Surgery Trial, 1991; Mayberg *et al.*, 1991; Barnett *et al.*, 1998) showing that carotid endarterectomy can reduce the risk of stroke for symptomatic carotid stenosis. More recent evidence (Yadav *et al.*, 2004) has shown that in certain subgroups of patients (high risk for carotid endarterectomy), carotid angioplasty and stenting may be an equally safe and effective treatment. This chapter will review the major clinical trials on carotid endarterectomy and carotid angioplasty and stenting and summarize the technique used by the authors for carotid endarterectomy. A brief review of the role for carotid angioplasty and stenting will shed light on the future that carotid endarterectomy may play in a rapidly changing environment.

Extracranial-intracranial (EC-IC) bypass as a technique to treat symptomatic internal carotid artery occlusion is less commonly employed following the results of the EC-IC bypass trial showing no benefit over the use of medical therapy (Failure of extracranial-intracranial bypass, 1985). That trial failed to select those patients with carotid occlusion who needed flow augmentation versus those that did not. Advances in technology have now made it possible to assess the cerebrovascular physiology of carotid occlusion patients; randomization of symptomatic carotid occlusion patients with diminished cerebrovascular reserve to either vascular bypass or best medical therapy comprises an ongoing study (Grubb *et al.*, 2003). These studies will be reviewed and current recommendations for the role of EC-IC for symptomatic carotid occlusion given.

Historical overview

Clinical trials have achieved a growing role in the contemporary practice of medicine, due in part to the advent of improved methodology for multicenter studies, increasing public awareness of

Carotid Disease: The Role of Imaging in Diagnosis and Management, ed. Jonathan Gillard, Martin Graves, Thomas Hatsukami and Chun Yuan. Published by Cambridge University Press. © Cambridge University Press 2007.

Table 6.1. Trials of carotid endarterectomy and carotid angioplasty and stenting for symptomatic carotid stenosis and extracranial-intracranial bypass for carotid occlusion

Trial	Inclusion criteria	Follow-up	Sample size	Primary endpoints	Results
European carotid surgery trial (ECST)	0–99% stenosis by angiography	5 yr	Prematurely terminated at 2200 pts.	Ipsilateral stroke	Surgical benefit for severe stenosis
North American symptomatic carotid endarterectomy trial (NASCET)	30–99% by angiography	5 yr	Prematurely terminated at 659 pts. with severe stenosis	Ipsilateral stroke, stroke-related death or death <30 d after randomization	Surgical benefit for severe stenosis
Veterans administration symptomatic stenosis trial (VASST)	50–99% by angiography	3 yr	Prematurely terminated at 193 pts.	Ipsilateral stroke or crescendo TIA; death <30 d after	Surgical benefit for stenosis >50%
Stent and angioplasty with protection for patients at high risk for endarterectomy (SAPPHIRE)	>50% by DUS and at least 1 high risk surgical criteria	1 yr	334 pts.	Cumulative death, stroke, MI within 30 d procedure or death or ipsilateral stroke 31 d–1 yr	CAS not inferior to CE
Carotid revascularization endarterectomy versus stent trial (CREST)	≥50% stenosis by DUS	4 yr	Ongoing study planned randomization of 2500 pts.	Stroke, MI death within 30 d of procedure or ipsilateral stroke during 4 yr follow-up	Ongoing study
Extracranial-intracranial (EC-IC) bypass study	Anterior circulation ischemia and MCA or ICA stenosis or occlusion	5 yr	1377 pts.	Fatal or nonfatal stroke	ECIC provided no benefit compared with medical therapy
Carotid occlusion surgery study (COSS)	Symptomatic ICA occlusion and ↑OEF	2 yr	372 pts.	Ipsilateral stroke through 2-yr follow-up or any stroke within 40 d of entry into trial	Ongoing study

Abbreviations: yr = year; pts. = patients; d = days; TIA = transient ischemic attack; DUS = Doppler ultrasound; MI = myocardial infarction; CAS = carotid angioplasty and stenting; CE = carotid endarterectomy; MCA = middle cerebral artery; ICA = internal carotid artery; OEF = oxygen extraction fraction.

clinical trials, the role of clinical trials in determining reimbursement policies and a general consensus in the medical community that any treatment administered should be proven effective according to rigorous scientific criteria.

The evolution of carotid endarterectomy, carotid angioplasty and stenting and EC-IC have been predicated on the results of clinical trials (Table 6.1), several of which are undergoing continued data collection to this day. The EC-IC bypass trial (Failure of extracranial-intracranial arterial bypass, 1985) introduced the concept of multicenter prospective randomized trials to the neurosurgical community. The widespread recognition of this trial and its consequences led in part to the development of several studies designed to test the efficacy of carotid endarterectomy. The studies evaluating the use of carotid endarterectomy for symptomatic stenosis are the North American symptomatic carotid endarterectomy trial (NASCET) (Beneficial effect of carotid endarterectomy, 1991), the European carotid surgery trial (ECST) (MRC European Carotid Surgery Trial, 1991) and the V.A. symptomatic stenosis trial (VASST). These trials (discussed below) published in the early 1990s demonstrated that in patients with symptomatic high-grade ($>70\%$) stenosis, carotid endarterectomy reduced stroke risk compared with medical therapy; the benefits of carotid endarterectomy, however, were only realized if the morbidity of surgery could be kept reasonably low (6%). Guidelines for carotid endarterectomy were published by the American Heart Association in 1995 (Moore et al., 1995) and the number of carotid endarterectomies performed in this country continued to rise.

At about the same time, however, endovascular technologic advances resulted in a self-expanding stent suitable for use in the carotid artery. The use of the stent for patients deemed high-risk candidates for carotid endarterectomy was increasing and it became evident that with increased operator experience, carotid angioplasty and stenting was safe and effective. The fact that the NASCET trial excluded many patients deemed to be at high risk for carotid endarterectomy further strengthened the interest in evaluation of carotid angioplasty and stenting for such patients. Clinical trials were initiated (Gray, 2005). The first trial comparing carotid angioplasty and stenting with carotid endarterectomy was published in 2001 and showed similar postprocedure stroke rates for the two procedures (Alberts et al., 1997). Additional studies comparing the two modalities followed quickly (Gray, 2004, 2005), the most important of

which showed equivalent success for high-risk patients when a distal embolic protection (DEP) device was employed (Yadav et al., 2004). This study resulted in FDA approval for carotid angioplasty and stenting with DEP; the procedure is now reimbursable. The ongoing carotid revascularization endarterectomy versus stent trial (CREST) (Hobson, 2000, 2002; Hobson et al., 2001) is prospectively randomizing patients with symptomatic carotid stenosis to either carotid endarterectomy or carotid angioplasty and stenting with DEP, regardless of perioperative risk stratification.

Prospective randomized trials for cerebral revascularization

Carotid endarterectomy and carotid angioplasty and stenting trials for symptomatic carotid stenosis

The ECST trial (MRC European Carotid Surgery Trial, 1991) entered patients with mild (defined as less than 30%), moderate (30–69%) or severe (70–99%) carotid stenosis, who were then randomized to surgical or nonsurgical treatment. Interim analysis of 2200 patients (mean follow-up = 2.7 years) led to premature termination of the trial for mild and severe stenosis groups. For mild stenosis, among 374 randomized patients there was no significant difference in ipsilateral stroke between the surgical and nonsurgical groups. There were more treatment failures in the surgery group, which was attributed to the 2.3% risk of death or disabling stroke during the first 30 days after surgery. For severe stenosis, however, surgery was shown to be beneficial in preventing stroke. There was a 7.5% risk of ipsilateral stroke or death within 30 days of surgery. At 3 years of follow-up, there was an additional 2.8% risk of stroke in the surgery group (total = 10.3%) compared to 16.8% in the nonsurgery group ($p < 0.0001$). More importantly, the risk of death or ipsilateral disabling stroke was reduced from 11% in the nonsurgery group to 6% in the surgery group.

The NASCET study (Beneficial effect of carotid endarterectomy, 1991) prematurely stopped randomizing patients with carotid stenosis greater than 70% due to the overwhelming stroke risk reduction observed in the surgical group. A total of 659 patients in this category of stenosis were randomized to surgical ($n=331$) or nonsurgical ($n=328$) therapy. At a mean follow-up of 24 months, ipsilateral stroke was noted in 26% of nonsurgical patients, compared to 9% of patients with endarterectomy, for an overall risk reduction of 17% (relative risk reduction = 71%). The benefit for surgical patients was highly significant ($p<$ 0.001) for a variety of outcomes, including stroke in any territory, major strokes and major stroke or death from any cause. A perioperative morbidity/ mortality of 5.8% was rapidly surpassed in the nonsurgical group, such that surgical benefit was apparent by 3 months. In addition, the protective effect of surgery was durable over time, with few strokes noted in the endarterectomy group beyond the perioperative period. There was a direct correlation between surgical benefit and the degree of angiographic stenosis.

Enrollment in the VASST study (Mayberg et al., 1991) was discontinued in early 1991 based upon preliminary data consistent with the NASCET findings. Subsequent analysis demonstrated a statistically-significant reduction in ipsilateral stroke or crescendo transient ischemic attack (TIA) for patients with carotid stenosis $>50\%$ (Mayberg et al., 1991). A total of 193 men aged 35–82 years (mean = 64.2 years) were randomized to surgical ($n=91$) and nonsurgical ($n=98$) treatment. Two-thirds of randomized patients demonstrated angiographic internal carotid artery stenosis greater than 70%.

At a mean follow-up of 11.9 months there was a significant reduction in stroke or crescendo TIA in patients receiving carotid endarterectomy (7.7%) compared to nonsurgical patients (19.4%), or a risk reduction of 11.7% (relative risk reduction = 60%; $p=0.028$). Among subgroups, the benefit of surgery was most prominent in TIA patients compared to transient monocular blindness (TMB) or stroke,

although these differences were not statistically significant. The benefit for surgery was apparent as early as 2 months after randomization, and persisted over the entire period of follow-up. The efficacy of carotid endarterectomy was durable with only one ipsilateral stroke beyond the 30-day perioperative period. Discounting one preoperative stroke, a perioperative morbidity of 2.2% and mortality of 3.3% (total = 5.5%) was achieved over multiple centers among relatively high-risk patients.

The Stenting and Angioplasty with Protection in Patients at High Risk for Endarterectomy (SAPPHIRE) trial was designed to test the hypothesis that carotid angioplasty and stenting was not inferior to carotid endarterectomy for patients deemed high risk for carotid endarterectomy – patients who theoretically would have been excluded from previous carotid endarterectomy trials. The premise was that with advances in endovascular capability to prevent embolic stroke during carotid angioplasty and stenting by using DEP, and given the cohort of patients in which morbidity has been shown to be quite high with carotid endarterectomy, a noninferiority hypothesis could be proven. Patients with symptomatic ($>50\%$ by Doppler ultrasound [DUS]) or asymptomatic ($>80\%$) carotid stenosis who met criteria for randomization (at least one of: congestive heart failure, abnormal stress test, need for open-heart surgery, severe pulmonary disease, contralateral carotid occlusion, contralateral laryngeal-nerve palsy, previous radical neck surgery or radiation therapy to the neck, recurrent stenosis after endarterectomy or age >80 years) were randomly assigned to either carotid endarterectomy ($n=167$) or carotid angioplasty and stenting ($n=167$) using a self-expanding nitinol stent with DEP. Patients had to be deemed suitable candidates for either carotid endarterectomy or carotid angioplasty and stenting prior to final randomization.

The primary endpoint of a composite of death, stroke, or myocardial infarction within 30 days of the procedure or death or ipsilateral stroke between 31 days and 1 year occurred in 12.2% of patients undergoing carotid angioplasty and stenting and 20.1% of patients undergoing carotid endarterectomy ($p=0.004$ for noninferiority). The majority of outcome difference could be attributed to a higher incidence of myocardial infarction in the surgery group; there were no significant differences in stroke or death between groups. Substratification of patients with symptomatic disease alone showed similar findings.

CREST (Hobson, 2000, 2002; Hobson et al., 2001) is an ongoing study in which patients with greater than 50% symptomatic carotid stenosis by DUS are undergoing randomization to either carotid endarterectomy or carotid angioplasty and stenting, irrespective of risk stratification. The primary outcome measures in the projected 2500 randomized patients are stroke, myocardial infarction, or death within 30 days of the procedure or ipsilateral stroke over a 4-year follow-up period.

Summary of trials for carotid endarterectomy and carotid angioplasty and stenting and proposed indications for intervention options

Based on the three major trials investigating carotid endarterectomy for symptomatic carotid stenosis, it is clear that carotid endarterectomy provided a profound protection against subsequent ipsilateral stroke or crescendo TIA in patients with high-grade symptomatic stenosis. In addition, carotid endarterectomy reduced stroke risk compared to medical therapy in patients with moderate-grade ($>50\%$) symptomatic carotid stenosis. The stroke risk reduction was realized early after surgery, persisted over extended periods of time and was independent of other risk factors. Efficacy for carotid endarterectomy, however, was only realized in these trials when an acceptable level of perioperative morbidity and mortality was achieved ($<6\%$).

A recent meta-analysis (Rothwell et al., 2003) of pooled data from the ECST, NASCET, and VASST trials was published and lends additional support to the 1995 guidelines by the American Heart Association (AHA) (Moore et al., 1995) for carotid endarterectomy. Data from 6092 patients with 35 000 patient-years of follow-up showed that surgery increased the 5-year risk of ipsilateral ischemic stroke in patients with less than 30% stenosis ($n=1746$, absolute risk reduction -2.2%, $p=0.05$), had no effect in patients with 30–49% stenosis (1429, 3.2%, $p=0.6$), was of slight benefit in those with 50–69% stenosis (1549, 4.6%, $p=0.04$), and was highly beneficial in those with 70% stenosis or greater without near-occlusion (1095, 16.0%, $p<0.001$). The AHA guidelines recommend carotid endarterectomy for patients with single or multiple TIAs and ipsilateral carotid stenosis $>70\%$ or for symptomatic carotid stenosis in patients with an ulcer on angiography and no other source of emboli. Patients with moderate stenosis remain an indeterminate indication for carotid endarterectomy.

Recognizing the emergence of new technology such as carotid angioplasty and stenting and DEP, a technology that continues to evolve in its ability to safely and efficaciously treat carotid occlusive disease (with the development of drug-eluting or radiation-laced stents or simpler and more reliable DEPs, for example), decisions to perform carotid endarterectomy must not only be made with best medical therapy as the alternative in mind. Patients who fall under the rubric of "high-risk" for carotid endarterectomy should be considered for carotid angioplasty and stenting and counseled regarding this option, given the exclusion of such patients from the major carotid endarterectomy trials such as NASCET, and the recent evidence showing the noninferiority of carotid angioplasty and stenting to carotid endarterectomy in this subgroup of patients (Mayberg, 2002; Brisman and Berenstein, 2003; Yadav et al., 2004). Carotid endarterectomy remains the treatment of choice for standard-risk patients with moderate- to high-grade symptomatic stenosis, with the understanding that the CREST trial is currently studying the comparative safety and efficacy of carotid endarterectomy versus carotid angioplasty and stenting for this more broader population of patients, and the results of this study may well alter this recommendation. In situations where carotid endarterectomy and carotid angioplasty and stenting appear equally efficacious in stroke reduction, more minor procedural risks, such as cranial nerve injury, which has recently been further quantified (Cunningham *et al.*, 2004), may play a greater role in decision making.

ECIC bypass trials

At 71 centers in the USA, Canada, Japan and Europe, 1377 patients with anterior circulation strokes, retinal infarction or TIA within 3 months of presentation were randomized to surgical ($n = 663$) or nonsurgical (714) treatment. Qualifying lesions included middle cerebral artery stenosis or occlusion, or cervical internal carotid artery occlusion or stenosis above the C2 vertebral body. Patients were followed for 5 years and primary endpoints were designated as fatal or nonfatal stroke (including all vascular distributions) (Failure of extracranial-intracranial arterial bypass, 1985).

At an average follow-up of 55.8 months, EC-IC bypass provided no significant protection against stroke in any distribution, ipsilateral stroke or stroke and death. Technical results of surgery were excellent, with 96% of anastomoses patent on postoperative angiogram. Perioperative major stroke and death was 4.5%; however, one-third (10 of 30) of these strokes occurred prior to surgery and were included in an intent-to-treat analysis. In the equivalent time period, 1.3% of nonsurgical patients had major strokes. By 60 months, there was no significant difference in stroke rate between surgical (20%) and nonsurgical (18%) groups. Outcome appeared to be worse after surgery in patients with middle cerebral artery stenosis or those with persistent ischemic symptoms after carotid occlusion. Analysis excluding surgical patients with preoperative stroke did not affect outcome. There was no benefit in terms of functional status for patients receiving EC-IC bypass. The authors concluded that EC-IC bypass surgery was ineffective in preventing cerebral ischemia in patients with atherosclerotic disease in the carotid and middle cerebral arteries (Failure of extracranial-intracranial arterial bypass, 1985).

The EC-IC bypass trial was widely criticized on several grounds (Ausman and Diaz, 1986; Awad and Spetzler, 1986; Day *et al.*, 1986; Goldring *et al.*, 1987). The ratio of persistently symptomatic versus asymptomatic patients studied was relatively low. A telephone survey (Sundt, 1987) of 57 participating centers revealed that during the time period of the trial, for 1255 patients entered into the study, more than twice as many patients (2572) received surgery outside of the trial. These data contradicted those in the published report, which described only 115 patients refusing entry and 52 patients with surgery outside of the trial. The ultimate fate of eligible nonrandomized patients represented a distinct subgroup (perhaps at lower risk) raising significant questions about the external validity of the conclusions of this study.

Additionally, and perhaps most importantly, the EC-IC study was nonselective in patient selection for randomization. The study made no effort to distinguish between patients with hemodynamic impairment and those without. Admittedly, techniques to assess cerebral hemodynamics did not exist. Patients with symptomatic carotid occlusions suffering from thrombo-embolic phenomena, for example, would not be expected to be alleviated with a vascular bypass. Yet such patients were randomized and on occasion bypassed, with the associated procedural risks.

Fortunately research since the EC-IC trial has expanded our understanding of cerebral blood flow and metabolism and technologic advances now permit a variety of techniques for the assessment of cerebral hemodynamics and vascular reserve. Neuronal metabolism depends on adequate cerebral blood flow (CBF), which in turn depends on the cerebral perfusion pressure (CPP). CBF is maintained over a wide range of CPPs by alterations in vascular resistance achieved by arterial and arteriolar vasoconstriction and vasodilatation, a process known as cerebral autoregulation. When CBF is adequate to maintain the metabolic demands of the brain, a steady state exists in which the cerebral oxygen extraction fraction (OEF) from the blood is relatively unchanged. If CBF begins to fall because of insufficient CPP, the OEF progressively increases to maintain cerebral oxygen metabolism (Grubb and Powers, 2001); once the OEF is maximized, further decreases in CBF result in cerebral ischemia or infarction.

A variety of relatively noninvasive tests (xenon computed tomography [CT], single positron emission computed tomography [SPECT], transcranial Doppler ultrasound [TCD], magnetic resonance angiography [MRA], and positron emission tomography [PET]) are now available that can measure CBF and using physiologic challenges assess both qualitatively and quantitatively the cerebrovascular reserve. The specifics of each method have been summarized elsewhere (Newell et al., 1994; Newell, 1995; Derdeyn et al., 1999, 2002; Grubb et al., 2003; Amin-Hanjani et al., 2005) and are beyond the scope of this chapter. In 1998, Grubb et al. published the results of a study (Grubb et al., 1998) in which they prospectively followed 81 patients with complete carotid occlusion and tested the hypothesis that increased OEF seen on PET was an independent risk factor for stroke in such patients treated medically. At 31.5 months mean follow-up, there were 13 ipsilateral ischemic strokes (15 total). In the patients with increased OEF ($n = 39$), there were 11 ipsilateral and 12 total strokes compared with two ipsilateral and three total strokes in the group with normal OEF ($n = 42$); the increased risk of stroke in patients with abnormally elevated OEF was significantly higher than those with normal OEF ($p = 0.005$). This prompted an NIH-funded multicenter prospective carotid occlusion surgery study (COSS) that is currently randomizing patients with symptomatic internal carotid occlusions (within 120 days of symptomatic TIA or stroke) and in whom have documented increased OEF on PET to either superficial temporal artery (STA)/middle cerebral artery (MCA) bypass or medial therapy (Grubb et al., 2003).

Summary of EC-IC bypass trials and proposed indications for intervention

Despite the results of the EC-IC bypass trial, sufficient evidence has accrued to show that STA/MCA when performed successfully can alleviate the symptoms of cerebral ischemia as a result of decreased CBF. The procedure is not without risk, both of technical failure (4%, by experienced operators in the EC-IC trial) and other significant perioperative morbidity (3%) (Mendelowitsch et al., 2004).

Patients suspected to suffer from cerebral ischemia from hemodynamic compromise, despite the use of anticoagulant and antiplatelet therapy and reasonable permissive hypertension (i.e. relaxation of antihypertensive medication), should undergo evaluation with cerebral angiography and at least one physiologic test (SPECT, xenon-CT, or PET) of cerebrovascular reserve. Angiography is required to confirm the occlusion, identify additional stenoses, and demonstrate the existence of a donor STA branch. Bypass is only undertaken if physiologic testing confirms lack of CBF reserve.

Preoperative evaluation of patients for carotid revascularization

History of presenting symptoms

Clinical and pathologic features of cerebral ischemia are described elsewhere in this volume. Symptoms of anterior circulation ischemia are typically classified as TIA, amaurosis fugax or TMB, or completed stroke (Pessin et al., 1977). Patients with chronic ischemia from carotid occlusion may present with a somewhat different constellation of symptoms including repetitive episodes of hemiparesis/hemisensory deficit, aphasia or visual disturbances and limb shaking, sometimes referred to as hemispheric claudication (Klempen *et al.*, 2002). Of interest, all three symptomatic carotid stenosis trials showed a high incidence of stroke in close temporal proximity to the presenting symptoms in nonsurgical patients, suggesting that patients with suspected cerebral ischemia should be evaluated with some urgency for potential surgical intervention.

Assessment of perioperative risk

Assessing perioperative risk is essential in the evaluation of patients in whom carotid endarterectomy, carotid angioplasty and stenting or EC-IC bypass is being considered. It not only permits appropriate discussion with patients regarding indications for and potential benefits of the three proposed procedures, but with recent data suggesting that for high-risk patients carotid angioplasty and stenting is as safe and as effective (at least in the short-term) as carotid endarterectomy, such risk profiling can help physicians decide which patients are most suitable for which treatment. We advocate cardiology consultation in all patients in whom such procedures are considered.

Imaging considerations

Multiple imaging modalities have been employed for the diagnosis of extracranial symptomatic carotid disease. Excellent sensitivities (SE) and specificities (SP) have been demonstrated with the three noninvasive imaging modalities: DUS, CT angiography (CTA), and MRA. Digital subtraction angiography (DSA) remains the gold standard, but carries a low risk of thromboembolic stroke or other minor injury relative to the noninvasive modalities. For stenosis, diagnostic accuracy relative to DSA is as follows: DUS (SE: 59.3–93%, SP: 90%) (Flanigan *et al.*, 1985; Stavenow *et al.*, 1987; Beneficial effect of carotid endarterectomy, 1991; Demchuk *et al.*, 2000; Bell *et al.*, 2002), CTA

(SE: 92.8%, SP: 100%) (Cumming and Morrow, 1994; Bell *et al.*, 2002), and MRA (SE: 92.2–100%, SP: 75.7–92%) (Bell *et al.*, 2002; Nederkoorn *et al.*, 2002; Wutke *et al.*, 2002; Butz *et al.*, 2004). For occlusion or deciphering between occlusion and near occlusion, diagnostic accuracy relative to DSA is: DUS (SE: 99–100%) (Flanigan *et al.*, 1985; El Saden *et al.*, 2001), CTA (SE: 100%, SP: 100%) (Cumming and Morrow, 1994) and MRA (SE: 92%, SP: 100%) (El Saden *et al.*, 2001).

There are no guidelines for the diagnostic evaluation of patients with suspected symptomatic carotid artery stenosis. Recommendations have recently been given by a panel that set out to review imaging work-up for 203 patients who subsequently underwent carotid endarterectomy as follows: DSA or two concordant noninvasive studies in patients with "moderate" symptomatic disease and one noninvasive modality in patients with "severe" symptomatic disease (Kennedy *et al.*, 2004). Reports have documented a 6–7.9% misclassification of degree of stenosis, even when two noninvasive imaging studies were used (Johnston and Goldstein, 2001; Patel *et al.*, 2002). DSA continues to play a role in the evaluation of symptomatic carotid stenosis, particularly in the face of discordant noninvasive data, ambiguity of diagnosis, contraindication to certain noninvasive tests, or suspected additional vascular lesions not well visualized by noninvasive modalities. For suspected symptomatic carotid occlusion in which bypass is entertained, DSA with at least one physiologic test to measure cerebrovascular reserve is requisite.

Operative technique

Carotid endarterectomy

We perform carotid endarterectomy under general anesthesia with electroencephalography (EEG) monitoring, although excellent results have been presented for individual series using regional anesthesia (Donato and Hill, 1992). The principal goals of anesthetic management are to maintain adequate cerebral and myocardial perfusion. The blood pressure should be maintained at or slightly above the patient's awake pressure.

The patient is placed in the supine position with the head turned away from the side of the operation. A small roll placed beneath the shoulders puts the neck in slight extension and facilitates full exposure of the carotid bifurcation. The operative field should extend from the mastoid process superiorly to the sternal notch inferiorly.

The procedure is performed using loupe magnification and headlight, although the operating microscope is an excellent alternative (Spetzler *et al.*, 1986). An incision is made along the anterior border of the sternocleidomastoid muscle, curving posteriorly toward the mastoid process about 1 cm below the angle of the mandible; this enables distal exposure of the internal carotid artery without injury to the mandibular ramus of the facial nerve. Attempts should be made to identify and protect the greater auricular nerve at the superior margin of the incision. Meticulous hemostasis is maintained throughout the procedure using bipolar cautery. The platysma is incised and the dissection is carried along the medial border of the sternocleidomastoid muscle. Generally an avascular plane is extant, and little cautery is required. At this point the ansa cervicalis is frequently encountered. Although it is safe to section this nerve, we prefer to mobilize it medially; this enables medial retraction of the hypoglossal nerve at its junction with ansa when dissecting the distal internal carotid artery.

Beneath the sternocleidomastoid muscle, the internal jugular vein is encountered. The common facial branch of this vein coursing medially is doubly ligated and divided and the vein is gently retracted laterally. At this point the carotid artery can be gently palpated and the carotid sheath is visible. Before manipulating the carotid artery in the region of the bifurcation, 2% xylocaine without epinephrine is instilled into the carotid sinus and along the course of the nerve of Hering to minimize bradycardia and hypotension resulting from stimulation of these structures. The carotid sheath is opened inferiorly along the anterior surface of the artery inferiorly to the level of the omohyoid muscle. Prior to further dissection, proximal control of the common carotid artery is obtained by carefully dissecting the posterior wall from the underlying vagus nerve and passing a vessel loop. Superiorly, the superior thyroid artery, external carotid artery and internal carotid artery are dissected in the region of the bifurcation.

Dissection is then carried distally along the internal carotid artery. Extreme care must be taken to identify the hypoglossal nerve early in dissection as it crosses the distal internal carotid artery. Dissection must be carried at least 1 cm distal to the end of the plaque to allow for posterior wall extension and placement of a shunt if necessary. A Rummel tourniquet is fashioned by placing the umbilical tapes on the internal carotid and common carotid arteries through a segment of rubber tubing. Dissection is then completed around the external carotid artery and superior thyroid artery which are isolated with vessel loops.

At this point the anesthesiologist is instructed to give heparin 100 U/kg as a bolus. The blood pressure is maintained at or slightly above awake baseline and the EEG is examined prior to clamping. The shunt tubing is filled with heparinized saline and clamped to ensure no intraluminal bubbles, and compared to the internal carotid artery to assure proper sizing.

The internal carotid artery is clamped first; we prefer to use an aneurysm clip since it has a lower profile and is less traumatic to the vessel. The common carotid artery is then clamped using an angled or straight Fogarty hydrogrip® clamp. External carotid artery and superior thyroid artery are then clamped with aneurysm clips. An arteriotomy is started about 1 cm proximal to the bifurcation in the midline of the common carotid artery. The incision is carried through the arterial wall until plaque is encountered and a smooth plane is developed between plaque and artery wall. At this point, the EEG is examined to determine whether shunt placement is necessary (see below). If no changes have occurred, dissection is carried distally along the plaque using a #4 Penfield dissector and the arteriotomy is completed with a Potts scissors (Figure 6.1). The arteriotomy should extend along the anterior midline of the internal carotid artery until normal intima beyond the plaque is reached. Circumferential dissection of the plaque is then accomplished at the proximal end, a curved clamp placed between plaque and artery wall, and the plaque sharply incised with a scalpel. Care must be taken to ensure that the remaining plaque in common carotid artery has a smooth edge. The plaque is then dissected free from arterial wall using the Penfield dissector to the bifurcation and into the external carotid artery (Figure 6.2).

A critical part of the dissection involves the distal attachment of the plaque to normal intima of the internal carotid artery. By gentle dissection and proximal traction on the plaque, it will usually tear away from its distal attachment leaving a firm, adherent normal intima. If the intima at this site is not adherent, it should be further resected, or less commonly, tacked to the arterial wall with a 6–0 proline suture.

Once the plaque is removed, the luminal surface is carefully inspected while the assistant continuously irrigates with heparinized saline. Small bits of debris apparent during this maneuver should be meticulously removed under magnified vision to create a lumen which is as smooth as possible. The arteriotomy is then closed with a running 6–0 proline suture from distal to proximal. Extreme care must be taken to approximate the edges with small equal bites so that no regions of stenosis are created. Just prior to final suturing at the proximal end of the arteriotomy, the internal carotid artery clamp is briefly released. The resulting back-flow of blood ensures that the artery is patent and flushes any residual debris from the lumen. The clamps are then removed in specific order; external carotid

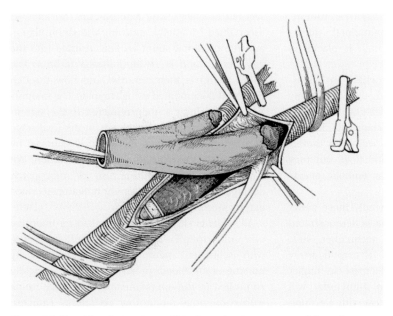

Figure 6.1 Carotid endarterectomy. The plaque has been separated from the outer wall of the common carotid and external carotid arteries and is now being removed from the internal carotid artery.

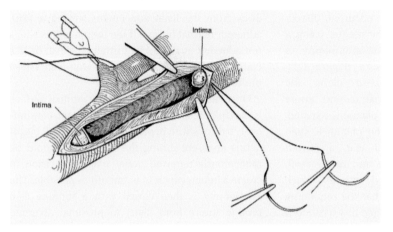

Figure 6.2 Carotid endarterectomy. Arteriotomy closure. Double-armed 6–0 proline sutures are placed at the distal end of the arteriotomy with care taken to suture both intimal and wall layers on both sides.

artery, common carotid artery, then internal carotid artery. This ensures that any potential embolic material will be flushed into the external artery circulation. The arteriotomy is covered with oxidized cellulose and gentle pressure applied to the wound with a sponge for about 1 minute. Meticulous hemostasis is maintained during closure; occasionally a small drain is placed in the superficial wound.

Intraoperative monitoring provides an assessment of cerebral blood flow during endarterectomy and may facilitate the decision whether to employ a shunt during carotid cross-clamping. EEG is widely available and correlates well with diminished hemispheric cerebral blood flow, but may not reflect regional ischemia or embolic events (Sundt, 1983).

We restrict use of a shunt to only those situations in which cerebral ischemia is demonstrated by EEG or other monitoring techniques. EEG changes occurring at the time of carotid artery cross-clamping (manifest by decrease in higher frequencies and/or decrease in amplitude) will occasionally spontaneously resolve with elevation of the blood pressure. When changes persist more than 60–90 seconds, the arteriotomy is extended through the plaque along its entire length using

Potts scissors to expose the normal intima of the distal internal carotid artery. The distal end of the saline-filled and clamped shunt tubing is carefully inserted into the internal carotid artery, which is briefly opened to permit shunt passage, then secured in place using a tourniquet. Backflow is ascertained by briefly removing the shunt clamp, and the proximal shunt is then inserted into the common carotid artery in a similar fashion. The shunt clamp is then removed and flow through the shunt documented using Doppler. The midportion of the shunt is then retracted to the side to enable plaque removal as above. At the final stage of arteriotomy suturing, the shunt is removed by reversing the steps listed above for insertion. We currently advocate routine use of vein patch angioplasty only for recurrent or radiation-induced carotid stenosis.

All patients should be observed in an intensive care unit setting for 4–6 hours after the procedure with sequential neurological examinations by nursing staff. Blood pressure should be rigidly controlled in the approximate preoperative range with continuous monitoring via arterial catheter. The cervical wound is sequentially examined for enlargement or superficial bleeding. Aspirin therapy is initiated immediately after surgery and stable patients are generally discharged home the following day.

EC-IC bypass

Operative technique for STA/MCA bypass has recently been described by various authors (Newell and Vilela, 2004; Wanebo *et al.*, 2004; Charbel *et al.*, 2005), with little variation, and is not repeated here. We employ the technique described by Newell and Vilela (2004). Additional EC-IC bypasses that might be necessary for symptomatic carotid artery occlusion, such as an interposition saphenous vein graft if an appropriate STA donor is not avaible, for example, are also well desribed (Newell and Vilela, 2004) and beyond the scope of this chapter.

Conclusions

Carotid endarterectomy remains an important part of the armamentarium in the treatment of symptomatic carotid stenosis. It is the preferred modality to treat standard-risk patients with symptomatic severe carotid stenosis (>70%); there is less compelling evidence supporting its use in patients with moderate (50–69%) stenosis. Evidence now supports the use of carotid angioplasty and stenting for high-risk patients. The results of the ongoing CREST trial, evaluating the relative safety and efficacy of carotid angioplasty and stenting versus carotid endarterectomy in standard-risk patients, may significantly alter the way carotid stenosis is treated in this country.

Patients with symptomatic carotid occlusions may benefit from EC-IC revascularization provided they suffer from diminished cerebrovascular reserve. Although the results of the early EC-IC bypass trial is of limited applicability to this subgroup of patients, due to its lack of selectivity, level 1 evidence supporting the use of EC-IC bypass is currently not available. The results of the COSS trial, prospectively randomizing such patients to bypass or medical therapy, will hopefully shed light on the best treatment for these patients.

Acknowledgement

The assistance of Lena Feld, medical librarian, in researching the literature is gratefully acknowledged.

REFERENCES

Alberts, M., McCann, R. and Smith, T. (1997). Schneider WALLSTENT EndoProsthesis Clinical Investigators: A randomized trial of carotid stenting versus endarterectomy in patients with symptomatic carotid stenosis – Study design. *Journal of Neurovascular Disease*, **2**, 228–34.

Amin-Hanjani, S., Du, X., Zhao, M., *et al.* (2005). Use of quantitative magnetic resonance angiography to stratify stroke risk in symptomatic vertebrobasilar disease. *Stroke*, **36**, 1140–5.

Ausman, J.I. and Diaz, F.G. (1986). Critique of the extracranial-intracranial bypass study. *Surgical Neurology*, **26**, 218–21.

Awad, I.A. and Spetzler, R.F. (1986). Extracranial-intracranial bypass surgery: a critical analysis in light of the International Cooperative Study. *Neurosurgery*, **19**, 655–64.

Barnett, H.J., Taylor, D.W., Eliasziw, M., *et al.* (1998). Benefit of carotid endarterectomy in patients with symptomatic moderate or severe stenosis. North American Symptomatic Carotid Endarterectomy Trial Collaborators. *New England Journal of Medicine*, **339**, 1415–25.

Bell, R., Armonda, R. and Noonan, P. (2002). Modern Imaging in the management of cervical carotid stenosis. In W. Fisher III and R. Armonda (eds.), *Seminars in Neurosurgery - Carotid Artery Disease: Contemporary Treatment*. New York: Thieme, pp. 217–28.

Beneficial effect of carotid endarterectomy in symptomatic patients with high-grade carotid stenosis. (1991). North American Symptomatic Carotid Endarterectomy Trial Collaborators. *New England Journal of Medicine*, **325**, 445–53.

Brisman, J. L. and Berenstein, A. (2003). Received wisdom vs evidence in stroke prevention: carotid stenting will soon replace endarterectomy for all patients requiring such revascularization. *Medical Genetics and Medicine*, **5**, 17.

Butz, B., Dorenbeck, U., Borisch, I., *et al.* (2004). High-resolution contrast-enhanced magnetic resonance angiography of the carotid arteries using fluoroscopic monitoring of contrast arrival: diagnostic accuracy and interobserver variability. *Acta Radiology*, **45**, 164–70.

Charbel, F. T., Meglio, G. and Amin-Hanjani, S. (2005). Superficial temporal artery-to-middle cerebral artery bypass. *Neurosurgery*, **56**, 186–90.

Cumming, M. J. and Morrow, I. M. (1994). Carotid artery stenosis: a prospective comparison of CT angiography and conventional angiography. *AJR. American Journal of Roentgenology*, **163**, 517–23.

Cunningham, E. J., Bond, R., Mayberg, M. R., *et al.* (2004). Risk of persistent cranial nerve injury after carotid endarterectomy. *Journal of Neurosurgery*, **101**, 445–8.

Day, A. L., Rhoton, A. L., Jr. and Little, J. R. (1986) The extracranial-intracranial bypass study. *Surgical Neurology*, **26**, 222–6.

Demchuk, A. M., Christou, I., Wein, T. H., *et al.* (2000). Accuracy and criteria for localizing arterial occlusion with transcranial Doppler. *Journal of Neuroimaging*, **10**, 1–12.

Derdeyn, C. P., Videen, T. O., Fritsch, S. M., *et al.* (1999). Compensatory mechanisms for chronic cerebral hypoperfusion in patients with carotid occlusion. *Stroke*, **30**, 1019–24.

Derdeyn, C. P., Videen, T. O., Yundt, K. D., *et al.* (2002). Variability of cerebral blood volume and oxygen extraction: stages of cerebral haemodynamic impairment revisited. *Brain*, **125**, 595–607.

Donato, A. T. and Hill, S. L. (1992). Carotid arterial surgery using local anesthesia: a private practice retrospective study. *American Surgery*, **58**, 446–50.

El Saden, S. M., Grant, E. G., Hathout, G. M., *et al.* (2001). Imaging of the internal carotid artery: the dilemma of total versus near total occlusion. *Radiology*, **221**, 301–8.

Failure of extracranial-intracranial arterial bypass to reduce the risk of ischemic stroke. (1985). Results of an international randomized trial. The EC/IC Bypass Study Group. *New England Journal of Medicine*, **313**, 1191–200.

Flanigan, D. P., Schuler, J. J., Vogel, M., *et al.* (1985) The role of carotid duplex scanning in surgical decision making. *Journal of Vascular Surgery*, **2**, 15–25.

Goldring, S., Zervas, N. and Langfitt, T. (1987) The Extracranial-Intracranial Bypass Study. A report of the committee appointed by the American Association of Neurological Surgeons to examine the study. *New England Journal of Medicine*, **316**, 817–20.

Gray, W. A. (2004). A cardiologist in the carotids. *Journal of the American College of Cardiology*, **43**, 1602–5.

Gray, W. A. (2005). Cervical carotid revascularization: indications from an endovascular perspective. *Neurosurgery Clinics of North America*, **16**, 259–61.

Grubb, R. L., Jr., Derdeyn, C. P., Fritsch, S. M., *et al.* (1998). Importance of hemodynamic factors in the prognosis of symptomatic carotid occlusion. *Journal of the American Medical Association*, **280**, 1055–60.

Grubb, R. L., Jr. and Powers, W. J. (2001). Risks of stroke and current indications for cerebral revascularization in patients with carotid occlusion. *Neurosurgical Clinics of North America*, **12**, 473–87.

Grubb, R. L., Jr., Powers, W. J., Derdeyn, C. P., *et al.* (2003) The carotid occlusion surgery study. *Neurosurgery Focus*, **14**, e9.

Hanel, R. A., Levy, E. I., Guterman, L. R., *et al.* (2005). Cervical carotid revascularization: the role of angioplasty with stenting. *Neurosurgical Clinics of North America*, **16**, 263–78, viii.

Hobson, R. W. (2000). CREST (Carotid Revascularization Endarterectomy versus Stent Trial): background, design, and current status. *Seminars in Vascular Surgery*, **13**, 139–43.

Hobson, R. W. (2002). Update on the Carotid Revascularization Endarterectomy versus Stent Trial (CREST) protocol. *Journal of American College of Surgery*, **194**, S9–14.

Hobson, R. W., Howard, V. J., Brott, T. G., *et al.* (2001). Organizing the Carotid Revascularization Endarterectomy versus Stenting Trial (CREST): National Institutes of Health, Health Care Financing Administration, and industry funding. *Current Control of Trials in Cardiovascular Medicine*, **2**, 160–4.

Johnston, D. C. and Goldstein, L. B. (2001). Clinical carotid endarterectomy decision making: noninvasive vascular imaging versus angiography. *Neurology*, **56**, 1009–15.

Kennedy, J., Quan, H., Ghali, W. A., *et al.* (2004). Importance of the imaging modality in decision making about carotid endarterectomy. *Neurology*, **62**, 901–4.

Klempen, N. L., Janardhan, V., Schwartz, R. B., *et al.* (2002). Shaking limb transient ischemic attacks: unusual presentation of carotid artery occlusive disease: report of two cases. *Neurosurgery*, **51**, 483–7.

Mayberg, M. R. (1996). Extracranial occlusive disease of the carotid artery. In J. R. Youmans (ed.), *Neurological Surgery*, 4th edn. Philadelphia: WB Saunders Company, pp. 1159–80.

Mayberg, M. R. (2002). Carotid artery stenting: fact or fiction. *Clinical Neurosurgery*, **49**, 247–60.

Mayberg, M. R., Wilson, S. E., Yatsu, F., *et al.* (1991). Carotid endarterectomy and prevention of cerebral ischemia in symptomatic carotid stenosis. Veterans Affairs Cooperative Studies Program 309 Trialist Group. *Journal of the American Medical Association*, **266**, 3289–94.

Mendelowitsch, A., Taussky, P., Rem, J. A., *et al.* (2004). Clinical outcome of standard extracranial-intracranial bypass surgery in patients with symptomatic atherosclerotic occlusion of the internal carotid artery. *Acta Neurochirurgica, (Wien.)*, **146**, 95–101.

Moore, W. S., Barnett, H. J., Beebe, H. G., *et al.* (1995). Guidelines for carotid endarterectomy. A multidisciplinary consensus statement from the Ad Hoc Committee, American Heart Association. *Circulation*, **91**, 566–79.

MRC European Carotid Surgery Trial. (1991). Interim results for symptomatic patients with severe (70–99%) or with mild (0–29%) carotid stenosis. European Carotid Surgery Trialists' Collaborative Group. *Lancet*, **337**, 1235–43.

Nederkoorn, P. J., Mali, W. P., Eikelboom, B. C., *et al.* (2002). Preoperative diagnosis of carotid artery stenosis: accuracy of noninvasive testing. *Stroke*, **33**, 2003–8.

Newell, D. W. (1995) Transcranial Doppler measurements. *New Horizons*, **3**, 423–30.

Newell, D. W., Aaslid, R., Lam, A., *et al.* (1994). Comparison of flow and velocity during dynamic autoregulation testing in humans. *Stroke*, **25**, 793–7.

Newell, D. W. and Vilela, M. D. (2004). Superficial temporal artery to middle cerebral artery bypass. *Neurosurgery*, **54**, 1441–8.

Patel, S. G., Collie, D. A., Wardlaw, J. M., *et al.* (2002). Outcome, observer reliability, and patient preferences if CTA, MRA, or Doppler ultrasound were used, individually or together, instead of digital subtraction angiography before carotid endarterectomy. *Journal of Neurology, Neurosurgery and Psychiatry*, **73**, 21–8.

Pessin, M. S., Duncan, G. W., Mohr, J. P., *et al.* (1977). Clinical and angiographic features of carotid transient ischemic attacks. *New England Journal of Medicine*, **296**, 358–62.

Rothwell, P. M., Eliasziw, M., Gutnikov, S. A., *et al.* (2003). Analysis of pooled data from the randomised controlled trials of endarterectomy for symptomatic carotid stenosis. *Lancet*, **361**, 107–16.

Spetzler, R. F., Martin, N., Hadley, M. N., *et al.* (1986). Microsurgical endarterectomy under barbiturate protection: a prospective study. *Journal of Neurosurgery*, **65**, 63–73.

Stavenow, L., Bjerre, P. and Lindgarde, F. (1987). Experiences of duplex ultrasonography of carotid arteries performed by clinicians–correlation to angiography. *Acta Medica Scandinavica*, **222**, 31–6.

Sundt, T. M., Jr. (1983). The ischemic tolerance of neural tissue and the need for monitoring and selective shunting during carotid endarterectomy. *Stroke*, **14**, 93–8.

Sundt, T. M., Jr. (1987). Was the international randomized trial of extracranial-intracranial arterial bypass representative of the population at risk? *New England Journal of Medicine*, **316**, 814–16.

Wanebo, J. E., Zabramski, J. M. and Spetzler, R. F. (2004). Superficial temporal artery-to-middle cerebral artery bypass grafting for cerebral revascularization. *Neurosurgery*, **55**, 395–8.

Wutke, R., Lang, W., Fellner, C., *et al.* (2002). High-resolution, contrast-enhanced magnetic resonance angiography with elliptical centric k-space ordering of supra-aortic arteries compared with selective X-ray angiography. *Stroke*, **33**, 1522–9.

Yadav, J. S., Wholey, M. H., Kuntz, R. E., *et al.* (2004). Protected carotid-artery stenting versus endarterectomy in high-risk patients. *New England Journal of Medicine*, **351**, 1493–1501.

7

Surgery for asymptomatic carotid stenosis

Stella Vig[1] and Alison Halliday[2]

[1]Mayday University Hospital, London Road, Croydon, CR7 7YE, UK
[2]St George's Hospital Medical School, Blackshaw Road, Tooting, London, SW17 0PT, UK

Introduction

Stroke is the third most common cause of death and a leading cause of disability in the Western world. In England and Wales, over 130 000 people will suffer a stroke annually. Of those who suffer from a stroke, a third are likely to die within the first 10 days, a third are likely to make a recovery within 1 month and a third are likely to be left disabled and need rehabilitation. Disability in those of working age prevents 80% of stroke survivors from continuing their normal job (Teasell *et al.*, 2000). In the United Kingdom, stroke affects over a quarter of a million people and is at present costing over £7 billion a year. Prevention of 10–15% of these strokes by judicial use of carotid surgery would benefit patients and the economy.

In the United States stroke mortality has fallen by 15% over 10 years (1988–98) (American Heart Association, 2000). Although the US Framingham study found that stroke severity and mortality decreased, stroke incidence and prevalence rates increased during the same time period (Wolf *et al.*, 1992). The British Government has set a target of reducing stroke incidence by 40% but as the percentage of the population over 65 years increases, the absolute number of stroke victims is likely to rise substantially by 2010 (Sacco *et al.*, 1997).

Improvement in stroke mortality may be due to control of hypertension, hypercholesterolemia and a decline in cigarette smoking. The British National Service Framework for Stroke states that "there have been recent improvements in general practitioners (family practitioners) identifying and advising people who, because they have high blood pressure or cholesterol levels, are at increased risk of having a stroke. Proposals to screen people over 40 could help identify those at high risk before they need treatment thereby allowing them to make lifestyle changes preventing stroke". Some of the reduction in stroke mortality may be due to early intervention in high-risk patients and some to secondary prevention measures in those who have already had strokes. The role of secondary prevention using carotid endarterectomy for symptomatic stenosis is now well established (as discussed in Chapter 20). Carotid endarterectomy as primary prevention for asymptomatic patients is now appropriate as more evidence has become available. The absolute number of patients who might be suitable for surgery is large, as many more patients have stenosis without symptoms; for them and for those who have missed having early intervention after minor symptoms, the 5-year benefits of endarterectomy are real.

In 1995, the US asymptomatic carotid atherosclerosis study first reported reduction in stroke rate after prophylactic carotid endarterectomy. These findings led to a huge increase in the number of prophylactic carotid endarterectomies performed in the US (Executive Committee for the Asymptomatic Carotid Atherosclerosis Study, 1995; Anderson, *et al.*, 2004). Indeed more than half

Carotid Disease: The Role of Imaging in Diagnosis and Management, ed. Jonathan Gillard, Martin Graves, Thomas Hatsukami and Chun Yuan. Published by Cambridge University Press. © Cambridge University Press 2007.

the carotid endarterectomies in the US are now performed for asymptomatic disease.

The publication of the much larger asymptomatic carotid surgery trial in 2004 has added considerable evidence supporting surgery for asymptomatic disease and the effect of this trial has already increased the proportion of prophylactic endarterectomies undertaken in the (much more conservative) UK from ∼10% to 20–25%.

Evidence for surgery in asymptomatic disease

Four large randomized trials have now been reported suggesting that carotid endarterectomy for asymptomatic disease can prevent stroke.

The US Veterans Administration hospitals' trial reported that 4 years after prophylactic carotid endarterectomy patients with asymptomatic carotid stenosis of 50–99% had significantly fewer transient ischemic attacks (TIA) and strokes than controls (8% vs. 20.6%, $p < 0.001$, 30-day surgical stroke and death rate 4.3%) (Hobson et al., 1993). After the (symptomatic) European carotid surgery trial (ECST), the European Carotid Trialists Collaborative Group also examined stroke risk in the asymptomatic carotid artery territory and found that 6% of patients with 70–90% stenosis had a stroke within 3 years (The European Carotid Trialists Collaborative Group, 1995).

The Asymptomatic Carotid Atherosclerosis Study (ACAS) multicenter trial randomized 1662 patients with 60–90% stenosis to endarterectomy plus medical treatment or to medical treatment alone (Executive Committee for the Asymptomatic Carotid Atherosclerosis Study, 1995; Anderson et al., 2004). The trial was stopped after a median follow-up of 2.7 years. The 5-year rate of ipsilateral stroke and death was halved in the endarterectomy group (11% vs. 5.1% for carotid endarterectomy patients). This included a very low rate of perioperative stroke and death of 2.3%. The reduction in cumulative risk of stroke was 53% (95% confidence interval [CI], 22–72).

The absolute reduction of major ipsilateral stroke, major perioperative stroke, or perioperative death was considerably smaller (estimated 5-year risk of 3.4% in the surgery group vs. 6% in the medical group, $p = 0.13$), and evident only in the fifth year of follow-up. Endarterectomy was apparently less effective in women compared to men (17% vs. 66% reduction, with wide CIs, in 5-year event rate), possibly due to higher perioperative complication rates (3.6% in women vs. 1.7% in men). The low perioperative stroke and death rate was thought to reflect careful selection of surgeons and might not be true in "real life". ACAS rejected 40% of initial applicants and subsequently barred some surgeons who had adverse operative outcomes during the trial (Rothwell and Goldstein 2004).

Although the trial suggested that the chances of having a stroke or dying over 5 years was halved, the absolute risk of having a stroke was very low and many European and Canadian neurologists waited for further evidence, feeling that surgery was inappropriate especially if the perioperative stroke and death was higher outside these centers.

The asymptomatic carotid surgery trial (ACST) is the largest vascular trial to date (3120 patients) (MRC Asymptomatic Carotid Surgery Trial [ACST] Collaborative Group, 2004). Patients were allocated to immediate versus delayed carotid endarterectomy (surgery only to be undertaken if clinically indicated). The baseline data, comorbidities and medical treatments were almost identical in both ACAS and ACST. Surgeons recruited to the trial had to have a perioperative stroke risk of ≤6% for their last 50 symptomatic carotid endarterectomies. During the trial no surgeon was excluded because of poor operative outcomes.

The risk of stroke or death within 30 days of carotid endarterectomy was 3.1% (95% CI 2.3–4.1), 2.5% in the immediate carotid endarterectomy group and 4.5% in the deferred group. Comparing all patients allocated immediate carotid endarterectomy versus all allocated deferral, but excluding such perioperative events, the 5-year stroke risks were 3.8% versus 11% (gain 7.2% [95% CI 5.0–9.4], $p < 0.0001$). This gain chiefly involved carotid

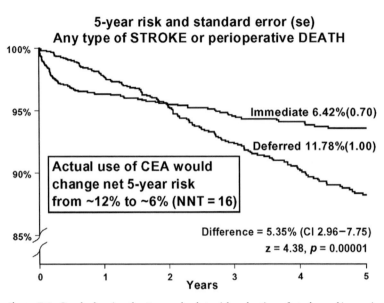

Figure 7.1 Graph showing the 5-year absolute risk reduction of stroke and/or perioperative death in the Asymptomatic Carotid Surgery Trial.

territory ischaemic strokes (2.7% vs. 9.5%; gain 6.8% [4.8–8.8], $p<0.0001$), of which half were disabling or fatal (1.6% vs. 5.3%; gain 3.7% [2.1–5.2], $p<0.0001$), as were half the perioperative strokes. Combining the perioperative events and the non-perioperative strokes, net 5-year risks were 6.4% versus 11.8% for all strokes (net gain 5.4% [3.0–7.8], $p<0.0001$) (Figure 7.1), 3.5% versus 6.1% for fatal or disabling strokes (net gain 2.5% [0.8–4.3], $p=0.004$), and 2.1% versus 4.2% just for fatal strokes (net gain 2.1% [0.6–3.6], $p=0.006$). The relative risk reduction of 46% was significant in favour of surgery and included the risks attached to surgery.

In men, there was an 8.2% reduction in 5-year stroke risk from 10.6% to 2.4% (CI 5.6–10.8, $p<0.00001$) (Figure 7.2). In women, the benefits from surgery were less clear with a 4.1% absolute decrease in 5-year stroke risk from 7.5% to 3.4% (CI 0.7–7.4) (Figure 7.3). There were fewer women in the trial but there was not a significantly higher operative risk in women. Women had a lower 5-year risk of stroke without surgery and both the trialists and reviewers felt that longer-term data

(10-year follow-up) would clarify benefit in both men and women (Rothwell, 2004a; Rothwell et al., 2004).

In asymptomatic patients, aged < 75, with carotid stenosis of 70% or greater, immediate carotid endarterectomy halved the net 5-year stroke risk from about 12% to about 6% (including the 3% perioperative hazard). In patients over the age of 75 years the potential benefits were uncertain with an absolute reduction of 3.3% in 5-year stroke risk (CI 1.9–8.4, $p=0.2$). This may be because more strokes occurred in both groups and half may have died within 5 years from unrelated causes.

There was no heterogeneity of benefit for patients with, for example, contralateral occlusion or soft plaque and no increased benefit with increasing stenosis beyond 70%. There was more benefit for patients with initial randomization cholesterol levels > 6.5 mmol/l but there is still a significant benefit for those with lower initial cholesterols.

Both ACST and ACAS have provided strong evidence of benefit from carotid surgery, with an absolute risk reduction of 5% and both studies reported a low surgical risk. Perioperative stroke

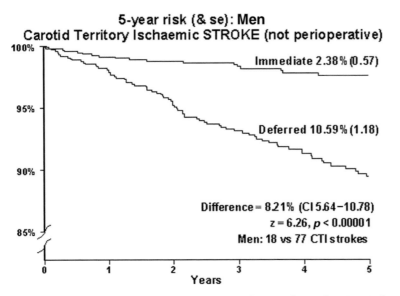

Figure 7.2 Graph showing the 5-year absolute risk reduction of carotid territory ischemic stroke in males within the Asymptomatic Carotid Surgery Trial.

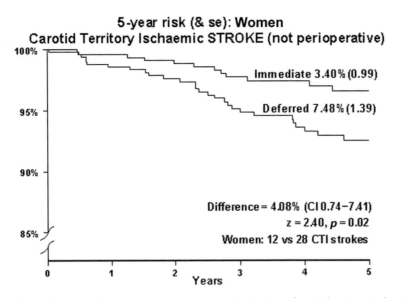

Figure 7.3 Graph showing the 5-year absolute risk reduction of carotid territory ischemic stroke in females within the Asymptomatic Carotid Surgery Trial.

and death rate may be higher in other centres as reported by ASA and carotid endarterectomy (ACE) trial. The complication rate in 70 American academic centers, among 1521 asymptomatic patients was 4.6%, comparable to the Veterans Study (The Veterans Affairs Cooperative Study Group, 1993; Taylor *et al.*, 1999). Another meta-analysis of 46 surgical case series reported an operative mortality eight times higher than that in ACAS (1.11% vs. 0.14%; $p = 0.01$) (Bond *et al.*, 2003). The risk of perioperative stroke and death was almost three times higher if outcome was assessed by a neurologist (4.3% vs. 1.5%; $p < 0.001$). ACAS selected participating surgeons with low surgical risk and ACST recruited surgeons whose declared perioperative stroke risks were similar to those suggested by the meta-analyses of large sympto-matic trials which should be widely applicable.

The ACST trialists suggest caution before apply-ing the results of the study to current practice. They and other authors suggest that careful audit of local results is necessary (Benavente *et al.*, 1998; Barnett, 2004). They concluded "that although the wider use of statins will reduce overall risk of carotid stroke, whatever risk remains should be avoidable by successful surgery", and warned that unsuc-cessful surgery with a high stroke and death risk will do harm.

Screening

Trials suggest that selected patients with asympto-matic disease will benefit from carotid endarter-ectomy. Selection could be by chance finding of carotid stenosis or by screening. The rationale for screening for carotid artery stenoses in these patients with asymptomatic stenoses are not only at increased risk for cerebrovascular disease but that early detection can reduce morbidity due to cardiovascular disease (Amarenco *et al.*, 1994; Warlow, 1995). A screening programme could be effective if a population with a 20% predicted prevalence of >60% carotid stenosis was identi-fied. Cost-effectiveness of carotid screening analyzed using the results of ACAS suggested that the cost was $120 000 per quality-adjusted life-year (assuming a survival advantage for 30 years) (Lee *et al.*, 1997).

Strokes may occur at any age, but the risk of stroke doubles in each successive decade of life starting at age 55 (Goldstein *et al.*, 2001). Screening an older population may therefore increase the pick up of asymptomatic disease but there is no proven benefit of prophylactic carotid endarterect-omy after the age of 75. Appropriate screening populations could include patients attending vascular clinics, patients with contralateral symp-tomatic stenoses or disease in another vascular bed. Hypertensive patients also have an increased incidence of asymptomatic carotid disease (Sutton-Tyrrell *et al.*, 1987). Other groups worth screen-ing include those over 60 years with aneurysms, hyperlipidemia and smokers (Constans, 2004).

Carotid bruits are not indicative of the degree of underlying carotid stenosis but may indicate a patient at higher risk of a stroke. In type 2 diabetic patients, an incidental carotid bruit increased the risk of first stroke within 2 years by a factor of 6 compared to patients without a bruit (Gillett *et al.*, 2003).

Surgery or angioplasty

Carotid angioplasty is gaining favor as radiological expertise increases as well as the technology of both stents and cerebral protection devices. Recommendations have been made for carotid endarterectomy for symptomatic and asympto-matic disease based on Level 1 evidence. Carotid endarterectomy has now been shown to be safe, durable, and effective in long-term stroke preven-tion of carotid endarterectomy (Ballotta *et al.*, 2004; LaMuraglia *et al.*, 2004). Carotid angioplasty is now increasingly practised as treatment for carotid stenosis and this might eventually supersede surgery (Brooks *et al.*, 2004). Level 1 evidence is needed, therefore, to allow any recommendations for carotid angioplasty in both symptomatic and asymptomatic disease.

Initial concerns about the risks and benefits of endovascular treatment led to the (mostly symptomatic) carotid and vertebral artery transluminal angioplasty study (CAVATAS, 2001). There was no difference in major outcome events between endovascular treatment and carotid endarterectomy, but the rate of procedural stroke or death was higher than desirable (10.0% vs. 9.9% for any stroke). The SAPPHIRE trial (stenting and angioplasty with protection in patients at high risk for endarterectomy) suggested that the major ipsilateral stroke rate was low at 3-year follow-up (Yadav et al., 2004). In North America, CREST (carotid revascularization endarterectomy versus stent trial) protocol is now completing its credentialing phase and randomization of cases has started (Hobson et al., 2004).

In Europe, the ICSS (International carotid stenting study) and EVA-3S (endarterectomy versus angioplasty in patients with symptomatic severe carotid stenosis) trials are recruiting symptomatic patients for randomization between carotid endarterectomy and carotid angioplasty (EVA-3S Investigators, 2004; Featherstone et al., 2004). SPACE (stent protected angioplasty versus carotid endarterectomy) has finished recruiting and will publish data this year (Ringleb et al., 2004). These three trials have prospectively agreed to combine individual patient data after completion of follow-up. This meta-analysis will provide more reliable results and should also allow informative subgroup analyses (Brown and Hacke, 2004).

No trial has yet been completed in asymptomatic patients. ACST-2 is about to commence randomization and it will be some years before any trial produces definitive results. Large numbers of patients are clearly required to successfully identify any real differences between stenting and surgery.

Patients with asymptomatic disease undergoing other surgery

The management of a patient with asymptomatic carotid disease undergoing other major vascular surgery is still to be determined. Carotid endarterectomy may be performed prophylactically or deferred until after the procedure.

A small study randomized patients with asymptomatic carotid disease undergoing major vascular surgery not (coronary artery bypass graft [CABG]) to prophylactic carotid endarterectomy (within 1 week before major surgery) or deferred carotid endarterectomy (between 30 days and 6 months after major surgery). There were no perioperative strokes in either group although the deferred group had a 5.1% risk of TIA prior to the deferred carotid endarterectomy (Ballotta et al., 2005).

Naylor et al. undertook a systematic review of 94 published series (7863 procedures) of synchronous carotid endarterectomy + CABG in patients with symptomatic and asymptomatic carotid disease (Naylor et al., 2003). The perioperative death/stroke/myocardial infarction rate was 11.5% of patients (95% CI 10.1–12.9). This is not an insignificant cardiovascular risk. However, recommendation for treatment of patients with carotid disease awaiting CABG is not possible as there are no comparable data available for similar patients undergoing CABG without prophylactic carotid endarterectomy.

A more recent study of combined or staged carotid endarterectomy and CABG in patients with asymptomatic carotid disease suggests that the perioperative stroke risk compares favorably with CABG alone (4%). Prophylactic carotid endarterectomy prior to CABG did not appear to confer any advantage over CABG alone for asymptomatic significant carotid disease (Ghosh et al., 2005).

Prophylactic carotid angioplasty prior to CABG has a lower perioperative stroke rate but reported series are small and multicenter randomized trials are needed to allow any recommendations (Randall et al., 2005; Kovacic et al., 2006).

The risk of death/stroke appeared to significantly diminish in studies published 1993–2002, compared with 1972–92 (7.2% [95% CI 6.5–9.1] vs. 10.7% [95% CI 8.9–12.5], $p = 0.03$) and may be a reflection of improving interventions (Naylor, 2003). With further improvements in technology, numbers of CABGs have decreased with increasing use of coronary angioplasty. Retrospective analyses of CABG populations of the 1980s and 1990s therefore may be an inappropriate reflection of intervention in the more complex remaining CABGs.

Summary

Appropriate medical management of patients with asymptomatic carotid disease will decrease stroke risk. Carotid endarterectomy halves the net 5-year stroke risk from about 12% to about 6% in selected patients with asymptomatic carotid disease.

In the future it may be appropriate for patients to undergo stenting instead of surgery but at present there is no evidence available in these patients and a new trial, ACST-2, has started to answer this question.

REFERENCES

Amarenco, P., Cohen, A., Tzourio, C., et al. (1994). Atherosclerotic disease of the aortic arch and the risk of ischemic stroke. *New England Journal of Medicine*, **331**, 1474–9.

American Heart Association. (2000). Stroke Statistics. In *2001 Heart and Stroke Statistical Update*. Dallas: American Heart Association.

Anderson, P. L., Gelijns, A., Moskowitz, A., et al. (2004). Understanding trends in inpatient surgical volume: vascular interventions, 1980–2000. *Journal of Vascular Surgery*, **39**, 1200–8.

Ballotta, E., Da Giau, G., Piccoli, A. and Baracchini, C. (2004). Durability of carotid endarterectomy for treatment of symptomatic and asymptomatic stenoses. *Journal of Vascular Surgery*, **40**, 270–8.

Ballotta, E., Renon, L., Da Giau, G., et al. (2005). Prospective randomized study on asymptomatic severe carotid stenosis and perioperative stroke risk in patients undergoing major vascular surgery: prophylactic or deferred carotid endarterectomy? *Annals of Vascular Surgery*, **19**, 876–81.

Barnett, H. J. M. (2004). Carotid endarterectomy. *Lancet*, **363**, 1486–7.

Benavente, O., Moher, D. and Pham, B. (1998). Carotid endarterectomy for asymptomatic carotid stenosis: a meta-analysis. *British Medical Journal*, **317**, 1477–80.

Bond, R., Rerkasem, K. and Rothwell, P. M. (2003). High morbidity due to endarterectomy for asymptomatic carotid stenosis. *Cerebrovascular Disease*, **16** (Suppl.), 65.

Brooks, W. H., McClure, R. R., Jones, M. R., Coleman, T. L. and Breathitt, L. (2004). Carotid angioplasty and stenting versus carotid endarterectomy for treatment of asymptomatic carotid stenosis: a randomised trial in a community hospital. *Neurosurgery*, **54**, 318–24.

Brown, M. M. and Hacke, W. (2004). Carotid artery stenting: the need for randomised trials. *Cerebrovascular Disease*, **18**, 57–61.

Constans, J. (2004) Is the screening of asymptomatic carotid stenosis worthwhile? *Annales de Cardiologie et Angéiologie (Paris)*, **53**, 39–43.

European Carotid Trialists Collaborative Group. (1995). Risk of stroke in the distribution of an asymptomatic carotid artery. *Lancet*, **345**, 209–12.

EVA-3S Investigators. (2004). Endarterectomy vs. Angioplasty in Patients with Symptomatic Severe Carotid Stenosis (EVA-3S) Trial. *Cerebrovascular Disease*, **18**, 62–5.

Executive Committee for the Asymptomatic Carotid Atherosclerosis Study. (1995). Endarterectomy for asymptomatic carotid artery stenosis. *Journal of the American Medical Association*, **273**, 1421–8.

Featherstone, R. L., Brown, M. M., Coward, L. J.; ICSS Investigators. (2004). International carotid stenting study: protocol for a randomised clinical trial comparing carotid stenting with endarterectomy in symptomatic carotid artery stenosis. *Cerebrovascular Disease*, **18**, 69–74.

Ghosh, J., Murray, D., Khwaja, N., Murphy, M. O. and Walker, M. G. (2005). The influence of asymptomatic significant carotid disease on mortality and morbidity in patients undergoing coronary artery bypass surgery. *European Journal of Vascular and Endovascular Surgery*, **29**, 88–90.

Gillett, M., Davis, W. A., Jackson, D., Bruce, D. G. and Davis, T. M. (2003). Fremantle Diabetes Study. Prospective evaluation of carotid bruit as a predictor of first stroke in type 2 diabetes: the Fremantle Diabetes Study. *Stroke*, **34**, 2145–51.

Goldstein, L. B., Adams, R., Becker, K., et al. (2001). Primary prevention of ischemic stroke: A statement for healthcare professionals from the Stroke Council of the American Heart Association. *Circulation*, **103**, 163–82.

Hobson, R.W., 2nd, Howard, V.J., Roubin, G.S., *et al.* (2004). CREST. Credentialing of surgeons as interventionalists for carotid artery stenting: experience from the lead-in phase of CREST. *Journal of Vascular Surgery*, **40**, 952–7.

Hobson, R.W., Weiss, D.G., Fields, W.S., *et al.* (1993). Efficacy of carotid endarterectomy for asymptomatic carotid stenosis. The Veterans Affairs Cooperative Study Group. *New England Journal of Medicine*, **328**, 221–7.

Kovacic, J.C., Roy, P.R., Baron, D.W. and Muller, D.W. (2006). Staged carotid artery stenting and coronary artery bypass graft surgery: Initial results from a single center. *Catheterization and Cardiovascular Interventions*, **67**, 142–8.

LaMuraglia, G.M., Brewster, D.C., Moncure, A.C., *et al.* (2004). Carotid endarterectomy at the millennium: what interventional therapy must match. *Annals of Surgery*, **240**, 535–44.

Lee, T.T., Solomon, N.A., Heidenreich, P.A., Oehlert, J. and Garber, A.M. (1997). Cost-effectiveness of screening for carotid stenosis in asymptomatic persons. *Annals of Internal Medicine*, **126**, 337–46.

MRC Asymptomatic Carotid Surgery Trial (ACST) Collaborative Group. (2004). Prevention of disabling and fatal strokes by successful carotid endarterectomy in patients without recent neurological symptoms: randomised controlled trial. *Lancet*, **363**, 1491–9.

Naylor, R., Cuffe, R.L., Rothwell, P.M., Loftus, I.M. and Bell, P.R. (2003). A systematic review of outcome following synchronous carotid endarterectomy and coronary artery bypass: influence of surgical and patient variables. *European Journal of Vascular and Endovascular Surgery*, **26**, 230–41.

No authors listed. (2001). Endovascular versus surgical treatment in patients with carotid stenosis in the Carotid and Vertebral Artery Transluminal Angioplasty Study (CAVATAS): a randomised trial. *Lancet*, **357**, 1729–37.

Randall, M.S., McKevitt, F.M., Cleveland, T.J., Gaines, P.A. and Venables, G.S. (2005). Is there any benefit from staged carotid and coronary revascularization using carotid stents? A single-center experience highlights the need for a randomized controlled trial. *Stroke*, Epub ahead of print.

Ringleb, P.A., Kunze, A., Allenberg, J.R., *et al.* (2004). The stent-supported percutaneous angioplasty of the carotid artery vs. endarterectomy trial. *Cerebrovascular Disease*, **18**, 66–8.

Rothwell, P.M. (2004). ACST: which subgroups will benefit most from carotid endarterectomy? *Lancet*, **364**, 1122–3.

Rothwell, P.M., Eliasziw, M., Gutnikov, S.A., *et al.*, for the Carotid Endarterectomy Trialists Collaboration. (2004). Effect of endarterectomy for symptomatic carotid stenosis in relation to clinical subgroups and to the timing of surgery. *Lancet*, **363**, 915–24.

Rothwell, P.M. and Goldstein, L.B. (2004). Carotid endarterectomy for asymptomatic carotid stenosis: asymptomatic carotid surgery trial. *Stroke*, **35**, 2425–7.

Sacco, R.L., Benjamin, E.J., Broderick, J.P., *et al.* (1997). American Heart Association Prevention Conference. IV. Prevention and rehabilitation of stroke risk factors. *Stroke*, **28**, 1507–17.

Sutton-Tyrrell, K.C., Alcorn, H.G., Wolfson, S.K., *et al.* (1987). Prediction of carotid stenosis in older adults with and without isolated systolic hypertension. *Stroke*, **18**, 817–22.

Taylor, D.W., Barnett, H.J., Haynes, R.B., *et al.* (1999). Low-dose and high-dose acetylsalicylic acid for patients undergoing carotid endarterectomy: a randomised controlled trial. ASA and Carotid Endarterectomy (ACE) Trial Collaborators. *Lancet*, **353**, 2179–84.

Teasell, R.W., McRae, M.P. and Finestone, H.M. (2000). Social issues in the rehabilitation of younger stroke patients. *Archives of Physical Medicine and Rehabilitation*, **81**, 205–9.

Warlow, C. (1995). Endarterectomy for asymptomatic stenosis? *Lancet*, **345**, 1254–5.

Wolf, P.A., D'Agostino, R.B., O'Neal, A., *et al.* (1992). Secular trends in stroke mortality. The Framingham study. *Stroke*, **23**, 1551–5.

Yadav, J.S., Wholey, M.H., Kuntz, R.E., *et al.* (2004). Stenting and Angioplasty with Protection in Patients at High Risk for Endarterectomy Investigators. Protected carotid-artery stenting versus endarterectomy in high-risk patients. *New England Journal of Medicine*, **351**, g1493–501.

8

Interventional management of carotid disease

Andrew G. Clifton

St George's Hospital, London SW17 0QT, UK

Surgical trials and the role of surgery

Stroke is the third most common cause of death in the Western world, and atherosclerotic stenosis of the carotid artery, close to the carotid bifurcation in the neck, causes about 10% of all strokes and transient ischemic attacks (TIA) (Clifton, 2002). For patients who have had recent symptoms associated with severe carotid stenosis the additional risk of stroke over the next 2 years is thought to be 20% or more if patients are treated medically and is thought to be greater in patients with very severe stenosis (Dennis *et al.*, 1990). It may be as high as 28% (North American Symptomatic Carotid Endarterectomy Trial Collaborators, 1991). Recent studies have shown, however, that the risks may be greater. The Oxford Community Stroke Project showed that much data looks at risk of stroke from either the date seen by a neurologist or from the date referred to at TIA service. They showed that the risk of stroke from the date of the first ever TIA was much greater in the first 30 days, in the region of 12%+ (Coull *et al.*, 2004). It has also been shown that the odds of having a stroke when the patient is found to have large artery disease, i.e. significant carotid stenosis, is much greater than if the cause is found to be secondary to small vessel disease or cardiac embolism (Lovett *et al.*, 2003). The benefits of secondary prevention in symptomatic patients have been convincingly established by the European carotid surgery trial (ECST) 1991 (European Carotid Surgery Trialists' Collaboration Group, 1991) and the North American

symptomatic carotid endarterectomy trial (NASCET) (North American Symptomatic Carotid Endarterectomy Trial Collaborators, 1991). These trials showed that stroke risk was significantly reduced by carotid surgery in suitable patients with recent symptoms and carotid stenosis narrowing the vessel by more than 70%. These trials established carotid endarterectomy as the standard treatment for severe symptomatic carotid artery stenosis, but the treatment is not without risks. NASCET and ECST reported perioperative stroke and death rates of 5.8% and 7.5%, respectively. The risks of surgery have been reported as higher in other reported series (Rothwell *et al.*, 1996a,b) which points out the complication rates are highest in series where patients have been assessed by an independent observer. Randomized prospective trials probably give the most accurate assessment of risk and benefits. For asymptomatic stenosis the risks and benefits of surgery are finely balanced and two recent trials, the asymptomatic carotid atherosclerosis study (ACAS) trial and the recent Medical Research Council (MRC) asymptomatic carotid surgery trial (ACST) have looked at this in great detail. ACAS enrolled 1662 patients at 39 centers, with a follow-up of about 2.7 years. An absolute risk reduction favoring endarterectomy of 5.9% was found, 30-day perioperative stroke and death rate was very low at 2.3%, but with more than half of these complications attributed to diagnostic cerebral angiography. There was a 5-year risk of ipsilateral stroke or death with a 60% or more carotid stenosis of 5.1% for the surgical arm and 11% for the medical arm (Executive Committee for the Asymptomatic Carotid Atherosclerosis Study, 1995). The recently published ACST looked at 3120 asymptomatic patients, between 1993 and 2003, with substantial carotid narrowing randomized between carotid endarterectomy and indefinite deferral of any carotid endarterectomy. The risk of stroke or death within 30 days of carotid endarterectomy was 3.1% and the interpretation of the study was that in asymptomatic patients, younger than 75 years of age with a carotid diameter reduction of about 70% or more on ultrasound (many of whom were on aspirin, antihypertensives and in recent years statin therapy), immediate carotid endarterectomy halved the net 5-year stroke risk from 12% to about 6% including the 3% perioperative hazard (Halliday et al., 2004). The benefit for women was less than men, however many stroke physicians feel too many patients are needed to be treated to prevent one stroke and feel that best medical therapy has progressed considerably since the major carotid endarterectomy trials. Two new trials are in the process of commencing: the asymptomatic carotid surgery trial II (ACST II), where appropriate patients with asymptomatic disease will be randomized between surgery and stenting and also the transatlantic asymptomatic carotid interventional trial (TACIT). TACIT will study all risk patients assigning these patients to one of three treatment arms: optimal medical therapy, including antiplatelet and antilipidemic and antihypertensive therapies as well as tight glycemic control and tobacco cessation efforts, the second arm will provide optimal medical therapy plus carotid endarterectomy and the third arm will provide optimal medical therapy plus carotid artery stenting with embolic protection. Enrollment for these studies will start in 2007.

Apart from the perioperative stroke risk associated with carotid endarterectomy other risks include myocardial infarction, pulmonary embolism, pneumonia, deep vein thrombosis (Sundt et al., 1975; Rothwell, 1995) and the side effects of general anaesthesia. Cranial nerve damage may

occur, most frequently involving the hypoglossal nerve, and has a significant morbidity. At least 10% of patents are affected by one of these complications. Furthermore some patients are not suitable for surgery because of concurrent medical conditions such as ischemic heart disease, recent myocardial infarction and uncontrolled hypertension. Patients that most benefit from carotid endarterectomy are those with hemispheric events, recurrent strokes, tight stenosis and plaque ulceration. There is decreased stroke risk in those patients with amarosis fugax and distal collapse of the vessel. There is increased surgical risk for females, hypertensive patients and those with peripheral vascular disease. Recent reanalysis of the NASCET and ECST data by Rothwell, looking at the effect of carotid endarterectomy, stratified by time from the last event to randomization in the trials shows there is significantly greater absolute risk reduction if surgery is carried out within the first 2 weeks (Rothwell et al., 2004). For example, an over 30% risk reduction treating a 70–99% stenosis in the first 2 weeks as compared to 9.4% risk reduction at over 12 weeks. Ideally surgical or endovascular treatment should be offered as part of a multidisciplinary team (MDT) comprising neurologist or stroke physician, carotid surgeon and interventionalist.

The most recent evidence concerning carotid angioplasty and stenting

Does angioplasty/stenting have a place in the routine management of carotid artery atherosclerosis? This question has not been adequately answered and, as I will detail, we are still awaiting the results of several ongoing randomized trials. The advantage of carotid stenting is that it is performed under local anaesthesia and thus avoids the complications of general anaesthesia and the discomfort of an incision in the neck at the same time as giving good angiographic results (Figure 8.1). Apart from the transient pain in the neck on dilatation of the balloon the

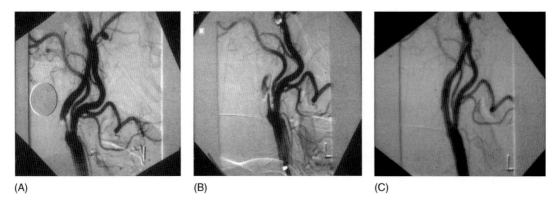

(A)   (B)   (C)

Figure 8.1 Demonstrates a tight stenosis of >70% (A), the stenosis has been crossed with a wire and an occlusion protection balloon is seen inflated in the distal ICA. (B), no residual stenosis is seen post stent insertion (C).

discomfort of successful stenting can be no more than that associated with diagnostic intraarterial angiography. Many of our patients require only mild sedation for perioperative discomfort and can be discharged from hospital 24 hours after the procedure. Angioplasty is generally cheaper than endarterectomy in monetary terms (Lambert, 1995). Although many, particularly interventional radiologists and neurologists, have enthusiastically promoted percutaneous transluminal angioplasty and stenting, it has not gained, as yet, general acceptance by vascular surgeons because of uncertainty about its risks and benefits. The technique has been widely criticized by both European and American surgeons at international meetings and in the literature (Beebe *et al.*, 1996; Brown *et al.*, 1996b, 1997; Hurst, 1996; Naylor *et al.*, 1997, 1998; Beebe, 1998). Published complication rates from carotid angioplasty alone vary from the extremes of 0–70% (Naylor *et al.*, 1998). However, data on carotid angioplasty available from several small series show the risks of procedural related stroke or death are similar to those reported in NASCET and ECST. The mean procedurally-related stroke rate amongst 477 patients treated by carotid tissue carotid angioplasty was 1.5% for minor or non-disabling stroke and 2.1% for major stroke or death, resulting in an overall stroke rate of 3.6% (Brown, 1996a; Crawley *et al.*, 1998). Rothwell *et al.* (1996a)

recently reviewed the risk of stroke and death due to endarterectomy in more than 50 published series that reported 16 000 surgical procedures for symptomatic stenosis. Combined mortality/ morbidity rates varied from 1 to 35%. Stroke and death rates correlated well with the method of assessment used, particularly when a neurologist performed postoperative assessment for complications. Complication rates (stroke) were three times higher (7.7%) when a neurologist assessed the patients than when they were assessed by a single surgeon (2.3%). Rothwell *et al.* (1996a) concluded that many perioperative strokes went undiagnosed. The same scenario can be extrapolated to endo-vascular case series. Michael Wholey has also published complication rates in a global survey of carotid stenting with complications in over 5000 patients being: minor stroke 2.8%, major stroke 1.6%, procedure-related death 0.9% and non-procedure-related death of 1.1% with a total 30-day stroke and death rate of 6.3% (Wholey *et al.*, 2000). However, this was a mix of symptomatic and asymptomatic patients. In recent years there have been many industry-sponsored case series of carotid stenting, usually of a single design of stent and protection device (Figure 8.2), such as the Boston scientific filter wire and the EndoTex Nex Stent (CABERNET) study, the Boston scientific EPI-A carotid stenting trial for high-risk surgical

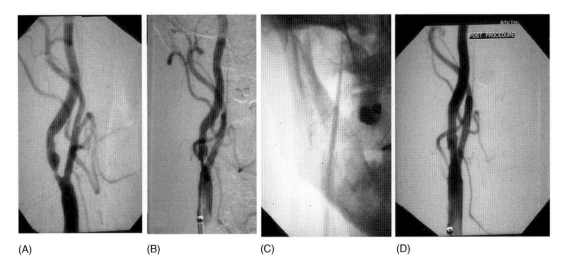

(A)   (B)   (C)   (D)

Figure 8.2 Demonstrates a 70% stenosis to the internal carotid origin with conventional angiography (A), with the filter deployed (B), with the filter being removed (C) and the postprocedure appearances (D).

patients (BEACH), the evaluation of the medtronic AVE self-expanding carotid stent system with distal protection in the treatment of carotid stenosis (MAVERIC) and the stenting of high-risk patients extracranial lesions trial with embolic removal (SHELTER) registries. There are also large European registers, such as the German carotid artery stenting registry, results presented by Mathias at the 16th International Symposium on Endovascular Therapy, Miami 2004, with 30-day stroke and death complications of 3.1% following 3267 attempted carotid artery stenting procedures.

However, there are problems with case series and registry data with uncertainty about the quality of data and the completeness of neurological follow-up. As stated above, symptomatic and asymptomatic patients are often mixed together and there is often selection bias by the operator and no-comparison group. There are several randomized trials that have been reported. Coward gives a very good summary of this in a review article in "Stroke" (Coward *et al.*, 2005). This was a Cochrane systemic review of the randomized evidence looking at the safety and efficacy of endovascular treatment of carotid artery stenosis compared with carotid endarterectomy.

Their conclusions, looking at the trials, which I will describe below, were that on looking at 30-day safety data there was no significant difference in the major risks between endovascular treatment and surgery but there were very wide confidence intervals surrounding the risks. They also concluded there was insufficient evidence currently to support a move away from carotid endarterectomy for treatment of carotid stenosis and importantly further randomized evidence of safety and efficacy of stenting was needed. They found three completed randomized studies, the carotid and vertebral artery transluminal angioplasty study (CAVATAS) 2001, (CAVATAS Investigators, 2001), the Kentucky study (Brooks *et al.*, 2001) and the Sapphire 2004 study (Yadav *et al.*, 2004). There were two others trials that stopped early: Leicester 1996 (Naylor *et al.*, 1998) and the Wallstent study (Alberts, 2001). I shall briefly summarize these trials and the relevant results. The main UK trial was CAVATAS 2001, which was an international, multicenter, randomized trial of endovascular treatment for extracranial cerebrovascular disease. Randomization started in 1992 and was completed in 1997; long-term follow-up is ongoing. Five hundred and five patients were randomized in the carotid stenosis suitable for surgery group, of which 96% were symptomatic. The majority of the patients had balloon angioplasty with stents only being deployed in 22%. No protection devices were employed and standard surgical techniques were used. There was no significant difference in the rates of stroke or death at 30 days, being approximately 10% in each arm. Confidence intervals were wide. Follow-up has been performed up to 8 years with no significant difference in fatal or disabling stroke or ipsilateral stroke up to this time between the two arms.

The Kentucky trial randomized 104 patients between stenting and endarterectomy. No patient in either group had a permanent stroke.

The Leicester trial randomized symptomatic patients between stenting and surgery. The trial was stopped after 23 patients due to the high morbidity in the angioplasty/stenting arm with five of the seven patients who underwent stenting/angioplasty having a stroke. No patients in the endarterectomy arm (ten) had a stroke. Six patients had not received their allocated treatment when the trial was suspended.

The Wallstent study randomized 219 patients with symptomatic internal carotid artery stenosis to stenting or endarterectomy. The study was stopped in view of the high 30-days complication rate in the stent group, being 12.1% against 3.6% in the endarterectomy group.

The Sapphire trial compared stenting (with cerebral protection) with endarterectomy in patients with symptomatic stenosis greater than 50% or asymptomatic stenosis greater than 80% and with coexisting conditions that potentially increased the risk of surgery. Three hundred and four patients were randomized and the primary analysis of stroke, myocardial infarction or death within 30 days plus ipsilateral stroke or death up to 1 year was 12.2% in the stent arm and 21% in the surgery arm.

As stated above the meta-analysis performed by the group at the international carotid stenting study (Coward *et al.*, 2005) showed insufficient evidence to support a move away from carotid endarterectomy but no significant difference in the major risks between the two techniques.

There are currently four ongoing trials comparing carotid stenting with carotid endarterectomy: the international carotid stenting study (ICSS) or CAVATAS II, the carotid revascularization endarterectomy versus stenting trial (CREST), the stent protected percutaneous angioplasty versus carotid endarterectomy trial (SPACE) and the endarterectomy versus angioplasty in patients with severe symptomatic carotid stenosis (EVA-3S).

The ICSS, CAVATAS II (www.cavatas.com), is an international study coordinated from London. This is a randomized trial to determine the risks and long-term benefits of carotid artery stenting in comparison to carotid endarterectomy. The inclusion criteria are symptomatic patients with an extracranial, internal bifurcation carotid artery stenosis greater than 50%. All centers must have a regular MDT meeting and follow-up by an independent neurologist or physician with a stroke interest. As of September 2005 there were 33 centers enrolled in 12 countries with over 650 patients recruited. The aim is to recruit 1500 patients with 95% confidence intervals for an equivalence trial with ±3% for 30-day disabling stroke or death and ±3.3% for stroke during follow-up. On current rates the trial will aim to finish recruiting during late 2007.

CREST (www.umdnj.edu/crestweb) compares stenting and surgery in both symptomatic and asymptomatic patients. The sample size is intended to be 2500 and as of May 2005 around 400 patients had been randomized.

There are also two European trials. SPACE is being carried out in Germany and Austria, with a projected sample size of 1900 with over 1000 patients randomized to date. In this trial cerebral protection is optional with 5–10% using it so far. There is also the EVA-3S trial from France, with a sample size of 1000 and 480 patients randomized. Cerebral protection with the PercuSurge balloon device is compulsory in this trial and there was a recent protocol amendment to this effect in 2004 (EVA-3S, 2004).

There has been agreement between the ICSS, EVA-3S and SPACE trials to perform a meta-analysis combining their results. All three trials collect identical baseline and follow-up data using the same definitions and measures of disability. The results in greater than 4000 patients will provide robust data and allow information subgroup analyses, particularly as to the use of protection devices, as will be discussed below.

In the USA there are several device-related registries of carotid stenting, as mentioned above including CABERNET, BEACH, MAVERIC and SHELTER. A useful website to look at carotid stent and stroke-related trials is www.stroketrials.org.

Evolution of endovascular treatment since first trials

It is useful to look at the evolution of endovascular treatment since the first registries and trials. Stenting is now the technique of choice that is generally thought to be superior to angioplasty. This is because any dissection or plaque rupture initiated by the balloon angioplasty is less likely to lead to complications as the stent maintains laminar flow across the stenosis and seals the site of dissection. Secondarily the stent mesh limits, at least in theory, the size of any thrombus or atheromatous debris that may be dislodged from the atheromatous plaque at the time of balloon dilatation.

The drawback to stenting was initially that stents specifically designed for use in the carotid were not available, however new stents, guidewires and delivery systems are now specifically designed for use in the carotid arteries. These began to appear during 2001 and most operators' use self-expanding stents and stents that are Conformité Européene (CE) marked are available from many manufacturers, such as the Boston carotid Wallstent and Cordis Precise stent.

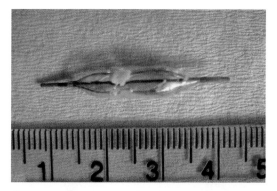

Figure 8.3 Demonstrates a filter device with an embolus *in situ*, without this filter this patient would almost certainly have suffered a large stroke.

Technique and patient selection has been improved and training schemes and proctoring are available for new stenters starting up carotid stenting. Guidelines are available both in the UK and in the USA (Sacks and Connors, 2005). Other factors which have improved are the use of dual antiplatelet therapy as discussed in the section on technique and the use of protection devices, also discussed below (Figure 8.3). The above is in comparison to, for instance CAVATAS I, where stents were only used in 22% of procedures, protection devices were not used, aspirin with intravenous heparin was used instead of dual antiplatelet agents which are far superior, and few centers had any experience before joining the trial.

Current indications for carotid stenting

Currently, until the above trials report, the indications for carotid stenting would be as part of a trial such as ICSS, high-surgical-risk patients with significant comorbidity, patients not suitable for surgery, such as patients with a high carotid bifurcation and stenosis necessitating dislocation of the jaw, restenosis postendarterectomy or postradiotherapy (Figure 8.4) and postcarotid dissection (Figure 8.5). As discussed above, stenting should be performed in centers

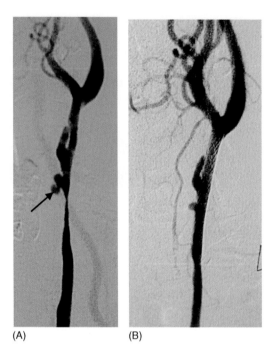

(A)   (B)

Figure 8.4 Demonstrates a postradiation stenosis (A) with some ulceration (arrow) as well as the appearances poststent insertion (B).

with relevant experience. Carotid stenting may also be useful to treat carotid dissection which is resistant to treatment with anticoagulants and antiplatelet treatment and to treat carotid pseudo-aneurysms postdissection which are symptomatic, i.e. expanding or embolizing despite maximum medical treatment.

Carotid stenting: technique

Patients are routinely placed on dual antiplatelet therapy. Patients should be placed on aspirin 75 mg per day and clopidogrel 75 mg per day for at least 7 days prior to the procedure. Alternatively a loading dose can be given of 600 mg aspirin and 600 mg clopidogrel and the patient commenced on 75 mg of each a minimum of 24 hours before the procedure with the 75 mg

doses being given on the day of procedure. It is my practice to perform the procedure with an anaesthetist present, although in most cases the procedure can be performed with little or no sedation, similar to the performance of a diagnostic angiogram.

Standard technique is used to access the femoral artery with local anaesthesia with lignocaine being given prior to this. A 6 French femoral sheath is placed in the right femoral artery and the appropriate common carotid artery accessed using standard technique. I use either a Mani or a Sidewinder catheter and I find a Simmons/ Sidewinder catheter most useful, particularly in the elderly patient with tortuous vessels. Selective angiography is performed to delineate both the anatomy of the common, internal and external carotid arteries and the degree of stenosis. Angled views are performed to achieve the best radiographic position to cross the stenosis. Full intracranial views of that circulation are also acquired.

Once the decision is made to proceed with stenting, the patient is heparinized with a standard dose of 5000 international units intravenously. Activated clotting time (ACT) measurements are made, with a target ACT of between 250 and 300 seconds, at least twice the baseline. Appropriate measurements are made of the common and internal carotid diameters as well as the length of the stenosis in order to size the protection device and the stent.

A Selectiva or Amplatz wire is then passed into the external carotid artery and a 7 French Cook or Arrow guiding sheath passed into the common carotid artery. Depending whether cerebral protection is to be used, I use the Filter device (a full discussion on cerebral protection will be made below). The lesion is either crossed with the filter, balloon or bare 014 wire. Predilatation is performed if necessary, the filter deployed, the stent deployed, postdilatation performed and the protection device if appropriate retrieved. The puncture site is then sealed with a protection device, either an Angioseal or Perclose.

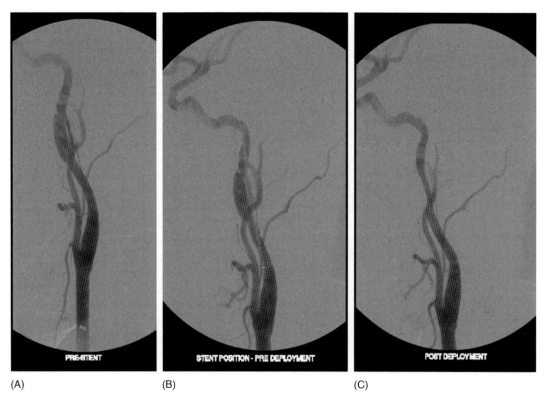

(A)   (B)   (C)

Figure 8.5 Demonstrates a carotid pseudoaneurysm postcarotid dissection (A). This was a dissection postangiography and access was required to retreat an intracranial aneurysm. A Symbiot-covered stent (Boston Scientific) was placed over the area of dissection (B) with an excellent angiographic result (C).

Monitoring, anaesthesia and premedication

An anaesthetist is present for minimal neuro-leptic analgesia and to monitor the patient. Electrocardiogram (ECG) and blood pressure monitoring are mandatory. Transcranial Doppler (TCD) monitoring is optional but is a useful tool to look at flow through the middle cerebral artery and the presence of emboli and is also useful for research. Atropine 0.6 mg or glycopyr-olate 0.2–0.5 mg is given prior to dilatation. Postprocedure aspirin 75 mg and clopidogrel 75 mg are continued for 1 month with aspirin for life. Our patients are routinely followed in the stent clinic with an ultrasound at 1 month and 6 months.

Cerebral protection. Should this be used routinely?

The major hazard of carotid stenting is dislodge-ment of, and distal embolization, of plaque mate-rial that can lead to stroke. It is logical to prevent this with a protection device. There are three types of device available: a filter system, a balloon occlu-sion system and systems that produce flow rever-sal. The use of protection devices is not proven; however most authorities, particularly in the UK and US, believe its use is mandatory. A review of the literature is as follows. There has been a recent systemic review of the literature by Kastrup (Kastrup *et al.*, 2003). This is a meta-analysis look-ing at 2537 stent procedures without protection devices and 896 procedures with protection devices. The meta-analysis showed combined 30-day stroke and death rate in symptomatic and asymptomatic cases of 1.8% with cerebral protection and 5.5% without, with the main effect being due to decrease in occurrence of minor strokes, 3.1% versus 0.5%. The death rates were identical at 0.8%. No difference was found between balloon and intravascular filter protection devices. The German registry showed little difference between centers using cerebral protection and those without, data presented by Mathias at the 16th International Symposium on Endovascular Therapy, Miami 2004. Use of cerebral protection in the EVA-3S trial is now mandatory. An article and commentary was published in "Stroke" (EVA-3S, 2004). The safety committee of this trial recommended stopping unprotected carotid angioplasty and stenting because the 30-day rate of stroke was 3.9 times higher than that of carotid angioplasty and stenting with cerebral protection. However, this decision has been criticized because of low numbers, high confidence intervals and the fact that a large number of patients treated without a protection device developed a stroke not during the procedure but during the first 30 days, which cannot be related to the nonuse of a protection device.

In unprotected carotid artery stenting procedural steps include guidewire passage, predilatation, stent placement and postdilatation. TCD studies show emboli occur at all stages but probably, depending on the study, most during primary wire passage and stent deployment. In protected carotid artery stenting, protection devices reduce (as shown on TCD and magnetic resonance diffusion weighted imaging [DWI] studies) but do not eliminate plaque embolization. The drawback of DWI studies is that high signal lesions can be seen postdiagnostic angiography, particularly in elderly patients with tortuous vessels. Flow reversal techniques may eliminate emboli completely. Vos *et al.* (2005) showed more microemboli in patients treated with filters than without, however more macroemboli in unprotected procedures

with, in their series, eight macroemboli and of these three had a TIA and two a major stroke. Cremonesi *et al.* (2003), has addressed the safety of these devices in his series of 442 patients. There was a 2.5% neurological event rate with a 30-day ipsilateral stroke and death rate of 1.1%. There was a low technical complication rate of 0.7% with only 0.2% needing surgical intervention with no clinical sequelae. In the past the following criticisms have been made of protected carotid artery stenting: that the devices are cumbersome, however new devices are very easy to use; that the filter fills with embolus and blocks flow, but they are easily removed, removing the embolus and restoring flow; and finally cost, however the cost of a stroke to the community is not usually taken into account in these calculations.

My own technique currently is to use protection when feasible, however if the vessels are extremely tortuous, particularly distal to the stenosis, I sometimes do not use protection for speed and simplicity of the procedure. However, where possible my current technique in 95%+ stenosis is to use the Emboshield, this device allows a very tight stenosis to be crossed by a bare wire, allows pre-dilatation and then filter deployment. The disadvantage is that the filter is not attached to the wire and can sometimes migrate up and down. If the stenosis is 95% or less I use the Boston or the Cordis filter devices, these are simple and one size fits all, but they are not as low profile as a balloon. In conclusion I favor routine but not mandatory use of protection devices, they are simple to use and have few risks, however, if appropriate it is totally acceptable to perform stenting without protection. The results of ongoing trials are awaited, particularly ICSS and SPACE in Germany as this will allow some analysis of data from procedures performed with and without protection following appropriate subgroup analysis.

Training

Currently in the UK there is no legislation to mandate postgraduate training in carotid stenting.

Successful management of carotid artery disease requires clinical neurological knowledge and experience to correctly identify suitable candidates, identify those with alternative disease processes and precisely document outcomes. Such a skill base may be best achieved in the UK by forming a clinical management team incorporating a clinical neurologist. Similar process may be of value in other countries. Understanding and experience of neuroimaging and neurophysiology and catheter skills to treat stenosis and salvage complications are mandatory.

Currently in the UK the carotid stent training program is that incorporated into the ICSS trial and includes a structured day of lectures with live cases, a visit by the entire MDT to observe cases at an experience center, a proctor then attends the hospital of the interventionalist to progressively teach the procedure on patients. The proctor trains the interventionalist to the satisfaction of the proctor. This current program is well received and copied elsewhere. In the UK it is recommended that this should be formally adopted as the template for all carotid artery stenting training. Similarly in the USA formal training in performing carotid stenting has not been part of many fellowship programs and a position statement on training was published in the *American Journal of Neuroradiology* in 2004 (Connors *et al.*, 2004).

Conclusion

Carotid stenting is now a mature technique and is being rapidly used by many centers as a first-line treatment for symptomatic and asymptomatic carotid stenosis, however as described in this article there is no clear evidence yet on the long-term efficiency of angioplasty and stenting available from any of the studies. The results of the ongoing randomized studies are essential. There is no real evidence to support a wholesale move away from carotid endarterectomy as the treatment of choice for carotid stenosis. Stenting should ideally be offered only within the ongoing trials of stenting versus surgery as well as for those conditions not suitable for carotid endarterectomy. Subanalysis will also show evidence for the efficacy or not of cerebral protection devices. It is essential that operators who have adequate competence perform carotid stenting as part of a MDT.

REFERENCES

Alberts, M. J. (2001). Results of a multi-centre prospective randomised trial of carotid artery stenting versus carotid endarterectomy. *Stroke*, **32**, 325 abstract.

Beebe, H. G. (1998). Scientific evidence demonstrating safety of carotid angioplasty and stenting: do we have enough to draw conclusions yet? *Journal of Vascular Surgery*, **27**, 788–90.

Beebe, H. G., Archie, J. P., Baker, W. H., *et al.* (1996). Concern about the safety of carotid angioplasty. *Stroke*, **27**, 788–90.

Brooks, W. H., Kleer, R. R., Jones, M. R., Coleman, T. L. and Ethet, L. (2001). Carotid angioplasty and stenting versus carotid endarterectomy, randomised trial in a community hospital. *Journal of the American College of Cardiology*, **38**, 1589–95.

Brown, M. M. (1996a). Balloon angioplasty for extracranial carotid disease. In *Advances in Vascular Surgery*, Vol. 4, ed. W.B Saunders. St Louis MO: Mosby Year Book, pp. 53–69.

Brown, M. M., Clifton, A. and Taylor, R. S. (1996b). Concern about the safety of carotid angioplasty. *Stroke*, **27**, 1435.

Brown, M. M., Vernables, G., Clifton, A., *et al.* (1997). Carotid endarterectomy versus carotid angioplasty. *Lancet*, **349**, 880–1.

CAVATAS Investigators (2001). Endovascular versus surgical treatment in patients with carotid stenosis and the Carotid and Vertebral Artery Transluminal Angioplasty Study (CAVATAS): a randomised trial. *Lancet*, **357**, 1729–37.

Clifton, A. (2002). Prevention of ischaemic stroke, the role of angioplasty and stenting in treatment of carotid and vertebral artery atherosclerotic disease. In *Interventional Neuroradiology*, ed. J. Byrne. Oxford: Oxford University Press, pp. 291–308.

Connors, J. J., Sacks, D., Furlan, A. J., *et al.* (2004). Training, competency and credentialing standards for diagnostic cervicocerebral angiography, carotid stenting and cerebrovascular intervention. *American Journal of Neuroradiology*, **25**, 1732–41.

Coull, A. J., Lovett, J. K. and Rothwell, P. M. (2004). Transient ischaemic attacks and minor strokes put patients at high risk for repeat stroke. *Journal of Clinical Outcomes Management*, **11**, 139.

Coward, L. J., Featherstone, R. L. and Brown, M. M. (2005). Safety and efficacy of endovascular treatment of carotid artery stenosis compared with carotid endarterectomy. A Cochrane systematic review of the randomised evidence. *Stroke*, **36**, 905–11.

Crawley, F., Brown, M. M. and Clifton, A. (1998). Angioplasty and stenting in the carotid and vertebral arteries. *Postgraduate Medical Journal*, **74**, 7–10.

Cremonesi, A., Manette, R. and Setalli, F. (2003). Protected carotid stenting: clinical advantages and complications of embolic protection devices in 442 consecutive patients. *Stroke*, **34**, 1936–43.

Dennis, M., Banford, J., Sandercock, P. and Warlow, C. (1990). Prognosis of transient ischaemic attacks in the Oxfordshire stroke project. *Stroke*, **21**, 848–51.

European Carotid Surgery Trialists Collaboration Group, MRC European Carotid Surgery Trial. (1991). Interim result for symptomatic patients with severe (70–79%) or with mild (0–29%) carotid stenosis. *Lancet*, **337**, 1235–43.

EVA-3S. (2004). Clinical alert from the endarterectomy versus angioplasty in patients with symptomatic severe carotid stenosis (EVA-3S) trial. *Stroke*, **35**, E18–E21.

Executive Committee for the Asymptomatic Carotid Atherosclerosis Study (1995). Endarterectomy for asymptomatic carotid stenosis. *Journal of the American Medical Association*, **273**, 1421–8.

Halliday, A., Mansfield, A., Marrow, J., *et al.* (2004). MRCA Asymptomatic carotid surgery trial (ACST) Collaborative Group. Prevention of disabling and fatal strokes by successful carotid endarterectomy in patients without recent neurological symptoms, randomised controlled trial. *Lancet*, **363**, 1491–502.

Hurst, R. E. (1996). Editorial. Carotid angioplasty. *Radiology*, **201**, 613–16.

Kastrup, A., Groschel, K., Krap, H., *et al.* (2003). Early outcome of carotid stenting with and without cerebral protection devices: a systemic review of the literature. *Stroke*, **34**, 813–19.

Lambert, M. (1995). Editorial. Should carotid endarterectomy be purchased? Purchasers need a broader perspective. *British Medical Journal*, **310**, 317–18.

Lovett, J. K., Coull, A. and Rothwell, P. M. (2003). Early risk of recurrent stroke by aetiological subtype; complications for stroke prevention. *Journal of Neurosurgery, Neurology and Psychiatry*, **74**, 1448.

Naylor, A. R., Bolier, A., Abbott, R. J., *et al.* (1998). Randomised study of carotid angioplasty and stenting versus carotid endarterectomy: a stopped trial. *Journal of Vascular Surgery*, **28**, 326–34.

Naylor, A. R., London, N. J. M. and Bell, P. R. F. (1997). Carotid endarterectomy versus carotid angioplasty. *Lancet*, **349**, 203–4.

North American Symptomatic Carotid Endarterectomy Trial Collaborators. (1991). Beneficial effects of carotid endarterectomy in symptomatic patients with high grade carotid stenosis. *New England Journal of Medicine*, **325**, 445–53.

Rothwell, P. (1995). Morbidity and mortality of carotid endarterectomy in the European Carotid Surgery Trial (abstract). *Cerebrovascular Diseases*, **4**, 226.

Rothwell, P., Eliasziw, M., Gutnusv, S. A., Warlow, C. P., *et al.* (2004). Endarterectomy for symptomatic carotid stenosis in relation to clinical subgroups and timing of surgery. *Lancet*, **363**, 915–24.

Rothwell, P., Slattery, J. and Warlow, C. (1996a). A systematic review of the risks of stroke and death due to endarterectomy for symptomatic carotid stenosis. *Stroke*, **27**, 260–5.

Rothwell, P., Slattery, J. and Warlow, C. (1996b). A systematic comparison of the risks of stroke and death due to endarterectomy for symptomatic and asymptomatic carotid stenosis. *Stroke*, **27**, 266–9.

Sacks, D. and Connors, J. J., III. (2005). Carotid stent placement, stroke prevention, and training. *Radiology*, **234**, 49–52.

Sundt, T. M., Sandok, B. and Whisnant, J. P. (1975). Carotid endarterectomy: complications and preoperative assessment of risk. *Mayo Clinic Proceedings*, **50**, 301–6.

Vos, A. J., van den Berg, J. C., Ernst, S. M. P. G., *et al.* (2005). Carotid angioplasty and stent placement: comparison of transcranial Doppler ultrasound data and clinical outcome with and without filtering in 509 patients. *Radiology*, **234**, 493–9.

Wholey, M. H., Mathias, H., Rubin, G. S., *et al.* (2000). Global experience in cervical carotid artery stent placement. *Catheterization and Cardiovascular Interventions*, **50**, 160.

Yadav, Y. S., Wholey, M. J. and Kunts, R. E. (2004). Protected carotid artery stenting versus endarterectomy in high risks patients. *New England Journal of Medicine*, **351**, 1493–501.

9

Conventional carotid Doppler ultrasound

Gregory Moneta

Oregon Health and Science University, Portland, OR, USA

Introduction

This chapter provides an overview of the traditional and evolving criteria used for grading carotid artery stenosis as well as the clinical relevance of sonography in the management of symptomatic and asymptomatic carotid disease. Additionally, discussions of carotid restenosis after endarterectomy as well as the diagnostic difficulties imposed by internal carotid coils and kinks, bilateral high-grade carotid stenosis and carotid stenting are included.

Technical points

Brachial systolic and diastolic blood pressures are measured in each arm. The carotid duplex ultrasound examination includes the carotid and vertebral arteries bilaterally, as stipulated by vascular laboratory accrediting organizations. Because the flow characteristics in one carotid artery may be influenced significantly by the status of the contralateral carotid artery, it is important to perform bilateral carotid examinations. A very high-grade stenosis or occlusion of one common or internal carotid artery can result in increased compensatory flow in the opposite vessel (Fujitani *et al.*, 1992). The velocity readings in the patent artery therefore are higher than expected and may suggest a greater degree of stenosis than is actually present.

The ultrasound examination should include both longitudinal and transverse views of the vessels. Vessel diameter measurements, visual assessment of stenosis severity, and plaque assessments should be done in the transverse plane. Doppler waveforms should be generated from the longitudinal plane. Gray-scale images alert the examiner to the presence of plaque in the arterial wall, while changes in the hue of the color flow pattern suggest the presence of stenosis.

Detailed characterization of carotid plaques for routine clinical duplex imaging is controversial. Advances in duplex imaging technology have allowed better elucidation and characterization of carotid plaque. Currently, however, no definite therapeutic recommendations may be made from ultrasound plaque characteristics.

Interpretative criteria for carotid stenosis are based primarily on the Doppler-derived velocity waveforms. Errors in Doppler position and errors in angle correction will therefore lead to serious errors in diagnosis. The Doppler waveform should be obtained with an angle of insonation not exceeding 60° and preferably as close to 60° as possible. Measurements obtained with an angle of insonation greater than 60° are likely to be inaccurate, even with the appropriate angle adjustment. In our department, we routinely obtain spectral Doppler waveforms from the common carotid artery (CCA) low in the neck; from the CCA just proximal to the carotid bifurcation; from the proximal, mid-, and distal (cervical) internal carotid artery (ICA); and from the origin of the external carotid artery (ECA). Additional waveforms are obtained from any areas of suspected stenosis,

Carotid Disease: The Role of Imaging in Diagnosis and Management, ed. Jonathan Gillard, Martin Graves, Thomas Hatsukami and Chun Yuan. Published by Cambridge University Press. © Cambridge University Press 2007.

as suggested by gray-scale or color flow images. When evaluating the CCA, a spectral waveform should always be generated from the most proximal, straight segment of the vessel that is accessible to the scan head. For calculating the systolic velocity ratio, the common carotid peak systolic velocity (PSV) should be measured at a standardized distance from the point at which the ICA and ECA divide. We also measure spectral Doppler waveforms across the transverse axis of the carotid bulb to document flow patterns indicating normality. Unidirectional flow is found along the flow divider of the bifurcation in normal carotid arteries. There is transient reversal of flow at peak systole near the center stream and at the outer wall opposite the flow divider, and the velocities along the outer wall may drop to zero at the end of diastole. These normal flow patterns are used in conjunction with the absence of visible plaque to indicate a normal carotid bulb.

Velocity measurements are recorded routinely from the proximal, mid-, and distal cervical portions of the ICA. The flow pattern should be that of a typical low-resistance vessel. Normal flow disturbances of the carotid bulb may extend into the mid-ICA and can be reflected in waveforms obtained at that level. The distal ICA includes the segment at least 3 cm above the bifurcation. Atherosclerosis usually develops within the first 2 cm of the bifurcation and rarely is isolated in the distal portion of the vessel. There are, however, a few circumstances, such as fibromuscular hyperplasia, where velocity increases are localized to the distal ICA without the presence of proximal ICA plaque.

Detecting and assessing stenosis

Doppler diagnosis of carotid stenosis focuses on three areas: the prestenotic region, the stenosis itself and the poststenotic region. Although the most important Doppler findings are observed within a carotid stenosis, diagnostically significant findings are present, as well, in the pre- and poststenotic regions.

CCA waveform findings

The character of the normal CCA Doppler velocity waveform is that of a low-resistance vessel, as 80% of the CCA flow is into the ICA. In normal individuals, the CCA end-diastolic velocity (EDV) should be above zero and should be similar to the EDV of the contralateral common carotid evaluated at approximately the same level in the neck.

In the majority of cases, carotid stenosis or occlusion occurs in the proximal ICA. As a result, the CCA exhibits Doppler waveform findings typical of the prestenotic region. In the presence of a very high-grade ICA stenosis or ICA occlusion, outflow is primarily through the higher-resistance external carotid circulation. The CCA waveform then takes on the high-flow resistance characteristics of an ECA (Figure 9.1), with flow to zero, or nearly zero, in end diastole. In addition, the PSV

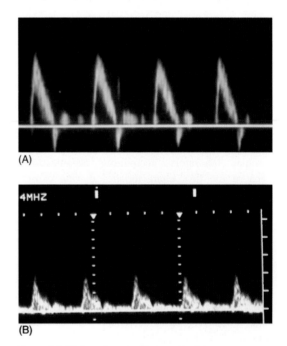

(A)

(B)

Figure 9.1 High resistance flow proximal to severe occlusive disease. (A) Common carotid Doppler has a high resistance, triphasic waveform secondary to ICA occlusion. (B) High resistance seen in this ICA waveform is due to distal ICA occlusion.

and the overall flow velocity may be substantially lower than normal due to reduced carotid artery flow. By observing these changes in the CCA, one can reliably predict the presence of high-grade stenosis or occlusion of the ICA. For this and other reasons, it is good practice to begin the interpretation of carotid ultrasound studies by comparing side to side the Doppler waveforms in the CCAs.

The CCA contralateral to an ICA stenosis or occlusion may demonstrate an increased flow velocity overall, with particular elevation of the EDV. These changes represent a compensatory increase in blood flow volume in the nonobstructed ICA in response to reduced cerebral perfusion. As this compensatory hemodynamic change can be substantial, stenosis-related flow velocities may be artificially elevated on the side with compensatory high-volume flow.

In the presence of a significant stenosis at the origin of the CCA or the right brachiocephalic artery, the ipsilateral CCA waveform may be dampened, with low velocity overall and a slower rise to peak systole when compared with the contralateral common carotid waveform (Figure 9.2). In these cases, the cervical CCA represents the poststenotic region, rather than the prestenotic region, as occurs in ICA stenosis. It is very important to take note of the CCA waveform caused by proximal stenosis, as it is often the only indicator of clinically significant carotid occlusive disease that may be treatable. The CCA flow changes seen with proximal stenosis are also important diagnostically because the overall reduction in flow velocity may artificially lower velocities in an ipsilateral ICA

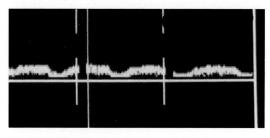

Figure 9.2 Markedly dampened waveforms due to proximal CCA occlusive disease.

stenosis, leading to underestimation of the severity of the stenosis. In some cases of proximal CCA or innominate artery stenosis, the ipsilateral common carotid waveform may exhibit poststenotic turbulence low in the neck, representing disturbed flow distal to the stenosis.

When low-velocity, dampened Doppler waveforms are seen in the CCA, initially it should be ascertained if the finding is unilateral or bilateral. If it is unilateral, the likely cause, as previously discussed, is a CCA origin or brachiocephalic artery stenosis. However, if the finding is bilateral, the etiology is cardiac, either in the form of critical aortic stenosis or severely diminished myocardial function with a low ejection fraction.

Doppler findings in the stenosis

Color-flow imaging permits rapid identification of the carotid vessels and allows for easier recognition of flow abnormalities that suggest the presence of stenosis. Additionally, color-flow imaging more accurately identifies ICA occlusion than does gray-scale imaging alone and is essential for distinguishing ICA occlusion from a very high-grade stenosis. The presence of color shifts, indicating high-velocity flow, and color mosaics, indicating poststenotic turbulence, aids in selecting potential areas for examination with the pulsed Doppler.

Although color flow and gray-scale imaging are important for identifying stenosis and for accurate placement of the Doppler sample volume, hemodynamic quantification of the severity of carotid stenosis is still primarily achieved by analysis of Doppler spectral waveforms. The specific measurements used for this purpose are the PSV, EDV and the systolic velocity ratio (Figure 9.3). As a stenosis develops, the PSV first becomes elevated; therefore, PSV is the principal measure of stenosis severity. EDV lags behind, relatively speaking, as stenosis severity progresses but rises rapidly as the stenosis becomes severe (diameter reduction of $\geq 60\%$). Thus, EDV is a good marker for high-grade stenosis. The systolic velocity ratio is a very important measure of stenosis severity, as it

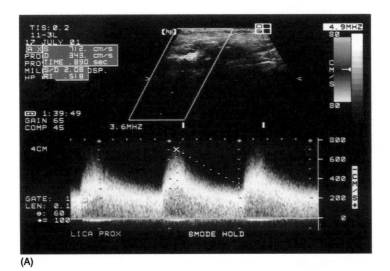

(A)

(B)

Figure 9.3 ICA stenosis with greater than 70% diameter reduction. (A) Color Doppler demonstrates narrowing of the ICA. Extremely high systolic and diastolic velocities are present in the stenosis (PSV 721 cm/s; EDV 343 cm/s). (B) In the poststenotic region, severely disturbed flow is identified and indicated by poor definition of the spectral border and simultaneous forward and reverse flow in systole. (C) ICA Doppler waveforms distal to the stenosis are dampened, with delayed acceleration to peak systolic velocity and disproportionate diastolic flow.

compensates for abnormally high and low-flow states that skew the PSV and EDV upward or downward.

To accurately measure flow velocity, the sample volume must be properly placed within the area of greatest stenosis. Originally, this meant placing the sample volume in the center of the vessel to minimize spectral broadening. Color flow, however, has demonstrated that the orientation of the stenotic jet within a stenosis is frequently

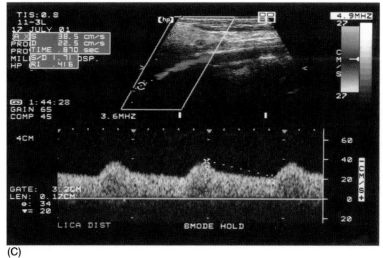

(C)

Figure 9.3 (*cont.*)

not along the longitudinal axis of the vessel. This finding has resulted in controversy with regard to the proper technique of obtaining velocity wave-forms at sites of stenosis. In areas of mild to moderate stenosis, use of a Doppler angle of 60 degrees to the long axis of the vessel is recommended. However, in areas of more severe stenosis and/or wall abnormalities, the Doppler angle of 60 degrees should be defined by the long axis of the stenotic flow jet, as demonstrated by color flow (Figure 9.3 A). The sample volume size should be kept as small as possible, usually 1.5 mm, to detect discrete changes in flow velocity. This is important as the highest velocities may be localized to a small area in the flow stream that emanate from the stenosis. In practice, the sonographer, having identified the stenosis, gently moves the sample volume around until the point of highest velocity is found.

Although color-flow sonography is not the primary means for measuring the severity of carotid stenosis, the flow image represents an important safeguard for preventing diagnostic error. In all cases, the Doppler and color-flow findings should be cross-checked for concordance. If there is disagreement between the impression obtained with the color and Doppler examinations (i.e. color Doppler suggests high-grade stenosis but velocities are only moderately elevated), the findings of both should be reviewed to resolve the discrepancy. Frequently, the cause of such discrepancies is abnormally high-or low-flow volume.

Doppler findings distal to the stenosis

Damping of Doppler velocity waveforms may be seen in the region distal to the carotid stenosis when the lesion is severe and flow reducing (Figure 9.3C). This finding was discussed previously with respect to carotid origin stenosis. Severely dampened Doppler signals may be seen distal to near-occlusive stenoses of the internal carotid.

The most common abnormality seen distal to carotid stenosis is spectral broadening caused by disturbed blood flow or frank turbulence. At best, poststenotic flow disturbance is a qualitative measure of arterial stenosis; nevertheless, its detection is important. Fill-in of the Doppler spectral waveform generally indicates the presence of carotid stenosis with diameter reduction of at least 50%, but this level of disturbed flow occasionally can be seen with nonstenotic disease. Diagnostically, the most significant poststenotic flow disturbance produces simultaneous forward and reverse spectral Doppler signal, accompanied by poor definition of the upper spectral border. This form of disturbed flow implies the presence of severe carotid stenosis and should not be disregarded. In patients with markedly calcified carotid plaque, the plaque may prevent direct insonation of the stenosis. Therefore, severely disturbed flow distal to the plaque may be the only substantial evidence for the presence of clinically significant stenosis.

The use of a large sample volume that incorporates flow from many points within the vessel in the generation of the spectral waveform may give the false impression of disturbed flow, potentially leading to the misdiagnosis of moderate disease in an otherwise normal vessel. This becomes particularly important when spectral broadening is a parameter in distinguishing normal arteries from those with mild or moderate degrees of atherosclerotic plaque. When spectral broadening is used to assess the degree of carotid artery stenosis, careful attention must also be paid to the gain settings. If the gain is set too high, spectral broadening will occur as an artifact.

Grading carotid stenosis

Many factors contribute to the clinical importance of a carotid plaque. These include plaque composition (Gray-Weale et al., 1988; Goes et al., 1990; Block and Lusby, 1992; El-Barghouty et al., 1995), hemorrhage (Lennihan et al., 1987), ulceration (Comerota et al., 1990), the state of the fibrous cap overlying the plaque, and the severity of lumen reduction. Of these factors, however, only the severity of stenosis has been unequivocally demonstrated to predict stroke. It is the ability of duplex imaging to accurately categorize carotid artery stenosis that has made duplex ultrasound the primary modality for evaluating carotid artery disease.

Duplex criteria for quantifying carotid artery stenosis have been developed primarily through comparisons of duplex-derived spectral waveforms and contrast arteriograms. Fine differences in the degree of stenosis, as measured by angiography, cannot be delineated with duplex imaging, and duplex-derived categories of stenosis are therefore relatively broad. Sensitivities and specificities for spectral analysis of duplex-derived waveforms for detecting an ICA stenosis of 50–99% or greater are between 90 and 95% (Colhoun and Macerlean, 1984; Eikelboom et al., 1983). At this time, detection of specific threshold levels of ICA stenosis appears to be most clinically important.

There are numerous spectral criteria for classifying stenosis in the ICA. Some focus on categories of stenosis, while others focus on threshold levels of stenosis. One of the most widely accepted classification schemes for categories for ICA stenosis was developed at the University of Washington. These criteria have been useful in the study of the natural history of carotid atherosclerosis and in clinical practice (Table 9.1). In the University of Washington system, velocity waveform analysis and spectral criteria are used to classify ICA angiographic stenosis as normal, 1–15%, 16–49%, 50–79%, 80–99% stenosis and occlusion (Strandness, 1990). Prospective validation of these criteria has demonstrated an overall agreement of 82% with contrast angiography. The ability of the criteria to detect carotid disease is 99% sensitive and the ability of the criteria to recognize normal arteries is 84% specific (Roederer et al., 1982, 1989).

NASCET/ACAS-based ICA stenosis criteria

Since the randomized carotid endarterectomy trials were completed, new duplex criteria have been developed for noninvasively determining ICA stenosis that are directly relevant to NASCET and ACAS (Moneta et al., 1993, 1995). These new criteria should not replace the University of Washington criteria that very accurately quantify atherosclerosis in the carotid bulb. Rather, they are

Table 9.1. University of Washington duplex criteria for internal carotid artery stenosis

Diameter reduction (%)	Velocity	Spectral characteristics
0	PSV < 125 cm/sec	No spectral broadening
1–15	PSV < 125 cm/sec	Spectral broadening in systolic deceleration
16–49	PSV > 125 cm/sec	Spectral broadening throughout systole
50–79	PSV > 125 cm/sec	Extensive spectral broadening
80–99	PSV > 125 cm/sec and EDV > 140 cm/sec	Extensive spectral broadening
Occluded	No ICA flow detected	Minimal diastolic flow or reversed flow in ipsilateral CCA

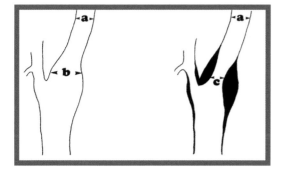

Figure 9.4 NASCET and ACAS stenosis measurement method. The smallest diameter of the stenosis (C) is compared with the postbulbar ICA diameter (A). Percent stenosis is S/C × 100. The University of Washington criteria were obtained by comparing the diameter of the residual stenotic lumen (A) with the diameter of the ICA bulb (B) estimated as if free of disease.

most useful in aiding selection of patients for carotid endarterectomy, because they are directly applicable to the threshold levels of carotid stenosis addressed in the NASCET and ACAS trials. Additionally, although the measurement methods for ICA stenosis used in the ACST and ECST were somewhat different than that used in NASCET and ACAS, conversion formulas have been devised so that the studies may be correlated and compared.

The initial studies addressing the issue of noninvasively determining ICA stenosis were performed at the Oregon Health & Science University

(OHSU). Duplex results in more than 300 internal carotid arteries were compared with angiograms, with angiographic stenosis calculated according to the NASCET and ACAS method (Figure 9.4). Using receiver-operator characteristics (ROC) curves and analysis of many duplex variables, it was determined that a systolic velocity ratio (the ratio of maximal ICA PSV to maximal CCA PSV) of 4.0 or more provided the highest accuracy in identifying a NASCET stenosis of 70–99% (Moneta et al., 1993). These data were later confirmed in a prospective study utilizing duplex scans and angiographic studies from OHSU and the University of Washington. In this study, duplex scans and angiograms were compared from 158 ICAs. Forty-two percent of the ICAs had an angiographic stenosis of 70–99% calculated according to the NASCET method. A systolic velocity ratio of 4.0 or higher was able to predict ICA stenosis of 70–99% with 91% sensitivity, 90% specificity, and an overall accuracy of 90% (Edwards et al., 1995).

Duplex velocity criteria were also initially proposed at OHSU for defining the ICA stenosis threshold of 60% or greater utilized by ACAS (Moneta et al., 1995). ICA angiograms and duplex examinations were again compared. ROC curves for many different duplex variables were derived, and the combination of a PSV of 260 cm/sec or greater and an EDV of 70 cm/sec or greater provided the highest accuracy for identifying an angiographic ICA stenosis of 60–99% (84% sensitivity, 94% specificity, 92% positive predictive value, overall accuracy of 90%). Similar results were obtained with a systolic velocity ratio of 3.2 or greater. Because a duplex scan suggesting ICA stenosis of 60–99% in an asymptomatic patient may lead to an angiogram or operation and noting the modest therapeutic benefit of carotid endarterectomy in asymptomatic patients, it was reasoned that under many clinical circumstances, criteria for asymptomatic patients should have an even higher positive predictive value than for symptomatic patients. A 95% positive predictive value for ICA angiographic stenosis of 60–99% could be achieved in the same patient database with a combination of an ICA PSV of 290 cm/sec or greater and an EDV of 80 cm/sec or greater. To provide maximal current clinical relevance to referring physicians, our vascular laboratory now reports the results of carotid artery duplex imaging using both the University of Washington criteria and these more recently derived threshold criteria for asymptomatic ICA stenosis of 60–99% and symptomatic ICA stenosis of 70–99%.

Different duplex devices are known to vary in their estimation of standardized velocities tested in a phantom model. Careful analysis of data by Fillinger and colleagues from several centers suggests that differences in patient composition at each center and slight variations in measured velocities from duplex devices of different manufacturers account for this finding (Fillinger et al., 1996). Clearly, no specific duplex criteria for a threshold level of angiographic carotid stenosis can be both 100% sensitive and specific. Proper interpretation of carotid artery duplex examinations requires recognition that criteria for predicting a specific level of angiographic ICA stenosis may vary with the duplex scanner utilized and that any given velocity criteria will be associated with some false negatives and some false positives.

Consensus committee ICA stenosis criteria

Recognizing that duplex criteria from different centers differ for the threshold levels of angiographic stenosis determined by ACAS and NASCET,

a panel of authorities from a variety of medical specialties assembled to review the carotid ultrasound literature. This group, which convened in 2002, focused on previously untreated atherosclerotic stenosis of the proximal ICA. The panel developed a consensus regarding the key components of the carotid ultrasound examination and reasonable criteria for stratification of ICA stenosis (Grant et al., 2003).

The consensus committee recommended that all carotid examinations be performed with gray-scale imaging, color Doppler, and spectral Doppler. The examination should be performed by a credentialed vascular technologist in accordance with the standards of one of the accrediting bodies. Doppler waveforms should be measured with an insonation angle as close to 60 degrees as possible but not exceeding 60 degrees, and the sample volumes should be placed within the area of maximal stenosis. The panelists also noted that reporting of the degree of ICA stenosis varies from laboratory to laboratory, among different readers within the same laboratory, and even with the same individual (Fillinger et al., 1996; Howard et al., 1996; Alexandrov et al., 1997; Kuntz et al., 1997; Ranke et al., 1999). The consensus panelists recommended that laboratories establish protocols for stratifying the degree of ICA stenosis based on Doppler measurements and that, once established, these criteria should apply to all readers within the laboratory. With the understanding that ultrasound is most accurate when lesions are classified as lying above or below a single level, such as above or below 60% stenosis or 70% stenosis, the panelists recommended the consistent use of relatively broad diagnostic strata to estimate the degree of ICA stenosis (Huston et al., 2000). They also recognized that Doppler is relatively inaccurate for subcategorizing stenoses of less than 50% and recommended that these stenoses be reported under a single category as stenosis of less than 50%. It was suggested that subcategories for minor degrees of stenosis not be used.

Based on extensive discussions and review of numerous studies (Tables 9.2A and 9.2B)

Table 9.2A. Review of literature for diagnosing internal carotid artery stenosis with Doppler thresholds

Author name	Year	N	% Stenosis[a]	PSV	EDV	Ratio[b]	% Sens	% Spec	% PPV	% NPV	% Acc
Huston J et al.	2000	915	50	130		1.6	92	90	90	91	91
Huston J et al.	2000	915	70	230	70	3.2	86	90	83	92	89
Soulez G et al.	1999		60			2.9	94	80	72	96	
AbuRahma AF et al.	1998		50	140			92	95	97	89	93
AbuRahma AF et al.	1998		60	150	65		82	97	96	86	90
AbuRahma AF et al.	1998		70	150	90		85	95	91	92	92
Carpenter JP et al.	1996	110	70	210			94	77	68	96	83
Carpenter JP et al.	1996	110	70		70		92	60	73	86	77
Carpenter JP et al.	1996	110				3.3	100	65	65	100	79
Hood DB et al.	1996	457	70	130	100		78	97	88	94	93
Carpenter JP et al.	1995		60	230			98	87	88	98	92
Carpenter JP et al.	1995		60		40		97	52	86	86	86
Carpenter JP et al.	1995		60			2.0	97	73	78	96	76
Carpenter JP et al.	1995		60	230	40	2.0	100	100	100	100	100
Browman MW et al.	1995	75	70	175			91	60			
Moneta GL et al.	1995	176	60	260	70	3.2–3.5	84	94	92	88	90
Neale ML et al.	1994	60	70	270	110		96	91			93
Moneta GL et al.	1993		70	325	130		83	90	80	92	88

[a]Degree of stenosis set as cutoff for diagnosis. [b]Ratio of ICA PSV to CCA PSV.
Abbreviations: Acc=accuracy; EDV=ICA end-diastolic velocity; N=number of patients; NPV=negative predictive value; PPV=positive predictive value; PSV=ICA peak systolic velocity; Ref=reference; sens=sensitivity; spec=specificity.

(Bluth et al., 1988; Hunink et al., 1993; Moneta et al., 1993; Neale et al., 1994; Browman et al., 1995; Carpenter et al., 1995, 1996; Moneta et al., 1995; Srinivasan et al., 1995; Derdeyn and Powers, 1996; Griewig et al., 1996; Hood et al., 1996; AbuRahma et al., 1998; Beebe et al., 1999; Grant et al., 1999, 2000; Ranke et al., 1999; Soulez et al., 1999; Huston et al., 2000; Perkins et al., 2000; Umemura and Yamada, 2000), the consensus panel recommended stratifying the degree of ICA stenosis, based on Doppler and imaging results, into the following strata: normal (no hemodynamic or gray-scale evidence of atherosclerosis); stenosis of less than 50%; stenosis of 50–69%; stenosis of 70% or more but less than near occlusion; near occlusion; and occlusion. The diagnosis of near occlusion and occlusion should be based on Doppler measurements of velocity as well as gray-scale and color Doppler findings. The stenosis thresholds of 50% and 70% were chosen because they were felt to be thresholds used by many surgeons for operative intervention.

The panel noted that many Doppler parameters are used for the evaluation of ICA stenosis, including ICA PSV, ICA EDV, the ICA/CCA PSV ratio, and the ICA/CCA EDV ratio. The panel recommended that the ICA PSV and the presence of plaque on gray-scale and/or color Doppler

Table 9.2B. Review of literature for diagnosing internal carotid artery stenosis with Doppler studies not providing sensitivities, specificities, and predictive values

Author			Threshold chosen			Performance	
Author name	Year	N	% Stenosis[a]	PSV	EDV	Ratio[b]	Assessment and Results
Umemura A & Yamada K	2000	60	Variable thresholds				Evaluated B flow without Doppler
Perkins JM et al.	2000						
Grant EG et al.	2000						Doppler performs poorly for estimating degree of stenosis, better for differentiating above and below a single degree of stenosis
Beebe HG et al.	1999						Color and gray-scale perform well alone; Doppler helps for mid-range lesions
Grant EG et al.	1999	303	60	200		3	Asymptomatic patients; outcome better than sensitivity/specificity/accuracy
Grant EG et al.	1999		70	175		2.5	Symptomatic patients; outcome better than sensitivity/specificity/accuracy
Ranke C et al.	1999		70				Ratio of ICA PSV at stenosis to ICA PSV distal to stenosis; sensitivity 94%, specificity 98%
Soulez G et al.	1999		70				Ratio of ICA PSV at stenosis to ICA PSV distal to stenosis; sensitivity 94%, specificity 98%
Derdeyn CP & Power WJ	1996		60	230			Simulator
Griewig B et al.	1996						Power Doppler better than color Doppler (not quantified)
Srinivasan J et al.	1995	164					Doppler poor for differentiating degree of stenosis for values <50%
Hunink MG et al.	1993	60					PSV best parameter for predicting stenosis > 70%
Bluth EI et al.	1988						EDV best, but did not use NASCET criteria for angiography

[a]Degree of stenosis set as cutoff for diagnosis. [b]Ratio of ICA peak systolic velocity to CCA peak systolic velocity.
Note: Abbreviations: EDV=ICA end diastolic velocity; ICA=internal carotid artery; N=number of patients; NASCET=North American Symptomatic Carotid Endarterectomy Trial; NPV=negative predictive value; PPV=positive predictive value; PSV=internal carotid artery peak systolic velocity; Ref=reference; sens=sensitivity; spec=specificity.

imaging should be the primary parameters used to diagnose and grade ICA stenosis.

ICA PSV is easy to obtain and seems reasonably reproducible. However, data suggest that the reproducibility of PSV, even among experienced vascular technologists, is sufficiently poor that PSVs should not be used as a continuous variable in clinical carotid duplex imaging (Hunink *et al.*, 1993). The degree of stenosis estimated by ICA

PSV and the degree of narrowing of the ICA lumen seen on gray-scale and color Doppler should correlate. Furthermore, additional parameters such as ICA/CCA PSV ratio and ICA EDV should be employed as internal checks and are especially useful when ICA PSV may not be representative of the extent of disease. Such situations include the presence of tandem lesions, contralateral high-grade stenosis, discrepancy between visual

Table 9.3. Consensus panel table of ultrasound and Doppler criteria for diagnosis of internal carotid artery stenosis

Primary parameters			Additional parameters	
Degree of stenosis	ICA PSV	Plaque estimate[a]	ICA/CCA PSV	ICA EDV
Normal	<125 cm/sec	None	<2.0	<40 cm/sec
<50%	<125 cm/sec	< 50% diameter reduction	<2.0	<40 cm/sec
50–69%	125–230 cm/sec	≥50% diameter reduction	2.0–4.0	40–100 cm/sec
≥70 but less than near occlusion	≥230 cm/sec	≥50% diameter reduction	>4.0	>100 cm/sec
Near occlusion	High, low or undetectable	Visible	Variable	Variable
Total occlusion	Undetectable	Visible, no detectable lumen	Not applicable	Not applicable

[a]Plaque estimate with the gray-scale ultrasound and the color Doppler imaging.

Abbreviations: CCA=common carotid artery; EDV=end-diastolic velocity; ICA=internal carotid artery; PSV=peak systolic velocity.

assessment of the plaque and ICA PSV, elevated CCA velocities, hyperdynamic cardiac states, or low cardiac output.

The consensus panel recommended the following criteria, stratifying ICA stenosis. These criteria have not been subjected to retrospective or prospective evaluation and do not represent the results of any one laboratory or study (Table 9.3).

The ICA is considered *normal* when the ICA PSV is less than 125 cm/sec and there is no visible plaque or intimal thickening. Normal arteries should also have an ICA/CCA ratio of less than 2.0 and ICA EDV of less than 40 cm/sec.

ICA stenosis of less than 50% is present when the ICA PSV is less than 125 cm/sec and there is visible plaque or intimal thickening. Such arteries should also have an ICA/CCA PSV ratio of less than 2.0 and an ICA EDV of less than 40 cm/sec.

ICA stenosis of 50–69% is present when the ICA PSV is 125–230 cm/sec and there is visible plaque. Such arteries should also have an ICA/CCA PSV ratio of 2.0–4.0 and an ICA EDV of 40–100 cm/sec.

ICA stenosis of 70% or more but less than near occlusion is present when the ICA PSV is more than 230 cm/sec and there is visible plaque with lumen narrowing on gray-scale and color Doppler imaging. The higher the PSV, the more likely (higher positive predictive value) it is to have severe disease. Such stenoses should also have an ICA/CCA ratio of more than 4 and an ICA EDV of more than 100 cm/sec.

In cases of *near occlusion* of the ICA, the velocity parameters may not apply. "Preocclusive" lesions may be associated with high, low, or undetectable velocity measurements. The diagnosis of near occlusion is therefore established primarily by demonstration of a markedly narrowed lumen with color Doppler. In some near occlusive lesions, color Doppler can distinguish between near occlusion and occlusion by demonstrating a thin wisp of color traversing the lesion.

Occlusion of the ICA is present when there is no detectable patent lumen on gray-scale imaging and no flow with spectral, color, and power Doppler. Near occlusive lesions

Table 9.4. Comparison of initial duplex parameters in ICAs progressing and not progressing from ICA stenosis of <60% to ICA stenosis of 60–99%

Initial duplex value	Non-progressing arteries (N = 587)	Progressing arteries	p value
Mean PSV	110 ± 47	166 + 55	<0.0001
Mean EDV	36 ± 15	55 + 22	<0.0001
Mean ICA/CCA PSV ratio	1.40 ± 0.68	2.21 + 1.00	<0.0001

Abbreviations: CCA = common carotid artery; EDV = end diastolic velocity; ICA = internal carotid artery; PSV = peak systolic velocity.

may be misdiagnosed as occlusions when only gray-scale ultrasound and spectral Doppler are used.

Other topics relevant to carotid artery duplex scanning

Surveillance of asymptomatic disease

A retrospective analysis performed at our institution of more than 300 patients determined that symptomatic patients with less than 60% diameter ICA stenosis and an ICA PSV of more than 175 cm/sec on initial duplex examination had a significantly higher rate of progression to ICA stenosis of 60–99% than asymptomatic patients with ICA PSVs of less than 175 cm/sec (Nehler et al., 1996). Based on this finding, a prospective evaluation of 407 patients was performed, representing 640 patent, nonoperated ICA stenoses less than 60% (Lovelace et al., 2001). Symptomatic progression of ICA stenosis was infrequent in this group. Only three patients, at a mean of 21 months, developed hemispheric symptoms (all had transient ischemic attacks) and had ipsilateral atherosclerosis progression. In addition, one ICA progressed to occlusion at 54 months, with a resulting transient ischemic attack. No patient had neurologic symptoms *without* ipsilateral progression of ICA stenosis.

Asymptomatic progression to ICA stenosis of 60–99% was detected in 10% of patients and 7% of

ICAs at a mean of 18 months, and such progression correlated with the patients' initial duplex examination. The mean PSV, mean EDV, and mean ICA/CCA PSV ratio were all higher initially in those whose plaque/stenosis subsequently progressed, versus those in whom the plaque/stenosis remained stable. Asymptomatic progression to ICA stenosis of 60–99% occurred in 4% of ICAs with initial PSVs of less than 175 cm/sec, while 26% of ICAs with initial PSVs of more than 175 cm/sec progressed to stenosis of 60–99% ($p < 0.0001$, Table 9.4). The mean time of progression to ICA stenosis of more than 60–99% was 21±10 months with initial PSVs of less than 175 cm/sec, as compared with 14±9 months in those with initial PSVs of more than 175 cm/sec. By life table analysis, freedom from progression to ICA stenosis of 60–99% was significantly higher for those patients with an initial ICA PSV of less than 175 cm/sec versus those with an initial ICA PSV of more than 175 cm/sec.

Thus, asymptomatic patients who have not had a previous ipsilateral endarterectomy and who have an ICA stenosis of less than 60% and duplex scan-determined ICA PSV of less than 175 cm/sec can be safely followed with serial scans at intervals of 1 year. Patients with ICA stenosis of less than 60% and PSVs of 175 cm/sec or higher on initial duplex examination are significantly more likely to progress asymptomatically to ICA stenosis of 60–99%. Progression in this subgroup is sufficiently frequent to warrant follow-up duplex studies at 6-month intervals.

Recurrent carotid stenosis

As with primary stenosis and occlusion, ultrasound can be used to demonstrate or rule out recurrent carotid stenosis after carotid endarterectomy, patch grafting, bypass surgery, and carotid stenting. Three patterns of ICA stenosis following carotid endarterectomy have been recognized. Lesions present within 1 month of carotid endarterectomy are likely to be residual lesions and represent a technically imperfect operation. Early recurrences following a technically adequate operation occur within the first 2 years after carotid endarterectomy, usually within the first 12 months, and result from myointimal hyperplasia. Late recurrences occur 2 years or more following endarterectomy and are due to recurrent atherosclerosis.

Over the past three decades, there have been more than 160 publications on recurrent carotid artery stenosis following carotid endarterectomy. These publications encompass more than 62 000 carotid endarterectomies. The incidence of carotid restenosis in these series averaged 6% (range: 0–50%). The mean incidence of asymptomatic carotid restenosis detected noninvasively is 9%, more than four times the 2% incidence of symptomatic recurrent stenosis. In recent years, the performance of routine patch angioplasty by many surgeons has lowered the rate of carotid restenosis. Restenosis develops in a mean of 12% of arteries closed primarily versus <5% of those closed with a patch. Overall, it appears that approximately 20% of carotid restenoses are due to residual stenosis at the time of surgery. Stenoses that occur within the first 2 years represent about 50% of carotid restenoses. The remaining 30% of restenoses occurs more than 2 years after the operation. Fewer than 25% of carotid restenoses ever become symptomatic, and only about 7% ever cause a stroke. One study of 380 patients followed up to 16 years or more found that the overall incidence of recurrent carotid stenosis equaling or exceeding 50% was 10.8%. Incidences at 1, 3, 5 and 10 years were 5.8%, 9.9%, 13.9%, and 23.4%,

respectively (Mattos *et al.*, 1993). Only 2.1% developed severe (>80%) recurrent stenosis.

Several studies have examined the optimal timing and frequency of duplex sonography after surgery to detect both recurrent carotid stenosis and contralateral atherosclerotic disease progression. The value of early duplex imaging after carotid endarterectomy in patients with a normal intraoperative completion study is limited, as shown by a retrospective study of 380 CEAs with intraoperative completion angiography, duplex scans, or both (Roth *et al.*, 1999; Pross *et al.*, 2001). Follow-up ICA duplex scans were normal in 95.8% of patients after carotid endarterectomy. There were no severe recurrent ICA stenoses. Overall, only 0.5% of the patients with operated ICAs developed even moderate restenosis within the first 6 months. This study demonstrated that when intraoperative completion studies are normal, duplex surveillance in the first 6 months postoperatively is unnecessary.

After carotid endarterectomy, contralateral progression of atherosclerosis is a much more important problem than ipsilateral ICA restenoses. In a study of 221 patients who underwent carotid endarterectomy, progression of contralateral disease, rather than restenosis, was the most common finding that resulted in the need for reintervention during a mean follow-up period of 27.4 months (Pross *et al.*, 2001). Only 2.7% of the patients with operated ICAs had asymptomatic recurrent stenosis of more than 50% diameter reduction by duplex imaging, and only one of 221 patients had recurrent stenosis of more than 75%, requiring reoperation. The yield for postcarotid endarterectomy surveillance in the operated artery was less than 1%, while progression of contralateral disease occurred in 12% of patients, leading to seven CEAs for high-grade stenosis. Importantly, disease progression to stenosis of more than 75% was five times as frequent in patients with ICA stenosis of more than 50% initially. All patients but one who eventually required contralateral endarterectomy for disease progression had ICA stenosis of more than 50% when first seen. The authors concluded that duplex imaging at 1- to 2-year intervals after carotid endarterectomy is adequate when an uncomplicated carotid endarterectomy is achieved (based on surgical completion studies) and when there is minimal contralateral disease (<50% stenosis).

These data show that following carotid endarterectomy, the likelihood of finding significant carotid restenosis requiring repair is quite low. If reoperation is indicated only for symptomatic recurrent lesions and selected high-grade asymptomatic restenoses, the frequency of subsequent follow-up examinations can be dictated primarily by the status of the contralateral, nonoperated carotid artery or by the development of neurologic symptoms. Generally, patients with carotid endarterectomy who have normal intraoperative completion studies and stenosis of less than 50% in the contralateral artery can be safely followed with carotid duplex imaging at 1-year intervals. Patients with less than technically perfect results of carotid endarterectomy or stenosis of more than 50% in the contralateral nonoperated ICA should undergo follow-up duplex imaging at 6 months.

Bilateral high-grade stenosis

Doppler-derived flow velocities from the ICA opposite an ICA occlusion or high-grade stenosis may suggest a higher degree of narrowing than is observed angiographically, due to compensatory flow. Several investigators have found that contralateral occlusion leads to overestimation of ICA stenosis with standard Doppler criteria (Hayes et al., 1988; Busuttil et al., 1996; van Everdingen et al., 1998). Until recently, no studies have addressed the effectiveness of carotid endarterectomy performed on the basis of ACAS-derived Doppler criteria for ICA stenosis contralateral to high-grade ICA stenosis or occlusion. This information is important in planning carotid endarterectomy when duplex imaging is used as the sole means of preoperative assessment.

A study conducted in our laboratory over an 8-year period determined the effects of unilateral carotid endarterectomy on the duplex scan findings in the contralateral ICA in patients with bilateral carotid stenosis (Abou-ZamZam et al., 2000). Four hundred and sixty patients underwent carotid endarterectomy for ICA stenosis of 60–99%, and 107 of these had an asymptomatic contralateral ICA stenosis of 50–99% by standard Doppler criteria (PSV > 125 cm/sec). When evaluating the nonoperated ICA postoperatively in these 107 patients, there was an overall decrease in PSV of 27±79 cm/sec (mean±SD) and a decrease of 19±42 cm/sec in EDV. Among the 107 asymptomatic stenoses, 38 met Doppler criteria for ICA stenosis of 60–99% preoperatively. Postoperatively, in these 38, there was a mean decrease of 48 cm/sec (10.1%) in PSV and 36 cm/sec (19.3%) in the EDV in the nonoperated, asymptomatic stenoses. In eight of 38 patients (21.1%), the nonoperated ICA lesions of 60–99% were reclassified as less than 60% on postoperative duplex imaging. Six of 69 patients with asymptomatic ICA stenosis who did not meet criteria for narrowing of 60–99% prior to contralateral carotid endarterectomy met these criteria on their first postoperative examination. All of these patients were close to the Doppler threshold on preoperative testing. It follows that when duplex imaging is used as the sole imaging modality before carotid endarterectomy, patients with severe bilateral carotid stenosis must have an additional duplex examination after the initial carotid endarterectomy to reassess stenosis severity and the need for surgery of the nonoperated ICA.

Our findings with respect to bilateral ICA stenosis were similar to those of Busuttil and coworkers, who found that duplex imaging, in comparison to angiography, overestimated the degree of stenosis in 27% of ICAs contralateral to a high-grade stenosis (Busuttil et al., 1996). These investigators observed an average decrease in peak systolic frequency of 1175 Hz (approximately 36 cm/sec) and end-diastolic frequency of 475 Hz (approximately 15 cm/sec) after contralateral carotid endarterectomy. Overall, 51% of patients had a one-category decrease in the Doppler-estimated severity of ICA stenosis following contralateral carotid endarterectomy. Fujitani and associates further noted that duplex scan overestimation of stenosis is more common in less-severe categories of stenosis than in higher-severity categories.

ICA coils and kinks

Tortuosity of the ICA is a common finding in elderly patients and may be difficult to distinguish from a carotid artery aneurysm on physical examination. Occasionally, ICA tortuosity is associated with fibromuscular dysplasia (Effeney *et al.*, 1979). In essence, tortuosity comes in two forms: coiling of the ICA and kinking, and they may occur together. Very unusual, marked ICA kinking, with an inside angle of less than 90 degrees, may result in neurologic symptoms if there is either flow reduction imposed by the kink or concomitant plaque formation at the site of the kink that results in distal embolization (Sarkari and Bickerstaff,

1973). A history of neurologic symptoms associated with head motion or the presence of an abnormal pulsation in the neck, should lead the clinician to suspect the presence of a kink. These observations are indications for further workup.

Internal carotid artery kinks and coils may cause problems with respect to duplex examination (Figure 9.5). The course of the tortuous ICA can usually be traced with color flow imaging, and real-time B-mode ultrasound can readily image concurrent atheromatous plaque in the tortuous segment. In addition, color flow can help distinguish a tortuous vessel from a carotid artery aneurysm in a patient with a pulsating neck mass. It is difficult, nonetheless, to interpret Doppler frequency shifts and spectral analysis findings in tortuous carotid arteries because of distorted flow patterns and angulations. Flow in the tortuous artery inevitably is quite disturbed, and marked turbulence may occur in kinked ICAs, yet the clinical importance of such disturbances is unknown. Color flow allows

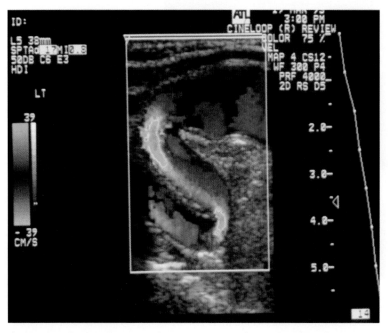

Figure 9.5 Color Doppler image of a tortuous ICA. By better identifying the course of the ICA with color flow, the Doppler angle can be more accurately determined, resulting in more reliable velocity measurements.

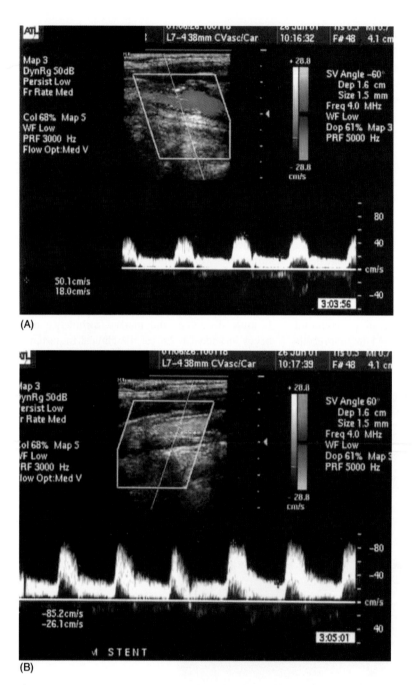

Figure 9.6 Carotid artery with stent in place. (A) Proximal ICA with stent. (B) Mid-ICA with higher velocities. (C) Distal ICA and outflow with slightly higher velocities. (D) ICA with stent in transverse view.

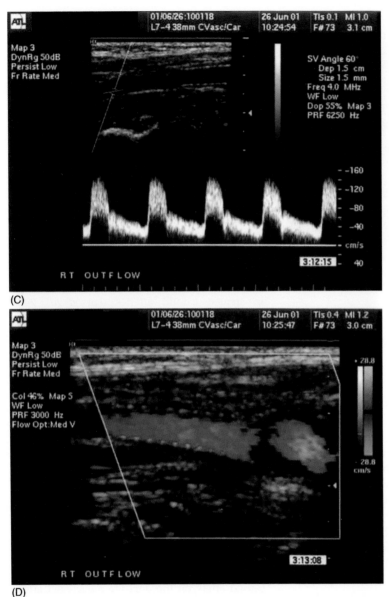

(C)

(D)

Figure 9.6 (*cont.*)

for reasonably accurate determination of the Doppler angle and placement of the sample volume, leading to more reliable velocity measurements when stenosis is suspected, but in some cases it is not clear that the ascribed Doppler angle is sufficiently accurate for diagnosis. A potential solution to these problems may lie with high-resolution, contrast-enhanced magnetic resonance or computed tomographic angiography. These methods now offer image resolution of 1 mm or less and the capacity to reconstruct the image in any plane of section. These capabilities are likely

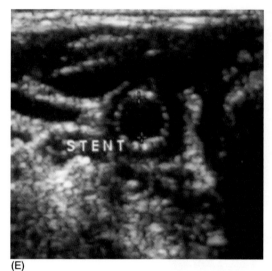

(E)

Figure 9.6 (*cont.*)

to provide the most accurate currently available assessment of tortuosity-related ICA stenosis.

CCA and ECA stenosis

The velocity criteria used for classifying disease in the internal carotid artery have not been tested for application to the ECA or the CCA. However, as with the ICA, relative degrees of stenosis may be determined by the presence of plaque with B-mode imaging, aberration in color flow on duplex examination, spectral broadening, and increases in PSV. Although not specifically tested, stenosis of more than 50% can be inferred by the presence of a focally increased velocity followed by poststenotic turbulence. Normally, the CCA has attributes of the ICA and ECA. The CCA will take on the quality of the "normal" vessel (ICA or ECA) when the other is occluded. If there is a proximal CCA (or right innominate artery) high-grade stenosis or occlusion, the ipsilateral CCA Doppler flow quality will be dampened with low PSVs, as compared with the contralateral side. Poststenotic turbulence also may be seen. There are no widely employed validated criteria to give a diameter reduction for stenosis in the CCA. Stenosis of greater than 50% is

inferred by PSV of more than 125 cm/sec associated with poststenotic turbulence. As noted previously, a focal high-grade stenosis or multiple lesions within the CCA can result in diminished PSVs and EDVs in the ICA, with resulting underestimation of the degree of stenosis within the ICA.

Carotid artery stenting

Carotid duplex studies have been used as the noninvasive standard to evaluate for carotid stenosis. Standardized criteria evaluating peak systolic velocities, end diastolic velocities, and the ICA/CCA ratio have been set and correlate to specific percentages of stenosis. With changes in blood flow through the stent as well as possible decreased compliance of the artery because of the stent, the velocities detected may be falsely elevated in stented carotid arteries (Lal *et al.*, 2004) (Figure 9.6). Several studies have been performed evaluating for early recurrent stenosis and the ultrasound criteria for those patients who have undergone carotid artery stenting (Groschel *et al.*, 2005). These studies have shown that the ultrasound criteria are unreliable for evaluating a stented carotid artery. Therefore, further studies have been undertaken to devise new thresholds for the stented carotid artery (Lal *et al.*, 2004; Stanziale *et al.*, 2005). These new criteria have only considered in-stent stenosis. Additionally, the number of patients in these studies that have had in-stent restenosis is small and therefore the data is not as reliable. None of these studies has correlated the degree of stenosis/increase in velocities with clinical symptoms or outcomes. These studies have also failed to evaluate the effect of the stented carotid artery on the opposite nonstented artery. The degree of stenosis and clinical symptoms need to be correlated to devise the best follow-up plan for these patients.

Conclusion

Duplex imaging remains the most accurate and clinically useful method to noninvasively evaluate the extracranial carotid artery. The addition of color flow to gray-scale imaging and pulse Doppler examination facilitates performance of the examination and, in some cases, improves accuracy. Performance and interpretation of duplex studies must, however, change with increased knowledge of carotid artery disease and its therapy. Only through continual reassessment and careful investigation will duplex imaging remain the preeminent noninvasive method for assessing the carotid artery.

REFERENCES

Abou-ZamZam, A. M. Jr, Moneta, G. L., Edwards, J. M., et al. (2000). Is a single preoperative duplex scan sufficient for planning bilateral carotid endarterectomy? *Journal of Vascular Surgery*, **31**, 282–8.

AbuRahma, A. F., Robinson, P. A., Stickler, D. L., et al. (1998). Proposed new duplex classification for threshold stenoses used in various symptomatic and asymptomatic carotid endarterectomy trials. *Annals of Vascular Surgery*, **12**, 349–58.

Alexandrov, A. V., Brodie, D. S., McLean, A., et al. (1997). Correlation of peak systolic velocity and angiographic measurement of carotid stenosis revisited. *Stroke*, **28**, 339–42.

Beebe, H. G., Salles-Cunha, S. X., Scissons, R. P., et al. (1999). Carotid arterial ultrasound scan imaging: A direct approach to stenosis measurement. *Journal of Vascular Surgery*, **29**, 838–44.

Block, R. W. and Lusby, R. J. (1992). Carotid plaque morphology and interpretation of echolucent lesion. *Diagnostic Vascular Imaging*, 225–36.

Bluth, E. I., Stavros, A. T., Marich, K. W., et al. (1988). Carotid duplex sonography: A multicenter recommendation for standardized imaging and Doppler criteria. *Radiographics*, **6**, 487–506.

Browman, M. W., Cooperberg, P. L., Harrison, P. B., et al. (1995). Duplex ultrasonography criteria for internal carotid stenosis of more than 70% diameter: Angiographic correlation and receiver operating characteristic curve analysis. *Canadian Association of Radiology Journal*, **46**, 291–5.

Busuttil, S. J., Franklin, D. P., Youkey, J. R., et al. (1996). Carotid duplex overestimation of stenosis due to severe contralateral disease. *American Journal of Surgery*, **172**, 144–8.

Carpenter, J. P., Lexa, F. J. and Davis, J. T. (1995). Determination of 60% or greater carotid artery stenosis by duplex Doppler ultrasonography. *Journal of Vascular Surgery*, **22**, 697–703.

Carpenter, J. P., Lexa, F. J. and Davis, J. T. (1996). Determination of duplex Doppler ultrasound criteria appropriate to the North American symptomatic carotid endarterectomy trial. *Stroke*, **27**, 695–9.

Colhoun, E. and Macerlean, D. (1984). Carotid artery imaging using duplex scanning and bi-directional arteriography: A comparison. *Clinical Radiology*, **35**, 101–6.

Comerota, A. J., Katz, M. L., White, J. V., et al. (1990). The pre-operative diagnosis of the ulcerated carotid atheroma. *Journal of Vascular Surgery*, **11**, 505–10.

Derdeyn, C. P. and Powers, W. J. (1996). Cost-effectiveness of screening for asymptomatic carotid artery disease. *Stroke*, **27**, 1944–50.

Edwards, J. M., Moneta, G. L., Papanicolaou, G., et al. (1995). Prospective validation of a new duplex ultrasound criteria for 70%–99% internal carotid stenosis. *Journal d'Echographie et de Médecine Ultrasonore*, **16**, 3–7.

Effeney, D. J., Ehrenfeld, W. K., Stoney, R. J., et al. (1979). Fibromuscular dysplasia of the internal carotid artery. *World Journal of Surgery*, **3**, 179.

Eikelboom, B. C., Ackerstaff, R. G., Ludwig, J. W., et al. (1983). Digital video subtraction angiography and duplex scanning in assessment of carotid artery disease: Comparison with conventional angiography. *Surgery*, **94**, 821–5.

El-Barghouty, N., Geroulakos, G., Nicolaides, A., et al. (1995). Computer assisted carotid plaque characterization. *European Journal of Vascular and Endovascular Surgery*, **9**, 389–93.

Fillinger, M. F., Baker, R. J. Jr, Zwolak, R. M., et al. (1996). Carotid duplex criteria for a 60% or greater angiographic stenosis: Variation according to equipment. *Journal of Vascular Surgery*, **24**, 856–64.

Fujitani, R. M., Mills, J. L., Wang, L. M. and Taylor, S. M. (1992). The effect of unilateral internal carotid arterial occlusion upon contralateral duplex study: Criteria for accurate interpretation. *Journal of Vascular Surgery*, **16**, 459–67.

Goes, E., Janssens, W., Maillet, B., et al. (1990). Tissue characterization of atheromatous plaques: Correlation between ultrasound image and histological findings. *Journal of Clinical Ultrasound*, **18**, 611–17.

Grant, E. G., Benson, C. B., Moneta, G. L., *et al.* (2003). Carotid artery stenosis: Gray-scale and Doppler us diagnosis — society of radiologists in ultrasound consensus conference (online). *Radiology*, **19**, 190–8.

Grant, E. G., Duerinckx, A. J., El Saden, S., *et al.* (1999). Doppler sonographic parameters for the detection of carotid stenosis. *American Journal of Roentgenology*, **172**, 1123–9.

Grant, E. G., Duerinckx, A. J., El Saden, S. M., *et al.* (2000). Ability to use duplex US to quantify internal carotid stenoses: Fact or fiction? *Radiology*, **214**, 247–52.

Gray-Weale, A. C., Graham, J. C., Burnett, J. R., *et al.* (1988). Carotid artery atheroma: comparison of pre-operative B-mode ultrasound appearance with carotid endarterectomy specimen. *Journal of Cardiovascular Surgery*, **29**, 115–23.

Griewig, B., Morganstern, C., Driesner, F., *et al.* (1996). Cerebrovascular disease assessed by color flow and power Doppler ultrasonography. Comparison with digital subtraction angiography in internal carotid artery stenosis. *Stroke*, **27**, 95–100.

Groschel, K., Riecker, A., Schulz, J. B., *et al.* (2005). Systematic review of early recurrent stenosis after carotid angioplasty and stenting. *Stroke*, **36**, 367–73.

Hayes, A. C., Johnson, K. W., Baker, W. H., *et al.* (1988). The effect of contralateral disease on carotid Doppler frequency. *Surgery*, **103**, 19–23.

Hood, D. B., Mattos, M. A., Mansour, A., *et al.* (1996). Prospective evaluation of new duplex criteria to identify 70% internal carotid artery stenosis. *Journal of Vascular Surgery*, **23**, 254–61.

Howard, G., Baker, W. H., Chambless, L. E., *et al.* (1996). An approach for the use of Doppler ultrasound as a screening tool for hemodynamically significant stenosis (despite heterogeneity of Doppler performance). A multicenter experience. Asymptomatic carotid atherosclerosis study investigators. *Stroke*, **27**, 1951–7.

Hunink, M. G., Polak, J. F., Barlan, M. M., *et al.* (1993). Detection and quantification of carotid artery stenosis: Efficacy of various Doppler velocity parameters. *American Journal of Roentgenology*, **160**, 619–25.

Huston, J. 3rd, James, E., Brown, R. D. Jr, *et al.* (2000). Redefined duplex ultrasonographic criteria for the diagnosis of carotid artery stenosis. *Mayo Clinic Proceedings*, **75**, 1133–40.

Kuntz, K. M., Polak, J. F., Whittermore, A. D., *et al.* (1997). Duplex ultrasound criteria for the identification of carotid stenosis should be laboratory specific. *Stroke*, **28**, 597–602.

Lal, B. K., Hobson, R. W. II, Goldstein, J., *et al.* (2004). Carotid artery stenting: Is there a need to revise ultrasound velocity criteria? *Journal of Vascular Surgery*, **39**, 58–66.

Lennihan, L., Krupsky, W. J., Mohr, J. P., *et al.* (1987). Lack of association between carotid plaque hematoma and ischemic cerebral symptoms. *Stroke*, **18**, 879–81.

Lovelace, T. D., Moneta, G. L., Abou-ZamZam, A. M. Jr, *et al.* (2001). Optimizing duplex follow-up in patients with an asymptomatic internal carotid artery stenosis of less than 60%. *Journal of Vascular Surgery*, **33**, 56–61.

Mattos, M. A., van Bemmelen, P. S., Barkmeier, I. D., *et al.* (1993). Routine surveillance after carotid endarterectomy: Does it affect clinical management? *Journal of Vascular Surgery*, **17**, 819–30.

Moneta, G. L., Edwards, J. M., Chitwood, R. W., *et al.* (1993). Correlation of North American Symptomatic Carotid Endarterectomy Trial (NASCET): Angiographic definition of 70% to 90% internal carotid artery stenosis with duplex scanning. *Journal of Vascular Surgery*, **17**, 152–9.

Moneta, G. L., Edwards, J. M., Papanicolaou, G., *et al.* (1995). Screening for asymptomatic internal carotid artery stenosis: Duplex criteria for discriminating 60% to 99% stenosis. *Journal of Vascular Surgery*, **21**, 989–94.

Neale, M. L., Chambers, J. L., Kelly, A. T., *et al.* (1994). Reappraisal of duplex criteria to assess significant carotid stenosis with special reference to reports from the North American symptomatic carotid endarterectomy trial and the European trial and the European carotid surgery trial. *Journal of Vascular Surgery*, **20**, 642–9.

Nehler, M. R., Moneta, G. L., Lee, R. W., *et al.* (1996). Improving selection of patients with less than 60% asymptomatic internal carotid stenosis for follow-up carotid artery duplex scanning. *Journal of Vascular Surgery*, **24**, 580–5.

Perkins, J. M., Galland, R. B., Simmons, M. J., *et al.* (2000). Carotid duplex imaging: Variation and validation. *British Journal of Surgery*, **87**, 320–2.

Pross, C., Shortsleeve, C. M., Baker, J. D., *et al.* (2001). Carotid endarterectomy with normal findings from a completion study: Is there need for early duplex scan? *Journal of Vascular Surgery*, **33**, 963–7.

Ranke, C., Creutzig, A., Becker, H., *et al.* (1999). Standardization of carotid ultrasound: A hemodynamic method to normalize for interindividual and interequipment variability. *Stroke*, **30**, 402–6.

Roederer, G. O., Langlois. Y. E., Chan, A. T., *et al.* (1982). Ultrasonic duplex scanning of the external carotid arteries: Improved accuracy using new features from the carotid artery. *Journal of Cardiovascular Ultrasonography*, **1**, 373–80.

Roederer, G. O., Langlois, Y. E., Jager, K. A., *et al.* (1989). A simple spectral parameter for accurate classification of severe carotid artery disease. *Bruit*, **3**, 174–8.

Roth, S. M., Back, M. R., Bandyk, D. F., *et al.* (1999). A rational algorithm for duplex scan surveillance after carotid endarterectomy. *Journal of Vascular Surgery*, **31**, 838–9.

Sarkari, N. B. and Bickerstaff, E. R. (1973). Neurological manifestations associated with internal carotid loops and kinks in children. *Journal of Neurology, Neurosurgery and Psychiatry*, **33**, 194.

Soulez, G., Therasse, E., Robillard, P., *et al.* (1999). The value of internal carotid systolic velocity ratio for assessing carotid artery stenosis with Doppler sonography. *American Journal of Roentgenology*, **172**, 207–12.

Srinivasan, J., Mayberg, M. R., Weiss, D. G., *et al.* (1995). Duplex accuracy compared with angiography in the veteran affairs cooperative studies trial for symptomatic carotid stenosis. *Neurosurgery*, **36**, 648–53.

Stanziale, S. F., Wholey, M. H., Boules, T. N., *et al.* (2005). Determining in-stent stenosis of carotid arteries by duplex ultrasound criteria. *Journal of Endovascular Therapy*, **12**, 346–53.

Strandness, D. E. Jr. (1990). *Duplex Scanning in Vascular Disorders*. New York: Raven Press, pp. 92–120.

Umemura, A. and Yamada, K. (2000). B-mode flow imaging of the carotid artery. *Stroke*, **32**, 2055–7.

van Everdingen, K. J. and Kapelle, L. J. (1998). Overestimation of a stenosis in the internal carotid artery by duplex sonography caused by an increase in flow volume. *Journal of Vascular Surgery*, **27**, 479–85.

10

Conventional digital subtraction angiography for carotid disease

Jean Marie U-King-Im and Jonathan H. Gillard

Addenbrooke's Hospital and the University of Cambridge, UK

Introduction

Carotid endarterectomy is now one of the most commonly performed vascular operations in the Western world, with significant increases in rates since the publication of large randomized trials such as the North American symptomatic carotid endarterectomy trial (NASCET) and the European carotid surgery trial [ECST], which have clearly demonstrated the benefits of surgery over medical therapy in recently symptomatic patients with severe carotid stenosis (randomized trial of endarterectomy for recently symptomatic carotid stenosis: final results of the MRC European carotid surgery trial (ECST), 1998; Barnett *et al.*, 1998; Tu *et al.*, 1998). In these trials, risk stratification was mainly based on severity of luminal stenosis and this has naturally highlighted the importance of accurate carotid imaging for patient selection. The gold standard method, in terms of diagnostic accuracy, for the measurement of stenosis remains conventional digital subtraction angiography (DSA), which was in routine use at the time of these trials. There are, however, several disadvantages associated with DSA. It is a relatively expensive and labor-intensive procedure whose costs may be up to 2.4 times that of alternative procedures such as magnetic resonance angiography (MRA) (U-King-Im *et al.*, 2004a). Moreover, patients, if given the choice, may tend to prefer less invasive modalities such as MRA (U. King-Im *et al.*, 2004c). More importantly, concerns about

potential risks of neurological complications associated with DSA, have generated strong interest in noninvasive modalities such as Doppler ultrasound (DUS), MRA or computerized tomography angiography (CTA) (Dawson *et al.*, 1997; Athanasoulis and Plomaritoglou, 2000; Long *et al.*, 2002). There is, however, strong ongoing controversy, regarding whether such noninvasive modalities, alone or in combination, can safely replace DSA as first-line modality in the routine work-up of the majority of patients with suspected carotid stenosis (Dawson *et al.*, 1997; Athanasoulis and Plomaritoglou, 2000; Long *et al.*, 2002; Norris *et al.*, 2003; Buskens *et al.*, 2004; U-King-Im *et al.*, 2005). Although there is no doubt that the routine use of DSA is generally declining, the catheter skills required to perform DSA remain crucial, especially as a prequel to carotid angioplasty or stenting, which are fast gaining acceptance and popularity (Langan *et al.*, 2005). This chapter reviews the current state of DSA in contemporary neurovascular imaging practice, including indications, techniques, complications and comparison with noninvasive techniques.

Indications and techniques

The main indication for carotid DSA in current practice remains the evaluation of carotid atherosclerotic disease and accurate measurement of stenosis. Other nonatherosclerotic indications such as fibromuscular dysplasia, dissection,

Carotid Disease: The Role of Imaging in Diagnosis and Management, ed. Jonathan Gillard, Martin Graves, Thomas Hatsukami and Chun Yuan. Published by Cambridge University Press. © Cambridge University Press 2007.

aneurysms or trauma are much less common and are outside the scope and objectives of this chapter. For atherosclerotic disease, DSA is usually performed as a confirmatory test, after a screening test, usually DUS, has suggested potentially significant carotid disease (Dawson *et al.*, 1997; Norris *et al.*, 2003). Because of the risks and costs associated with DSA, it is generally not thought cost-effective to perform DSA as first-line modality in unscreened patients with a stroke or a transient ischemic attack (Vanninen *et al.*, 1995). The threshold for proceeding to DSA after screening by DUS varies from institution to institution and may range from 30 to 70% stenosis by the NASCET criteria. DSA is routinely performed either as day-case procedure with between 4 and 6 hours of bed rest and monitoring or as an "overnight admission" procedure.

The techniques of cerebral angiography have significantly evolved since the pioneering days of Egas Moniz in the 1920s. In his initial series of nine cases, Moniz attempted direct carotid artery puncture through both the percutaneous method and through surgical exposure of the vessel, with varying degrees of success (Wolpert, 1999). Because of the subsequent initial use of thoroplast as contrast agent, with its high incidence of complications, cerebral angiography, however, took many years to slowly become accepted by the medical community as a viable and useful diagnostic procedure (Wolpert, 1999). Today, carotid angiography is most commonly performed through percutaneous puncture of the femoral artery under local anaesthetic. Although access through the upper extremity vessels is frequently used for coronary angiography, both carotid and cerebral angiography can also be safely performed through trans-radial, trans-brachial or trans-ulnar arterial punctures and there are recent reports of some centers advocating these approaches on the basis of decreased puncture-site-related complications and improved patient comfort (Matsumoto *et al.*, 2001; Nohara and Kallmes, 2003; Lee *et al.*, 2004). In addition, the trans-radial approach may be particularly suited to catheterization and

interventions in the right carotid and vertebral systems (Nohara and Kallmes, 2003). Attempts have also been made in the past to perform DSA through intravenous injections: two decades ago, there was enthusiasm for intravenous DSA as a replacement for conventional intraarterial DSA, with promising initial reports, but the technique was rapidly abandoned because of inaccuracy and complications (Turner and Murie, 1989).

If the common carotid arteries or brachiocephalic trunk are selectively catheterized, then two to four views of each carotid bifurcation are acquired, usually after injection of typically 5–7 ml of iodinated contrast medium. Although powered injectors can be used, and are probably more common place in the USA, manual injection is generally sufficient for high-quality images. With newer diagnostic DSA machines with biplane capabilities, the amount of contrast medium necessary is reduced as two perpendicular views can be achieved during the same injection. Meticulous attention to technique is essential throughout the procedure with emphasis on minimal manipulation of the arch and carotid vessels and careful catheter flushing to avoid potential embolization of thrombus which may have formed within the catheter. Alternatively, some centers now routinely use the technique of arch aortography, with the tip of the catheter parked in the ascending aorta and typically using antero-posterior and 30-degree left and right anterior oblique positions (Berczi *et al.*, 2006). This is thought to be safer than selective carotid angiography although a power injector is essential and a large volume of contrast material is rapidly injected, resulting in potential cardiovascular complications (Berczi *et al.*, 2005). In addition to the carotid bifurcation, standard views of each cerebral hemisphere are usually performed, to look for incidental intracranial pathology or tandem lesions, especially at the carotid siphon. Indeed, patients with coexisting intracranial atherosclerotic disease may have a worse prognosis and arguably medical therapy may need to be more intensive (Executive Committee for the Asymptomatic

Carotid Atherosclerosis Study, 1995). In symptomatic patients with moderate stenosis, the presence of tandem lesions has been shown to increase the benefit of surgery over medical therapy (Kappelle et al., 1999). Detection of tandem lesions is often quoted as a significant argument in favor of routine use of DSA, as DUS alone is obviously unable to provide such information and there is currently limited data regarding the ability and accuracy of MRA or CTA to do so. It remains unclear, however, to what extent such tandem lesions influence management decisions regarding proceeding to carotid endarterectomy (Rouleau et al., 1999).

Because of the common occurrence of noncircular stenotic lumens, the optimal projection to visualize the maximum stenosis may be missed with standard views of the carotid bifurcation. This is generally regarded as a limitation of DSA and may lead to underestimation of stenosis, especially if additional projections are not acquired at the discretion of the angiographer (Porsche et al., 2001). To overcome this problem, DSA machines with rotational capabilities have been introduced over the past few years and have been used to image the carotid artery during both common carotid artery catheterization and arch aortography (Pozzi Mucelli et al., 2005). Rotational DSA allows a 3D volume angiographic acquisition during injection of a single bolus of contrast medium. Studies can subsequently be viewed in 3D on workstations using image reconstruction algorithms such as volume rendering with unlimited projections possible and the optimal projection depicting the most severe stenosis can be reliably chosen for measurement purposes. As shown by Elgersma et al. in a sample of 47 stenotic internal carotid arteries, rotational DSA frequently depicted more severe stenosis compared to conventional DSA in two or three projections, with an additional seven cases regraded as severe (70–99% stenosis) with the use of 3D acquisitions (Elgersma et al., 1999). Similarly, the issue of noncircular lumens has also surfaced during discussions of comparisons between conventional 2D DSA and noninvasive modalities such as MRA and CTA which are essentially 3D volume acquisitions. It has thus been suggested that part of the reasons behind misclassification is the difference in the number of projections available. For instance, Elgersma et al. showed that the apparent overestimation of carotid stenosis at 3D time-of-flight MR angiography versus conventional DSA may be partly explained by the greater number of projection images available at MRA (Elgersma et al., 2000). Similarly, Anzalone et al. showed the best correlation between rotational DSA and contrast-enhanced MR angiography, with conventional DSA resulting in underestimation of stenosis (Anzalone et al., 2005). However, U-King-Im et al., recently compared DSA and MRA and found that, despite using identical projections, there was still a tendency toward overestimation of stenosis with MRA, suggesting that differences in resolution may also be partly responsible for misclassification (U-King-Im et al., 2004c).

Complications of DSA

Complications related to DSA can be classified as puncture-site-related, contrast-medium-related (allergic or nephrotoxic reactions) or neurological. Puncture-site complications such as minor hematomas have been reported with incidences up to 8% although it is rare that these delay hospital discharge (Willinsky et al., 2003; Berczi et al., 2006). More problematic complications such as pseudoaneurysms or large hematomas requiring surgical intervention are more infrequent (Willinsky et al., 2003).

There have been several published series of the risks of neurological complications after DSA (Mani et al., 1978; Faught et al., 1979; Eisenberg et al., 1980; Earnest et al., 1984; Dion et al., 1987; Skalpe, 1988; Grzyska et al., 1990; Hankey et al., 1990a; Waugh and Sacharias, 1992; Davies and Humphrey, 1993; Heiserman et al., 1994; Eliasziw et al., 1995; Leffers and Wagner, 2000; Johnston et al., 2001; Willinsky et al., 2003;

Table 10.1. Summary of main published data regarding the overall risks of neurological complications after cerebral angiography. The population of studies marked * included solely patients with suspected carotid stenosis or cerebrovascular disease

Design	Number of patients	Permanent neurological complications (%)	Transient neurological complications (%)	Reference
Prospective	5000	0.16	1.24	(Mani *et al.*, 1978)
Retrospective	147	5.20	7.00	(Faught *et al.*, 1979)*
Retrospective	85	0.00	1.30	(Eisenberg *et al.*, 1980)*
Prospective	1517	0.33	2.27	(Earnest *et al.*, 1984)
Prospective	1002	0.40	2.70	(Dion *et al.*, 1987)
Retrospective	2509	0.16	1.60	(Skalpe, 1988)
Prospective	2770	0.09	0.45	(Grzyska *et al.*, 1990)
Prospective	382	1.30	1.30	(Hankey *et al.*, 1990a)*
Prospective	2475	0.30	1.80	(Waugh and Sacharias, 1992)
Prospective	200	4.00	6.00	(Davies and Humphrey, 1993)*
Prospective	1000	0.50	0.50	(Heiserman *et al.*, 1994)
Prospective	2320	0.78	Not applicable	(Eliasziw *et al.*, 1995)*
Retrospective	483	0.40	1.90	(Leffers and Wagner, 2000)
Retrospective	569	0.50	0.40	(Johnston *et al.*, 2001)*
Prospective	2899	0.50	0.90	(Willinsky *et al.*, 2003)
Retrospective	311	0.00	0.90	(Berczi *et al.*, 2006)*

Berczi *et al.*, 2006). These are summarized in Table 10.1. For all indications included (i.e. excluding studies in which DSA was performed exclusively for cerebrovascular disease), the risks of permanent neurological complications can be seen to range from 0.09 to 0.50% and that of transient neurological complications from 0.45 to 2.70%. However, some of the series reporting complications rates at the higher end of the reported spectrum clearly date from more than two decades ago. Hankey *et al.* reviewed eight prospective and seven retrospective studies published prior to 1990 and found that the overall combined risk of transient ischemic attack (TIA)/stroke was 4.0%, including a 1.0% risk of disabling permanent stroke and a 0.1% mortality rate (Hankey *et al.*, 1990b). It is frequently argued that current advances in catheter technology, contrast medium and operator experience may currently have resulted in reduced procedural morbidity. If only studies from 1990 onwards are included for analysis, the rates of permanent neurological complications can be adjusted to range from 0.09 to 0.50% and that of transient neurological complications from 0.45 to 1.90% (Grzyska *et al.*, 1990; Hankey *et al.*, 1990a; Waugh and Sacharias, 1992; Davies and Humphrey, 1993; Heiserman *et al.*, 1994; Eliasziw *et al.*, 1995; Leffers and Wagner, 2000; Johnston *et al.*, 2001; Willinsky *et al.*, 2003; Berczi *et al.*, 2006). These rates are probably a more accurate reflection of contemporary practice but are, arguably, not significantly different from the figures quoted by Hankey *et al.*, suggesting that even in modern-day era, cerebral angiography remains associated with low but potentially significant morbidity and mortality.

The complication rates quoted in the series above, however, refer to cerebral angiography in general, which may be performed for a variety of indications other than carotid atherosclerotic disease. When DSA is performed for suspected carotid stenosis, there is evidence to suggest that complication rates may, in fact, be higher. Indeed, a meta-analysis by Cloft *et al.* clearly demonstrated that the overall combined neurological complication rate was significantly higher for TIA/stroke patients compared to patients with subarachnoid hemorrhage, aneurysms or arteriovenous malformations (3.9% vs. 0.8%), as was the risk of permanent neurological complications (0.7% vs. 0.07%) (Cloft *et al.*, 1999). In the individual studies included in this meta-analysis, Heiserman *et al.* reported that all their neurological complications occurred in patients presenting with stroke/TIA (Heiserman *et al.*, 1994). Moreover, the presence of carotid stenosis was also associated with higher incidence of neurological complications compared to the overall population studied but not to the subset of patients with previous stroke. Similarly, in the study by Dion *et al.* the risk of total neurological complications within the first 24 hours was 2.5% for patients being investigated for cerebrovascular disease compared to 1.3% overall (Dion *et al.*, 1987). These figures are consistent with the rate of permanent neurological complication rates of 0.78% reported in the NASCET study (Eliasziw *et al.*, 1995). In the most recent and largest series by Willinsky *et al.*, the overall rate of neurological complications was found to be only slightly higher in the stroke/carotid stenosis subgroup compared to the whole population (1.8% vs. 1.3%), as was the rate of permanent stroke (0.6% vs. 0.5%) (Willinsky *et al.*, 2003). Differences were clinically small and not statistically significant. Whether this reflects the particular expertise and skill of the angiographers at this institution is unclear.

The complication rates of two small studies by Davies *et al.* (4.0% permanent and 6.0% transient neurological complications) and by Faught *et al.* (5.20% permanent and 7.0% transient neurological complications), have to be highlighted as remarkably high and perhaps out of keeping with the remainder of the published literature, even accounting for the fact that they were performed exclusively in patients with suspected carotid stenosis (Faught *et al.*, 1979; Davies and Humphrey, 1993). The reasons behind this are unclear but this raises the possibility that published complication rates may reflect those of specialist centers with substantial angiography expertise and that actual complication rates in the average community or district general hospital may, in fact, be higher. Finally, the series by Berczi *et al.*, in whom all patients had arch aortography, reported the lowest complication rates of 0.90% TIA, with no permanent complications, findings consistent with the argument that arch aortography may be safer than selective carotid artery catheterization (Berczi *et al.*, 2006). However, this was a relatively small retrospective study and conclusions may perhaps need to be tempered until the results of larger series become available.

Moreover, although the apparent neurological complication rates quoted in the series above refer to clinically detectable complications, a number of studies have suggested that the incidence of silent embolic events may, actually, be much higher (Bendszus *et al.*, 1999; Britt *et al.*, 2000; Chuah *et al.*, 2004). Thus, Bendszus *et al.* showed, using pre- and postprocedural diffusion-weighted magnetic resonance imaging (MRI) in a series of 66 patients undergoing diagnostic cerebral angiography, that the incidence of new ischemic lesions may be as high as 26% (Bendszus *et al.*, 1999). Furthermore, in patients, with a history of vasculopathy, the frequency of radiological ischemic lesions was much higher compared to patients without vascular risk factors (44% vs. 13%). Whether such silent embolic events may have subtle long-term clinical effects such as mild effects on cognitive function is debatable but clearly within the realms of possibility.

Several mechanisms have been postulated to account for the occurrence of neurological complications. The most common cause is thought to be thrombus forming inside the catheters during manipulation of the guide wire or during guide wire withdrawal into the catheter, leaving blood to stagnate in this dead space. Disruption of plaque in the arch or bifurcation, as well as arterial dissection, has also been implicated. Meticulous attention to technique, as previously discussed, therefore remains a sine qua non to limit complication rates. It is noteworthy that in most series, complications happened within the first 24 hours of the procedure but Dion *et al.* showed that in a proportion of cases, symptoms can also occur between 24 and 72 hours (Dion *et al.*, 1987). It is debatable whether these relatively late events are directly attributable to DSA or whether they form part of the natural history of the disease (Willinsky *et al.*, 2003). In addition to a history of stroke/TIA, there have been a number of other identifiable risk factors associated with the occurrence of neurological complications. Willinsky *et al.* found a relative increase in risk of 22% for each 10-year increase in age, with significantly higher rates in patients aged 55 or above (Willinsky *et al.*, 2003). Long procedure times, which often reflected the difficulty of the procedure, have been found to have a direct correlation with increased complications (Heiserman *et al.*, 1994). Finally, increased rates of complications have been reported when trainees perform the procedure as opposed to more experienced angiographers (Davies and Humphrey, 1993).

Measurement systems for carotid stenosis

In clinical practice worldwide, several established measurement methods are used to quantify the severity of internal carotid artery (ICA) stenosis prior to revascularization (Figure 10.1). The NASCET method is most widely used in North America, while the ECST method tends to be frequently used in Europe (Randomised trial of endarterectomy for recently symptomatic carotid stenosis: final results of the MRC European Carotid Surgery Trial (ECST), 1998; Barnett *et al.*, 1998;

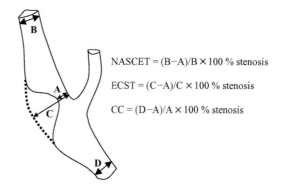

$$NASCET = (B-A)/B \times 100 \% \text{ stenosis}$$

$$ECST = (C-A)/C \times 100 \% \text{ stenosis}$$

$$CC = (D-A)/A \times 100 \% \text{ stenosis}$$

Figure 10.1 Diagram of an internal carotid artery stenosis illustrating different measurement methods. (A): Luminal diameter at the site of maximal narrowing; (B): diameter of normal distal internal carotid artery (ICA) beyond the bulb where the artery walls are parallel; (C): diameter of estimated original width of the ICA at the site of maximal narrowing; and (D): diameter of normal common carotid artery proximal to the bulb where artery walls are parallel.

Rothwell *et al.*, 2003a). There are several technical pitfalls which need to be highlighted to avoid inaccuracies (Eliasziw *et al.*, 1994a; Rothwell *et al.*, 1994a; Young *et al.*, 1996a). For the NASCET method, it is important that, for the denominator, the diameter of the ICA is measured well distal to the bulb, where the artery walls have become parallel to avoid overestimation of stenosis. For the ECST method, the denominator is measured as the diameter of the estimated original width of the ICA at the site of maximal stenosis rather than as the maximal diameter of the bulb, or otherwise again, stenosis will be overestimated. Moreover, a minority of centers use the common carotid (CC) method, which uses the proximal common carotid artery (CCA) as denominator, on the basis that it has previously been shown to be more reproducible (Rothwell *et al.*, 1994b; Wardlaw *et al.*, 2001). This increased interobserver agreement with the CC method has, however, not been confirmed subsequently (Young *et al.*, 1996a; U-King-Im *et al.*, 2004b).

Despite initial confusion generated by use of these different methods when the trials were first published, their equivalences as well as differences are now well understood. All these methods have been shown to have similar prognostic value, and as such, are acceptable means of risk stratification (Rothwell *et al.*, 1994b). Indeed, reanalysis of the results of ECST by the NASCET measurement method has shown that the two trials were largely consistent with each other (Rothwell *et al.*, 2003b). Both the ECST and CC methods generally result in a higher percentage stenosis compared to NASCET, given that the denominator used in NASCET, the distal ICA is generally smaller than the proximal ICA or CCA (Rothwell *et al.*, 1994a). To account for this, Rothwell *et al.* demonstrated the mathematical equivalence of the three methods through analysis of a large number of angiograms and mathematical regression techniques (Rothwell *et al.*, 1994a; Rothwell *et al.*, 2003a). For centers using the NASCET method, the pooled analysis of individual patient data from NASCET, ECST and Veteran Affairs Trial has confirmed that surgery is associated with a significant risk reduction in severe (70–99%) stenosis and a more marginal risk reduction in moderate stenosis (50–69%) (Rothwell *et al.*, 2003a). These cut-off points of 50% and 70% stenosis with NASCET method have been shown to roughly be equivalent to 65% and 82%, respectively, for both ECST and CC methods (Rothwell *et al.*, 1994a, 2003a). While such mathematical conversions are useful as an approximate guide, it should be noted that, in practice, even allowing for different thresholds for severity of stenosis, at an individual level, a patient may be classified in different categories of severity if different measurement methods are used (U-King-Im *et al.*, 2004b). Thus, a proportion of patients may be managed differently according to the measurement method used, supporting arguments that call for a universal measurement method to be adopted worldwide (Rothwell *et al.*, 2003b; U-King-Im *et al.*, 2004b).

Whatever the measurement method used, it should moreover be noted that determination of carotid stenosis is subject to significant inter-observer and intraobserver variability, even when performed by experts (Young *et al.*, 1996a). For instance, Young *et al.* compared inter-observer variability for each of the measurement methods. While typical measurement errors amongst different observers were on the order of ±5%, each method produced some sizable individual differences for the same angiogram, with resultant-wide 95% Bland-Altman limits of agreement, which ranged up to ±20%. A recent meta-analysis of published data regarding measurement error associated with carotid DSA revealed a standard deviation of 8% for the average error observed at 60% stenosis, implying a misclassification of approximately 4% overall (Heiserman, 2005). This raises the issue that, in fact, DSA is not a true gold standard and that this variability may need to be taken into consideration when noninvasive modalities are validated against DSA, as it may account for part of the misclassification (U-King-Im *et al.*, 2004d).

Angiographic determination of plaque surface morphology

The hypothesis that carotid plaque ulceration or surface irregularity may increase the risk of stroke originally initiated from analogies with coronary atherosclerosis pathophysiology; stable angina is usually associated with uncomplicated plaques with a smooth intact fibrous cap whereas unstable angina and myocardial infarction are almost invariably associated with irregular, fissured or ruptured fibrous cap, large necrotic lipid core with hemorrhage or thrombus formation (Imparato *et al.*, 1979; Falk, 1989; Fuster *et al.*, 1992; Spagnoli *et al.*, 2004).

Several studies have subsequently demonstrated that plaque surface irregularity or ulceration on DSA indicates a particularly high risk of stroke on medical treatment and increased benefit from carotid endarterectomy (Figure 10.2). Analysis of data from NASCET showed that the presence of angiographic ulceration in medically treated patients with severe stenosis increased the risk of

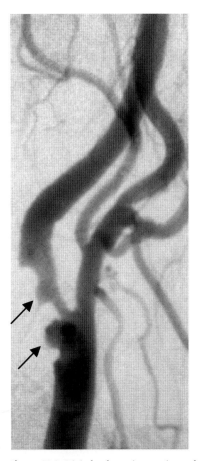

Figure 10.2 Digital subtraction angiography of a right internal carotid artery in a symptomatic patient with three episodes of transient ischemic attacks. There is a 68% stenosis, as measured by the NASCET criteria, as well as major surface irregularity with the presence of two large ulcer craters into the atheromatous plaque (arrows). The presence of such ulceration has been shown to be an independent predictor of increased risk of stroke in patients on medical therapy.

degrees of stenosis (hazard ratio = 1.80; 95% CI, 1.14−2.83) (Rothwell *et al.*, 2000a).

Distinction between an ulcer and irregularity on carotid DSA can be subjective, although definitions for an ulcer include a crater at least 2 mm deep on the profile view and a clear double density on the ''en face'' view (Streifler *et al.*, 1994; Eliasziw *et al.*, 1994b; Rothwell *et al.*, 2000a). The prevalence of such ulcers in the NASCET population was 14% and they have been shown to be more common proximal rather than distal to the point of maximal stenosis, correlating to points of maximal mechanical stress (Lovett and Rothwell, 2003). However, there has been controversy regarding the ability of DSA to resolve plaque surface morphology. For instance, Streifler *et al.* found little agreement between angiographic ulceration and surgical observations of carotid endarterectomy specimens in detecting plaque ulceration in the first 500 patients recruited into NASCET. Sensitivity and specificity of DSA for detection of ulcerated plaques were as low as 45.9% and 74.1%, respectively, with a positive predictive value of 71.8% (Streifler *et al.*, 1994). The inaccuracy of DSA for detection of ulceration was also shown by Eikelboom *et al.*, who compared radiological and morphological findings in 155 carotid endarterectomies (Eikelboom *et al.*, 1983). Diagnostic performance included a sensitivity of 73% and a specificity of 62%, with high interobserver variability: independent readers disagreed as to the presence of ulceration on DSA in up to 24% of cases.

These initial studies may however have been limited by the fact that the reference standard used was macroscopic evaluation of the endarterectomy specimens rather than detailed histological analysis. More recently, in contrast to these initial studies, Lovett *et al.* demonstrated strong and significant associations between the angiographic presence of ulceration and the presence of histological markers of vulnerable plaques such as large lipid cores, thin fibrous caps, intraplaque hemorrhage or plaque rupture (Lovett *et al.*, 2004). With the current trend toward noninvasive imaging, more data regarding the diagnostic performance

ipsilateral stroke at 24 months by a factor ranging from 1.24 to 3.43 (Eliasziw *et al.*, 1994b). These findings were confirmed by the European carotid surgery trialists, who demonstrated that angiographic plaque irregularity was an independent predictor of ipsilateral ischemic stroke on medical treatment not only for severe stenosis, but at all of noninvasive lumen-based modalities such as MRA and CTA for detection of ulceration are required. In one study, the sensitivity of contrast-enhanced MRA to detect DSA-defined ulceration was found to be only 65%, a fact accounted for by the current lower spatial resolution of MRA (U-King-Im et al., 2004d). More recently, as opposed to lumen-based angiographic modalities such as DSA or MRA, there is currently strong research interest in the ability of high-resolution axial multispectral MRI to directly characterize the vulnerable features of the carotid plaque including rupture and ulceration (Yuan et al., 2001; Trivedi et al., 2004). High-resolution MRI can easily be combined with an MRA examination, providing both luminal and detailed plaque morphological information at the same time. Although clearly, MRI is very likely to be superior to DSA with respect to plaque morphology, its exact role as a clinical tool still remains to be defined in practice.

Current trends and controversies

Although there have been an abundant number of studies dealing with carotid imaging in the literature, there is still ongoing debate regarding whether DSA is still necessary in the routine work-up of patients with suspected carotid stenosis (Davis and Donnan, 2003). Part of the problem may lie in that many of these studies are undermined by methodological factors such as poor design, inadequate sample size and inappropriate analysis and presentation of data, with the consequences that clinicians are often confused from measures of diagnostic accuracy for noninvasive tests that range from perfect to disturbingly poor (Rothwell et al., 2000b). For example, many centers base their decision-making prior to carotid endarterectomy on the results of DUS alone and there have been several reports in the surgical literature advocating the safety of this approach (Loftus et al., 1998; Logason et al., 2002). On the other hand, Johnston et al. found that DUS had a specificity of 46% only for detection of severe stenosis and that DSA would

have altered the decision to proceed to surgery in up to 28% of cases when compared to DUS alone. Similar confusing and conflicting reports can be found for both MRA (Johnston et al., 2002; U-King-Im et al., 2004d) and CTA (Berg et al., 2002; Alvarez-Linera et al., 2003) in the published literature. However, whatever the respective merits or flaws of each of these individual studies, it is clear that the performance of noninvasive tests will vary from institution to institution. Although traditionally, DUS is associated with high inter-observer variability, it is important to realize that the performance of both MRA and CTA will also vary significantly depending on the spatial resolution achieved, machines, equipment, imaging protocols, techniques as well as the experience of the readers (Murphy, 2005). It is thus, perhaps more important to determine the choice of imaging protocol prior to carotid endarterectomy at a local level, based on institutional choice, local expertise and complications related to DSA and internal validation of the performance of noninvasive tests such DUS, MRA or CTA.

Nonetheless, it is undeniable that the routine use of DSA for carotid imaging worldwide has now considerably decreased since its heyday in the 1980s. In the UK, a postal survey revealed that nearly 100% of centers use DUS as first-line modality and for up to 64% of centers, CTA or MRA was their preferred method for confirming equivocal DUS results (Osarumwense et al., 2005). Analysis of data from participants of the asymptomatic carotid surgery trial showed a significant trend occurring from 1993 to 1997: the proportion of centers using routine preoperative DSA had decreased from 77 to 26%, in parallel with an increase in the proportion using DSA selectively from 23 to 70% (Robless and Halliday, 1999). These trends have also been confirmed in the USA as well as in France (Dawson et al., 1997; Athanasoulis and Plomaritoglou, 2000; Long et al., 2002). These surveys also reveal a wide range of existing carotid imaging practices either with DUS alone, or with screening DUS and confirmatory DUS, MRA or CTA as the most popular noninvasive strategies. There is moreover strong emphasis on reducing the misclassification rates by using combinations of noninvasive strategies; for example decision-making can be based on DUS and MRA if the results are concordant but proceed to confirmatory DSA if the results disagree (U-King-Im *et al.*, 2004d).

The diagnostic performance of these individual modalities and strategies are reviewed in their corresponding chapters and is outside the scope of this discussion. However, the crux of the controversy resides in whether the misclassification associated with these noninvasive tests outweigh the benefits of more accurate imaging with DSA incurring the small risks of neurological complications. Results of recent cost-effectiveness analyses, which have modelled the complexities of this issue while taking into account the true costs of each strategy, tend to suggest that this is probably the case. Buskens *et al.* found that DUS alone resulted in less long-term morbidity than DSA and was more cost-effective (Buskens *et al.*, 2004). U-King-Im *et al.* recommended screening DUS and confirmatory contrast-enhanced MRA, with DSA reserved for discordant cases as the least morbid and most cost-effective strategy (U-King-Im *et al.*, 2005). The probability that DSA was most cost-effective was 4.1% or less. Similarly, the systematic review and cost-effectiveness modelling exercise by the United Kingdom Health and Technology Assessment Panel found that the combination of DUS and contrast-enhanced MRA was the most cost-effective strategy (Wardlaw *et al.*, 2006). Although, there was some disagreement in these studies about which noninvasive strategy was optimal, probably related to variability in diagnostic performance, there was general consensus that the risks of DSA were outweighed by use of noninvasive strategies.

Conclusions

Even in the modern-day era, DSA remains associated with a small but potentially significant risk of neurological complications. Its use in the routine assessment of patients with suspected carotid stenosis is declining in parallel with the increased popularity of noninvasive alternatives such as MRA and CTA. With further technological improvement in the quality of these noninvasive modalities, this trend is likely to continue. Nonetheless, DSA is still the gold standard method in terms of diagnostic accuracy and remains important as a confirmatory test when noninvasive tests are equivocal or disagree. Moreover, with the increasing acceptance of carotid angioplasty and stenting as a viable treatment strategy, the trend regarding the declining use of DSA may become reversed in the future and it is crucial that we continue to maintain the catheter skills required to perform DSA effectively and safely.

REFERENCES

Alvarez-Linera, J., Benito-Leon, J., Escribano, J., Campollo, J. and Gesto, R. (2003). Prospective evaluation of carotid artery stenosis: elliptic centric contrast-enhanced MR angiography and spiral CT angiography compared with digital subtraction angiography. *AJNR. American Journal of Neuroradiology*, **24**, 1012–19.

Anzalone, N., Scomazzoni, F., Castellano, R., *et al.* (2005). Carotid artery stenosis: intraindividual correlations of 3D time-of-flight MR angiography, contrast-enhanced MR angiography, conventional DSA, and rotational angiography for detection and grading. *Radiology*, **236**, 204–13.

Athanasoulis, C.A. and Plomaritoglou, A. (2000). Preoperative imaging of the carotid bifurcation. Current trends. *International Angiology*, **19**, 1–7.

Barnett, H.J., Taylor, D.W., Eliasziw, M., *et al.* (1998). Benefit of carotid endarterectomy in patients with symptomatic moderate or severe stenosis. North American Symptomatic Carotid Endarterectomy Trial Collaborators. *New England Journal of Medicine*, **339**, 1415–25.

Bendszus, M., Koltzenburg, M., Burger, R., *et al.* (1999). Silent embolism in diagnostic cerebral angiography and neurointerventional procedures: a prospective study. *Lancet*, **354**, 1594–7.

Berczi, V., Elfleet, E., Turner, D., Cleveland, T. J. and Gaines, P. A. (2005). Adverse cardiac events as a result of high volume contrast injection during rotational arch aortography. *Journal of Vascular and Interventional Radiology*, **16**, 558–9.

Berczi, V., Randall, M. and Balamurugan, R. (2006). Safety of arch aortography for assessment of carotid arteries. *European Journal of Vascular and Endovascular Surgery*, **31**, 3–7.

Berg, M. H., Manninen, H. I., Rasanen, H. T., Vanninen, R. L. and Jaakkola, P. A. (2002). CT angiography in the assessment of carotid artery atherosclerosis. *Acta Radiologica*, **43**, 116–24.

Britt, P. M., Heiserman, J. E., Snider, R. M., *et al.* (2000). Incidence of postangiographic abnormalities revealed by diffusion-weighted MR imaging. *AJNR. American Journal of Neuroradiology*, **21**, 55–9.

Buskens, E., Nederkoorn, P. J., Der Woude, T. B., *et al.* (2004). Imaging of carotid arteries in symptomatic patients: cost-effectiveness of diagnostic strategies. *Radiology*, **233**, 101–12.

Chuah, K. C., Stuckey, S. L. and Berman, I. G. (2004). Silent embolism in diagnostic cerebral angiography: detection with diffusion-weighted imaging. *Australasian Radiology*, **48**, 133–8.

Cloft, H. J., Joseph, G. J. and Dion, J. E. (1999). Risk of cerebral angiography in patients with subarachnoid hemorrhage, cerebral aneurysm, and arteriovenous malformation: a meta-analysis. *Stroke*, **30**, 317–20.

Davies, K. N. and Humphrey, P. R. (1993). Complications of cerebral angiography in patients with symptomatic carotid territory ischaemia screened by carotid ultrasound. *Journal of Neurology, Neurosurgery and Psychiatry*, **56**, 967–72.

Davis, S. M. and Donnan, G. A. (2003). Is carotid angiography necessary? Editors disagree. *Stroke*, **34**, 1819.

Dawson, D. L., Roseberry, C. A. and Fujitani, R. M. (1997). Preoperative testing before carotid endarterectomy: a survey of vascular surgeons' attitudes. *Annals of Vascular Surgery*, **11**, 264–72.

Dion, J. E., Gates, P. C., Fox, A. J., Barnett, H. J. and Blom, R. J. (1987). Clinical events following neuroangiography: a prospective study. *Stroke*, **18**, 997–1004.

Earnest, F. T., Forbes, G., Sandok, B. A., *et al.* (1984). Complications of cerebral angiography: prospective assessment of risk. *AJR. American Journal of Roentgenology*, **142**, 247–53.

Eikelboom, B. C., Riles, T. R., Mintzer, R., *et al.* (1983). Inaccuracy of angiography in the diagnosis of carotid ulceration. *Stroke*, **14**, 882–5.

Eisenberg, R., Bank, W. and Hedgcock, M. (1980). Neurologic complications of angiography for cerebrovascular disease. *Neurology*, **30**, 895–7.

Elgersma, O. E., Buijs, P. C. and Wust, A. F. (1999). Maximum internal carotid arterial stenosis: assessment with rotational angiography versus conventional intra-arterial digital subtraction angiography. *Radiology*, **213**, 777–83.

Elgersma, O. E., Wust, A. F., Buijs, P. C., *et al.* (2000). Multidirectional depiction of internal carotid arterial stenosis: three-dimensional time-of-flight MR angiography versus rotational and conventional digital subtraction angiography. *Radiology*, **216**, 511–16.

Eliasziw, M., Rankin, R. N., Fox, A. J., Haynes, R. B. and Barnett, H. J. (1995) Accuracy and prognostic consequences of ultrasonography in identifying severe carotid artery stenosis. North American Symptomatic Carotid Endarterectomy Trial (NASCET) Group. *Stroke*, **26**, 1747–52.

Eliasziw, M., Smith, R. F., Singh, N., *et al.* (1994a). Further comments on the measurement of carotid stenosis from angiograms. North American Symptomatic Carotid Endarterectomy Trial (NASCET) Group. *Stroke*, **25**, 2445–9.

Eliasziw, M., Streifler, J. Y. and Fox, A. J. (1994b). Significance of plaque ulceration in symptomatic patients with high-grade carotid stenosis. North American Symptomatic Carotid Endarterectomy Trial. *Stroke*, **25**, 304–8.

Executive Committee for the Asymptomatic Carotid Atherosclerosis Endarterectomy for asymptomatic carotid artery stenosis. (1995). Executive Committee for the Asymptomatic Carotid Atherosclerosis Study. *Journal of the American Medical Association*, **273**, 1421–8.

Falk, E. (1989). Morphologic features of unstable atherothrombotic plaques underlying acute coronary syndromes. *American Journal of Cardiology*, **63**, 114E–20E.

Faught, E., Trader, S. D. and Hanna, G. R. (1979). Cerebral complications of angiography for transient ischemia and stroke: prediction of risk. *Neurology*, **29**, 4–15.

Fuster, V., Badimon, L., Badimon, J. and Chesebro, J. (1992). The pathogenesis of coronary artery disease and the acute coronary syndromes. *New England Journal of Medicine*, **326**, 242–50.

Grzyska, U., Freitag, J. and Zeumer, H. (1990). Selective cerebral intraarterial DSA. Complication rate and control of risk factors. *Neuroradiology*, **32**, 296–9.

Hankey, G. J., Warlow, C. P. and Molyneux, A. J. (1990a). Complications of cerebral angiography for patients with mild carotid territory ischaemia being considered for carotid endarterectomy. *Journal of Neurology, Neurosurgery and Psychiatry*, **53**, 542–8.

Hankey, G. J., Warlow, C. P. and Sellar, R. J. (1990b). Cerebral angiographic risk in mild cerebrovascular disease. *Stroke*, **21**, 209–22.

Heiserman, J. (2005). Measurement error of percent diameter carotid stenosis determined by conventional angiography: implications for noninvasive evaluation. *American Journal of Neuroradiology*, **26**, 2102–7.

Heiserman, J. E., Dean, B. L., Hodak, J. A., *et al.* (1994). Neurologic complications of cerebral angiography. *AJNR. American Journal of Neuroradiology*, **15**, 1401–7; discussion 1408–11.

Imparato, A. M., Riles, T. S. and Gorstein, F. (1979). The carotid bifurcation plaque: pathologic findings associated with cerebral ischemia. *Stroke*, **10**, 238–45.

Johnston, D. C., Chapman, K. M. and Goldstein, L. B. (2001). Low rate of complications of cerebral angiography in routine clinical practice. *Neurology*, **57**, 2012–14.

Johnston, D. C., Eastwood, J. D., Nguyen, T. and Goldstein, L. B. (2002). Contrast-enhanced magnetic resonance angiography of carotid arteries: utility in routine clinical practice. *Stroke*, **33**, 2834–8.

Kappelle, L. J., Eliasziw, M., Fox, A. J., Sharpe, B. L. and Barnett, H. J. (1999). Importance of intracranial atherosclerotic disease in patients with symptomatic stenosis of the internal carotid artery. The North American Symptomatic Carotid Endarterectomy Trial. *Stroke*, **30**, 282–6.

Langan, E. M., 3rd, Gray, B. H. and Sullivan, T. M. (2005). Carotid angiography in contemporary vascular surgery practice. *Seminars in Vascular Surgery*, **18**, 83–6.

Lee, D. H., Ahn, J. H., Jeong, S. S., Eo, K. S. and Park, M. S. (2004). Routine transradial access for conventional cerebral angiography: a single operator's experience of its feasibility and safety. *British Journal of Radiology*, **77**, 831–8.

Leffers, A. M. and Wagner, A. (2000). Neurologic complications of cerebral angiography. A retrospective study of complication rate and patient risk factors. *Acta Radiologica*, **41**, 204–10.

Loftus, I. M., Mccarthy, M. J. and Pau, H. (1998). Carotid endarterectomy without angiography does not compromise operative outcome. *European Journal of Vascular and Endovascular Surgery*, **16**, 489–93.

Logason, K., Karacagil, S. and Hardermark, H. (2002). Carotid endarterectomy soley based on duplex scan findings. *European Journal of Vascular and Endovascular Surgery*, **36**, 9–15.

Long, A., Lepoutre, A., Corbillon, E., Branchereau, A. and Kretz, J. G. (2002). Modalities of preoperative imaging of the internal carotid artery used in France. *Annals of Vascular Surgery*, **16**, 261–5.

Lovett, J. K. and Rothwell, P. M. (2003). Site of carotid plaque ulceration in relation to direction of blood flow: an angiographic and pathological study. *Cerebrovascular Diseases*, **16**, 369–75.

Lovett, J. K., Gallagher, P. J., Hands, L. J., Walton, J. and Rothwell, P. M. (2004). Histological correlates of carotid plaque surface morphology on lumen contrast imaging. *Circulation*, **110**, 2190–7.

Mani, R. L., Eisenberg, R. L., Mcdonald, E. J., Jr., Pollock, J. A. and Mani, J. R. (1978). Complications of catheter cerebral arteriography: analysis of 5,000 procedures. I. Criteria and incidence. *AJR. American Journal of Roentgenology*, **131**, 861–5.

Matsumoto, Y., Hongo, K., Toriyama, T., Nagashima, H. and Kobayashi, S. (2001). Transradial approach for diagnostic selective cerebral angiography: results of a consecutive series of 166 cases. *AJNR. American Journal of Neuroradiology*, **22**, 704–8.

Murphy, K. (2005). Simplicity, voxels and finding the signal in the noise. *Annals of Neurology*, **58**, 493–4.

Nohara, A. M. and Kallmes, D. F. (2003). Transradial cerebral angiography: technique and outcomes. *AJNR. American Journal of Neuroradiology*, **24**, 1247–50.

Norris, J. W., Morriello, F., Rowed, D. W. and Maggisano, R. (2003). Vascular imaging before carotid endarterectomy. *Stroke*, **34**, E16.

Osarumwense, D., Pararajasingham, R., Wilson, P., Abraham, J. and Walker, S. (2005). Carotid artery imaging in the United Kingdom: a postal questionnaire of current practice. *Vascular*, **13**, 173–7.

Porsche, C., Walker, L., Mendelow, D. and Birchall, D. (2001). Evaluation of cross-sectional luminal morphology in carotid atherosclerotic disease by use of spiral CT angiography. *Stroke*, **32**, 2511–15.

Pozzi Mucelli, F., Calgaro, A., Bruni, S., Bottaro, L. and Pozzi Mucelli, R. (2005). Three-dimensional rotational angiography of the carotid arteries with high-flow injection from the aortic arch. Preliminary experience. *La Radiologia Medica*, **109**, 108–17.

Randomised trial of endarterectomy for recently symptomatic carotid stenosis: final results of the MRC European Carotid Surgery Trial (ECST). (1998). *Lancet*, **351**, 1379–87.

Robless, P. and Halliday, A. (1999). Vascular Surgical Society of Great Britain and Ireland: carotid angiography is used more selectively in the Asymptomatic Carotid Surgery Trial. *British Journal of Surgery*, **86**, 690–1.

Rothwell, P. M., Gibson, R. J., Slattery, J., Sellar, R. J. and Warlow, C. P. (1994a). Equivalence of measurements of carotid stenosis. A comparison of three methods on 1001 angiograms. European Carotid Surgery Trialists' Collaborative Group. *Stroke*, **25**, 2435–9.

Rothwell, P. M., Gibson, R. J., Slattery, J. and Warlow, C. P. (1994b). Prognostic value and reproducibility of measurements of carotid stenosis. A comparison of three methods on 1001 angiograms. European Carotid Surgery Trialists' Collaborative Group. *Stroke*, **25**, 2440–4.

Rothwell, P. M., Gibson, R. and Warlow, C. P. (2000a). Interrelation between plaque surface morphology and degree of stenosis on carotid angiograms and the risk of ischemic stroke in patients with symptomatic carotid stenosis. On behalf of the European Carotid Surgery Trialists' Collaborative Group. *Stroke*, **31**, 615–21.

Rothwell, P. M., Pendlebury, S. T., Wardlaw, J. and Warlow, C. P. (2000b). Critical appraisal of the design and reporting of studies of imaging and measurement of carotid stenosis. *Stroke*, **31**, 1444–50.

Rothwell, P. M., Eliasziw, M., Gutnikov, S. A., *et al.* (2003a). Analysis of pooled data from the randomised controlled trials of endarterectomy for symptomatic carotid stenosis. *Lancet*, **361**, 107–16.

Rothwell, P. M., Gutnikov, S. A. and Warlow, C. P. (2003b). Reanalysis of the final results of the European Carotid Surgery Trial. *Stroke*, **34**, 514–23.

Rouleau, P. A., Huston, J., 3rd, Gilbertson, J., *et al.* (1999). Carotid artery tandem lesions: frequency of angiographic detection and consequences for endarterectomy. *AJNR. American Journal of Neuroradiology*, **20**, 621–5.

Skalpe, I. O. (1988). Complications in cerebral angiography with iohexol (Omnipaque) and meglumine metrizoate (Isopaque cerebral). *Neuroradiology*, **30**, 69–72.

Spagnoli, L. G., Mauriello, A., Sangiorgi, G., *et al.* (2004). Extracranial thrombotically active carotid plaque as a risk factor for ischemic stroke. *Journal of the American Medical Association*, **292**, 1845–52.

Streifler, J. Y., Eliasziw, M., Fox, A. J., *et al.* (1994). Angiographic detection of carotid plaque ulceration. Comparison with surgical observations in a multicenter study. North American Symptomatic Carotid Endarterectomy Trial. *Stroke*, **25**, 1130–2.

Trivedi, R. A., U-King-Im, J. M., Graves, M. J., *et al.* (2004). MRI-derived measurements of fibrous-cap and lipid-core thickness: the potential for identifying vulnerable carotid plaques in vivo. *Neuroradiology*, **46**, 738–43.

Tu, J. V., Hannan, E. L., Anderson, G. M., *et al.* (1998). The fall and rise of carotid endarterectomy in the United States and Canada. *New England Journal of Medicine*, **339**, 1441–7.

Turner, W. H. and Murie, J. A. (1989). Intravenous digital subtraction angiography for extracranial carotid artery disease. *British Journal of Surgery*, **76**, 1247–50.

U-King-Im, J., Hollingworth, W., Trivedi, R., *et al.* (2005). Cost-effectiveness of diagnostic strategies prior to carotid endarterectomy. *Annals of Neurology*, **58**, 506–15.

U-King-Im, J., Hollingworth, W., Trivedi, R. A., *et al.* (2004a). Contrast-enhanced MR angiography vs intra-arterial digital subtraction angiography for carotid imaging: activity-based cost analysis. *European Radiology*, **14**, 730–5.

U-King-Im, J., Trivedi, R. A., Cross, J. J., *et al.* (2004b). Measuring carotid stenosis on contrast-enhanced magnetic resonance angiography. Diagnostic performance and reproducibility of 3 different methods. *Stroke*, **35**, 2083–8.

U.-King-Im, J., Trivedi, R., Cross, J., *et al.* (2004c). Conventional digital subtraction x-ray angiography versus magnetic resonance angiography in the evaluation of carotid disease: patient satisfaction and preferences. *Clinical Radiology*, **59**, 358–63.

U-King-Im, J., Trivedi, R. A., Graves, M. J., *et al.* (2004d). Contrast-enhanced MR angiography for carotid disease: diagnostic and potential clinical impact. *Neurology*, **62**, 1282–90.

Vanninen, R., Manninen, H. and Soimakallio, S. (1995). Imaging of carotid artery stenosis: clinical efficacy and cost-effectiveness. *AJNR. American Journal of Neuroradiology*, **16**, 1875–83.

Wardlaw, J. M., Chappell, F. M., Stephenson, M., *et al.* (2006). Accurate, practical and cost-effective assessment of carotid stenosis in the UK. *Health Technology Assessments*, **10**, 1–200.

Wardlaw, J. M., Lewis, S. C., Humphrey, P., *et al.* (2001). How does the degree of carotid stenosis affect the accuracy and interobserver variability of magnetic resonance angiography? *Journal of Neurology, Neurosurgery and Psychiatry*, **71**, 155–60.

Waugh, J. R. and Sacharias, N. (1992). Arteriographic complications in the DSA era. *Radiology*, **182**, 243–6.

Willinsky, R. A., Taylor, S. M., Terbrugge, K., *et al.* (2003). Neurologic complications of cerebral angiography: prospective analysis of 2,899 procedures and review of the literature. *Radiology*, **227**, 522–8.

Wolpert, S. M. (1999). Neuroradiology classics. *AJNR. American Journal of Neuroradiology*, **20**, 1752–3.

Young, G. R., Humphrey, P. R., Nixon, T. E. and Smith, E. T. (1996a). Variability in measurement of extracranial internal carotid artery stenosis as displayed by both digital subtraction and magnetic resonance angiography: an assessment of three caliper techniques and visual impression of stenosis. *Stroke*, **27**, 467–73.

Young, G. R., Sandercock, P. A., Slattery, J., *et al.* (1996b). Observer variation in the interpretation of intra-arterial angiograms and the risk of inappropriate decisions about carotid endarterectomy. *Journal of Neurology, Neurosurgery and Psychiatry*, **60**, 152–7.

Yuan, C., Mitsumori, L. M., Beach, K. W. and Maravilla, K. R. (2001). Carotid atherosclerotic plaque: noninvasive MR characterization and identification of vulnerable lesions. *Radiology*, **221**, 285–99.

11

Magnetic resonance angiography of the carotid artery

Martin J. Graves, Jean Marie U-King-Im and Jonathan H. Gillard

University of Cambridge, Cambridge CB2 2QQ, UK

Introduction

Magnetic resonance angiography (MRA) has emerged as one of the leading noninvasive modalities used to image the carotid artery. The core of MRA is its ability to portray blood vessels in a projective format similar to the gold standard, conventional digital subtraction angiography (DSA). The potential advantages of MRA over DSA are, however, numerous and compelling: MRA is less expensive, is the modality that patients tend to prefer, does not require iodinated contrast medium, is an outpatient procedure and more significantly, does not incur the 1–2% risks of neurological complications generally associated with intra-arterial catheterization (Willinsky et al., 2003; U-King-Im et al., 2004a,b). Recent advances in MRA technology, resulting from fast gradients and use of contrast agents has allowed substantial improvement in the quality of MRA examinations, leading to increased confidence of both radiologists and clinicians in the modality. Not surprisingly, this has been followed by the widespread use of MRA in the routine clinical work-up of patients with suspected carotid stenosis. This chapter summarizes the current state of carotid MRA. The first sections deal with the technical aspects of the various types of MRA, including time-of-flight (TOF), phase-contrast and contrast-enhanced MRA and highlight promising future developments as well as potential novel contrast agents. The current utility and efficacy of MRA in clinical practice is then discussed from an evidence-based perspective.

Time-of-flight (TOF) MRA

TOF MRA utilizes gradient-echo sequences with short repetition times (TR) to saturate the signal from stationary spins, whilst unsaturated spins flowing into the imaging slice with full magnetization yield a high signal (Wehrli et al., 1986). TOF MRA can be performed as either multiple 2D single slice acquisitions or as a 3D volumetric flow compensated acquisition. These sequences usually include additional gradient pulses to compensate for the phase shifts induced by moving spins (Nishimura et al., 1986; Laub and Kaiser, 1988). Postprocessing methods such as the maximum intensity projection (MIP) algorithm are used to accentuate these differences and produce an angiographic-type display (Laub, 1990), although the limitations of data presented in this manner should be appreciated (Anderson et al., 1990; Brown and Riederer, 1992). To maximize the in-flow effect the slices are usually acquired perpendicular to the major flow direction. For the carotid arteries the flow direction is primarily in the superior-inferior direction, implying the use of axial slices. It is important to always review the axial source data and not rely

Carotid Disease: The Role of Imaging in Diagnosis and Management, ed. Jonathan Gillard, Martin Graves, Thomas Hatsukami and Chun Yuan. Published by Cambridge University Press. © Cambridge University Press 2007.

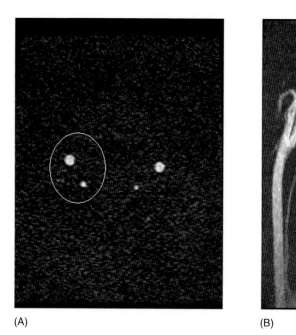

(A)   (B)

Figure 11.1 2D time-of-flight (TOF) magnetic resonance angiography. (A) shows a single 1.5-mm thick slice from a multiple slice axial 2D TOF acquisition; (B) shows the maximum intensity projection (MIP) in a perpendicular plane from the elliptical region shown in (A). A superior saturation slab is used to eliminate the venous signal.

only on the MIPs for measuring stenoses (Anderson *et al.*, 1994).

2D TOF

2D TOF MRA involves the sequential acquisition of many thin (approximately 1–2 mm) 2D slices, followed by MIP of the stacked slices (Keller *et al.*, 1989) (Figure 11.1). The advantage of this technique is that the saturation of background tissue is quite effective since high-flip angles can be used (typically 60°). The sequence is also sensitive to slow flow since the velocity threshold for complete replacement of spins (v = z/TR) is low because of the small slice thickness (z). Selectivity to a particular flow direction (i.e. arterial or venous) can be obtained by applying tracking presaturation bands either above or below the imaging slice, depending on the direction of flow to be suppressed. The disadvantages of 2D TOF include relatively long echo times (TE) associated with selecting thin slices, which can result in signal loss from turbulent or complex flow, and poor through-plane resolution compared with the in-plane resolution (Patel *et al.*, 1994). Clinical evaluations have shown reasonable agreement with contrast angiography (Litt *et al.*, 1991; Anderson *et al.*, 1992; Heiserman *et al.*, 1992; Huston *et al.*, 1993), with regions of flow gap correlating particularly well with significant stenosis (Heiserman *et al.*, 1996; Demarco *et al.*, 2001). Since TOF MRA relies on differences in the longitudinal magnetization for contrast a potential problem can arise when a luminal thrombus contains short T1 blood break-down products such as methamoglobin. Due to the shortened T1 relaxation times the thrombus may appear hyperintense on TOF MRA potentially mimicking vessel patency.

Using ECG or peripheral pulse gating in combination with short-TR gradient echoes can reduce the problem of pulsatility artefacts in 2D TOF; for example, in the aortic arch. By acquiring data only during peak systole, the vascular contrast is increased and ghosting artefacts are reduced (de Graaf and Groen, 1992), alternatively acquiring data in diastole when flow velocities are smaller has been shown to improve the depiction of carotid stenosis (Anderson *et al.*, 1994). 2D TOF methods are best used as rapid vascular localizers, or for screening.

3D TOF

3D TOF methods acquire a volume of data. A relatively thick slab of tissue is excited and then subdivided into thin slices or partitions by a second phase-encoding process in the slice-selection direction. Image reconstruction is achieved with a 3D Fourier transform (FT) instead of the usual 2D FT (Dumoulin *et al.*, 1989a; Obuchowski *et al.*, 1999). The advantage of slice encoding using this method is that much thinner slices can be reconstructed (typically as little as 0.7 mm), which improves the resolution and hence vessel conspicuity by reducing the partial volume effect and intravoxel phase dispersion due to complex/turbulent flow. The SNR in individual images is also significantly improved compared to 2D methods due to the excitation of a thick slab of tissue. However, this improvement in SNR also applies to the background tissue that limits the contrast and visibility of some small vessels in the final MIP, particularly in intracranial vessels. Magnetization transfer techniques are commonly used to reduce the background tissue signal (Pike *et al.*, 1992; Lin *et al.*, 1993).

Clinical comparisons with conventional angiography have demonstrated good agreement (Wagle *et al.*, 1989; Obuchowski *et al.*, 1999) for the measurement of carotid stenosis. Flow gaps on 3D MRA of the carotids have also been shown to correlate with severe stenosis (Nederkoorn *et al.*, 2002b), however this is critically dependent upon

the TE of the sequence (Lev *et al.*, 2003). A further problem with 3D TOF studies is the progressive saturation of slow flow. Repeatedly exciting a thick slab of tissue means that the signal from flowing spins gradually saturates as the spins penetrate more distally into the volume, i.e. spins progressively experience more radiofrequency (RF) pulses the longer they remain within the volume. Although the signal loss can be reduced through the use of small imaging flip angles, e.g. 25°, this is at the expense of an overall reduction in vascular contrast. Various approaches have been adopted to try and reduce this effect including ramped excitation pulses and the use of multiple, overlapping, thin slabs. Ramped RF pulses are specially designed excitation pulses that increase the flip angle across the 3D acquisition volume (Nagele *et al.*, 1995; Priatna and Paschal, 1995; Ikushima *et al.*, 1997). Instead of exciting a flat-topped rectangular slab profile, the profile is a trapezoid with a linear variation of flip angle with position through the slab. The ramp direction is set so that the higher flip angles are used more distally in the slab, i.e. downstream of the blood flow to help compensate for the saturation, whilst the lower flip angles are proximally in the slab to ensure that the inflowing spins are not saturated. The second improvement is the use of a 2D/3D hybrid technique, often termed MOTSA (Multiple Overlapping Thin Slab Acquisition) (Blatter *et al.*, 1993) (Figure 11.2). This method aims to reduce the saturation effect by reducing the thickness of the 3D slabs, but maintains the volume coverage by using multiple slabs. Continuity is maintained by slightly overlapping the slabs, and discarding the overlapping slices when doing the final MIP. This can sometimes cause a slab boundary artefact (SBA) commonly known as the "venetian blind" effect (Figure 11.2). Various methods have been used to try and reduce this effect including the optimization of imaging parameters together with postprocessing of data in the overlap region (Blatter *et al.*, 1993), the use of ramped excitation pulses (Ding *et al.*, 1994) and sliding interleaved kY (SLINKY) acquisition (Liu and Rutt, 1998).

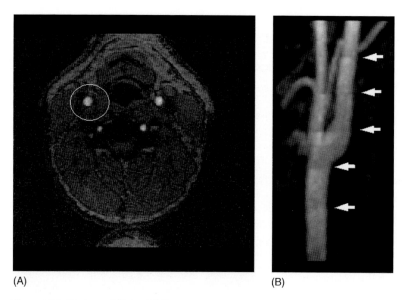

(A)   (B)

Figure 11.2 3D time-of-flight (TOF) magnetic resonance angiography. (A) shows a single 0.7-mm thick slice from an axial six slab 3D TOF acquisition; (B) shows the maximum intensity projection (MIP) in a perpendicular plane from the elliptical region shown in (A). Note the slab boundary artefact. A superior saturation slab is used to eliminate the venous signal.

Phase contrast

Phase-contrast MRA relies on detecting changes in the phase of blood's transverse magnetization as it moves along a magnetic field gradient. A bipolar imaging gradient will give a zero phase shift for stationary spins, but a nonzero phase shift for moving spins (Moran, 1982). In a phase-contrast pulse sequence additional bipolar gradients are used to create a known linear relationship between blood velocity and the phase of the MR signal. The constant linking velocity and phase angle is known as the velocity encoding or "venc". The venc is the maximum velocity that will be properly encoded by the sequence (Pelc *et al.*, 1991b).

Phase-contrast MRI is most commonly used with gradient-echo acquisitions. This means that variations in static magnetic field homogeneity produce nonuniform phase shifts even for stationary spins. Therefore, two acquisitions are performed with the bipolar velocity-encoding gradients reversed in

polarity for the second acquisition. The phase images for each acquisition are then calculated and subtracted. Since the background phase variation due to the inhomogeneous magnetic field is constant, after subtraction the background is zero with positive and negative values (phase shifts) only where the spins are moving. Finally to suppress background pixels, e.g. air, where the phase is essentially random, the phase subtraction image is multiplied, pixel-by-pixel, with the conventional magnitude image (Pelc *et al.*, 1991b).

Phase-contrast MRA is also directionally sensitive, which means only blood moving in the same direction, as a bipolar flow-encoding gradient will result in a phase shift. Therefore, it is necessary to match the flow-encoding axes to the direction of blood flow. In most cases blood vessels follow a fairly tortuous path throughout the body and we have to flow-sensitize in the slice select, phase encoding and frequency encoding directions. Although this means that in principle six acquisitions are required, it is usual to reduce this to four, e.g. one in each direction and one with no velocity sensitizing, although in practice there are more efficient schemes, that can improve the signal-to-noise ratio (SNR) (Dumoulin *et al.*, 1991; Hausmann *et al.*, 1991; Pelc *et al.*, 1991a). Even so, this means that a phase-contrast MRA study with velocity sensitization in all three directions will take at least four times as long as an equivalent TOF study. Even if velocity sensitization is only required in a single direction, e.g. for through-plane flow quantification, we still need two acquisitions. In order to produce an angiogram the individual phase images for each flow direction are combined. This involves calculating for each pixel the resultant flow magnitude from the three vector directions x, y and z using the expression:

$$|v| = \sqrt{x^2 + y^2 + z^2} \qquad (11.1)$$

The resultant magnitude image has no directional information and is best termed a "speed" image (Figure 11.3). Also since each velocity value is squared in the calculation, all the positive and negative velocity information is eliminated and thus any aliasing that might have occurred disappears from the speed image. The result is an image with a background value of zero (black) and positive values only for pixels with flow. Since this processing avoids the problems of flow aliasing, the venc can be set to the average velocity within a vessel, which for laminar flow is about half the peak velocity. This has the effect of increasing the signal from spins near the vessel wall that are travelling more slowly, giving a more realistic visualization of the true diameter of the vessels. Finally, since only moving spins give signals on phase-contrast MRA images, they do not have the same problems with short-T1 blood-breakdown products as TOF MRA images.

2D PC

2D phase contrast (2D PC) is a single-slice method, usually used to provide a projection angiogram through a thick slice, i.e. visualization of all vessels

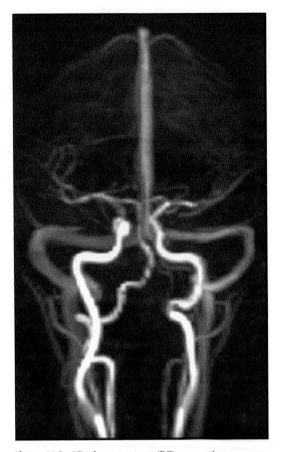

Figure 11.3 3D phase contrast (PC) magnetic resonance angiography. Coronal maximum intensity projection from a 3D PC acquisition acquired in the sagittal plane. Note the different signal intensities in the arteries and veins due to the different blood velocities.

within the slab – very similar to an X-ray angiogram. Signal cancellation can occur in regions where vessels with flow in opposite directions overlap along the projection direction. The use of thick slices, however, requires two slight modifications to the technique. First, because blood vessels will only occupy a small proportion of the slice volume, an additional dephasing gradient is applied in the slice-select direction (Dixon *et al.*, 1986). This has the effect of reducing the large signal from stationary tissue. Second, instead of a phase subtraction, a "complex" subtraction is performed, i.e. a vector rather than a phase subtraction is performed. Complex subtraction produces a better quality image in this situation, compared with phase subtraction (Bernstein and Ikezaki, 1991). Because 2D PC is a single-slice technique, angiograms can be produced quite quickly (Little *et al.*, 1988). Alternatively the sequence can be combined with cardiac triggering to obtain multiphase cardiac images, producing dynamic angiograms. Depending on the choice of venc, images of either slow or fast flow may be acquired. The speed of acquisition also means that they can be used as "venc localizers" to choose the optimal venc for a more time-consuming 3D PC study.

Thin section 2D PC techniques using phase difference processing can be used to produce phase contrast images that show flow direction and also permit the quantification of flow velocity and volume flow rate, particularly when combined with ECG triggering to produce cine images. Although not an angiographic technique these methods can be used to provide additional hemodynamic information, for example, in differentiating critical stenosis from total occlusion (Vanninen *et al.*, 1995a).

3D PC

3D PC MRA is a thin-slice volumetric technique with each slice having velocity sensitization in the required directions, usually all three (Dumoulin *et al.*, 1989b). This means that 3D PC studies are quite time-consuming and usually we have to sacrifice some resolution in the phase-encoding direction for a reduction in scan times. The MIP algorithm processes the speed images from each 3D slice as usual in order to produce an angiogram.

Despite of the longer acquisition times, 3D PC produces better quality images than thick-slab projection 2D PC methods since much thinner slices are possible. The use of a low venc means that good 3D images of slow flow can be obtained, which are not possible with 3D TOF techniques due to slow flow saturation. One of the disadvantages of 3D PC is the requirement for all the additional bipolar flow-encoding gradients, which increases the TE resulting in poorer image quality in areas of complex flow or magnetic susceptibility. However, the presence of a flow gap and poststenotic signal loss has been shown to be a reliable marker of severe (>80%) stenosis (Iseda *et al.*, 2000). Furthermore, since PC methods are by definition not flow-compensated, there is increased artefact seen around vessels with pulsatile flow.

Contrast-enhanced MRA

Gadolinium-based contrast agents have been used with TOF MRA in order to improve the SNR of carotid angiograms (Cloft *et al.*, 1996). However, the term "contrast-enhanced (CE) MRA" generally refers to MR angiograms acquired during the first pass of a paramagnetic contrast agent, usually a Gd-chelate, which reduces the T1 relaxation time of tissue (Korosec *et al.*, 1999). CE MRA can be considered to be a variant of 3D TOF techniques since we are exploiting differences in the longitudinal magnetization to yield vascular contrast. However, unlike TOF methods, these differences arise because of the shortening of the blood's T1 relaxation time by the contrast agent, rather than the TOF phenomenon. This means that vascular contrast is relatively independent of flow dynamics and problems associated with saturation effects are considerably reduced. CE MRA can therefore be used to acquire large field-of-view 3D angiograms in coronal or sagittal planes without the problems of spin saturation (Figure 11.4). A fast 3D gradient-echo sequence, with short TE and TR, is used to capture the first-pass transit of the contrast agent bolus through the area of interest. The TE is usually minimized by not using flow-compensation methods and by employing fractional echo data collection.

The reduction in T_1 achievable with a paramagnetic contrast agent is given by:

$$\frac{1}{T_{1,\text{post}}} = \frac{1}{T_{1,\text{pre}}} + R_1 \cdot [C_A] \qquad (11.2)$$

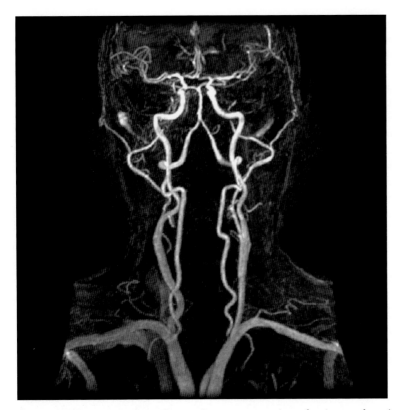

Figure 11.4 3D contrast enhanced magnetic resonance angiography. A coronal maximum intensity projection obtained in 40 s. Note the extended coverage achievable using a dedicated neurovascular coil.

where $T_{1,\text{pre}}$ is the T_1 of blood prior to administration of the agent (typically 1200 ms), $T_{1,\text{post}}$ is the T_1 of blood following administration, R_1 is the relaxivity of the contrast agent and $[C_A]$ is the concentration of the agent. Standard Gd-DTPA has a concentration of 0.5 molL^{-1} and an R_1 of approximately 4.5 mM^{-1}s^{-1} at 1.5 T.

For first-pass studies the dynamic contrast agent concentration $[C_A]$ is given (Prince *et al.*, 2003):

$$[C_A] = \frac{\text{injection rate } \left(\text{mls}^{-1}\right)}{\text{cardiac output } \left(\text{Ls}^{-1}\right)} \qquad (11.3)$$

The objective is to reduce the T_1 of blood to below that of the most hyperintense tissue on T_1-weighted imaging, typically fat with a T_1 of around 270 ms at 1.5 T. Using Equations (11.2) and

(11.3) above it can be seen that an injection rate of 2–3 mls^{-1} the T_1 of blood can be reduced to around 20 ms over a wide range of cardiac outputs.

Practically CE MRA is performed by injecting the contrast agent as a bolus, usually using an MR-compatible power injector and imaging during the first pass of the contrast agent through the anatomy of interest. Synchronization of the injection and the initiation of the scan are critically important and the relevant issues of scan timing and phase-encode ordering are discussed in detail below. Carotid MRA usually involves imaging from the aortic arch to the middle cerebral arteries necessitating the use of a coil that provides extended coverage over this region. Most MR system vendors provide dedicated multielement neurovascular coils that can provide this coverage with good SNR. Breath-holding has been shown to provide significantly sharper images of the arch and great vessel origins but to have no effect on the carotid vessels themselves (Carr *et al.*, 2002). An imaging protocol for CE MRA will generally involve the use of the shortest possible TE, ideally <1 ms, to minimize intravoxel spin dephasing and T_2^* decay, and the shortest possible TR, ideally <5 ms, to keep the overall acquisition time as short as possible. The optimal flip angle is dependent upon the blood T_1 and the TR but a value of 45° is good for a TR of 5 ms and an injection rate of 2 mls^{-1}. A target spatial resolution of $1 \times 1 \times 1$ mm is desirable (Fain *et al.*, 1999), with zero-filling interpolation techniques used to trade-off acquisition time with anterior-posterior coverage (Bernstein *et al.*, 2001), although reports have shown that decreasing the voxel size may improve the depiction of the stenosis compared to conventional angiography but does not improve diagnostic yield (Cosottini *et al.*, 2003). Once acquired the images may be subtracted from a baseline acquisition acquired without contrast to eliminate residual background signals making the vessels more conspicuous (Korosec *et al.*, 1999).

Timing

Timing is critical in CE MRA studies; the scan acquisition has to be timed to coincide with peak contrast agent concentration in the area of interest. Otherwise image quality can be significantly impaired (Slosman *et al.*, 1998). In order to maximize arterial contrast it is important to ensure that the centre of MR raw data space (*k*-space), which primarily contributes to the contrast in an image, is acquired when the arterial contrast agent concentration is at its peak in the area of interest. Since there is a delay between peak arterial and venous enhancement it is possible, with appropriate sequences and phase-encode ordering, to capture only the arterial phase. The importance of the phase-encode ordering is discussed below. Acquiring data too early with respect to the injection can result in poor arterial

enhancement and vessel edge artefacts (Maki *et al.*, 1996) whist acquiring data too late not only gives poor arterial enhancement but also unwanted venous enhancement. Whilst the circulation time can be estimated for each patient or standardized for all patients (Levy and Prince, 1996), the best and most consistent results are obtained by optimizing the timing, either retrospectively or prospectively.

The retrospective method involves the injection of a small test bolus, typically 2 ml, of contrast. Rapid repeat (multiphase dynamic) imaging of a slice through the vessel at the level of interest is performed during the injection. Analysis of the multiphase images shows a peak in the signal intensity when the contrast reaches the area of interest. Thus the circulation time of the contrast through the patient can be determined (Kim *et al.*, 1998).

There are currently two prospective triggering methods. The first uses a rapid one-dimensional (1D) monitoring sequence that detects the increase in signal intensity as the contrast agent arrives in the area of interest (or lower in the arterial path) and starts the 3D MRA sequence automatically (Yuan *et al.*, 1994; Isoda *et al.*, 1998). The second method uses rapid "fluoroscopic" imaging at the level of interest so that the operator can see the contrast arrive and then manually start the MRA sequence (Wilman *et al.*, 1998). This technique has been reported as being 97.3% reliable in 330 cases (Riederer *et al.*, 2000). For both triggering methods the MR system also needs to provide a rapid switch over between the monitoring sequence and the actual 3D CE MRA sequence.

Phase-encode ordering

A major factor in the optimization of CE MRA of the extracranial arterial circulation is to minimize the signal within the venous circulation. In the abdomen and peripheral circulation this is relatively easy given the difference in circulation time between the arteries and veins. However, in the head and neck the rapid transit of the contrast agent from arteries to veins, typically 6 or 7 s, means that it is very difficult to obtain purely arterial angiograms without some degree of venous enhancement. In order to overcome this problem researchers have developed new strategies for the ordering of data acquisition (Wilman *et al.*, 1998; Watts *et al.*, 2002; Willinek *et al.*, 2002).

We know that the center of k-space is the most important for controlling the contrast within an image. In a conventional encoded 3D sequence the entire slice-encoding (k_{SS}) loop is acquired before the k_{PE} phase-encoding step is changed. So even if the phase-encoding were centrically ordered (i.e. starting at zero and increasing to the maximum, alternating between positive and negative) we would be acquiring central k_{SS} lines right through the acquisition. The elliptic centric ordering acquires the k_{SS} and k_{PE} lines in a spiral fashion starting from the center and moving outward depending upon the actual spacing in k-space for each k_{PE} and k_{SS} step. In this way all the central k-space lines are acquired together. This ordering is known as elliptic centric (Wilman *et al.*, 1998). This ordering means that the center of k-space is acquired almost a factor of 10 times faster than a conventional centric acquisition. Therefore scans with a much higher spatial resolution can be obtained even though the overall scan time will be many times longer than the arterial-venous transit (Fain *et al.*, 1999).

Elliptic centric ordering together with a test bolus has shown to be more effective than MOTSA (De Marco *et al.*, 2001) and single-detector spiral computerized tomography angiography (CTA) (Alvarez-Linera *et al.*, 2003), whilst its use in combination with fluoroscopic triggering has demonstrated excellent agreement with conventional angiography, ultrasound and endarterectomy specimens (Fellner *et al.*, 2000; Huston *et al.*, 2001; Phan *et al.*, 2001).

Recently parallel imaging techniques such as sensitivity encoding (SENSE) (Pruessmann *et al.*, 1999), simultaneous acquisition of spatial harmonics (SMASH) (Sodickson and Manning, 1997)

and generalized autocalibrating partially parallel acquisition (GRAPPA) (Anderson *et al.*, 1992) have been developed that exploit multichannel coil arrays to allow reductions in MR imaging times without sacrificing spatial resolution, albeit at a reduction in SNR. When applied in combination with elliptic centric acquisitions SENSE has been demonstrated to reduce venous contamination by 20% (Hu *et al.*, 2004) and to produce higher SNR with reduced ringing artefacts at higher injection rates (Riedy *et al.*, 2005).

Dynamic CE MRA

In comparison to conventional angiography, CE MRA is generally a static imaging technique and gives very little information on flow dynamics. There are a number of methods by which multiphase 2D single-slice projection (Wang *et al.*, 1996; Hennig *et al.*, 1997) or 3D volume (Levy and Prince, 1996; Melhem *et al.*, 1999) CE MRA acquisitions can be performed. A 3D volume could be repeated multiple times but the temporal resolution would be quite poor unless the time for an individual volume is reduced. The most common methods for reducing scan time in 3D CE MRA are to use the shortest possible TR, to use partial Fourier acquisitions and to decrease the resolution, particularly in the phase-encoding and slice-selection directions. The reduction in acquisition resolution can be partly offset through the use of zero-filling interpolation methods. If repeated fast enough then a pure arterial phase volume should occur in at least one of the acquisitions (Levy and Prince, 1996). Alternatively only the central k-space data can be repeatedly acquired, a technique known as keyhole imaging. This has been demonstrated to acquire 3D volumes of the carotid at a rate of 3.6 per second (Melhem *et al.*, 1999). As discussed above, parallel imaging techniques such as SENSE can also be employed to reduce the acquisition time for an individual volume (Golay *et al.*, 2001). Alternatively methods that leverage the relationship between the bulk of the image contrast and the acquisition of the centre of k-space can be used to acquire volumes

DSA reserved for disparate results may reduce the number of diagnostic misclassifications (U-King-Im et al., 2004c). Such combination strategies have also been found to be cost-effective when the true costs of these diagnostic pathways are incorporated (U-King-Im et al., 2005).

MRA generally tends to overestimate stenosis compared to DSA. It was initially thought that this was due to the use of different projections in the measurement process when stenosed lumens were noncircular; MRA being a 3D technique with unlimited number of projections possible while conventional DSA is a 2D modality with 2–4 projections usually acquired (Nederkoorn et al., 2002a). It has subsequently been shown that, even with similar projections, there is still a tendency toward overestimation with MRA (U-King-Im et al., 2004c). Another explanation is that the submillimeter spatial resolution currently achieved by MRA is still lagging behind that of DSA (0.32×0.32 mm) by a factor of 2–3 times (Figure 11.7). Finally, it is noteworthy that there will be wide variations in the spatial resolution achieved by MRA across different centers, depending on the type and make of MR machine, imaging protocols and coils (Nederkoorn et al., 2003). This means that, like ultrasound, individual centers may need to be aware about how their MRA technique compares to DSA at a local level through audit and internal validation.

Conclusion

MRA of the carotid vessels is a well-established technique that is becoming accepted for the diagnosis of clinically significant stenosis and appears likely to replace contrast angiography. Amongst the various types of MRA available, 2D TOF and PC techniques are suitable for screening but they suffer from a number of technical limitations. Targeted 3D TOF may still have slightly higher spatial resolution, but CE MRA is slowly emerging as the most effective technique for obtaining large coverage, high contrast vascular

images for the overall detection of carotid disease. High resolution imaging with intravascular contrast agents represent promising technical developments which will further enhance the quality of MRA and thus its acceptability in the clinical arena.

REFERENCES

Alvarez-Linera, J., Benito-Leon, J., Escribano, J., Campollo, J. and Gesto, R. (2003). Prospective evaluation of carotid artery stenosis: elliptic centric contrast-enhanced MR angiography and spiral CT angiography compared with digital subtraction angiography. AJNR. American Journal of Neuroradiology, 24, 1012–19.

Anderson, C. M., Lee, R. E., Levin, D. L., De La Torre Alonso, S. and Saloner, D. (1994). Measurement of internal carotid artery stenosis from source MR angiograms. Radiology, 193, 219–26.

Anderson, C. M., Saloner, D., Lee, R. E., et al. (1992). Assessment of carotid artery stenosis by MR angiography: comparison with x-ray angiography and color-coded Doppler ultrasound. AJNR. American Journal of Neuroradiology, 13, 989–1003; discussion 1005–8.

Anderson, C. M., Saloner, D., Tsuruda, J. S., Shapeero, L. G. and Lee, R. E. (1990). Artifacts in maximum-intensity-projection display of MR angiograms. AJR. American Journal of Roentgenology, 154, 623–9.

Athanasoulis, C. A. and Plomaritoglou, A. (2000). Pre-operative imaging of the carotid bifurcation. Current trends. International Angiology, 19, 1–7.

Bernstein, M. A. and Ikezaki, Y. (1991). Comparison of phase-difference and complex-difference processing in phase-contrast MR angiography. Journal of Magnetic Resonance Imaging, 1, 725–9.

Bernstein, M. A., Fain, S. B. and Riederer, S. J. (2001). Effect of windowing and zero-filled reconstruction of MRI data on spatial resolution and acquisition strategy. Journal of Magnetic Resonance Imaging, 14, 270–80.

Blatter, D. D., Bahr, A. L., Parker, D. L., et al. (1993). Cervical carotid MR angiography with multiple overlapping thin-slab acquisition: comparison with conventional angiography. AJR. American Journal of Roentgenology, 161, 1269–77.

Bluemke, D. A., Stillman, A. E., Bis, K. G., et al. (2001). Carotid MR angiography: phase II study of safety and efficacy for MS-325. Radiology, 219, 114–22.

Bossuyt, P. M., Reitsma, J. B., Bruns, D. E., *et al.* (2003). Towards complete and accurate reporting of studies of diagnostic accuracy: the STARD initiative. *British Medical Journal*, **326**, 41–4.

Brown, D. G. and Riederer, S. J. (1992). Contrast-to-noise ratios in maximum intensity projection images. *Magnetic Resonance in Medicine*, **23**, 130 7.

Carr, J. C., Ma, J., Desphande, V., *et al.* (2002). High-resolution breath-hold contrast-enhanced MR angiography of the entire carotid circulation. *AJR. American Journal of Roentgenology*, **178**, 543–9.

Catalano, C., Pediconi, F., Nardis, P., *et al.* (2004). MR angiography with MultiHance for imaging the supra-aortic vessels. *European Radiology*, **14** (Suppl. 7), O45–51; discussion O61–2.

Cloft, H. J., Murphy, K. J., Prince, M. R. and Brunberg, J. A. (1996). 3D gadolinium-enhanced MR angiography of the carotid arteries. *Magnetic Resonance Imaging*, **14**, 593–600.

Cosottini, M., Calabrese, R., Puglioli, M., *et al.* (2003). Contrast-enhanced three-dimensional MR angiography of neck vessels: does dephasing effect alter diagnostic accuracy? *European Radiology*, **13**, 571–81.

Davis, S. M. and Donnan, G. A. (2003). Is carotid angiography necessary? Editors disagree. *Stroke*, **34**, 1819.

Dawson, D. L., Roseberry, C. A. and Fujitani, R. M. (1997). Preoperative testing before carotid endarterectomy: a survey of vascular surgeons' attitudes. *Annals of Vascular Surgery*, **11**, 264–72.

De Graaf, R. G. and Groen, J. P. (1992). MR angiography with pulsatile flow. *Magnetic Resonance Imaging*, **10**, 25–34.

De Marco, J. K., Schonfeld, S., Keller, I. and Bernstein, M. A. (2001). Contrast-enhanced carotid MR angiography with commercially available triggering mechanisms and elliptic centric phase encoding. *AJR. American Journal of Roentgenology*, **176**, 221–7.

Demarco, J. K., Rutt, B. K. and Clarke, S. E. (2001). Carotid plaque characterization by magnetic resonance imaging: review of the literature. *Topics in Magnetic Resonance Imaging*, **12**, 205–17.

Ding, X., Tkach, J. A., Ruggieri, P. R. and Masaryk, T. J. (1994). Sequential three-dimensional time-of-flight MR angiography of the carotid arteries: value of variable excitation and postprocessing in reducing venetian blind artifact. *AJR. American Journal of Roentgenology*, **163**, 683–8.

Dixon, W. T., Du, L. N., Faul, D. D., Gado, M. and Rossnick, S. (1986). Projection angiograms of blood labeled by adiabatic fast passage. *Magnetic Resonance in Medicine*, **3**, 454–62.

Dumoulin, C. L., Cline, H. E., Souza, S. P., Wagle, W. A. and Walker, M. F. (1989a). Three-dimensional time-of-flight magnetic resonance angiography using spin saturation. *Magnetic Resonance in Medicine*, **11**, 35–46.

Dumoulin, C. L., Souza, S. P., Walker, M. F. and Wagle, W. (1989b). Three-dimensional phase contrast angiography. *Magnetic Resonance in Medicine*, **9**, 139–49.

Dumoulin, C. L., Souza, S. P., Darrow, R. D., *et al.* (1991). Simultaneous acquisition of phase-contrast angiograms and stationary-tissue images with Hadamard encoding of flow-induced phase shifts. *Journal of Magnetic Resonance Imaging*, **1**, 399–404.

Fain, S. B., Riederer, S. J., Bernstein, M. A. and Huston, J., 3rd (1999). Theoretical limits of spatial resolution in elliptical-centric contrast-enhanced 3D-MRA. *Magnetic Resonance in Medicine*, **42**, 1106–16.

Fellner, F. A., Fellner, C., Wutke, R., *et al.* (2000). Fluoroscopically triggered contrast-enhanced 3D MR DSA and 3D time-of-flight turbo MRA of the carotid arteries: first clinical experiences in correlation with ultrasound, x-ray angiography, and endarterectomy findings. *Magnetic Resonance Imaging*, **18**, 575–85.

Fellner, C., Lang, W., Janka, R., Wutke, R., Bautz, W. and Fellner, F. A. (2005). Magnetic resonance angiography of the carotid arteries using three different techniques: accuracy compared with intraarterial x-ray angiography and endarterectomy specimens. *Journal of Magnetic Resonance Imaging*, **21**, 424–31.

Golay, X., Brown, S. J., Itoh, R. and Melhem, E. R. (2001). Time-resolved contrast-enhanced carotid MR angiography using sensitivity encoding (SENSE). *AJNR. American Journal of Neuroradiology*, **22**, 1615–19.

Goyen, M., Herborn, C. U., Vogt, F. M., *et al.* (2003). Using a 1 M Gd-chelate (gadobutrol) for total-body three-dimensional MR angiography: preliminary experience. *Journal of Magnetic Resonance Imaging*, **17**, 565–71.

Grist, T. M., Korosec, F. R., Peters, D. C., *et al.* (1998). Steady-state and dynamic MR angiography with MS-325: initial experience in humans. *Radiology*, **207**, 539–44.

Hausmann, R., Lewin, J. S. and Laub, G. (1991). Phase-contrast MR angiography with reduced acquisition time: new concepts in sequence design. *Journal of Magnetic Resonance Imaging*, **1**, 415–22.

Heiserman, J. E., Drayer, B. P., Fram, E. K., *et al.* (1992). Carotid artery stenosis: clinical efficacy of two-dimensional time-of-flight MR angiography. *Radiology*, **182**, 761–8.

Heiserman, J. E., Zabramski, J. M., Drayer, B. P. and Keller, P. J. (1996). Clinical significance of the flow gap in carotid magnetic resonance angiography. *Journal of Neurosurgery*, **85**, 384–7.

Hennig, J., Scheffler, K., Laubenberger, J. and Strecker, R. (1997). Time-resolved projection angiography after bolus injection of contrast agent. *Magnetic Resonance in Medicine*, **37**, 341–5.

Hu, H. H., Madhuranthakam, A. J., Kruger, D. G., Huston, J., 3rd and Riederer, S. J. (2004). Improved venous suppression and spatial resolution with SENSE in elliptical centric 3D contrast-enhanced MR angiography. *Magnetic Resonance in Medicine*, **52**, 761–5.

Huston, J., 3rd, Fain, S. B., Wald, J. T., *et al.* (2001). Carotid artery: elliptic centric contrast-enhanced MR angiography compared with conventional angiography. *Radiology*, **218**, 138–43.

Huston, J., 3rd, Lewis, B. D., Wiebers, D. O., *et al.* (1993). Carotid artery: prospective blinded comparison of two-dimensional time-of-flight MR angiography with conventional angiography and duplex US. *Radiology*, **186**, 339–44.

Ikushima, I., Korogi, Y., Hirai, T. and Takahashi, M. (1997). Variable tip angle slab selection pulses for carotid and cerebral time-of-flight MR angiography. Theory and experimental analysis. *Acta Radiologica*, **38**, 275–80.

Iseda, T., Nakano, S., Miyahara, D., *et al.* (2000). Poststenotic signal attenuation on 3D phase-contrast MR angiography: a useful finding in haemodynamically significant carotid artery stenosis. *Neuroradiology*, **42**, 868–73.

Isoda, H., Takehara, Y., Isogai, S., *et al.* (1998). Technique for arterial-phase contrast-enhanced three-dimensional MR angiography of the carotid and vertebral arteries. *AJNR. American Journal of Neuroradiology*, **19**, 1241–4.

Kallmes, D. F., Omary, R. A., Dix, J. E., Evans, A. J. and Hillman, B. J. (1996). Specificity of MR angiography as a confirmatory test of carotid artery stenosis. *American Journal of Neuroradiology*, **17**, 1501–6.

Keller, P. J., Drayer, B. P., Fram, E. K., *et al.* (1989). MR angiography with two-dimensional acquisition and three-dimensional display. Work in progress. *Radiology*, **173**, 527–32.

Kim, J. K., Farb, R. I. and Wright, G. A. (1998). Test bolus examination in the carotid artery at dynamic gadolinium-enhanced MR angiography. *Radiology*, **206**, 283–9.

Korosec, F. R., Frayne, R., Grist, T. M. and Mistretta, C. A. (1996). Time-resolved contrast-enhanced 3D MR angiography. *Magnetic Resonance in Medicine*, **36**, 345–51.

Korosec, F. R., Turski, P. A., Carroll, T. J., Mistretta, C. A. and Grist, T. M. (1999). Contrast-enhanced MR angiography of the carotid bifurcation. *Journal of Magnetic Resonance Imaging*, **10**, 317–25.

Laub, G. (1990). Displays for MR angiography. *Magnetic Resonance in Medicine*, **14**, 222–9.

Laub, G. A. and Kaiser, W. A. (1988). MR angiography with gradient motion refocusing. *Journal of Computer Assisted Tomography*, **12**, 377–82.

Lev, M. H., Romero, J. M. and Gonzalez, R. G. (2003). Flow voids in time-of-flight MR angiography of carotid artery stenosis? It depends on the TE! *AJNR. American Journal of Neuroradiology*, **24**, 2120.

Levy, R. A. and Prince, M. R. (1996). Arterial-phase three-dimensional contrast-enhanced MR angiography of the carotid arteries. *AJR. American Journal of Roentgenology*, **167**, 211–15.

Li, W., Tutton, S., Vu, A. T., *et al.* (2005). First-pass contrast-enhanced magnetic resonance angiography in humans using ferumoxytol, a novel ultrasmall superparamagnetic iron oxide (USPIO)-based blood pool agent. *Journal of Magnetic Resonance Imaging*, **21**, 46–52.

Lin, W., Tkach, J. A., Haacke, E. M. and Masaryk, T. J. (1993). Intracranial MR angiography: application of magnetization transfer contrast and fat saturation to short gradient-echo, velocity-compensated sequences. *Radiology*, **186**, 753–61.

Litt, A. W., Eidelman, E. M., Pinto, R. S., *et al.* (1991). Diagnosis of carotid artery stenosis: comparison of 2DFT time-of-flight MR angiography with contrast angiography in 50 patients. *AJNR. American Journal of Neuroradiology*, **12**, 149–54.

Little, W. C., Constantinescu, M., Applegate, R. J., *et al.* (1988). Can coronary angiography predict the site of a subsequent myocardial infarction in patients with mild-to-moderate coronary artery disease? *Circulation*, **78**, 1157–66.

Liu, K. and Rutt, B. K. (1998). Sliding interleaved kY (SLINKY) acquisition: a novel 3D MRA technique with suppressed slab boundary artifact. *Journal of Magnetic Resonance Imaging*, **8**, 903–11.

Long, A., Lepoutre, A., Corbillon, E., Branchereau, A. and Kretz, J. G. (2002). Modalities of preoperative imaging of the internal carotid artery used in France. *Annals of Vascular Surgery*, **16**, 261–5.

Maki, J. H., Prince, M. R., Londy, F. J. and Chenevert, T. L. (1996). The effects of time varying intravascular signal intensity and k-space acquisition order on three-dimensional MR angiography image quality. *Journal of Magnetic Resonance Imaging*, **6**, 642–51.

Melhem, E. R., Caruthers, S. D., Faddoul, S. G., Tello, R. and Jara, H. (1999). Use of three-dimensional MR angiography for tracking a contrast bolus in the carotid artery. *AJNR. American Journal of Neuroradiology*, **20**, 263–6.

Moran, P. R. (1982). A flow velocity zeugmatographic interlace for NMR imaging in humans. *Magnetic Resonance Imaging*, **1**, 197–203.

Naganawa, S., Koshikawa, T., Fukatsu, H., *et al.* (2001). Contrast-enhanced MR angiography of the carotid artery using 3D time-resolved imaging of contrast kinetics: comparison with real-time fluoroscopic triggered 3D-elliptical centric view ordering. *Radiation Medicine*, **19**, 185–92.

Nagele, T., Klose, U., Grodd, W., Nusslin, F. and Voigt, K. (1995). Nonlinear excitation profiles for three-dimensional inflow MR angiography. *Journal of Magnetic Resonance Imaging*, **5**, 416–20.

Nederkoorn, P. J., Elgersma, O. E., Mali, W. P., *et al.* (2002a). Overestimation of carotid artery stenosis with magnetic resonance angiography compared with digital subtraction angiography. *Journal of Vascular Surgery*, **36**, 806–13.

Nederkoorn, P. J., Van Der Graaf, Y., Eikelboom, B. C., *et al.* (2002b). Time-of-flight MR angiography of carotid artery stenosis: does a flow void represent severe stenosis? *AJNR. American Journal of Neuroradiology*, **23**, 1779–84.

Nederkoorn, P. J., Van Der Graaf, Y., Hunink, M. G., Forsting, M. and Wanke, I. (2003). Duplex ultrasound and magnetic resonance angiography compared with digital subtraction angiography in carotid artery stenosis: a systematic review. *Stroke*, **34**, 1324–32.

Nishimura, D. G., Macovski, A. and Pauly, J. M. (1986). Magnetic resonance angiography. *IEEE Transactions on Medical Imaging*, **5**, 140–51.

Obuchowski, N. A., Lieber, M. L., Magdenic, M., *et al.* (1999). Small but quantifiable patient preference for MRA versus catheter angiography. *Stroke*, **30**, 2247–8.

Patel, M. R., Klufas, R. A., Kim, D., Edelman, R. R. and Kent, K. C. (1994). MR angiography of the carotid bifurcation: artifacts and limitations. *AJR. American Journal of Roentgenology*, **162**, 1431–7.

Pelc, N. J., Bernstein, M. A., Shimakawa, A. and Glover, G. H. (1991a). Encoding strategies for three-direction phase-contrast MR imaging of flow. *Journal of Magnetic Resonance Imaging*, **1**, 405–13.

Pelc, N. J., Herfkens, R. J., Shimakawa, A. and Enzmann, D. R. (1991b). Phase contrast cine magnetic resonance imaging. *Magnetic Resonance Quarterly*, **7**, 229–54.

Phan, T., Huston, J., 3rd, Bernstein, M. A., Riederer, S. J. and Brown, R. D., Jr. (2001). Contrast-enhanced magnetic resonance angiography of the cervical vessels: experience with 422 patients. *Stroke*, **32**, 2282–6.

Pike, G. B., Hu, B. S., Glover, G. H. and Enzmann, D. R. (1992). Magnetization transfer time-of-flight magnetic resonance angiography. *Magnetic Resonance in Medicine*, **25**, 372–9.

Powers, W. J. (2004). Carotid arteriography: still golden after all these years? *Neurology*, **62**, 1246–7.

Priatna, A. and Paschal, C. B. (1995). Variable-angle uniform signal excitation (VUSE) for three-dimensional time-of-flight MR angiography. *Journal of Magnetic Resonance Imaging*, **5**, 421–7.

Prince, M. R., Grist, T. M. and Debatin, J. F. (2003). *3D Contrast MR Angiography*. Berlin: Springer.

Pruessmann, K. P., Weiger, M., Scheidegger, M. B. and Boesiger, P. (1999). SENSE: sensitivity encoding for fast MRI. *Magnetic Resonance in Medicine*, **42**, 952–62.

Riederer, S. J., Bernstein, M. A., Breen, J. F., *et al.* (2000). Three-dimensional contrast-enhanced MR angiography with real-time fluoroscopic triggering: design specifications and technical reliability in 330 patient studies. *Radiology*, **215**, 584–93.

Riedy, G., Golay, X. and Melhem, E. R. (2005). Three-dimensional isotropic contrast-enhanced MR angiography of the carotid artery using sensitivity-encoding and random elliptic centric k-space filling: technique optimization. *Neuroradiology*, **47**, 668–73.

Rothwell, P. M., Pendlebury, S. T., Wardlaw, J. and Warlow, C. P. (2000). Critical appraisal of the design and reporting of studies of imaging and measurement of carotid stenosis. *Stroke*, **31**, 1444–50.

Slosman, F., Stolpen, A. H., Lexa, F. J., *et al.* (1998). Extracranial atherosclerotic carotid artery disease: evaluation of non-breath-hold three-dimensional gadolinium-enhanced MR angiography. *AJR. American Journal of Roentgenology*, **170**, 489–95.

Sodickson, D. K. and Manning, W. J. (1997). Simultaneous acquisition of spatial harmonics (SMASH): fast imaging with radiofrequency coil arrays. *Magnetic Resonance in Medicine*, **38**, 591–603.

U-King-Im, J., Hollingworth, W., Trivedi, R.A., *et al.* (2004a). Contrast-enhanced MR angiography vs intra-arterial digital subtraction angiography for carotid imaging: activity-based cost analysis. *European Radiology*, **14**, 730–5.

U-King-Im, J., Hollingworth, W., Trivedi, R.A., *et al.* (2005). Cost-effectiveness of diagnostic strategies prior to carotid endarterectomy. *Annals of Neurology*, **58**, 506–15.

U-King-Im, J., Trivedi, R., Cross, J., *et al.* (2004b). Conventional digital subtraction x-ray angiography versus magnetic resonance angiography in the evaluation of carotid disease: patient satisfaction and preferences. *Clinical Radiology*, **59**, 358–63.

U-King-Im, J., Trivedi, R.A., Graves, M.J., *et al.* (2004c). Contrast-enhanced MR angiography for carotid disease: diagnostic and potential clinical impact. *Neurology*, **62**, 1282–90.

Unterweger, M., Froehlich, J.M., Kubik-Huch, R.A., et al. (2005). Dose optimization of contrast-enhanced carotid MR angiography. *European Radiology*, **15**, 1797–805.

Vanninen, R.L., Manninen, H.I., Partanen, P.L., Vainio, P.A. and Soimakallio, S. (1995a). Carotid artery stenosis: clinical efficacy of MR phase-contrast flow quantification as an adjunct to MR angiography. *Radiology*, **194**, 459–67.

Vanninen, R., Manninen, H. and Soimakallio, S. (1995b). Imaging of carotid artery stenosis: clinical efficacy and cost-effectiveness. *AJNR. American Journal of Neuroradiology*, **16**, 1875–83.

Wagle, W.A., Dumoulin, C.L., Souza, S.P. and Cline, H.E. (1989). 3DFT MR angiography of carotid and basilar arteries. *AJNR. American Journal of Neuroradiology*, **10**, 911–19.

Wang, Y., Johnston, D.L., Breen, J.F., *et al.* (1996). Dynamic MR digital subtraction angiography using contrast enhancement, fast data acquisition, and complex subtraction. *Magnetic Resonance in Medicine*, **36**, 551–6.

Wardlaw, J.M., Chapell, F.M., Best, J.J., Wartolowska, K. and Berry, E. (2006). Non-invasive imaging compared with intra-arterial angiography in the diagnosis of symptomatic carotid stenosis: a meta-analysis. *Lancet*, **367**, 1503–12.

Watts, R., Wang, Y., Redd, B., *et al.* (2002). Recessed elliptical-centric view-ordering for contrast-enhanced 3D MR angiography of the carotid arteries. *Magnetic Resonance in Medicine*, **48**, 419–24.

Wehrli, F.W., Shimakawa, A., Gullberg, G.T. and Macfall, J.R. (1986). Time-of-flight MR flow imaging: selective saturation recovery with gradient refocusing. *Radiology*, **160**, 781–5.

Westwood, M.E., Kelly, S., Berry, E., *et al.* (2002). Use of magnetic resonance angiography to select candidates with recently symptomatic carotid stenosis for surgery: systematic review. *British Medical Journal*, **324**, 198.

Willinek, W.A., Gieseke, J., Conrad, R., *et al.* (2002). Randomly segmented central k-space ordering in high-spatial-resolution contrast-enhanced MR angiography of the supraaortic arteries: initial experience. *Radiology*, **225**, 583–8.

Willinsky, R.A., Taylor, S.M., Terbrugge, K., *et al.* (2003). Neurologic complications of cerebral angiography: prospective analysis of 2,899 procedures and review of the literature. *Radiology*, **227**, 522–8.

Wilman, A.H., Riederer, S.J., Huston, J., 3rd, Wald, J.T. and Debbins, J.P. (1998). Arterial phase carotid and vertebral artery imaging in 3D contrast-enhanced MR angiography by combining fluoroscopic triggering with an elliptical centric acquisition order. *Magnetic Resonance in Medicine*, **40**, 24–35.

Yuan, C., Tsuruda, J.S., Beach, K.N., *et al.* (1994). Techniques for high-resolution MR imaging of atherosclerotic plaque. *Journal of Magnetic Resonance Imaging*, **4**, 43–9.

12

Computed tomographic angiography of carotid artery stenosis

Paul J. Nederkoorn, Charles B. L. M. Majoie and Jan Stam

Academic Medical Center, Amsterdam, The Netherlands

Introduction

In large randomized trials carotid endarterectomy was shown to be beneficial in symptomatic patients (transient ischemic attack [TIA] or minor stroke in the past 6 months) with a severe stenosis (70–99%) of the internal carotid artery (ICA) (Rothwell *et al.*, 2003). Subgroups of patients with a symptomatic stenosis of 50–69% also benefit from carotid endarterectomy. Recently, even for asymptomatic patients, a small effect of carotid endarterectomy was reported (Halliday *et al.*, 2004). The discussion whether this effect was sufficiently large to advise surgery to (subgroups of) asymptomatic patients is still ongoing (Barnett, 2004). A more recent development is treatment of the carotid artery stenosis with endovascular stenting (Cambria, 2004). Randomized trials are still ongoing to assess the efficacy of this treatment. In the trials with symptomatic patients, an increasing degree of stenosis yielded increasing benefit from surgery. Therefore, precise estimation of the degree of stenosis is crucial for decisions on interventions for carotid artery atherosclerotic disease.

In the trials the degree of stenosis was assessed with intraarterial digital subtraction angiography (DSA), which consequently has become the standard of reference in the selection of patients for carotid endarterectomy. However, DSA has a nonnegligible morbidity and mortality, which decreases the potential overall benefit of endarterectomy (Hankey *et al.*, 1990; Willinsky *et al.*, 2003). Therefore, computerized tomography angiography (CTA) is increasingly used in the diagnosis of carotid artery stenosis, along with other noninvasive tests such as duplex ultrasound (DUS) or magnetic resonance angiography (MRA) (Anderson *et al.*, 2000; Binaghi *et al.*, 2001; Hirai *et al.*, 2001; Randoux *et al.*, 2001; Patel *et al.*, 2002; Alvarez-Linera *et al.*, 2003; Hollingworth *et al.*, 2003; Feasby and Findlay, 2004; Josephson *et al.*, 2004; Koelemay *et al.*, 2004; Nonent *et al.*, 2004; Berg *et al.*, 2005). In contrast with DSA, these non- or minimally invasive tests do not carry the potential risk of thromboembolic complications. However, if a new test is to be used in the diagnosis of carotid artery stenosis, it is essential that the stenosis measurements are related to DSA, in order to reliably apply the trial-results to individual patients.

CTA in carotid artery stenosis

Imaging of vessels with CT techniques has been used since 1982. With the introduction of spiral CT systems, selective imaging of blood vessels became widely available (Dillon *et al.*, 1993). The use of intravenous iodinated contrast in CTA allows excellent images of the lumen of the arteries (Vieco, 1998). To date, CTA offers high spatial resolution

Carotid Disease: The Role of Imaging in Diagnosis and Management, ed. Jonathan Gillard, Martin Graves, Thomas Hatsukami and Chun Yuan. Published by Cambridge University Press. © Cambridge University Press 2007.

and contrast resolution, and it is a very fast technique (Kaufmann and Kallmes, 2005). With further improvements, such as faster data acquisition and a larger scan volume, pure arterial phase imaging from the aortic arch to the circle of Willis is possible. Currently, the quality of imaging of the lumen of the artery with CTA may be comparable to DSA. Whereas DSA provides pure "luminology" only, CTA also visualizes the wall of the arteries and the morphology of the atherosclerotic plaque (Zhang et al., 2005). Although plaque morphology is not yet routinely taken into account in the decision on carotid endarterectomy, it might become an important feature in the near future (Gillard, 2003).

CT-based imaging of vessels has been available for quite a long time. With the use of intravenous contrast, angiography of the (remaining) lumen in a stenosed carotid artery first became really accurate. However, the timing of contrast arrival in relation to the start of the data acquisition remains difficult and is an important drawback of this technique. Compared to other parts of the body, such as the liver or the kidneys, there is a smaller time-window before venous overprojection of the vessels in the head and neck occurs. The jugular vein overlapping the carotid bifurcation is one of the main technical problems that can interfere with an exact assessment of the degree of stenosis. Another disadvantage of the use of intravenous contrast in CTA is that its application in patients with renal insufficiency or cardiac failure is limited.

Bone and calcification artefacts create a second limitation of CTA. With the subtraction technique used in DSA, this seldom causes problems in imaging the carotid bifurcation. With MRA, this problem does not occur either. Extensive calcification causes artefacts in CTA, especially in arteries with circumferentially calcified plaques. In patients with severe atherosclerosis these artefacts may obscure a clear image of the lumen of the ICA. Recent developments may limit this drawback and will be discussed below. Contrary to the problems caused by bone and calcification, the total volume of calcium at the carotid bifurcation, measured

with CT, is significantly correlated to the presence of a stenosis ($>40\%$) in the ICA (McKinney et al., 2005).

Finally, in contrast to DUS or MRA, CTA uses ionizing radiation which is potentially harmful. The absorbed dose during a diagnostic CT examination is, however, relatively low and typically estimated to be in the range of 1–4 mSv. The effective dose we receive from natural background radiation is approximately 2 mSv per year in Western-European countries.

Postprocessing techniques

From the cross-sectional source images, computer reconstructions can produce 2D or 3D images with different protocols (Figures 12.1 and 12.2). More than the cross-sectional images, such a postprocessed angiographic display is useful for the identification of the maximal stenosis, and for the visualization of overall vascular anatomy (Dix et al., 1997; Wise et al., 1998). In addition, these reconstructions enable stenosis measurements according to the criteria of the North American symptomatic carotid endarterectomy trial (NASCET), as will be discussed below (NASCET collaborators, 1991).

Multiplanar (MPR) or curved planar reconstructions (CPR) provide 2D images of any predefined surface; mostly longitudinal with the arteries in the neck. A disadvantage in MPR is that the structure of interest should lie in one plane. In CPR, the surface can be constructed in such a way that it exactly follows the anatomic curvatures of the carotid artery. In MPR or CPR, interactive MPR reformatting allows the selection of the plane revealing the most severe stenosis, enabling precise stenosis measurements. It is important to recognize, however, that this process remains operator-dependent.

The different postprocessing techniques used to construct a 3D angiographic display of the artery each have their particular strengths and weaknesses in imaging carotid artery stenosis

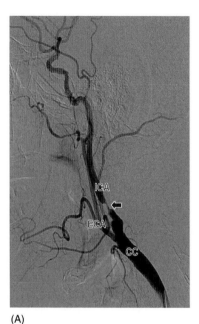

(A)

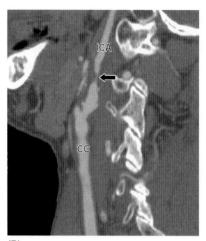

(B)

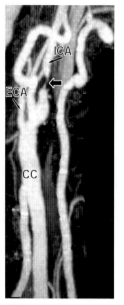

(C)

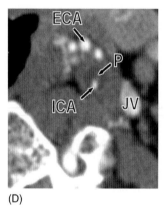

(D)

Figure 12.1 Example of a severe internal carotid artery (ICA) stenosis estimated at 90%. (A): digital subtraction angiography; (B): multiplanar reformat; and (C): maximum intensity projection, respectively. Large arrow represents point of maximum stenosis. ECA = external carotid artery, CC = common carotid artery. (D): cross-sectional source image. P indicates soft plaque. Contrast in the remaining lumen is visible indicated by ICA. JV = jugular vein.

(Takhtani, 1998; Vieco, 2005). In shaded surface display (SSD), densities below a certain threshold of Hounsfield units are excluded and the remaining data are viewed as if the surfaces of these data are illuminated by a point source (Vieco, 1998). These reconstructions give a good 3D image of the outer vessel wall, but no information about the residual lumen. As a consequence, SSD images tend to underestimate stenoses, which makes this technique less useful in the assessment of carotid artery stenosis (Papp *et al.*, 1997). Another SSD protocol depicts the inner vessel wall as a shaded

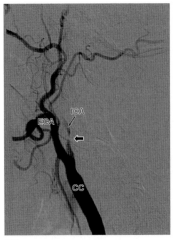

(A)

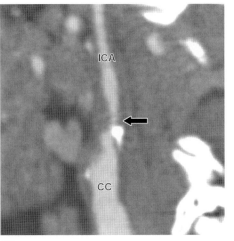

(B)

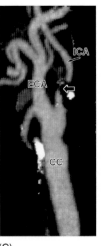

(C)

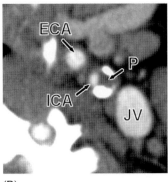

(D)

Figure 12.2 Example of a severe ICA stenosis estimated at 99%. A,B,C: images of DSA, MPR, and MIP respectively. Large arrow represents point of maximum stenosis. ICA = internal carotid artery, ECA = external carotid artery, CC = common carotid artery. D: cross-sectional source image. P indicates soft plaque. Contrast in the remaining lumen is visible indicated by ICA. JV = jugular vein.

surface, but the accuracy of this technique is not known. Volume rendering (VR) allows for 3D reconstructions quite similar to SSD images and can differentiate between the arterial wall and surrounding structures.

Maximum intensity projection (MIP) reconstructions are often used in CTA because they can rapidly automatically be generated. MIP images are processed by projection of the maximum intensity pixels from the 3D data set on predefined 2D planes. However, the maximum value along a line in the direction of projection is often that of bone, which obscures vessels. Calcification artifacts can be removed by thresholding, but this introduces possible error. If the manually defined threshold is not precise, parts of the lumen of the artery may be distracted from the images as well. Thus, stenosis can be overestimated.

Stenosis measurements

In symptomatic carotid surgery trials, DSA was performed in two or three projections (lateral, posteroanterior, and/or oblique). As a result, carotid artery stenosis is now often measured in a comparable way, according to the NASCET criteria (NASCET collaborators, 1991). In these criteria the degree of stenosis is defined as the remaining lumen at the stenosis as percentage of the normal lumen distal to the stenosis. The projection, lateral, posteroanterior, or oblique, which shows the most severe stenosis, is used for establishing the degree of stenosis. Measurements with CTA should preferably be done in a comparable manner, in order to correctly apply the trial data to the clinical decisions about carotid endarterectomy. Thus, for a valid comparison with DSA, we should only use the percentage of stenosis measured on postprocessed images of the three projections mentioned above. Measurements of the remaining lumen at the point of maximum stenosis and the normal lumen distal to the stenosis are easily performed on postprocessed images, by hand with calipers, or automatically. The different postprocessing techniques may introduce different errors in stenosis measurements (Hirai *et al.*, 2001). In general with SSD the degree of stenosis is underestimated, whereas MIP reconstructions tend to overestimate, based on the technical limitations (Vieco, 1998). Preferably, MPR or CPR reconstructions should be used when the NASCET stenosis measurement is applied.

In contrast with traditional DSA in three directions, CTA and MRA allow projections in any predefined (3D) plane. 3D images by CTA or MRA therefore provide more information on the morphology of the stenosis than conventional DSA. Several studies with MRA and CTA have demonstrated that the residual stenotic lumen is almost never circular, and that DSA performed in a limited number of projections does not always reveal the narrowest residual lumen (Pan *et al.*, 1995;

Serfaty *et al.*, 2000; Nederkoorn *et al.*, 2002; Zhang *et al.*, 2005). Automated analysis of 3D information provides an even more realistic model of the true luminal area or morphology (Zhang *et al.*, 2004). Therefore, it is likely that postprocessed images and the use of 3D techniques in CTA or MRA reveal a more precise estimate of the actual degree of stenosis. However, with a potentially more precise estimate of the stenosis, the relation with DSA-based trial results becomes more remote. DSA may not be the gold standard anymore with respect to state-of-the-art imaging and postprocessing techniques, however, it does remain the standard of reference with respect to clinical decision-making on carotid endarterectomy based upon what we know from the trials. Ideally, new 3D techniques should be compared with conventional DSA in sufficient large consecutive patient series. However, in clinical practice DSA is not routinely used anymore in all patients in whom carotid endarterectomy is considered. Therefore, such a diagnostic study would be unethical.

Diagnostic accuracy

More data are available on the diagnostic accuracy of DUS and MRA than of CTA and these techniques have been better validated (Westwood *et al.*, 2002; Nederkoorn *et al.*, 2003; Koelemay *et al.*, 2004). Several studies which compare CTA with DSA in the assessment of carotid artery studies have been reported. In a recent systematic review summarizing the literature between January 1990 and July 2003, the pooled sensitivity and specificity for detection of a 70–99% stenosis were 85% and 93%, respectively. For detection of an occlusion the sensitivity and specificity were 97% and 99% (Koelemay *et al.*, 2004). The accuracy of CTA for detecting severe (70–99%) stenosis lies in between the diagnostic accuracy of MRA, which performed slightly better, and DUS, which has the least diagnostic accuracy when used as a sole imaging test. The accuracy of CTA to detect occlusions (100%) is very good and comparable to MRA and DUS. Meaningful subgroup analysis, for example for the diagnostic accuracy of the different scan-protocols and postprocessing techniques, was not possible. In the future, multi-slice CT-scanning together with other technical developments will probably further improve the diagnostic accuracy of CTA. Furthermore, the best preoperative test strategy in which CTA is used, could very well be a combination of non- and minimally-invasive tests, for example DUS followed by CTA; discussion about this issue is beyond the scope of this chapter.

In general the quality of design and reporting of results of diagnostic imaging studies of the carotid arteries needs improvement (Rothwell, 2000). Another important issue is the fact that almost all studies on carotid artery imaging included the asymptomatic contralateral carotid artery in the analysis (Westwood *et al.*, 2002; Nederkoorn *et al.*, 2003; Koelemay *et al.*, 2004). Generally, the clinical decision to perform carotid endarterectomy is made solely on the basis of the stenosis in the symptomatic artery. As a result the specificity in these studies will be overestimated, because of the relatively high proportion of arteries without significant stenosis that are likely to be correctly identified by the test under study. This methodological shortcoming is not unique for studies of CTA, but is also common in evaluations of MRA and DUS.

Finally, to decide whether CTA, or any non-invasive test or combination of tests, could replace DSA, reporting the false positive and false negative rates only is not sufficient. To completely understand and evaluate the consequences of implementing a new diagnostic test in clinical practice, the results of a cost-effectiveness analysis should be taken into account. For MRA these analyses have been published, but for CTA such data are still unavailable but needed (Buskens *et al.*, 2004; King-Im *et al.*, 2005).

New developments

Possible solutions for bone and calcification artefacts have been developed. Removal of bone and calcification pixels from conventional CTA is time consuming and operator-dependent. Automatic removal remains difficult because the CT values of bone and calcification are comparable with the contrast in the lumen (van Straten *et al.*, 2004). Matched mask bone elimination (MMBE) is a new development for the automated removal of bone pixels from CTA data sets (Venema *et al.*, 2001). In MMBE bone pixels are identified in a low-dose non-enhanced data set and the corresponding pixels in the CTA data set are given an arbitrarily low value. After registration of the CTA scan and the nonenhanced scan, the bone in the CTA scan is masked. With this method it is possible to obtain MIP images of the cervical arteries free of over projecting bone in a fully automatic and reproducible way. However, the removal of arterial wall calcification still might introduce error in stenosis estimates. Because a small additional strip of approximately 1 mm is removed together with the calcification, the stenosis might be overestimated. A promising development solving this problem is a technique that combines automatic removal of large bone structures with an additional subtraction technique for the small calcification nearby the artery wall (van Straten *et al.*, 2004).

CTA techniques will keep on improving because of the introduction of faster machines. Recent studies suggest that true arterial phase imaging from the aortic arch to the circle of Willis will be possible with the use of 16-, 32- or 64-slice-spiral-CT machines, with improved spatial resolution, and lower doses of contrast material (Fleischmann, 2002; de Monye *et al.*, 2005). The faster acquisitions, possible with these multiple detector-row CT scanners, will give better understanding of the dynamics of contrast medium and thus will help to overcome problems with over-projections. The future will show which CTA protocols will help us to evaluate patients suspected of carotid artery disease with the best accuracy and cost-effectiveness.

REFERENCES

Alvarez-Linera, J., ito-Leon, J., Escribano, J., Campollo, J. and Gesto, R. (2003). Prospective evaluation of carotid artery stenosis: elliptic centric contrast-enhanced MR angiography and spiral CT angiography compared with digital subtraction angiography. *AJNR. American Journal of Neurorodiology*, **24**, 1012–19.

Anderson, G. B., Ashforth, R., Steinke, D. E., Ferdinandy, R. and Findlay, J. M. (2000). CT angiography for the detection and characterization of carotid artery bifurcation disease. *Stroke*, **31**, 2168–74.

Barnett, H. J. (2004). Carotid endarterectomy. *Lancet*, **363**, 1486–7.

Berg, M., Zhang, Z., Ikonen, A., *et al.* (2005). Multi-detector row CT angiography in the assessment of carotid artery disease in symptomatic patients: comparison with rotational angiography and digital subtraction angiography. *AJNR. American Journal of Neuroradiology*, **26**, 1022–34.

Binaghi, S., Maeder, P., Uske, A., *et al.* (2001). Three-dimensional computed tomography angiography and magnetic resonance angiography of carotid bifurcation stenosis. *European Neurology*, **46**, 25–34.

Buskens, E., Nederkoorn, P. J., Buijs-Van Der, W. T., *et al.* (2004). Imaging of carotid arteries in symptomatic patients: cost-effectiveness of diagnostic strategies. *Radiology*, **233**, 101–12.

Cambria, R. P. (2004). Stenting for carotid-artery stenosis. *New England Journal of Medicine*, **351**, 1565–7.

de Monye, C., Cademartiri, F., de Weert, T. T., *et al.* (2005). Sixteen-detector row CT angiography of carotid arteries: comparison of different volumes of contrast material with and without a bolus chaser. *Radiology*, **237**, 555–62.

Dillon, E. H., van Leeuwen, M. S., Fernandez, M. A., Eikelboom, B. C. and Mali, W. P. (1993). CT angiography: application to the evaluation of carotid artery stenosis. *Radiology*, **189**, 211–19.

Dix, J. E., Evans, A. J., Kallmes, D. F., Sobel, A. H. and Phillips, C. D. (1997). Accuracy and precision of CT angiography in a model of carotid artery bifurcation stenosis. *AJNR. American Journal of Neuroradiology*, **18**, 409–15.

Feasby, T. E. and Findlay, J. M. (2004). CT angiography for the assessment of carotid stenosis. *Neurology*, **63**, 412–13.

Fleischmann, D. (2002). Present and future trends in multiple detector-row CT applications: CT angiography. *European Radiology*, **12** (Suppl. 2), S11–S15.

Gillard, J. H. (2003). Imaging of carotid artery disease: from luminology to function? *Neuroradiology*, **45**, 671–80.

Halliday, A., Mansfield, A., Marro, J., *et al.* (2004). Prevention of disabling and fatal strokes by successful carotid endarterectomy in patients without recent neurological symptoms: randomised controlled trial. *Lancet*, **363**, 1491–502.

Hankey, G. J., Warlow, C. P. and Molyneux, A. J. (1990). Complications of cerebral angiography for patients with mild carotid territory ischaemia being considered for carotid endarterectomy. *Journal of Neurology, Neurosurgery and Psychiatry*, **53**, 542–8.

Hirai, T., Korogi, Y., Ono, K., *et al.* (2001). Maximum stenosis of extracranial internal carotid artery: effect of luminal morphology on stenosis measurement by using CT angiography and conventional DSA. *Radiology*, **221**, 802–9.

Hollingworth, W., Nathens, A. B., Kanne, J. P., *et al.* (2003). The diagnostic accuracy of computed tomography angiography for traumatic or atherosclerotic lesions of the carotid and vertebral arteries: a systematic review. *European Journal of Radiology*, **48**, 88–102.

Josephson, S. A., Bryant, S. O., Mak, H. K., *et al.* (2004). Evaluation of carotid stenosis using CT angiography in the initial evaluation of stroke and TIA. *Neurology*, **63**, 457–60.

Kaufmann, T. J. and Kallmes, D. F. (2005). Utility of MRA and CTA in the evaluation of carotid occlusive disease. *Seminars in Vascular Surgery*, **18**, 75–82.

King-Im, J. M., Hollingworth, W., Trivedi, R. A., *et al.* (2005). Cost-effectiveness of diagnostic strategies prior to carotid endarterectomy. *Annals of Neurology*, **58**, 506–15.

Koelemay, M. J., Nederkoorn, P. J., Reitsma, J. B. and Majoie, C. B. (2004). Systematic review of computed tomographic angiography for assessment of carotid artery disease. *Stroke*, **35**, 2306–12.

McKinney, A. M., Casey, S. O., Teksam, M., *et al.* (2005). Carotid bifurcation calcium and correlation with percent stenosis of the internal carotid artery on CT angiography. *Neuroradiology*, **47**, 1–9.

Nederkoorn, P. J., Elgersma, O. E., Mali, W. P., *et al.* (2002). Overestimation of carotid artery stenosis with magnetic resonance angiography compared with digital subtraction angiography. *Journal of Vascular Surgery*, **36**, 806–13.

Nederkoorn, P. J., van der, Graaf. Y. and Hunink, M. G. (2003). Duplex ultrasound and magnetic resonance angiography compared with digital subtraction angiography in carotid artery stenosis: a systematic review. *Stroke*, **34**, 1324–32.

Nonent, M., Serfaty, J. M., Nighoghossian, N., *et al.* (2004). Concordance rate differences of 3 noninvasive imaging techniques to measure carotid stenosis in clinical routine practice: results of the CARMEDAS multicenter study. *Stroke*, **35**, 682–6.

North American Symptomatic Carotid Endarterectomy Trial Collaborators. (1991). Beneficial effect of carotid endarterectomy in symptomatic patients with high-grade carotid stenosis. *New England Journal of Medicine*, **325**, 445–53.

Pan, X. M., Saloner, D., Reilly, L. M., *et al.* (1995). Assessment of carotid artery stenosis by ultrasonography, conventional angiography, and magnetic resonance angiography: correlation with ex vivo measurement of plaque stenosis. *Journal of Vascular Surgery*, **21**, 82–8.

Papp, Z., Patel, M., Ashtari, M., *et al.* (1997). Carotid artery stenosis: optimization of CT angiography with a combination of shaded surface display and source images. *AJNR. American Journal of Neuroradiology*, **18**, 759–63.

Patel, S. G., Collie, D. A., Wardlaw, J. M., *et al.* (2002). Outcome, observer reliability, and patient preferences if CTA, MRA, or Doppler ultrasound were used, individually or together, instead of digital subtraction angiography before carotid endarterectomy. *Journal of Neurology, Neurosurgery and Psychiatry*, **73**, 21–8.

Randoux, B., Marro, B., Koskas, F., *et al.* (2001). Carotid artery stenosis: prospective comparison of CT, three-dimensional gadolinium-enhanced MR, and conventional angiography. *Radiology*, **220**, 179–85.

Rothwell, P. M. (2000). Analysis of agreement between measurements of continuous variables: general principles and lessons from studies of imaging of carotid stenosis. *Journal of Neurology*, **247**, 825–34.

Rothwell, P. M., Eliasziw, M., Gutnikov, S. A., *et al.* (2003). Analysis of pooled data from the randomised controlled trials of endarterectomy for symptomatic carotid stenosis. *Lancet*, **361**, 107–16.

Serfaty, J. M., Chirossel, P., Chevallier, J. M., *et al.* (2000). Accuracy of three-dimensional gadolinium-enhanced MR angiography in the assessment of extracranial carotid artery disease. *AJR. American Journal of Roentgenology*, **175**, 455–63.

Takhtani, D. (2005). CT neuroangiography: a glance at the common pitfalls and their prevention. *AJR. American Journal of Roentgenology*, **185**, 772–83.

Van Straten. M., Venema, H. W., Streekstra, G. J., *et al.* (2004). Removal of bone in CT angiography of the cervical arteries by piecewise matched mask bone elimination. *Medical Physics*, **31**, 2924–33.

Venema, H. W., Hulsmans, F. J. and den Heeten, G. J. (2001). CT angiography of the circle of Willis and intracranial internal carotid arteries: maximum intensity projection with matched mask bone elimination-feasibility study. *Radiology*, **218**, 893–8.

Vieco, P. T. (1998). CT angiography of the carotid artery. *Neuroimaging Clinics of North America*, **8**, 593–605.

Westwood, M. E., Kelly, S., Berry, E., *et al.* (2002). Use of magnetic resonance angiography to select candidates with recently symptomatic carotid stenosis for surgery: systematic review. *British Medical Journal*, **324**, 198.

Willinsky, R. A., Taylor, S. M., TerBrugge. K., *et al.* (2003). Neurologic complications of cerebral angiography: prospective analysis of 2,899 procedures and review of the literature. *Radiology*, **227**, 522–8.

Wise, S. W., Hopper, K. D., Ten, H. T. and Schwartz, T. (1998). Measuring carotid artery stenosis using CT angiography: the dilemma of artifactual lumen eccentricity. *AJR. American Journal of Roentgenology*, **170**, 919–23.

Zhang, Z., Berg, M. H., Ikonen, A. E., Vanninen, R. L. and Manninen, H. I. (2004). Carotid artery stenosis: reproducibility of automated 3D CT angiography analysis method. *European Radiology*, **14**, 665–72.

Zhang, Z., Berg, M., Ikonen, A., *et al.* (2005). Carotid stenosis degree in CT angiography: assessment based on luminal area versus luminal diameter measurements. *European Radiology*, **15**, 2359–65.

13

Cost-effectiveness analysis for carotid imaging

Jean Marie U-King-Im[1], William Hollingworth[2] and Jonathan H. Gillard[1]

[1]Addenbrooke's Hospital and the University of Cambridge, UK
[2]University of Washington, Seattle, WA 98103, USA

Introduction

The pooled analysis of data from large randomized trials such as the North American symptomatic carotid trial (NASCET) and the European carotid surgery trial (ECST) has confirmed the significant benefits of surgery for severe (70–99%) carotid stenosis in recently symptomatic patients (Rothwell *et al.*, 2003). Moreover, in asymptomatic patients, 60% stenosis is generally used as a cut-off for surgery based on the results of the asymptomatic carotid atherosclerosis study (ACAS) (Endarterectomy for asymptomatic carotid artery stenosis. Executive Committee for the Asymptomatic Carotid Atherosclerosis Study, 1995). In most of these trials, intraarterial digital subtraction angiography (DSA) has been used to measure the degree of stenosis and as such, remains the gold standard method in terms of diagnostic accuracy, against which alternative imaging modalities need to be validated. Concerns about the small but potentially significant risks of neurological complications associated with DSA have generated a strong trend toward the use of noninvasive modalities such as Doppler ultrasound (DUS), magnetic resonance angiography (MRA) or computerized tomography angiography (CTA) alone or in combination (Dawson *et al.*, 1997; Athanasoulis and Plomaritoglou, 2000; Long *et al.*, 2002).

In current clinical practice, there is ongoing controversy whether noninvasive strategies can replace DSA as the preoperative imaging modality of choice (Derdeyn and Powers, 1996; Davis and Donnan, 2003). This lack of consensus is reflected by a wide variety of existing practices worldwide (Dawson *et al.*, 1997; Athanasoulis and Plomaritoglou, 2000; Long *et al.*, 2002; Willinsky *et al.*, 2003). Although practices may differ from country to country, up to 50% of centers still use and consider DSA to be routinely necessary in the majority of patients (Robless and Halliday, 1999; Norris *et al.*, 2003). While DUS is portable, relatively inexpensive, potentially very accurate in experienced hands and frequently used as sole diagnostic modality, it is subject to significant interobserver variability and a proportion of centers prefer to use it as an initial screening tool prior to an additional confirmatory test (Perkins *et al.*, 2000). Multislice CTA is promising but remains limited by radiation dose, plaque calcifications which may obscure the actual stenosis, as well as a relative paucity of published rigorous studies (Alvarez-Linera *et al.*, 2003; Randoux *et al.*, 2004). Surveys suggest that the combination of screening DUS with MRA, especially contrast enhanced MRA (CE MRA), has emerged as the noninvasive imaging strategy of choice for preoperative evaluation (Dawson *et al.*, 1997; Berry *et al.*, 2002; Long *et al.*, 2002).

While numerous studies report on the diagnostic accuracy of noninvasive modalities compared to DSA, little consideration has been given to the

Carotid Disease: The Role of Imaging in Diagnosis and Management, ed. Jonathan Gillard, Martin Graves, Thomas Hatsukami and Chun Yuan. Published by Cambridge University Press. © Cambridge University Press 2007.

associated medical and economic repercussions (Kent *et al.*, 1995; Berry *et al.*, 2002). Because DSA is used as the gold standard and, as such, is considered 100% accurate, and because the measurement of carotid stenosis is, in itself, subject to significant interobserver variability, noninvasive tests will never completely agree with DSA (U-King-Im *et al.*, 2004b). Therefore, to determine the optimal imaging strategy with the least long-term morbidity and mortality, the consequences of diagnostic misclassification with noninvasive tests (i.e. inappropriately denying or referring patients for surgery) need to be closely balanced against the risks associated with DSA. Moreover, from a societal or hospital perspective, it is also essential for the true costs of using these various imaging strategies to be addressed. In theory, large trials randomizing patients to alternative imaging strategies prior to treatment could be used to determine the most cost-effective carotid imaging strategy. However, due to the large number of permutations in imaging modality and the small differences in diagnostic accuracy, such trials would have to be prohibitively large in order to demonstrate a difference in patient outcomes. In practice, no such cost-effectiveness trials have been conducted. Instead, cost-effectiveness modelling techniques have been used to clearly identify the relevant diagnostic alternatives, synthesize the vast amount of relevant data present in the literature and derive conclusions on the cost and outcomes of carotid imaging strategies. This chapter provides a brief overview of basic cost-effectiveness analysis methodology and terminology and summarizes the main studies published to date.

Cost-effectiveness decision analysis models: methodology and terminology

Cost-effectiveness analysis is a systematic technique for comparing alternative health care strategies in terms of patient outcomes and the resources used to achieve those outcomes.

This is important because, in some circumstances, minimal increases in diagnostic accuracy and marginal improvements in patient outcomes may not justify large increases in health care spending. Many healthcare authorities now evaluate both effectiveness and cost-effectiveness before issuing guidance on medical technologies (Devlin and Parkin, 2004). Often, this evaluation requires researchers to project from the available data examining intermediate outcomes (e.g. sensitivity, specificity, short-term survival) to estimate the likely lifetime costs and outcomes using decision analysis modelling.

Decision analysis modelling combines clinical and economic data from a number of primary sources and thus is especially useful in reducing complex and inherently difficult decisions into simpler more manageable ones (Philips *et al.*, 2004). In general, decision analyses of diagnostic imaging studies are slightly more difficult than assessments of therapeutic interventions, mainly because of uncertainty about the relation between accurate diagnosis and the outcome of care. Nonetheless, with the growing demands on imaging technology and the limited availability of resources, the number of cost-effectiveness studies that focus on diagnostic imaging has nearly quadrupled over the past 20 years (Blackmore and Smith, 1998).

In asymptomatic patients, the main focus of economic analyses has been the cost-effectiveness of screening programmes for more than 60% stenosis based on the results of the ACAS trial (Derdeyn and Powers, 1996; Lee *et al.*, 1997; Yin and Carpenter, 1998). On the other hand, in patients with recent neurological symptoms, cost-effectiveness analysis studies have generally concentrated on modelling the process of assessing patients with symptomatic carotid disease, and then mathematically comparing the effect of replacing the gold standard, DSA, with less-invasive diagnostic strategies (Kent *et al.*, 1995; Buskens *et al.*, 2004; U-King-Im *et al.*, 2005). The cost-effectiveness analysis model typically starts with the reference case, which would usually be a typical hypothetical patient who has suffered from a minor stroke or a transient ischemic attack. The criteria for treatment decisions then need to be defined: for instance, depending on the objectives of the study, the model may assume that all patients may receive optimal medical therapy but are only referred for carotid endarterectomy if test results show a severe stenosis.

There are several mathematical tools that researchers may use to simulate the clinical pathway of diagnosis, treatment, and patient outcomes. These tools include "Decision-trees", "Markov models" and "Monte-Carlo simulation", all three of these tools might be used in combination to describe the pathway from identification of carotid artery stenosis to subsequent stroke, quality of life and mortality. For further understanding, readers are referred to a series of articles by Detsky *et al.* in "Medical Decision Making" that describe these tools well (Detsky *et al.*, 1997a,b; Krahn *et al.*, 1997; Naglie *et al.*, 1997; Naimark *et al.*, 1997). The exact tools used to model the clinical pathway will depend on the clinical question to be answered, the depth of available data, the intended audience for the model and the personal preferences of the modeller.

In its simplest form, a decision-tree model is essentially a horizontal flow chart that depicts all the decisions, chance events and outcomes that stem from an initial set of imaging options. It is essential that the pathways being investigated bear close relevance to clinical practice. For instance, routinely, many centers use DUS as a screening modality rather than as sole imaging modality. Patients may then proceed to an additional confirmatory test such as MRA, CTA or DSA above a predefined threshold, for example, a stenosis of 50% or more, as shown by DUS. Moreover, there have also been several studies suggesting that combinations of noninvasive tests may reduce the degree of inaccuracy with respect to DSA when compared to a noninvasive test in isolation. Under such strategies, clinical decision-making is based on the results of two noninvasive tests alone, e.g. DUS and MRA or DUS and CTA, with DSA reserved

for patients with discordant noninvasive imaging results. All practical imaging strategies need to be examined in the cost-effectiveness analysis model to maximize clinical credibility and relevance. For asymptomatic patients, it is important to evaluate a "no imaging" strategy in order to exclude the possibility that preemptive screening and therapy may harm patients. An example of a truncated decision-tree for carotid imaging studies is illustrated in Figure 13.1. Decision trees are particularly adept at handling one-off chance events that happen within a short period of time. For example, the patient with symptomatic carotid stenosis can be rapidly referred for imaging which will result in either a true positive, false positive, true negative or false negative diagnosis. Decision-trees are less well-suited for predicting the path of chronic disease where important multiple clinical events evolve over a long period of time.

In order to address this shortcoming, many decision analyses combine decision-trees with Markov models. Markov models track patients as they transition among predefined health states over time (Sonnenberg and Beck, 1993). In carotid artery imaging, these states might include: healthy, nondisabling stroke, disabling stroke, fatal stroke, and death from causes other than stroke. Representing such clinical settings with conventional decision-trees is difficult and may require unrealistic simplifying assumptions. Markov models assume that a patient is always in one of the mutually exclusive health states, called Markov states (Figure 13.2). In order for the Markov model to function, the researcher must define the probability of patient transition from one health state to another at any given time point or "cycle" of the model. The researcher selects the appropriate "cycle length" for the model based on the available data. For carotid stenosis, a 1-year cycle length is frequently used because most trials report patient outcomes at yearly intervals after medical or surgical intervention. Markov models may be evaluated deterministically by matrix algebra or as a single cohort simulation. However, Monte Carlo simulation is most frequently used to estimate the

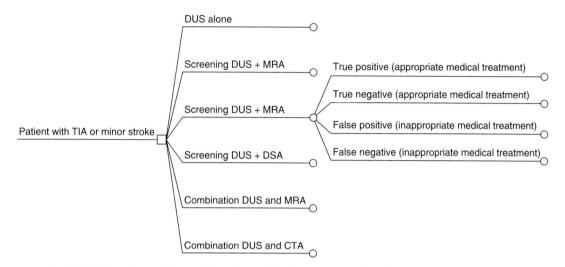

Figure 13.1 Typical decision-tree for carotid imaging studies. Screening Doppler ultrasound (DUS) implies that patients are referred for additional confirmatory tests such as magnetic resonance angiography (MRA), computerized tomography angiography (CTA) or CTA only above a predefined DUS stenosis threshold. With combination strategies, decision-making is based on the results of noninvasive tests alone if they agree but patients proceed to a third confirmatory test, digital subtraction angiography (DSA), if noninvasive results are discordant.

likely influence of transition probability uncertainty on the predictions of the model (Sonnenberg and Beck, 1993; Naimark *et al.*, 1997).

Once the structure of the model has been created, a number of probabilities and model parameters need to be input. These data can be derived from a combination of primary studies, literature syntheses or expert opinion. For example, in Figure 13.1, the proportion of true-positives, true-negatives, false-positives and false-negatives for each pathway may be estimated from accuracy estimates of sensitivity and specificity as well as the prevalence of severe stenosis in the population of interest. Furthermore, the probabilities of transition from one health state to another also have to be estimated at each cycle of the Markov model. For carotid studies, these transition probabilities have generally been estimated from large randomized controlled trials of carotid endarterectomy versus medical therapy such as NASCET, ECST or ACAS which still guide clinical practice today (Randomised trial of endarterectomy for recently symptomatic carotid stenosis: final results of the

MRC European Carotid Surgery Trial [ECST], 1998; Beneficial effect of carotid endarterectomy in symptomatic patients with high-grade carotid stenosis. North American Symptomatic Carotid Endarterectomy Trial Collaborators, 1991). However, these trials only have a finite follow-up period. Modellers can either choose to curtail their cost-effectiveness analysis model at the end of trial follow-up or extrapolate further based on assumptions that morbidity and mortality differences between medical and surgical management diminish, remain constant, or diverge after the end of the trial follow-up.

There are several potential outcome measures which can be used to gauge the effectiveness of different imaging strategies. These include number of stroke cases prevented, life-years saved or quality-adjusted-life-years (QALYs). QALYs remain one of the most popular measures of effectiveness used in cost-effectiveness analysis studies as they incorporate both length and quality-of-life (Singer and Applegate, 2001). The QALY approach assigns each health state a quality-of-life weight.

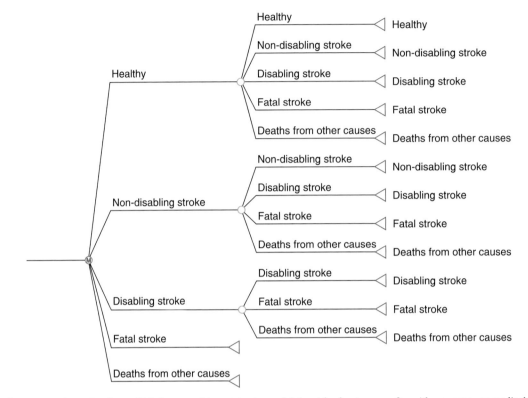

Figure 13.2 Example of use of Markov transition states to model the risk of outcomes after either surgery or medical therapy. The Markov node is represented by M and terminal nodes by the red triangles. It is assumed that a patient can either stay in the same health state or progress to a more severe health state but cannot move to a less severe state.

These weights are anchored at 0 (for a health state considered equivalent to death) and 1 (for an optimal health state). To calculate QALYs, the number of years that the average patient spends in a particular health state is multiplied by the quality-of-life weight assigned to that health state. Particularly useful in carotid imaging studies, the quality-of-life weights for different health states after stroke have been systematically reviewed by Post *et al.* (2001).

Costs need to be included in the model. These, for instance, include cost of noninvasive imaging tests, costs of DSA, costs of carotid endarterectomy and medical therapy as well as acute and long-terms costs of caring for stroke-related functional impairment (Benade and Warlow, 2002a,b). The most obvious portion of this cost burden falls on health care payers. However, there may be significant out-of-pocket costs for the patient and their family. Furthermore, from the most inclusive, societal, perspective, stroke-related disability will also result in productivity losses, also known as indirect costs. Therefore, the perspective of the study is crucial in determining the type of costs included in the model. It is essential for cost-effectiveness analysis studies to explicitly state the perspective from which they are conducted and therefore which costs are included. For instance, if the societal perspective is adopted, then all costs including lost productivity due to absence from work must be considered. If the perspective of the health care provider is adopted, then such costs could be excluded as they are not part of the hospital's financial responsibility. Costs can be calculated or estimated in a number of ways (Cohen, 2001). For instance, they may be derived from hospital charges after adjustment via the cost-to-charge ratio. Another method, activity-based costing (ABC), in which every resource item is identified and quantified into a unit cost, is considered by many health economists to be the most appropriate way of costing a radiological procedure although it is relatively labour-intensive (Cohen *et al.*, 2000). An example of ABC analysis is the study by U-King-Im *et al.*, which compared the costs of CE MRA and DSA in the assessment of patients with carotid stenosis (U-King-Im *et al.*, 2004a).

Discounting is usually applied to both costs and utilities because society places more importance on benefits gained and costs incurred in the present rather than at some point in the future. Discounting is particularly influential for screening and preventative interventions where costs occur early, and benefits and savings accumulate in later years. The choice of discount rate may vary according to local jurisdictions. For example, discount rates recommended by the UK National Institute of Clinical Excellence are 3.5% for both costs and utilities while in the USA, the Panel on Cost-effectiveness in Health and Medicine recommends rates of 3.0% for both (Siegel *et al.*, 1997; Berry *et al.*, 2002).

Once the model is completed, analysis can be performed to determine the mean cost and mean effectiveness of each strategy (Weinstein and Stason, 1977). Imaging strategies which are both more costly and less effective than others can be immediately rejected; in economic parlance these strategies are "dominated". Likewise if one strategy is cheaper and more effective than all alternatives (dominant) it can be selected without the need for further analysis. However, in many situations a small increase in diagnostic accuracy and effectiveness will come at the expense of increased costs. This trade-off can be quantified in the incremental cost effectiveness ratio (ICER). The ICER is the ratio of the increase in costs, or incremental costs, divided by the increase in

effectiveness, or incremental effectiveness. The ICER is especially useful in determining which of several strategies is the most cost-effective, yielding the most incremental benefits for acceptable incremental costs.

Finally, sensitivity analyses are necessary to determine the robustness of the conclusions of the model with regards to its assumptions and parameter uncertainty. For example, the sensitivity of DUS will not be known with complete certainty, but rather is thought very likely to lie within the bounds of a confidence interval. In one of its simplest forms, one-way sensitivity analysis, all the parameter values including probabilities, utilities and costs are varied one by one, from the upper to the lower clinically plausible bounds while other parameters are kept constant (Briggs *et al.*, 1994). In a robust model, plausible variations in parameter values will not alter the conclusions of the study. It is accepted practice to then proceed to simultaneously vary the most sensitive parameters in pairs or threes (two-way or three-way sensitivity analyses) to again determine the effect on the conclusions. Sensitivity analyses are also important to determine which variables carry more weight than others and hence, which are the most important variables in the model that drive the results and conclusions. For more detailed description of more complex sensitivity analyses, such as probabilistic sensitivity analyses, in which all parameters are varied simultaneously, readers are referred to Briggs *et al.* (Briggs *et al.*, 2002; Briggs, 2005).

Cost-effectiveness studies in symptomatic patients

There have been several studies reporting on the cost-effectiveness of carotid imaging modalities prior to surgery (Hankey and Warlow, 1990; Kent *et al.*, 1995; Vanninen *et al.*, 1995; Buskens *et al.*, 2004; U-King-Im *et al.*, 2005). Their main features are summarized in Table 13.1.

Table 13.1. Summary of main features of cost-effectiveness studies for carotid imaging in symptomatic patients

	Hankey and Warlcw, 1990	Vanninen et al., 1995	Kent et al., 1995	Buskens et al., 2004	U-King-Im et al., 2005	Wardlaw et al., 2006
Year	1990	1995	1995	2004	2005	2006
Study design	Scenario setting	Scenario setting	Decision-tree with Markov Model	Decision-tree with Markov model	Decision-tree with Markov model	Decision-tree with Markov model
Objective	Patient selection for DSA	Patient selection for surgery	Patient selection for surgery	Patient selection for surgery	Patient selection for surgery	Patient selection for surgery
Strategies compared	Auscultation, DUS, combination	DUS, MRA, DSA, combinations	DUS, MRA, DSA, combinations	DUS, MRA, DSA, combinations	DUS, DSA, CE MRA, combinations	DUS, CTA, CE MRA, DSA, combinations
Source of diagnostic accuracy data	Prospective 296 patients	Prospective 45 patients	Prospective 81 patients	Prospective 350 patients	Prospective 186 patients	Meta-analysis of individual patient data from 12 studies (2416 patients)
Source of clinical outcomes data	NA	NASCET (preliminary)	NASCET	NASCET	ECST	Oxford vascular study, NASCET, ECST
Duration	Not specified Short-term?	Not specified	Lifetime	Lifetime	10.8 years	20 years
Sensitivity analyses	One-way	Not performed	One-way and multiway	One-way	One-way probabilistic	One-way and multiway
Main outcome measures	Cost/case detected	Costs per stroke prevented	ICER Cost/QALY	ICER Cost/QALY	ICER Cost/QALY	Cost/QALY
Baseline results	For 75% stenosis, screening DUS and confirmatory DSA in all patients, regardless of carotid bruits	Screening DUS and DSA most cost-effective compared to DSA in all patients. Confirmatory MRA may also be cost-effective	Combination of screening DUS and MRA, with DSA for disparate results most cost-effective	DUS alone most cost-effective	Confirmatory DSA not cost-effective. Combinations of DUS and CE MRA, with DSA for disparate results most cost-effective	For early presentation, strategies including DUS as first or repeat, not DSA. For late presentation, DUS and CE MRA recommended

Abbreviations: NA: not available; CE MRA: contrast-enhanced magnetic resonance angiography; ICER: incremental cost-effectiveness ratio; QALY: Quality-adjusted-life-years

Hankey *et al.* investigated the safest and most cost-effective way to select patients for DSA prior to carotid endarterectomy by comparing different strategies involving clinical examination and DUS, in a cohort of 296 symptomatic patients (Hankey and Warlow, 1990). Main outcome measures were costs and number of disabling strokes after DSA. Their conclusions were that the optimal way to select patients for DSA was dependent on the degree of stenosis that the strategy aimed to detect. Thus, to detect stenosis of 50% or more, the most cost-effective method was to proceed directly to DSA in all patients with bruits and perform screening DUS in the remainder. For detection of 75% or more stenosis, screening all patients with ultrasound irrespective of bruits was shown to be least expensive while resulting in the least number of strokes after DSA. This study is somewhat limited as it antedated the final results of NASCET and ECST, and therefore the objectives were restricted to the selection of patients for DSA. This study did not examine outcomes after carotid endarterectomy. More importantly, it assumed that the sensitivity of duplex ultrasound was 100%, which is clearly unrealistic. The clinical relevance of this model is, however, perhaps outdated in modern day era where little emphasis is now placed on examination for carotid bruits before referring symptomatic patients for imaging.

Vanninen *et al.* also used a type of modelling technique to investigate the most cost-effective imaging protocol for patient selection prior to surgery (Vanninen *et al.*, 1995). They compared several imaging strategies which included DSA in all patients, screening DUS and confirmatory DSA, MRA in all patients and screening DUS and confirmatory MRA. Estimates of diagnostic accuracy were derived from a sample of 45 symptomatic patients. Main outcome measures were costs and number of prevented strokes. The conclusions were that strategies combining screening DUS and proceeding to either time-of-flight MRA or DSA in cases where DUS showed a moderate or severe stenosis were the most cost-effective. Strategies involving MRA or DSA as first-line modality

without screening DUS were clearly not cost-effective. Major limitations of this study however include absence of sensitivity analyses, small sample size, crude analysis of outcomes after surgery based on preliminary results of NASCET over a 12-month period only and limited description of the analysis of clinical efficacy.

Kent *et al.* used a decision-analytical model with Markov transition states to evaluate the least morbid and most cost-effective strategy for detection of severe stenosis. The combination of DUS and time-of-flight MRA, with DSA reserved for disparate results was found to be more cost-effective than DSA alone. Although methodologically sound from an economic point of view, limitations include accuracy estimates based on a small sample of patients, and inclusion of the asymptomatic side for calculation of estimates of diagnostic sensitivity and specificity. This inclusion may artificially inflate the specificity of the diagnostic tests as shown by Kallmes *et al.* (1996). Moreover, only short to moderate term outcomes of NASCET were available at the time of publication and long-term results had to be estimated from expert opinion.

Two more recent studies have also investigated the cost-effectiveness of diagnostic strategies in detection of severe carotid stenosis using decision-analytical models with Markov transition states. Buskens *et al.* found that DUS alone without MRA was the most cost-effective strategy (Buskens *et al.*, 2004). The strengths of the study included a large sample size of 350 symptomatic patients for calculations of estimates of accuracy. However, a time-of-flight MRA technique was used rather than the CE technique which is generally thought to result in technically superior quality MRA studies (Leclerc and Pruvo, 2000). On the other hand, in a study based on diagnostic accuracy results from 186 patients, U-King-Im *et al.* found that a combination of DUS and CE MRA, with DSA reserved for disparate results, was the most cost-effective strategy (U-King-Im *et al.*, 2005). The strengths of this study included prospectively acquired costs data as well as transition probabilities derived from individual patient data from the ECST study. This study defined a more selective combination of noninvasive imaging whereby patients only proceeded to DSA if the CE MRA was positive and the DUS negative for severe stenosis. This was the most cost-effective strategy as the marginal loss in diagnostic accuracy incurred by this strategy was outweighed by the reduced number of DSA procedures necessary compared to traditional combination strategies.

The most important point to highlight is the fact that in both these studies, there was consensus that routine DSA was no longer cost-effective in the routine work-up of the majority of patients after screening DUS. There was however discrepancy as to which noninvasive strategy was most-cost-effective. The main reason behind this apparent discrepancy probably resides in the diagnostic accuracy of DUS. Indeed, the specificity of DUS was 76% in the study by Buskens *et al.* compared to 66% in the study by U-King-Im *et al.* (Buskens *et al.*, 2004; U-King-Im *et al.*, 2005). This clearly highlights one of the most significant limitations of DUS, i.e. its interobserver variability. In fact, sensitivity analysis by U-King-Im *et al.* also showed that DUS was most cost-effective provided that its specificity exceeded 75%, although it needs to be stressed that this referred to a population of symptomatic arteries only (U-King-Im *et al.*, 2005). This also suggests that while cost-effectiveness analysis models are extremely useful in setting up guidelines, these guidelines cannot be universal; rather, they should be flexible and based on the accuracies of DUS and MRA at each institution as well as the local risks associated with DSA and carotid endarterectomy.

Finally, the most comprehensive cost-effectiveness analysis model on carotid imaging to date is the United Kingdom Health and Technology Assessment report, which comprised the work of a panel of UK experts in stroke, imaging, vascular surgery, statistics and health economic modelling (Wardlaw *et al.*, 2006). This model was based on a systematic review of the accuracy of less-invasive carotid imaging using STARD (standards for reporting of diagnostic accuracy) methodology, supplemented by individual patient data from primary research and audit studies in the UK. Costs of less-invasive tests, outpatient clinics, endarterectomy, and of stroke were also systematically reviewed and a microcosting exercise was performed. A key strength of the model was that it took into account the fact that emerging data now suggests that speed from symptom onset to definitive treatment, either surgery or medical therapy, is essential as the risk of subsequent stroke is highest in the first few weeks after a first transient ischemic attack and then declines thereafter (Coull *et al.*, 2004; Rothwell *et al.*, 2004; Fairhead and Rothwell, 2005). Therefore, for patients who present early (first few weeks) after a transient ischemic attack, both moderate and severe stenosis groups benefited from surgery and it was therefore less essential for imaging to accurately distinguish between moderate and severe stenosis. Thus strategies allowing more patients to reach endarterectomy quickly prevented most strokes and produced greatest net benefit. This included most strategies with DUS as first or repeat, not those with DSA. On the other hand, in patients investigated late after TIA, accuracy of imaging was much more crucial, as patients with moderate stenosis had lesser benefit with surgery, and CE MRA, following screening DUS was advocated prior to surgery.

Cost-effectiveness studies in asymptomatic patients

In asymptomatic patients, cost-effectiveness analysis studies have generally focussed on the cost-effectiveness of screening for the identification of more than 60% stenosis based on the results of the ACAS trial. Derdeyn *et al.* found that a one-time screening programme, with DUS and confirmatory DSA, in an asymptomatic population may be cost-effective only if the prevalence of disease was at least 20% in the population to be screened (Derdeyn and Powers, 1996). Results were however sensitive to the long-term risk of stroke after surgery as well as annual discount rates and QALYs. Annual screening programmes were not cost-effective. On the other hand, Lee *et al.* concluded that screening with DUS and confirmatory DSA in an asymptomatic population costs more per QALY than society generally considers acceptable (Lee *et al.*, 1997). For screening, compared to DUS alone, the use of confirmatory DSA after DUS was shown by Yin *et al.* to offer few additional QALYs at additional costs and was not advocated (Yin and Carpenter, 1998). Overall, the evidence for a routine screening programme for asymptomatic population is not compelling although in selected high-risk populations, it is possible that screening may be cost-effective.

Discussion

The quality of economic studies with respect to preoperative carotid imaging studies in symptomatic patients has significantly increased over the past decade. The two earlier studies published by Hankey *et al.* in 1990 and Vanninen *et al.* in 1994, although based on scenario setting, did not use recognized decision analysis methodology (Hankey and Warlow, 1990; Vanninen *et al.*, 1995). Since then, there have been several high-quality studies regarding the cost-effectiveness of preoperative carotid imaging. These recent studies seem to agree that confirmatory DSA is not cost-effective and not routinely indicated in the work-up of the majority of symptomatic patients prior to surgery. Thus, the benefits of imaging with noninvasive strategies (DUS alone, MRA, especially CE MRA, or combination strategies of DUS and MRA, with DSA reserved for disparate results) appear to outweigh the consequences of diagnostic misclassification with such noninvasive tests. It is also clear that there are only minimal differences between many noninvasive imaging strategies. Therefore, every institution need not rigidly apply guidelines based on one single study. Indeed, which noninvasive strategy is optimal, will vary at a local level based

on the accuracy of DUS and MRA as well as the risks of DSA and surgery. Local protocols may thus need to be defined on the basis of local expertise and preferences.

The report of the UK Health and Technology assessment panel needs to be highlighted as the most comprehensive study to date (Wardlaw *et al.*, 2006). Diagnostic accuracy estimates were based on a systematic review as well as individual patient data from 12 specialist centers as opposed to a single-center trial as in most other studies. Furthermore, other strengths are that most of the data and parameters input were based on clearly defined systematic reviews of the literature, representing the best published evidence to date. Finally, this report raises the issue that the most cost-effective imaging protocol may vary depending on whether the patient presents early or late after initial symptom onset. As shown by subgroup analysis of the major trials of carotid endarterectomy, for patients presenting within a few weeks of initial transient ischemic attack, both moderate and severe stenosis appear to derive significant benefit from surgery (Rothwell *et al.*, 2004). Therefore, accurate imaging to distinguish between moderate and severe stenosis may be less crucial than the speed to which these examinations can be practically conducted in order to precipitate rapid definitive treatment. The risk following initial symptom onset however appears to decline rather rapidly with time, and in patients presenting late, only severe stenosis derives significant benefit from surgery (Rothwell and Warlow, 2005). In patients presenting late, accurate preoperative imaging to distinguish between moderate and severe stenosis, such as DUS and MRA rather than DUS alone, may therefore be optimal.

There are several issues which warrant further study and need therefore to be discussed. First, all of the cost-effectiveness analysis studies attempted to define the optimal strategy prior to carotid endarterectomy, usually based on NASCET or ECST. However, with advances in experience and technology, carotid angioplasty and stenting are fast emerging as credible and safe alternatives to surgery (Yadav *et al.*, 2004). While several cost-effectiveness analysis models have addressed the issue of cost-effectiveness of stenting compared to surgery, none have yet studied the cost-effectiveness of imaging protocols prior to stenting (Gray *et al.*, 2002). It remains to be seen whether differences in costs as well as both short and long-term risks of strokes after stenting would affect the above conclusions. More prospective long-term data is however necessary for credible and relevant cost-effectiveness analysis models. Finally, with stenting, a potential new strategy whereby patients may proceed directly to DSA with a view to proceeding to stenting at the same sitting in DUS-screened patients, may also be contemplated, which may perhaps render MRA or CTA obsolete in routine patients.

Second, most of the cost-effectiveness analysis studies have used data from NASCET or ECST to model the risks of stroke and death after either surgery or medical therapy. While these large-scale studies still guide clinical practice today, the results of these trials were published at least 8 years ago and at that time best medical therapy comprised mainly of aspirin alone. It is suggested that, currently, the advent of newer medical therapies such as aggressive lipid lowering with high-dose statins or folate supplements may reduce the risk benefit of carotid endarterectomy compared to medical therapy. However, this still remains to be conclusively proven and results of trials such as the Intensive Carotid Artery Stenosis Treatment Trial which aims to evaluate such advances are currently awaited (Chaturvedi, 2003; Chaturvedi *et al.*, 2004).

Third, apart from the Health Technology Assessment report, few studies have dealt with the cost-effectiveness of CTA for carotid imaging. With the advent of multislice technology, initial studies had suggested a promising role for CTA (Cinat *et al.*, 1998). This probably reflects the paucity of rigorous published data regarding the accuracy of CTA in practice, as well as its limitations such as radiation exposure and inaccuracy in the presence of calcifications (Hollingworth *et al.*,

2003). Finally, studies have concentrated on the detection of severe stenosis and few have addressed the issue of cost-effectiveness of imaging for detection of moderate stenosis. This is due to the fact that it is debatable whether patients with moderate stenosis as a whole significantly benefit from surgery (Rothwell *et al.*, 2003). Risk assessment for such patients need to be taken at an individual level taking into account other clinical or angiographic risk factors, e.g. plaque ulceration, and this uncertainty clearly would make any cost-effectiveness analysis model highly complex.

Conclusions

Cost-effectiveness analysis is an invaluable tool in the setting of general guidelines and decision-making with regards to carotid imaging. Results of recent studies suggest that DSA is not cost-effective in the routine work-up of the majority of symptomatic patients prior to carotid endarterectomy but is still important as a definitive test when noninvasive tests disagree. There is debate as to which noninvasive strategy, amongst which DUS or MRA alone or in combination are most popular, is the optimal strategy but this is clearly dependent on individual center expertise. For asymptomatic patients, the evidence demonstrating the cost-effectiveness of screening programmes with either DUS alone or DUS and DSA is not very robust. Future work is necessary to evaluate the cost-effectiveness of imaging prior to new treatment strategies such as carotid stenting in symptomatic patients.

REFERENCES

Alvarez-Linera, J., Benito-Leon, J., Escribano, J., Campollo, J. and Gesto, R. (2003). Prospective evaluation of carotid artery stenosis: elliptic centric contrast-enhanced MR angiography and spiral CT angiography compared with digital subtraction angiography. *AJNR. American Journal of Neuroradiology*, **24**, 1012–19.

Athanasoulis, C. A. and Plomaritoglou, A. (2000). Pre-operative imaging of the carotid bifurcation. Current trends. *International Angiology*, **19**, 1–7.

Benade, M. M. and Warlow, C. P. (2002a). Cost of identifying patients for carotid endarterectomy. *Stroke*, **33**, 435–9.

Benade, M. M. and Warlow, C. P. (2002b). Costs and benefits of carotid endarterectomy and associated preoperative arterial imaging: a systematic review of health economic literature. *Stroke*, **33**, 629–38.

Beneficial effect of carotid endarterectomy in symptomatic patients with high-grade carotid stenosis. North American Symptomatic Carotid Endarterectomy Trial Collaborators (1991). *New England Journal of Medicine*, **325**, 445–53.

Berry, E., Kelly, S., Westwood, M. E., *et al.* (2002). The cost-effectiveness of magnetic resonance angiography for carotid artery stenosis and peripheral vascular disease: a systematic review. *Health Technology Assessment*, **6**, 1–155.

Blackmore, C. C. and Smith, W. J. (1998). Economic analyses of radiological procedures: a methodological evaluation of the medical literature. *European Journal of Radiology*, **27**, 123–30.

Briggs, A. (2005). Probabilistic analysis of cost-effectiveness models: statistical representation of parameter uncertainty. *Value Health*, **8**, 1–2.

Briggs, A. H., Goeree, R., Blackhouse, G. and O'Brien, B. J. (2002). Probabilistic analysis of cost-effectiveness models: choosing between treatment strategies for gastroesophageal reflux disease. *Medical Decision Making*, **22**, 290–308.

Briggs, A., Sculpher, M. and Buxton, M. (1994). Uncertainty in the economic evaluation of health care technologies: the role of sensitivity analysis. *Health Economics*, **3**, 95–104.

Buskens, E., Nederkoorn, P. J., Buijs-Van Der Woude, T., *et al.* (2004). Imaging of carotid arteries in symptomatic patients: cost-effectiveness of diagnostic strategies. *Radiology*, **233**, 101–12.

Chaturvedi, S. (2003). Should the multicenter carotid endarterectomy trials be repeated? *Archives of Neurology*, **60**, 774–5.

Chaturvedi, S., Clagett, P., Cote, R., Dillon, W., Findlay, M. and Flack, J. (2004). Intensive carotid artery stenosis treatment trial. Proceedings of the 29th International Stroke Conference.

Cinat, M., Lane, C. T., Pham, H., *et al.* (1998). Helical CT angiography in the preoperative evaluation of carotid artery stenosis. *Journal of Vascular Surgery*, **28**, 290–300.

Cohen, M. D. (2001). Determining costs of imaging services. *Radiology*, **220**, 563–5.

Cohen, M. D., Hawes, D. R., Hutchins, G. D., *et al.* (2000). Activity-based cost analysis: a method of analyzing the financial and operating performance of academic radiology departments. *Radiology*, **215**, 708–16.

Coull, A. J., Lovett, J. K. and Rothwell, P. M. (2004). Population based study of early risk of stroke after transient ischaemic attack or minor stroke: implications for public education and organisation of services. *British Medical Journal*, **328**, 326.

Davis, S. M. and Donnan, G. A. (2003). Is carotid angiography necessary? Editors disagree. *Stroke*, **34**, 1819.

Dawson, D. L., Roseberry, C. A. and Fujitani, R. M. (1997). Preoperative testing before carotid endarterectomy: a survey of vascular surgeons' attitudes. *Annals of Vascular Surgery*, **11**, 264–72.

Derdeyn, C. P. and Powers, W. J. (1996). Cost-effectiveness of screening for asymptomatic carotid atherosclerotic disease. *Stroke*, **27**, 1944–50.

Detsky, A. S., Naglie, G., Krahn, M. D., Naimark, D. and Redelmeier, D. A. (1997a). Primer on medical decision analysis: Part 1–Getting started. *Medical Decision Making*, **17**, 123–5.

Detsky, A. S., Naglie, G., Krahn, M. D., Redelmeier, D. A. and Naimark, D. (1997b). Primer on medical decision analysis: Part 2–Building a tree. *Medical Decision Making*, **17**, 126–35.

Devlin, N. and Parkin, D. (2004). Does NICE have a cost-effectiveness threshold and what other factors influence its decisions? A binary choice analysis. *Health Economics*, **13**, 437–52.

Endarterectomy for asymptomatic carotid artery stenosis. Executive Committee for the Asymptomatic Carotid Atherosclerosis Study (1995). *JAMA: the Journal of the American Medical Association*, **273**, 1421–8.

Fairhead, J. F. and Rothwell, P. M. (2005). The need for urgency in identification and treatment of symptomatic carotid stenosis is already established. *Cerebrovascular Diseases*, **19**, 355–8.

Gray, W. A., White, H. J., Jr., Barrett, D. M., *et al.* (2002). Carotid stenting and endarterectomy: a clinical and cost comparison of revascularization strategies. *Stroke*, **33**, 1063–70.

Hankey, G. J. and Warlow, C. P. (1990). Symptomatic carotid ischaemic events: safest and most cost effective way of selecting patients for angiography, before carotid endarterectomy. *British Medical Journal*, **300**, 1485–91.

Hollingworth, W., Nathens, A. B., Kanne, J. P., *et al.* (2003). The diagnostic accuracy of computed tomography angiography for traumatic or atherosclerotic lesions of the carotid and vertebral arteries: a systematic review. *European Journal of Radiology*, **48**, 88–102.

Kallmes, D. F., Omary, R. A., Dix, J. E., Evans, A. J. and Hillman, B. J. (1996). Specificity of MR angiography as a confirmatory test of carotid artery stenosis. *American Journal of Neuroradiology*, **17**, 1501–6.

Kent, K. C., Kuntz, K. M., Patel, M. R., *et al.* (1995). Perioperative imaging strategies for carotid endarterectomy. An analysis of morbidity and cost-effectiveness in symptomatic patients. *JAMA: the Journal of the American Medical Association*, **274**, 888–93.

Krahn, M. D., Naglie, G., Naimark, D., Redelmeier, D. A. and Detsky, A. S. (1997). Primer on medical decision analysis: Part 4–Analyzing the model and interpreting the results. *Medical Decision Making*, **17**, 142–51.

Leclerc, X. and Pruvo, J. P. (2000). Recent advances in magnetic resonance angiography of carotid and vertebral arteries. *Current Opinion in Neurology*, **13**, 75–82.

Lee, T. T., Solomon, N. A., Heidenreich, P. A., Oehlert, J. and Garber, A. M. (1997). Cost-effectiveness of screening for carotid stenosis in asymptomatic persons. *Annals of Internal Medicine*, **126**, 337–46.

Long, A., Lepoutre, A., Corbillon, E., Branchereau, A. and Kretz, J. G. (2002). Modalities of preoperative imaging of the internal carotid artery used in France. *Annals of Vascular Surgery*, **16**, 261–5.

Naglie, G., Krahn, M. D., Naimark, D., Redelmeier, D. A. and Detsky, A. S. (1997). Primer on medical decision analysis: Part 3–Estimating probabilities and utilities. *Medical Decision Making*, **17**, 136–41.

Naimark, D., Krahn, M. D., Naglie, G., Redelmeier, D. A. and Detsky, A. S. (1997). Primer on medical decision analysis: Part 5–Working with Markov processes. *Medical Decision Making*, **17**, 152–9.

Norris, J. W., Morriello, F., Rowed, D. W. and Maggisano, R. (2003). Vascular imaging before carotid endarterectomy. *Stroke*, **34**, E16.

Perkins, J. M., Galland, R. B., Simmons, M. J. and Magee, T. R. (2000). Carotid duplex imaging: variation and validation. *British Journal of Surgery*, **87**, 320–2.

Philips, Z., Ginnelly, L., Sculpher, M., *et al.* (2004). Review of guidelines for good practice in decision-analytic modelling in health technology assessment. *Health Technology Assessment*, **8**, iii-iv, ix-xi, 1–158.

Post, P. N., Stiggelbout, A. M. and Wakker, P. P. (2001). The utility of health states after stroke: a systematic review of the literature. *Stroke*, **32**, 1425–9.

Randomised trial of endarterectomy for recently symptomatic carotid stenosis: final results of the MRC European Carotid Surgery Trial (ECST) (1998). *Lancet*, **351**, 1379–87.

Randoux, B., Marro, B. and Marsault, C. (2004). Carotid artery stenosis: competition between CT angiography and MR angiography. *AJNR. American Journal of Neuroradiology*, **25**, 663–4; author reply 664.

Robless, P. and Halliday, A. (1999). Vascular Surgical Society of Great Britain and Ireland: carotid angiography is used more selectively in the Asymptomatic Carotid Surgery Trial. *British Journal Surgery*, **86**, 690–1.

Rothwell, P. M., Eliasziw, M., Gutnikov, S. A., *et al.* (2003). Analysis of pooled data from the randomised controlled trials of endarterectomy for symptomatic carotid stenosis. *Lancet*, **361**, 107–16.

Rothwell, P. M., Eliasziw, M., Gutnikov, S. A., Warlow, C. P. and Barnett, H. J. (2004). Endarterectomy for symptomatic carotid stenosis in relation to clinical subgroups and timing of surgery. *Lancet*, **363**, 915–24.

Rothwell, P. M. and Warlow, C. P. (2005). Timing of TIAs preceding stroke: time window for prevention is very short. *Neurology*, **64**, 817–20.

Siegel, J. E., Torrance, G. W., Russell, L. B., *et al.* (1997). Guidelines for pharmacoeconomic studies. Recommendations from the panel on cost effectiveness in health and medicine. Panel on cost Effectiveness in Health and Medicine. *Pharmacoeconomics*, **11**, 159–68.

Singer, M. E. and Applegate, K. E. (2001). Cost-effectiveness analysis in radiology. *Radiology*, **219**, 611–20.

Sonnenberg, F. A. and Beck, J. R. (1993). Markov models in medical decision making: a practical guide. *Medical Decision Making*, **13**, 322–38.

U-King-Im, J., Hollingworth, W., Trivedi, R. A., *et al.* (2005). Cost-effectiveness of diagnostic strategies prior to carotid endarterectomy. *Annals of Neurology*, **58**, 506–15.

U-King-Im, J., Hollingworth, W., Trivedi, R. A., *et al.* (2004a). Contrast-enhanced MR angiography vs intra-arterial digital subtraction angiography for carotid imaging: activity-based cost analysis. *European Radiology*, **14**, 730–5.

U-King-Im, J., Trivedi, R. A., Graves, M. J., *et al.* (2004b). Contrast-enhanced MR angiography for carotid disease: diagnostic and potential clinical impact. *Neurology*, **62**, 1282–90.

Vanninen, R., Manninen, H. and Soimakallio, S. (1995). Imaging of carotid artery stenosis: clinical efficacy and cost-effectiveness. *AJNR. American Journal of Neuroradiology*, **16**, 1875–83.

Wardlaw, J. M., Chappell, F. M., Stephenson, M., *et al.* (2006). Accurate, practical and cost-effective assessment of carotid stenosis in the UK. *Health Technology Assessment*, **10**, 1–200.

Weinstein, M. C. and Stason, W. B. (1977). Foundations of cost-effectiveness analysis for health and medical practices. *New England Journal of Medicine*, **296**, 716–21.

Willinsky, R. A., Taylor, S. M., Terbrugge, K., *et al.* (2003). Neurologic complications of cerebral angiography: prospective analysis of 2,899 procedures and review of the literature. *Radiology*, **227**, 522–8.

Yadav, J. S., Wholey, M. H., Kuntz, R. E., *et al.* (2004). Protected carotid-artery stenting versus endarterectomy in high-risk patients. *New England Journal of Medicine*, **351**, 1493–501.

Yin, D. and Carpenter, J. P. (1998). Cost-effectiveness of screening for asymptomatic carotid stenosis. *Journal of Vascular Surgery*, **27**, 245–55.

14

MR plaque imaging

Chun Yuan and Tom Hatsukami

University of Washington, Seattle WA, USA

Introduction

The progression of atherosclerosis, from its initial state to the formation of "high risk" advanced lesions, is in most cases a complex, indolent process. Noninvasive techniques for imaging the diseased vessel wall will play an increasingly important role in the assessment of atherosclerotic disease status, so that optimized treatment schemes, from lifestyle changes to surgery or stenting, can be individualized for each patient.

In this chapter, the state-of-the-art noninvasive magnetic resonance imaging (MRI) techniques used to monitor atherosclerosis of the carotid artery are introduced and summarized. The clinical value of these techniques will be assessed and the future role of MR in vascular imaging will be considered.

Role of MRI

Clinically, the degree of lumen stenosis is used as a marker for atherosclerosis severity. Vulnerable plaques, however, often elude detection by techniques that rely on measuring the size of the vessel lumen alone. One reason this occurs is due to expansive arterial remodeling, in which the artery increases only its external wall boundary in response to the development of an atherosclerotic plaque (Glagov et al., 1997). The other reason is that plaque tissue constituents are closely linked

to not only lumen size but also plaque vulnerability (Fuster et al., 2005). Thus, an ideal imaging technique should be able to demarcate the vessel lumen and outer wall boundary, distinguish the main atherosclerotic plaque components, and determine luminal surface conditions. High-resolution MRI is an ideal plaque imaging technique because it is noninvasive and able to create excellent soft tissue contrast and distinguish flowing blood from surrounding stationary tissues.

MR carotid plaque imaging technique

Surface coil

Histological evaluation of carotid endarterectomy specimens has demonstrated that the mean values for the volume of major plaque components (the lipid-rich necrotic core [LRNC], intraplaque hemorrhage [IPH], fibrous tissue, and calcification) ranges from 0.3 mm³ and up (Hatsukami et al., 1997). In order to achieve submillimeter voxel sizes with whole body 1.5 T machines, the use of a phase-array surface coil, pioneered by Hayes et al. (1996), has been widely deployed in carotid plaque imaging. This phased-array design improves the signal-to-noise ratio (SNR) for imaging the common, internal and external carotid arteries with a best voxel size of $0.25 \times 0.25 \times 2.0$ mm³. In addition to the carotid phased-array assembly, a custom designed head holder was constructed

Carotid Disease: The Role of Imaging in Diagnosis and Management, ed. Jonathan Gillard, Martin Graves, Thomas Hatsukami and Chun Yuan. Published by Cambridge University Press. © Cambridge University Press 2007.

using vacuum-formed PVC plastic. The head holder provides support for the occiput and neck, which not only improves patient comfort, but also facilitates repeatable scan positioning and reduces patient movement.

Multicontrast weighted imaging

Most recent literature supports the use of a multi-contrast weighted imaging technique to study the in vivo morphology of carotid plaques (Yuan *et al.*, 1994; Toussaint *et al.*, 1996; Shinnar *et al.*, 1999; Hatsukami *et al.*, 2000; Yuan *et al.*, 2001; Mitsumori *et al.*, 2003). A key element of plaque imaging is to combine the use of "bright blood" and "black blood" techniques, which either enhance or suppress signals from flowing blood. Black blood techniques can be combined with regular spin echo (or fast spin echo) sequences to acquire cross-sectional images of the artery with T_1-weighting, T_2-weighting and other contrast-weighted images. This technique is particularly useful to visualize the vessel lumen and outer wall boundaries. A multicontrast weighted imaging protocol, based on extensive testing with normal volunteers and carotid endarterectomy patients, can be found in (Yarnykh and Yuan, 2003a). This protocol: (1) provides an oblique view of the carotid artery to better visualize the location of the carotid bifurcation and to demonstrate plaque distribution; (2) uses the bifurcation as an internal landmark to reproducibly prescribe slice locations for serial studies; and (3) maintains the total exam time to an average of 40 minutes. This protocol has been used in a series of validation studies and multicenter clinical trials (Kang *et al.*, 2000; Yuan *et al.*, 2001; Cai *et al.*, 2002; Luo *et al.*, 2003; Chu *et al.*, 2004; Saam *et al.*, 2005a,b) (Figure 14.1). Chemical selective fat saturation is used to reduce the signal from the subcutaneous tissues (Yarnykh and Yuan, 2003a) in all sequences. Cardiac gating was found to reduce flow and motion artifacts and is incorporated with the long echo time (TE) and repetition time (TR) sequences.

Histological validation

Over the past decade, the accuracy of MRI for characterizing carotid atherosclerosis has been extensively validated by comparing preoperative carotid MRI findings to matched histological sections of the excised plaque.

MRI to determine atherosclerotic plaque lesion type

The objective of the American Heart Association (AHA) histological classification of atherosclerosis, first published in 1995, was to provide a clinically relevant categorization of human atherosclerotic lesions based on their histological composition and structure (Stary *et al.*, 1995). The types of lesions that constitute this histological classification are perceived as characteristic gradations or stages from initial minimal changes to lesions associated with clinical manifestations. The resulting classification reflects the temporal natural history of the disease. Therefore, a noninvasive method for determining lesion types in vivo using imaging would be important for clinical staging of athero-sclerosis. A recent study demonstrated the ability of multicontrast weighted carotid MRI to determine these lesions types. Using a modified AHA lesion type definition, Cai *et al.* studied the agreement between histology and MRI for classifying lesion types in 60 patients scheduled for carotid endar-terectomy. Preoperative carotid MRI imaging was performed within 1 week prior to surgery. The MR images and histological specimens were reviewed and classified by independent readers who were blinded to each other's findings. Overall, the classification obtained by MRI and histology showed good agreement, with Cohen's κ (95% CI, 0.74 [0.67–0.82]) and weighted $\kappa = 0.79$ (Cai *et al.*, 2002) (Table 14.1).

MRI to measure diseased vessel wall size

The ability of MRI to delineate both the luminal surface and outer wall boundary (adventitia) was

Table 14.1. Classification of carotid atherosclerotic plaque by multicontrast weighted magnetic resonance imaging (MRI) and histological examination

Classification by MRI	Classification by histological examination						
	I–II	III	IV–V	VI	VII	VIII	Total
I–II	8	...	...	...	...	...	8
III	4	30	...	...	...	...	34
IV–V	...	7	47	8	2	2	66
VI	...	...	6	75	7	1	89
VII	...	...	3	9	37	1	50
VIII	...	...	...	...	...	5	5
Total	12	37	56	92	46	9	252

Source: Cohen's (95% CI = 0.74 [0.67 − 0.82]; weighted κ = 0.79.

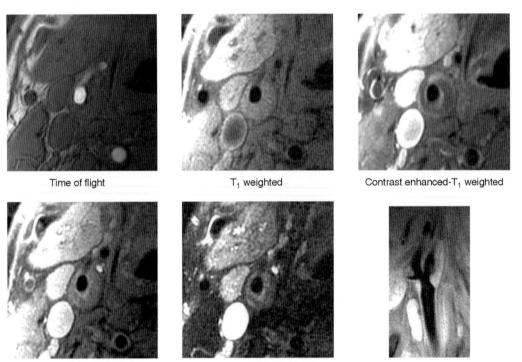

Time of flight T_1 weighted   Contrast enhanced-T_1 weighted

Proton density weighted T_2 weighted T_1 weighted

Figure 14.1 Multiple contrast imaging. There is an atherosclerotic plaque in the right carotid artery. This lesion demonstrates a slightly hyperintense signal on T_1, proton density, and T_2. This lesion shows no contrast enhancement on contrast enhanced T_1 weighted. Note: luminal surface demonstrates isointense signal on T_1-weighted, hyperintense signal on proton density and T_2. It shows contrast enhancement on contrast enhanced T_1. (Courtesy of J. M. Cai of PLA General Hospital in Beijing.)

first validated by a study that compared the maximum wall areas measured from MR images of the carotid artery in vivo to those from the carotid endarterectomy specimen ex vivo (Yuan *et al.*, 1998). This study demonstrated that black blood (T_1-weighting and proton density weighted) MRI is highly accurate for in vivo measurement of artery wall area in patients with advanced carotid atherosclerosis. The intraobserver and interobserver variability was small, with intraclass correlation coefficients ranging from 0.90 to 0.98. A series of studies have followed this work in (1) developing automated boundary detection techniques to trace the lumen and outer vessel wall area accurately and efficiently (Chao *et al.*, 2003) (discussed further in Chapter 30 on image postprocessing); (2) introducing improved image acquisition techniques aimed at improving spatial resolution, coverage, and flow suppression (Yarnykh and Yuan, 2003b); and (3) conducting reproducibility and inter- or intrarater variability studies. In an early study assessing the precision of quantitative measurements of the diseased vessel wall with MRI, the error for wall volume measurement ranged from 4 to 6% across different contrast methods (Kang *et al.*, 2000). In a more recently published multicenter study involving individuals undergoing repeated MRI studies, measurement error for assessing wall volume was 5.8%, lumen volume was 4.3%, and outer wall volume (also known as total wall volume) was 3.3% (Saam *et al.*, 2005b). Measurement error for assessing percent atheroma volume, defined as the wall volume divided by total wall volume, was 3.2%. As described in more detail in Chapter 30, vessel wall volume has been used in a number of clinical trials as the primary endpoint to evaluate the effect of LDL-cholesterol-lowering drugs in patients with carotid and aortic atherosclerosis.

MRI to detect and quantitate plaque composition

Major plaque components include fibrous connective tissue (including the fibrous cap), the lipid-rich necrotic core, intraplaque hemorrhage, and calcification. Over the years, a significant number of studies have evaluated the ability of MRI to detect these atherosclerotic tissues (Fayad and Fuster, 2000; Yuan and Kerwin, 2004), and many have noted the need to use both bright and black blood techniques with different contrast weightings. In particular, black blood T_1-weighted, T_2-weighted, or bright blood time-of-flight (TOF) or the combination of these different contrast-weighted imaging techniques have all been proven to be useful (Yuan *et al.*, 1995; Toussaint *et al.*, 1996; Hatsukami *et al.*, 1997; Cai *et al.*, 2002; Saam *et al.*, 2005a). Based on ex vivo studies, diffusion-weighted imaging has also been shown to be useful for identifying the lipid-rich necrotic core (Shinnar *et al.*, 1999; Clarke *et al.*, 2003). The four categories of studies summarized below reflect the current state of plaque tissue characterization that is based on multicontrast weighting and the use of gadolinium contrast enhancement.

Study 1: Quantitative evaluation of carotid plaque composition by in vivo MRI: (Saam et al., *2004, 2005a)*

This study evaluated the ability of MRI to quantify all major carotid atherosclerotic plaque components in vivo, using a histological goldstandard for comparison. Thirty-one subjects, scheduled for carotid endarterectomy were imaged with a 1.5 T machine using TOF, T_1-weighted, proton density-weighted, and T_2-weighted images. Two hundred and fourteen MRI locations were matched to corresponding histology sections. For both MRI and histology, area measurements of the major plaque components, such as the LRNC, calcification, loose extracellular matrix and dense (fibrous) tissue were recorded as percentages of the total wall area. Intraclass correlation coefficients (ICC) were computed to determine intra- and interreader reproducibility. MRI measurements of plaque composition were statistically equivalent to those of histology for the LRNC (23.7 vs. 20.3%; $p = 0.1$), loose matrix (5.1 vs. 6.3%; $p = 0.1$) and dense

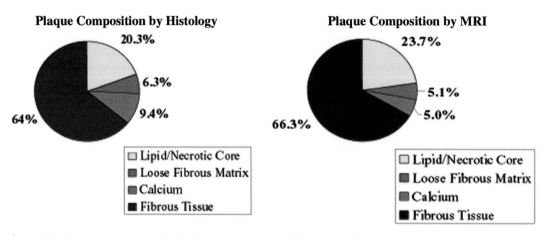

Figure 14.2 Plaque composition calculated as the percentage of the vessel wall area, calculated per artery, and then averaged across all arteries for magnetic resonance imaging (MRI) and histology (Saam, T. *et al.* (2004), *JCMR.* 2004).

(fibrous) tissue (66.3% vs. 64%; $p = 0.4$). Calcification differed significantly when measured as a percentage of wall area (9.4 vs. 5%; $p < 0.001$). Intra- and interreader reproducibility was good to excellent for all tissue components, with ICC ranging from 0.73 to 0.95. Findings from this study demonstrate that MRI-based tissue quantification of carotid plaque composition is accurate and reproducible (Figure 14.2).

In another recently published study by Trivedi and colleagues (Trivedi *et al.*, 2004), 25 recently symptomatic patients with severe internal carotid artery stenosis underwent preoperative in vivo multisequence MRI of the carotid artery using a 1.5 T system. Individual plaque constituents were characterized on axial MR images according to net signal intensities. Analysis of fibrous cap and lipid core content was quantified proportional to overall plaque area. Similar to the aforementioned study, there was good agreement between readers, with intraclass correlation coefficients of 0.94 and 0.88 for quantifying fibrous cap and lipid core components, respectively. Furthermore, there was good agreement between MR and histology-derived quantification of both fibrous cap and lipid core content. The mean % difference for fibrous cap was 0.75% (±2.86%) and for lipid core was 0.86% (±1.76%).

Study 2: Fibrous cap status as assessed by MRI

A report published in 2000 described the use of a 3D-TOF bright-blood imaging technique to identify unstable fibrous caps in atherosclerotic human carotid arteries in vivo (Hatsukami *et al.*, 2000). Based on the preoperative images of 22 consecutive endarterectomy patients, the state of the fibrous cap was categorized as intact/thick, intact/thin, or ruptured. Intact/thick fibrous caps on 3D-TOF images appeared as a continuous hypointense band near the bright lumen (from flowing blood). In plaques where the hypointense band could not be visualized, the cap was categorized as intact/thin. Fibrous cap rupture was identified by the absence or discontinuity of the hypointense band, juxtaluminal hyperintense signal in the TOF and T_1-weighting images (consistent with recent hemorrhage), and/or irregular lumen surface. The authors found a high level of agreement between the MRI findings and the histological state of the fibrous cap, with a kappa (95% CI) value of 0.83 (0.67–1.0) and a weighted kappa value of 0.87. In a follow-up study, the accuracy of fibrous cap detection based on a multicontrast approach (including 3D-TOF) was assessed by comparing preoperative MRI findings in patients scheduled for carotid endarterectomy to histology

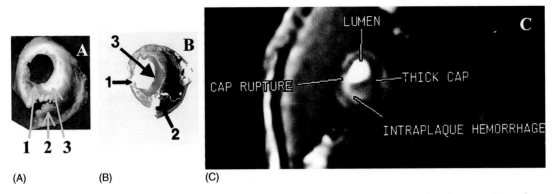

Figure 14.3 Example of plaque with fibrous cap rupture on gross section histology (Masson's trichrome stain), and magnetic resonance imaging (MRI). On gross and histological sections, there is an area of cap rupture (arrow 1) next to a region where fibrous cap is thick (arrow 3). Cap rupture site corresponds to region where dark band is absent, and hyperintense, bright region is seen adjacent to lumen on MRI. Hyperintense region in plaque core on MRI corresponds to region of recent intraplaque hemorrhage on gross and histological cross sections (arrow 2). (Hatsukami, T. S. *et al.* (2000) Circulation, **102**, 959–64.)

(Mitsumori *et al.*, 2003). The sensitivity and specificity for identifying a thin or ruptured cap in vivo, were 81% and 90%, respectively. Figure 14.3 illustrates the multicontrast appearance of the fibrous cap.

Study 3: Gadolinium contrast-enhanced MRI improves the quantitative measurement of lipid-rich necrotic core size and the fibrous cap

Previous studies using contrast-enhanced MRI (CE MRI) have shown that the fibrous cap (FC) in atherosclerotic carotid plaque enhances with gadolinium-based contrast agents (Wasserman *et al.*, 2002; Yuan *et al.*, 2002a). Conversely, the lipid-rich necrotic core, lacking both vasculature and matrix shows no or slight enhancement. In a recently published study (Cai *et al.*, 2005), the ability of CE MRI to accurately measure the dimensions of intact FC and the lipid-rich necrotic core was assessed. Twenty-one patients scheduled for carotid endarterectomy were imaged with a 1.5 T machine. Precontrast images and CE MRI were obtained. One hundred and eight locations with an intact FC were matched between MRI and the excised histology specimen. The quantitative measurements of FC length along the lumen circumference, FC area and LRNC area were collected from CE MRI images and histology sections. Blinded comparison of corresponding MR images and histology slices showed moderate to good correlation for length ($r = 0.73$, $p < 0.001$) and area ($r = 0.80$, $p < 0.001$) of the intact FC. The mean percentage LRNC areas (LRNC area/wall area) measured by CE MRI and histology were 30.1% and 32.7%, respectively, and were strongly correlated ($r = 0.87$, $p < 0.001$). The investigators concluded that in vivo high resolution CE MRI is capable of quantitatively measuring the dimensions of intact FC and LRNC, and provides continuous variables for characterizing intact FC and LRNC in progression and regression studies.

Study 4: Differentiation of intraplaque versus juxtaluminal hemorrhage in advanced atherosclerotic lesions by MRI (Kampschulte et al., 2004)

Intraplaque hemorrhage, deep within the core of the lesion, and juxtaluminal hemorrhage may differ in etiology and clinical implications. A recent study tested the hypothesis that MRI can distinguish between deep intraplaque hemorrhage and juxta-luminal hemorrhage in 26 patients scheduled for carotid endarterectomy. Hemorrhages were identified using previously established MRI criteria, and their locations were differentiated between intraplaque and juxtaluminal. Corresponding histology was used to confirm the MR findings. Matched sections ($n = 190$) contained 144 areas of hemorrhage by histology, of which MRI correctly detected 132 areas. The sensitivity and specificity for MRI to correctly identify cross-sections containing hemorrhage were 96% and 82%, respectively. Furthermore, MRI was able to distinguish juxtaluminal hemorrhage/thrombus from intraplaque hemorrhage with an accuracy of 96%. The authors concluded that in vivo high resolution MRI can detect and differentiate intraplaque hemorrhage from juxtaluminal hemorrhage with good accuracy, and that noninvasive MRI provides a possible tool for prospectively studying differences in etiology of plaque hemorrhage and its association of plaque progression and instability.

Clinical studies with MRI

Factors associated with more rapid progression in plaque burden

Noninvasive MRI provides an opportunity to prospectively study factors that influence the rate of progression of atherosclerotic plaque burden, as well as vessel wall remodeling. In a recent study, Saam *et al.* analyzed 68 asymptomatic subjects with ≥50% stenosis, as measured by duplex ultrasound, who underwent serial carotid MRI examinations over an 18-month period (Saam *et al.*, 2006). Clinical risk factors for atherosclerosis and medications were also documented prospectively. The wall and outer wall areas, matched across time-points, were measured from cross-sectional images using a custom-designed image analysis tool. The wall/outer wall ratio was calculated and used as a marker of disease severity. Multiple regression analysis was used to correlate risk

factors and morphological features of the plaque with the rate of progression/regression. Averaged across the 68 subjects, the wall area increased by 2.3% per year ($p = 0.004$). Multiple regression analysis demonstrated that statin therapy ($p = 0.02$) and lesions with a wall/outer wall ratio >0.6 at baseline ($p = 0.002$), were associated with a significantly reduced rate of progression in mean wall area. The rate of mean wall area progression amongst subjects on statins ($n = 47$) was 1.2% per year, compared to 4.4% per year for those not on statin therapy ($n = 21$). Amongst arteries with a wall/outer wall ratio of ≤0.6 at baseline ($n = 32$), the mean wall area increased by 4.6% per year, compared to 0.0% per year for those with a wall/outer wall ratio >0.6 ($n = 36$). Furthermore, the study demonstrated that earlier stage lesions, as defined by a wall/outer wall ratio <0.6, exhibited expansive remodeling without reduction in mean lumen area, whereas more advanced lesions (wall/outer wall ratio >0.6) showed progression in luminal narrowing, but no expansive remodeling.

Another interesting recent study provides in vivo support for histological studies suggesting that intraplaque hemorrhage into the necrotic core may be a driving force in the progression of atherosclerosis (Takaya *et al.*, 2005a). In this case-control study, 29 subjects (14 cases with intraplaque hemorrhage and 15 controls with comparably sized plaques without intraplaque hemorrhage at baseline) underwent serial carotid MRI examination with a multicontrast weighted protocol over a period of 18 months. The volumes of wall, lumen, lipid-rich necrotic core, calcification, and intraplaque hemorrhage were measured with a custom-designed image analysis tool. The percent change in wall volume (6.8% vs. −0.15%; $p = 0.009$) and lipid-rich necrotic core volume (28.4% versus −5.2%; $p = 0.001$) was significantly higher in the hemorrhage group than in controls over the course of the study. Furthermore, those with intraplaque hemorrhage at baseline were much more likely to have new plaque hemorrhages at 18 months compared with controls (43% vs. 0%; $p = 0.006$).

Table 14.2. Status of the fibrous cap as determined by magnetic resonance imaging (MRI) versus symptomatic status of patient

Cap status by MRI	Symptomatic	Asymptomatic	% With symptoms	Odds ratio for symptoms	95% CI
Intact thick (I)	1	10	9	1	…
Intact thin (II)	6	6	50	10	1.0, 104
Ruptured (III)	21	9	70	23	3, 210

Source: $p = 0.001$ Mann-Whitney test for cap status versus symptoms. Patients were considered symptomatic if they had a transient ischemic attack or stroke appropriate to the distribution of the index carotid artery within 90 days before carotid endarterectomy.

Association between plaque characteristics and transient ischemic attack or stroke

In a cross-sectional study aimed at determining whether MRI identification of fibrous cap rupture is associated with recent transient ischemic attack (TIA) or stroke, MRI scans were performed on 53 patients (28 symptomatic, 25 asymptomatic), and the fibrous cap was categorized as thick, thin, or ruptured (Yuan *et al.*, 2002b). There was a highly significant trend showing a higher percentage of symptomatic patients for ruptured caps (70%) compared with thick caps (9%) ($p = 0.001$ Mann-Whitney test for cap status vs. symptoms). Compared with patients with thick fibrous caps, patients with ruptured caps were 23 times more likely to have had a recent ipsilateral carotid-distribution TIA or stroke (Table 14.2).

More recently, these findings were given further support by a prospective study examining the association between baseline carotid plaque characteristics and the development of future ipsilateral TIA or stroke (Takaya *et al.*, 2005b, 2006). Patients ($n = 154$) who initially had an asymptomatic 50–79% carotid stenosis by ultrasound underwent a baseline multicontrast weighted carotid MRI and were followed clinically every 3 months to identify symptoms of TIA or stroke. Over a mean follow-up period of 38.2 months, 12 carotid cerebrovascular events occurred ipsilateral to the index carotid artery. Cox regression analysis demonstrated a significant association between baseline MRI identification of the following plaque characteristics and subsequent symptoms during follow-up: presence of a thin or ruptured fibrous cap (hazard ratio, 17.0; $p < 0.001$), intraplaque hemorrhage (hazard ratio, 5.2; $p = 0.005$), larger mean intraplaque hemorrhage area (hazard ratio for 10 mm^2 increase, 2.6; $p = 0.006$), larger maximum % lipid-rich/necrotic core (hazard ratio for 10% increase, 1.6; $p = 0.004$), and larger maximum wall thickness (hazard ratio for a 1 mm increase, 1.6; $p = 0.008$). This prospective study provided the first evidence that baseline plaque characteristics, as identified by MRI, are significantly associated with the development of future ischemic events.

Clinical implications and future directions

In two recently published consensus reports by a group of experts in atherosclerosis research, including pathologists, clinicians, molecular biologists and imaging scientists, the key features of the vulnerable plaque were redefined (Naghavi *et al.*, 2003a,b). The report argues that knowledge of the luminal diameter is not sufficient to determine the risk of an atherosclerotic lesion, and proposed five major and five minor criteria for the detection of vulnerable plaque. These plaque features included thin caps with large necrotic core, active inflammation, fissured plaque, stenosis >90%, superficial calcified nodules, intraplaque hemorrhage, glistening yellow color by angioscopy, endothelial denudation or dysfunction and outward remodeling.

MRI is capable of identifying many of the key vulnerable plaque features defined by the expert panel with a high level of accuracy and reproducibility. This capability is further substantiated by recently published prospective studies that demonstrate significant associations between MRI-identified plaque features and more rapid progression as well as risk for future ischemic events.

In order to use this technique effectively, it is critical to establish efficient, automated image analysis tools that will provide quantitative data on plaque morphology and composition accurately and reproducibly. Novel strategies for quantitative analysis are discussed in Chapter 30. Furthermore, there is a need for standardized criteria for describing MRI findings of the complex atherosclerotic plaque, ideally in the form of a simple scoring system that provides predictive value for rapid plaque progression and future ischemic events.

Another important development is targeted imaging, which potentially will permit identification of specific tissues, cells and molecules not currently visible with MR technology.

Conclusions

MRI is able to noninvasively identify the critical features of the vulnerable plaque, and provides an opportunity to prospectively examine in vivo, the association between plaque characteristics, rapid progression, and the development of ischemic events. Furthermore, there is increasing recognition of the importance of systemic factors, such as the inflammatory and thrombogenic state of the patient, and MRI provides an essential tool to examine the effect of both systemic and local processes on the development of the high-risk atherosclerotic lesion. Improved methods of detecting the individual at greatest risk will permit more

selective aggressive therapy, and ultimately provide benefits in terms of improved quality of life and reduced health-care costs.

REFERENCES

Cai, J. M., Hatsukami, T. S., Ferguson, M. S., et al. (2005). In vivo quantitative measurement of intact fibrous cap and lipid rich necrotic core size in atherosclerotic carotid plaque: a comparison of high resolution contrast enhanced MRI and histology. *Circulation*, **112**, 3437–44.

Cai, J. M., Hatsukami, T. S., Ferguson, M. S., Small, R., Polissar, N. L. and Yuan, C. (2002). Classification of human carotid atherosclerotic lesions with in vivo multicontrast magnetic resonance imaging. *Circulation*, **106**, 1368–73.

Chao, H., Kerwin, W. S., Hatsukami, T. S., Hwang, J. N. and Yuan, C. (2003). Detecting objects in image sequences using rule-based control in an active contour model. *IEEE Transactions on Bio-Medical Engineering*, **50**, 705–10.

Chu, B., Hatsukami, T. S., Polissar, N. L., et al. (2004). Determination of carotid artery atherosclerotic lesion type and distribution in hypercholesterolemic patients with moderate carotid stenosis using noninvasive magnetic resonance imaging. *Stroke*, **35**, 2444–8.

Clarke, S. E., Hammond, R. R., Mitchell, J. R. and Rutt, B. K. (2003). Quantitative assessment of carotid plaque composition using multicontrast MRI and registered histology. *Magnetic Resonance in Medicine*, **50**, 1199–208.

Fayad, Z. A. and Fuster, V. (2000). Characterization of atherosclerotic plaques by magnetic resonance imaging. *Annals of the New York Academy of Sciences*, **902**, 173–86.

Fuster, V., Moreno, P. R., Fayad, Z. A., Corti, R. and Badimon, J. J. (2005). Atherothrombosis and high-risk plaque: part I: evolving concepts. *Journal of the American College of Cardiology*, **46**, 937–54.

Glagov, S., Bassiouny, H. S., Sakaguchi, Y., Goudet, C. A. and Vito, R. P. (1997). Mechanical determinants of plaque modeling, remodeling and disruption. *Atherosclerosis*, **131** (Suppl.), S13–4.

Hatsukami, T. S., Ferguson, M. S., Beach, K. W., et al. (1997). Carotid plaque morphology and clinical events. *Stroke*, **28**, 95–100.

Hatsukami, T. S., Ross, R., Polissar, N. L. and Yuan, C. (2000). Visualization of fibrous cap thickness and rupture in human atherosclerotic carotid plaque in vivo with high-resolution magnetic resonance imaging. *Circulation*, **102**, 959–64.

Hayes, C. E., Mathis, C. M. and Yuan, C. (1996). Surface coil phased arrays for high resolution imaging of the carotid arteries. *Journal of Magnetic Resonance Imaging*, **1**, 109–12.

Kampschulte, A., Ferguson, M. S., Kerwin, W. S., *et al.* (2004). Differentiation of intraplaque versus juxtaluminal hemorrhage/thrombus in advanced human carotid atherosclerotic lesions by in vivo magnetic resonance imaging. *Circulation*, **110**, 3239–44.

Kang, X., Polissar, N. L., Han, C., Lin, E. and Yuan, C. (2000). Analysis of the measurement precision of arterial lumen and wall areas using high-resolution MRI in Process Citation. *Magnetic Resonance in Medicine*, **44**, 968–72.

Luo, Y., Polissar, N., Han, C., *et al.* (2003). Accuracy and uniqueness of three in vivo measurements of atherosclerotic carotid plaque morphology with black blood MRI. *Magnetic Resonance in Medicine*, **50**, 75–82.

Mitsumori, L. M., Hatsukami, T. S., Ferguson, M. S., *et al.* (2003). In vivo accuracy of multisequence MR imaging for identifying unstable fibrous caps in advanced human carotid plaques. *Journal of Magnetic Resonance Imaging*, **17**, 410–20.

Naghavi, M., Libby, P., Falk, E., *et al.* (2003a). From vulnerable plaque to vulnerable patient: a call for new definitions and risk assessment strategies: Part I. *Circulation*, **108**, 1664–72.

Naghavi, M., Libby, P., Falk, E., *et al.* (2003b). From vulnerable plaque to vulnerable patient: a call for new definitions and risk assessment strategies: Part II. *Circulation*, **108**, 1772–8.

Saam, T., Ferguson, M. S., Yarnykh, V., *et al.* (2004). Accuracy of in vivo quantitative characterization of atherosclerotic carotid plaque: A high-resolution, multicontrast magnetic resonance imaging study. *Journal of Cardiovascular Magnetic Resonance*, **6**, 96–7.

Saam, T., Ferguson, M. S., Yarnykh, V. L., *et al.* (2005a). Quantitative evaluation of carotid plaque composition by in vivo MRI. *Arteriosclerosis, Thrombosis, and Vascular Biology*, **25**, 234–9.

Saam, T., Kerwin, W. S., Chu, B., *et al.* (2005b). Sample size calculation for clinical trials using magnetic resonance imaging for the quantitative assessment of carotid atherosclerosis. *Journal of Cardiovascular Magnetic Resonance*, **7**, 799–808.

Saam, T., Yuan, C., Chu, B., *et al.* (2006). Predictors of carotid plaque progression as measured by non-invasive magnetic resonance imaging. *Atherosclerosis*, in press.

Shinnar, M., Fallon, J. T., Wehrli, S., *et al.* (1999). The diagnostic accuracy of ex vivo MRI for human athero-sclerotic plaque characterization. *Arteriosclerosis, Thrombosis, and Vascular Biology*, **19**, 2756–61.

Stary, H. C., Chandler, A. B., Dinsmore, R. E., *et al.* (1995). A definition of advanced types of atherosclerotic lesions and a histological classification of atherosclerosis. *Circulation*, **92**, 1355–74.

Takaya, N., Yuan, C., Chu, B., *et al.* (2005a). Presence of intraplaque hemorrhage stimulates progression of carotid atherosclerotic plaques: a high-resolution magnetic resonance imaging study. *Circulation*, **111**, 2768–75.

Takaya, N., Yuan, C., Chu, B., *et al.* (2005b). Association between carotid plaque characteristics and subsequent ischemic cerebrovascular events: A prospective assess-ment with magnetic resonance imaging. *Circulation*, **112** (Suppl.), II–383.

Takaya, N., Yuan, C., Chu, B., *et al.* (2006). Association between carotid plaque characteristics and subsequent ischemic cerebrovascular events: A prospective assess-ment with magnetic resonance imaging – initial results. *Stroke*, **37**, 818–23.

Toussaint, J. F., Lamuraglia, G. M., Southern, J. F., Fuster, V. and Kantor, H. L. (1996). Magnetic resonance images lipid, fibrous, calcified, hemorrhagic, and thrombotic components of human atherosclerosis in vivo. *Circulation*, **94**, 932–8.

Trivedi, R. A., J, U. K.-I., Graves, M. J., Horsley, J., *et al.* (2004). Multi-sequence in vivo MRI can quantify fibrous cap and lipid core components in human carotid atherosclerotic plaques. *European Journal of Vascular and Endovascular Surgery*, **28**, 207–13.

Wasserman, B. A., Smith, W. I., Trout, H. H., 3rd, *et al.* (2002). Carotid artery atherosclerosis: in vivo morpho-logic characterization with gadolinium-enhanced double-oblique MR imaging initial results. *Radiology*, **223**, 566–73.

Yarnykh, V. and Yuan, C. (2003a). High resolution multi-contrast MRI of the carotid artery wall for evaluation of atherosclerotic plaques. *Current Protocols in Magnetic Resonance Imaging*, **1**, A1.4.1–A1.4.17.

Yarnykh, V. L. and Yuan, C. (2003b). Multislice double inversion-recovery black-blood imaging with simultaneous slice reinversion. *Journal of Magnetic Resonance Imaging*, **17**, 478–83.

Yuan, C., Beach, K. W., Smith, L. H. and Hatsukami, T. S. (1998). Measurement of atherosclerotic carotid plaque size in-vivo using high resolution magnetic resonance imaging. *Circulation*, **98**, 2666–71.

Yuan, C. and Kerwin, W. S. (2004). MRI of atherosclerosis. *Journal of Magnetic Resonance Imaging*, **19**, 710–9.

Yuan, C., Kerwin, W. S., Ferguson, M. S., *et al.* (2002a). Contrast enhanced high resolution MRI for atherosclerotic carotid artery tissue characterization. *Journal of Magnetic Resonance Imaging*, **15**, 62–7.

Yuan, C., Mitsumori, L. M., Ferguson, M. S., *et al.* (2001). In vivo accuracy of multispectral magnetic resonance imaging for identifying lipid-rich necrotic cores and intraplaque hemorrhage in advanced human carotid plaques. *Circulation*, **104**, 2051–6.

Yuan, C., Murakami, J. W., Hayes, C. E., *et al.* (1995). Phased-array magnetic resonance imaging of the carotid artery bifurcation: Preliminary results in healthy volunteers and a patient with atherosclerotic disease. *Journal of Magnetic Resonance Imaging*, **5**, 561–5.

Yuan, C., Tsuruda, J. S., Beach, K. N., *et al.* (1994). Techniques for high-resolution MR imaging of atherosclerotic plaque. *Journal of Magnetic Resonance Imaging*, **4**, 43–9.

Yuan, C., Zhang, S., Polissar, N. L., *et al.* (2002b). Identification of fibrous cap rupture with magnetic resonance imaging is highly associated with recent TIA or stroke. *Circulation*, **105**, 181–5.

15

CT plaque imaging

Thomas T. de Weert, Mohamed Ouhlous, Marc R. H. M. van Sambeek and Aad van der Lugt

Erasmus MC, University Medical Center, Rotterdam, The Netherlands

Introduction

Stroke is the most common cause of disability in adults in Western societies. Infarction and ischemia account for 80% of all strokes and about 20–30% of ischemic stroke can be linked to carotid artery stenosis (Caplan, 1991). The degree of carotid luminal stenosis is used in therapeutic decision-making: patients with symptomatic or asymptomatic carotid stenosis above a certain degree are considered candidates for carotid intervention, such as carotid endarterectomy or stent placement.

However, the fact that most symptomatic patients have only mild stenotic lesions and that most patients with severe carotid stenosis are asymptomatic (North American Symptomatic Carotid Endarterectomy Trial Collaborators, 1991; Randomised trial of endarterectomy, 1998), show that apart from the degree of stenosis, other features may play a role in an acute ischemic event and in the assessment of stroke risk.

Morphology studies on carotid and coronary atherosclerotic plaque have lead to the consensus opinion that atherosclerotic plaque morphology and luminal plaque surface could be these important features (Naghavi et al., 2003). An atherosclerotic plaque with specific morphological features (e.g. a large lipid core with a thin fibrous cap; outward remodeling) is more prone to rupture, and irregular luminal plaque surfaces (caused by ruptured or eroded plaques) are more prone to thrombus formation, thromboembolization and consequent acute events (Figure 15.1) (Naghavi et al., 2003).

Because computerized tomography angiography (CTA) can accurately grade the severity of carotid luminal stenosis (Koelemay et al., 2004) computerized tomography (CT) is increasingly used in the evaluation of stroke patients. The question then arises whether CT can also provide detailed information about atherosclerotic plaque morphology and luminal plaque surface.

History

Single-slice CT

In 1984 it was demonstrated that single-slice CTA was able to detect the presence of intimal atherosclerotic disease in the carotid bifurcation (Heinz et al., 1984). Later studies showed that CTA had a high degree of correlation with results of digital subtraction angiography (DSA) in the evaluation of carotid luminal stenosis (Cumming and Morrow, 1994; Link et al., 1996). In addition, CTA more frequently depicted luminal surface irregularities than either DSA or magnetic resonance angiography (MRA) (Randoux et al., 2001). It was also shown that electron-beam CT (EBCT) was an excellent tool for detecting and quantifying

Carotid Disease: The Role of Imaging in Diagnosis and Management, ed. Jonathan Gillard, Martin Graves, Thomas Hatsukami and Chun Yuan. Published by Cambridge University Press. © Cambridge University Press 2007.

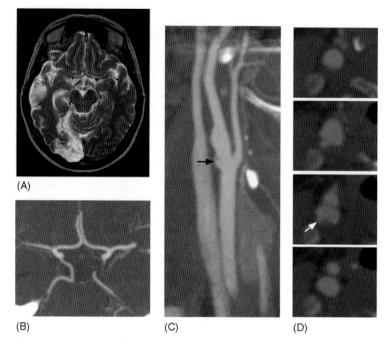

Figure 15.1 MR image of a 37-year-old woman with infarcts in the territory of the medial and posterior cerebral artery (A). MDCT image, showing the circle of Willis with a fetal origin of the posterior cerebral artery demonstrating that both infarcts are in the territory of the right internal carotid artery (B). MDCT image of the right carotid artery shows mild atherosclerotic plaque formation at the level of the carotid bifurcation. In addition, it shows an ulcer with extension of contrast material beyond the vascular lumen into the surrounding plaque (arrow) (C). Four axial MDCT images at the level of the right carotid bifurcation with an eccentric plaque and confirmation of the presence of an ulcer (arrow) (D).

vessel wall calcifications in the coronary arteries (Agatston *et al.*, 1990) as well as in the carotid arteries (Arad *et al.*, 1998).

Validation studies compared 3-mm thick CT images with histologic sections of carotid endarterectomy specimens. The results were, however, confusing. Two studies reported that the major plaque components could be differentiated based on differences in measured density expressed in Hounsfield units (HU): hyperdense structures correspond with calcification, hypodense regions with lipid, and isodense regions with fibrosis (Estes *et al.*, 1998; Oliver *et al.*, 1999). However, another study concluded that CT failed to reliably indicate the presence of lipid or fibrous tissue and suggested the need of multislice technology (Walker *et al.*, 2002).

Multidetector CT

Multidetector CT (MDCT) allows full vascular imaging (from the aorta to the circle of Willis). By providing this large coverage with an evaluation of other important atherosclerotic predilection sites, MDCTA can now compete with DSA and MRA in the evaluation of stroke patients. However, the main advantage of MDCT for carotid atherosclerotic plaque evaluation is the increased in-plane resolution, the decreased slice thickness (<0.75 mm) and the subsequent ability to obtain near isotropic voxels. More detailed analysis of atherosclerotic plaque morphology (based on differences in HU) and luminal plaque surface may now be possible.

Influence of imaging and reconstruction parameters

Slice thickness

In single-slice CT, slice thickness and detector collimation (defined as the width of the individual detector) are the same; however, the effective slice thickness is larger than the reconstructed slice thickness. In MDCT the reconstructed slice thickness is independent of the detector collimation and is equal to or larger than the single detector collimation. In addition, the effective slice thickness reaches the reconstructed slice thickness. Reconstruction of thin slices is important in plaque imaging for two reasons. First, with thinner slices true volumetric data sets can be acquired which allows reconstruction in other planes (Figure 15.2). Second, as atherosclerotic plaques are very small and heterogeneous, thinner slices lead to less volume averaging and may therefore enhance the differentiation of plaque components. This is especially important for differentiation of lipid and fibrous tissue.

The latter phenomenon has been confirmed in a phantom study in which silicon tubes with two different plaque types (resembling lipid and fibrous tissue) were scanned with two different detector widths (4 × 1.0 mm vs. 4 × 2.5 mm). A larger slice thickness increased the density measurements of both plaque types; an effect that was even more evident in the plaques with lower densities (resembling lipid) (Schroeder *et al.*, 2001a).

Tube energy (kVp)

The potential difference across the X-ray tube determines the effective energy of the X-ray beam, which influences the type and amount of interactions of the X-ray beam in the tissue. The most commonly used tube energy is 120 kVp, although current MDCT machines allow other tube energy settings in the range of 60–140 kVp. With higher kVp almost all interaction in the tissue occurs by Compton scattering. Lowering the kVp

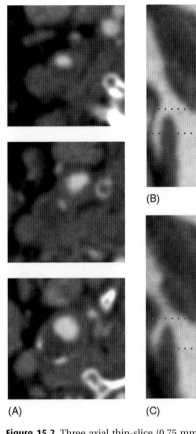
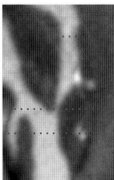
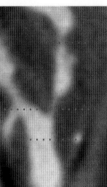

(A)   (C)

Figure 15.2 Three axial thin-slice (0.75 mm) MDCT images of the internal carotid artery (A). The true volumetric data sets with (nearly) isotropic voxels allow reconstruction in other planes, like the sagittal and coronal plane. One-mm multiplanar reformat (B) and 2-mm maximum intensity projection (C) in the sagittal plane depicts the carotid bifurcation with an eccentric plaque.

from 140 to 80 will increase the number of photoelectric interactions. Therefore for calcium and contrast material, lowering the tube energy will increase the X-ray attenuation coefficient, as reflected by the measured density.

The high density calcifications normally lead to overestimation of the true volume of the calcium and can lead to overestimation of plaque size with an increase in the severity of luminal stenosis. This so-called blooming artifact is caused by the large difference in density between calcifications and surrounding tissue. This difference causes partial volume averaging effects due to the finite spatial resolution of CT.

The main problem of this blooming artifact is hampering of the optimal characterization of the noncalcified part of the plaque. Increasing the tube energy will reduce the size of the already over-estimated calcifications. An ex vivo study in which carotid specimens were scanned with MDCT revealed that the calcium volume decreased by 14.0%, 17.3% and 20.2% with 100-, 120-, and 140-kVp settings, respectively, as compared with the volume measured with 80-kVp acquisition (Hoffmann *et al.*, 2003). The same results were found in a second ex vivo study (Figure 15.3) (de Weert *et al.*, 2005). The effects on plaque analysis of an increase in the density values of the contrast material in the lumen with lower tube energy are discussed below (see section entitled "Contrast material").

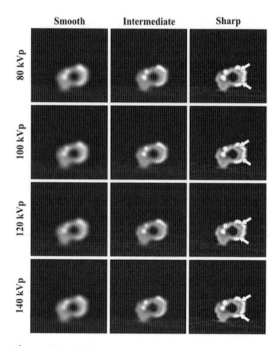

Figure 15.3 MDCT images of a carotid endarterectomy specimen. All images are obtained at the same location in the specimen, but with different kVp settings (80 kVp, 100 kVp, 120 kVp, or 140 kVp) and different reconstruction algorithms (smooth, intermediate or sharp). Higher kVp settings decrease the calcium volume up to 20.2% (140 kVp). Furthermore, the evaluation of plaque composition is influenced by the reconstruction algorithm. Sharp algorithms produce low-intensity rings around calcifications (white arrows) that hamper plaque characterization. (Reprinted with permission from De Weert *et al.* (2005). *European Radiology*, **15**, 1906.)

Tube current (mAs)

Radiographic exposure (the product of tube current and exposure time) is the main determinant of image quality, more specifically the signal-to-noise ratio (SNR) in the CT image. Normally, the small size of the neck region leads to sufficient SNR in the CT image for clinical evaluation. However, the size of the atherosclerotic plaque (<10 mm) means that a reconstructed CT image needs a thin slice thickness and a small field-of-view. The resultant decrease in SNR demands a higher exposure since only a high SNR allows differentiation of tissues with a small difference in density.

Contrast material

To differentiate lumen from plaque, contrast material in the patent lumen is a prerequisite (Figure 15.4). In CTA, in which assessment of the severity of stenosis was the main indication, the aim is to have a high dose of contrast material in the artery under study. To achieve this high dose a high concentration of iodine is injected with a high injection rate into the anticubital vein (Cademartiri *et al.*, 2002). With higher densities in the contrast-filled lumen, the cut-off point for the differentiation of lumen from plaque is subsequently higher. Therefore, fixed cut-off points will lead to an underestimation of the size of the atherosclerotic plaque and the severity of stenosis.

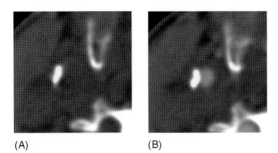

(A)   (B)

Figure 15.4 Two MDCT images of an atherosclerotic carotid artery of the same patient at the same level, one without (A) and one with contrast material in the lumen (B). Contrast material in the patent lumen is a prerequisite to visualize the atherosclerotic wall thickening.

Higher densities in the lumen may also influence the density measurements in the atherosclerotic plaque, especially in small arteries. A phantom study in which silicon tubes with two different plaque types (resembling lipid and fibrous tissue) were scanned with different contrast medium concentrations (258 HU, 280 HU and 336 HU) revealed an increase in the measured plaque density with higher contrast medium concentrations (Schroeder et al., 2001a). This was explained by the presence of partial volume effects, a problem that might be reduced by further technical improvements in collimation width (e.g. thinner). An ex vivo study in which coronary arteries filled with different contrast material concentrations were scanned, demonstrated that the intraluminal attenuation significantly modifies the attenuation of plaques (Cademartiri et al., 2005a). Based on this study, Cademartiri and colleagues concluded that it is difficult to identify absolute ranges of attenuation that relate to specific plaque characteristics. They suggested that when plaque density measurements are performed, intraluminal attenuation should be reported, and that a calibration factor should be introduced to address this issue (Cademartiri et al., 2005a).

Whether this is also a problem in the evaluation of the carotid atherosclerotic plaque has not yet been explored. Since the size of the plaque in carotid arteries is much larger than in coronary arteries, partial volume effects will only influence the density measurements in plaque near the luminal border. However, another explanation for the increased density in the plaque in the presence of intraluminal contrast, is that the plaque may be enhanced by the entrance of contrast material via the vasa vasorum. In that case plaque evaluation will not be hampered but improved, since perfusion studies may provide additional information on the plaque composition.

Reconstruction algorithms

In CT, raw data are collected from multiple directions. In the reconstruction of a CT image from the raw data a convolution back projection procedure is used together with a mathematical function, the convolution kernel. The choice and design of the convolution kernel influences image characteristics, i.e. a smooth algorithm will reduce spatial resolution as well as SNR, whereas a sharp algorithm has the opposite effect.

Plaque characterization and quantification of the different plaque components based on measured densities is strongly influenced by the type of convolution kernel used in the reconstruction algorithm. "Smooth" kernels decrease SNR but also lead to less interpretability due to averaging of contrast differences. This is especially important when the density differences between tissues are small, which is the case for lipid and fibrous tissue (de Weert et al., 2005). "Sharp" kernels increase the contrast differences between these tissues, but they also lead to an increase in calcium size and low intensity rings around calcifications (edge-enhancement artifacts) which hamper interpretation (Cademartiri et al., 2005b; de Weert et al., 2005). Therefore, CT images reconstructed with an intermediate kernel will lead to an optimal CT image (Figure 15.3).

Window-level setting

In the CT image, density values are represented as grey scale values. With windowing, the density range of diagnostic relevance is assigned the whole range of discernible grey values. With window-level setting, it is first defined by which density (expressed in HU) the central grey scale value is to be assigned to. By setting the window width, it is then defined by which densities above and below the central grey value can still be discriminated by varying shades of grey, with black representing tissue of the lowest density and white representing tissue of the highest density. Normally, in evaluation of CTA a large window width (±500 to 1000 HU) is used to differentiate the contrast-filled

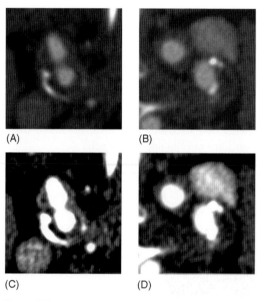

(A)   (B)

(C)   (D)

Figure 15.5 Four MDCT images, two with a large window setting and two with a small window setting. With the large window width setting (500/200) (A, B) the contrast-filled lumen can more easily be differentiated from calcifications. Calcifications appear (often) brighter. However, the noncalcified plaque looks rather homogenous. For evaluation of the plaque smaller window widths (120/50) (C, D) are more optimal to discern the small differences in densities inside the noncalcified part of the plaque.

lumen from the plaque with calcifications. In such images the noncalcified plaque looks rather homogenous. For evaluation of the plaque, smaller windows are more optimal to discern the small differences in densities inside the noncalcified part of the plaque (Figure 15.5). Drawbacks are the effects on differentiation of contrast-filled lumen and calcification, and the size of the patent lumen and subsequently the size of the plaque.

Imaging protocol

Because the plaque density measurements are affected by scanning and image reconstruction parameters it is essential that scanning and reconstruction protocols are standardized. Normally, a carotid plaque imaging protocol is part of a carotid CTA protocol which is used in the work-up of patients with a transient ischemic attack or stroke (de Monye *et al.*, 2005). This protocol requires an injection of 80 cc of contrast material and 40 cc bolus chaser at an injection rate of 4 cc/sec. The contrast material is injected using a double-head power injector in an antecubital vein. The CTA scan range reaches from the ascending aorta to the intracranial circulation. Scan direction is craniocaudal to reduce perivenous artifacts (de Monye *et al.*, 2006). Typical imaging parameters are: number of detector rows = 16, individual detector width = 0.75 mm, table feed per rotation = 12 mm (pitch 1), gantry rotation time = 0.37−0.5 sec, kVp = 120, effective mAs = 180, and scan time = 10−14 sec (depending on the individual patient's size and anatomy). Synchronization between the passage of contrast material and data acquisition is achieved by real-time bolus tracking. With this protocol a relatively homogenous luminal attenuation is reached (368 ± 92 HU) with a small density difference between the lumen attenuation at the proximal and distal border of the plaque (5 ± 17 HU). CT images are reconstructed with slice width of 1 mm, reconstruction interval of 0.6 mm, field-of-view of q120 mm, and intermediate convolution kernel.

Validation

Lumen surface morphology

CTA allows the surface of the atherosclerotic plaque to be analyzed whereby a differentiation can be made between plaque irregularities and plaque ulceration (Figure 15.6). A plaque ulcer is defined as an ulcer niche with extension of contrast material beyond the vascular lumen into the surrounding plaque (Walker *et al.*, 2002). The accuracy of DSA in the detection of ulceration, with surgical observations as reference, has been reported to be low (sensitivity 46% and specificity 74%) (Streifler *et al.*, 1994). However, with microscopic evaluation of the plaque it became clear that plaque surface morphology assessed on DSA is strongly associated with the presence of plaque rupture, plaque hemorrhage, lipid core size and proportion of fibrous tissue, i.e. features that are all closely related with the concept of a vulnerable plaque (Lovett *et al.*, 2004).

The first reports on the accuracy of CTA compared with DSA in the assessment of plaque ulcers were disappointing, but this might be explained by the thick slice thickness used with single section CT (Oliver *et al.*, 1999). A later report demonstrated that MDCTA was superior to DSA in the detection of plaque irregularities and ulcerations (Randoux *et al.*, 2001). Walker and colleagues evaluated 165 CTA studies, compared them with endarterectomy specimens, and reported

a sensitivity of 60% and a specificity of 74% (Walker *et al.*, 2002).

Calcification

The presence of calcification in atherosclerotic plaques can easily be detected with CT due to the high attenuation of the X-rays by calcium hydroxyapatite which leads to a high density structure in the plaque. Agatston and colleagues were the first to show that coronary calcifications could be detected and quantified with EBCT (Agatston *et al.*, 1990). Later on this principle of calcium quantification was also used in the carotid arteries (Arad *et al.*, 1998; Allison *et al.*, 2004). The threshold for calcification is normally set at a density of 130 HU having an area ≥ 1 mm^2. Calcification can be detected and quantified without the presence of intraluminal contrast media. In the presence of intraluminal contrast media the threshold value has to be higher to differentiate between calcifications and contrast media (Hong *et al.*, 2003). The main problem with the Agatston score for coronary calcification is the substantial measurement variability (up to 30%); the variability for carotid calcification is not yet known. Calcification can also be quantified with MDCT using the Agatston score or new alternative scorings methods (volume or mineral mass score). Phantom studies and an ex vivo study with atherosclerotic carotid specimens have shown that the mineral mass score

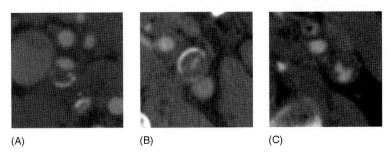

(A)   (B)   (C)

Figure 15.6 Three MDCT images with atherosclerotic carotid plaque formation. The plaque surface appears smooth (A), irregular (B), or ulcerated (C).

Table 15.1. Results of validation studies in carotid/coronary arteries using histology/IVUS as reference

Reference	Type of artery	Type of study	Number of patients	Histology (reference)		p-value
				Lipid-rich	Fibrous-rich	
(Estes *et al.*, 1998)	Carotid	in vivo	21	39 ± 12 ($n = 11$)	90 ± 24 ($n = 15$)	<0.001
(de Weert *et al.*, 2005)	Carotid	ex vivo	15	45 ± 21 ($n = 35$)	79 ± 20 ($n = 28$)	<0.001
(de Weert *et al.*, 2006)	Carotid	in vivo	15	25 ± 19 ($n = 31$)	88 ± 18 ($n = 53$)	<0.001
(Becker *et al.*, 2003)	Coronary	ex vivo	11	47 ± 9 ($n = 15$)	104 ± 28 ($n = 16$)	<0.01
(Schroeder *et al.*, 2004)	Coronary	ex vivo	12	42 ± 22 ($n = 6$)	71 ± 21 ($n = 6$)	<0.001
(Nikolaou *et al.*, 2004)	Coronary	ex vivo	13	47 ± 13 ($n = 10$)	87 ± 29 ($n = 11$)	<0.01
				IVUS (reference)		
				Soft (hypoechoic)	Intermediate (hyperechoic)	
(Schroeder *et al.*, 2001)	Coronary	in vivo	15	14 ± 26 ($n = 12$)	91 ± 21 ($n = 5$)	<0.0001
(Leber, *et al.*, 2004)	Coronary	in vivo	58	49 ± 22 ($n = 62$)	91 ± 22 ($n = 87$)	<0.02

Abbreviations: n = number of measurements; IVUS = intravascular ultrasound.
Data, expressed in Hounsfield units (HU), are mean ± SD.

is the most precise and best reproducible scoring method (Hoffmann *et al.*, 2003; Hong *et al.*, 2003).

Noncalcified plaque components

Because the presence of noncalcified parts of the atherosclerotic plaque is considered to be important for the (in)stability of the plaque, much attention has been given to the ability of MDCT to further classify the plaques. Several studies have compared the density values obtained in different type of plaques (Table 15.1). The classification scheme normally used for these studies is based on the (modified) criteria set by the American Heart Association Committee on vascular lesions (Stary *et al.*, 1994; Stary *et al.*, 1995; Stary, 2000) which is sometimes simplified to predominantly lipid-rich plaques, intermediate (fibrous) plaques, and predominantly calcified plaques. These studies have mainly been performed in coronary arteries.

Because the atherosclerotic plaques in the carotid artery are larger than those in the coronary arteries, it should be possible not only to characterize a whole plaque as lipid-rich, fibrous-rich or calcified, but also to characterize regions within

the plaque as predominantly lipid-rich, fibrous-rich or calcified and then to measure the density of that region. The second advantage of carotid studies compared with coronary studies is the possibility to perform the MDCT in vivo and to acquire the surgical carotid endarterectomy specimen for histological correlation, whereas coronary studies in vivo are correlated with intravascular ultrasound (IVUS).

With single-slice CT (3-mm slice thickness) it was already possible to differentiate between lipid and fibrous tissue in the carotid atherosclerotic plaque. Density measurements revealed a significant difference for lipid and fibrous tissue (39 ± 13 HU and 90 ± 24 HU, respectively) (Estes *et al.*, 1998).

De Weert and colleagues performed an ex vivo study in which carotid endarterectomy specimens were scanned and the MDCT images were compared with histological sections (Figure 15.7) (de Weert *et al.*, 2005). Lipid-rich and fibrous-rich regions within plaques had significantly different density values (45 ± 21 HU and 79 ± 20 HU, respectively). The histograms revealed a small overlap in the distribution of the lipid and fibrous

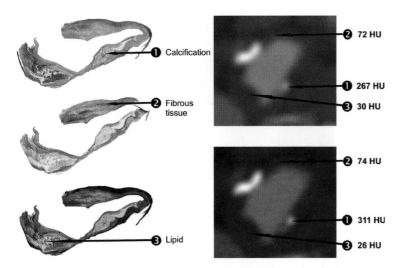

Figure 15.7 Three differently stained histologic sections (HE = hematoxylin eosin; SR = Sirius Red; EVG = elastic van Gieson) and two corresponding differently reconstructed MDCT images (intermediate smooth, intermediate sharp) of atherosclerotic carotid plaque. The Hounsfield value was measured in the MDCT images in regions with one predominant plaque component on histology.

tissue density measurements (Figure 15.8). Based on this distribution a receiver-operating-characteristic curve was created, which revealed 60 HU as the optimal cut-off point to differentiate lipid-rich from fibrous-rich tissue, with a sensitivity and specificity of 89% and 93%, respectively (de Weert *et al.*, 2005).

Such a validation study was subsequently performed with MDCT images acquired in vivo, and the density values for lipid-rich and fibrous-rich regions in the plaques were 25 ± 19 HU and 88 ± 18 HU, respectively. The distribution of density values of lipid-rich and fibrous-rich regions again showed an optimal cut-off point at 60 HU to differentiate lipid from fibrous tissue, with 100% sensitivity and specificity (de Weert *et al.*, 2006).

The density values of lipid-rich regions measured in vivo are lower than those measured ex vivo, and some of them reached values below zero (Figure 15.9). Prospective analysis of the MDCT images in which all hypodense (<60 HU) regions were detected based on thresholding, revealed that

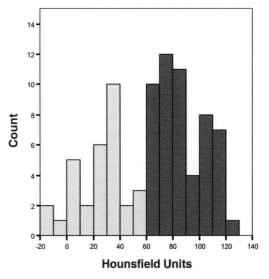

Figure 15.8 Frequency distribution of measured density values of lipid-rich regions (yellow bars) and fibrous-rich regions (red bars) in MDCT images. The most optimal cut-off point to differentiate lipid-rich from fibrous-rich tissue in MDCT images was 60 HU, with 100% sensitivity and specificity.

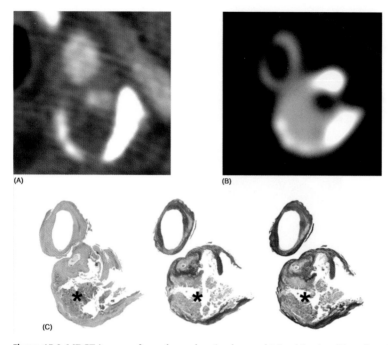

Figure 15.9 MDCT images of an atherosclerotic plaque obtained in vivo (A) and ex vivo (B). The density value of a lipid-rich region measured in vivo (5 HU) was lower than measured ex vivo (32 HU). The lipid-rich region is highlighted with an asterisk in three histologic sections (Haematoxylin Eosin, Sirus Red, and Elastic-Van Gieson, respectively) (C).

the positive predictive value of a hypodense region in the plaque with a density value <30 HU for a lipid-rich region was 97%, while the positive predictive value of a hypodense region with a density value between 30 and 60 HU was 23% (de Weert *et al.*, 2006).

The results of the carotid validation studies are confirmed by the results of several ex vivo coronary validation studies (Table 15.1). All these studies showed a significant difference in density values between lipid-rich plaques and fibrous-rich plaques (Becker *et al.*, 2003; Nikolaou *et al.*, 2004; Schroeder *et al.*, 2004). Other coronary studies used IVUS as a reference and found a significant difference in the density values of soft (hypoechoic) and intermediate (hyperechoic) plaques (Schroeder *et al.*, 2001b; Leber *et al.*, 2004).

Due to the relatively small size of the atherosclerotic plaques in coronary arteries, plaques have

to be characterized by their predominant tissue which ignores the fact that atherosclerotic disease is often very heterogenic and that a solitary plaque might contain areas with different morphology. Furthermore, some studies revealed a considerable overlap in density values of lipid-rich and fibrous-rich plaques, which decreases the accuracy of MDCT in coronary plaque analysis (Schroeder *et al.*, 2001a; Leber *et al.*, 2004).

Quantification

Plaque volume quantification

The cross-sectional nature of CT allows the measurement of both luminal and vessel area. Plaque area is calculated by subtracting luminal area from vessel area. Plaque volumes are

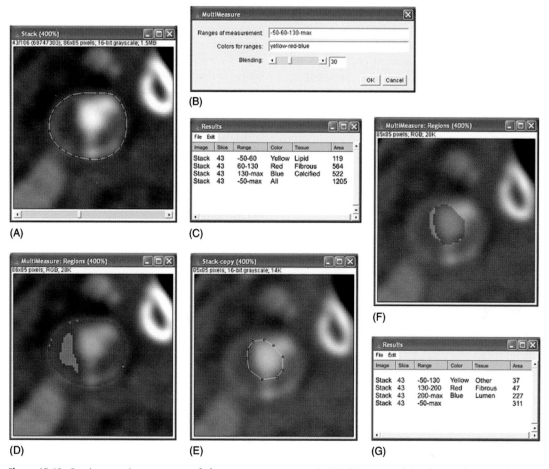

Figure 15.10 Semiautomatic assessment of plaque component areas in MDCT images. This software allows an observer to draw a region of interest (ROI) (= vessel outline) (A). After the input of specific ranges of Hounsfield values (HV) (B), which should represent specific plaque components, it assesses the amount of pixels within each range of HV (C). Each range of HV is given a different color and an MDCT-based plaque morphology image is produced (D). To differentiate lumen from the atherosclerotic plaque and from calcified tissue, a second ROI is drawn (E). A second morphology image is produced (F), and the number of lumen pixels are calculated (G). The exact number of fibrous and calcified pixels can now be determined. Fibrous = fibrous measurement-1 (60–130 HU) plus fibrous measurement-2 (130–200 HU); calcified = calcified measurement-1 (>130 HU) minus lumen measurement-2 (>200 HU) minus fibrous measurement-2 (130–200 HU).

calculated by multiplying plaque area and slice increment. Outlining the luminal area can be performed by (semi-)automated measures based on a threshold to separate lumen from plaque. Calcification (which also has a high density) near the lumen may be included in the lumen but then

manual correction should be performed. The vessel area is currently drawn manually because the carotid vessel is not surrounded circumferentially by a tissue with a homogenous lower or higher density to allow a threshold-based semiautomated technique to outline this boundary.

Semiautomated measurements are influenced by the thresholds, which should vary depending on the density of the intraluminal contrast. The main problem with manually-assessed contours is the influence of window-level setting on the visualization of the boundaries between lumen and plaque, and between vessel wall and surrounding tissues. Validation of plaque area measurements with histology are hampered by the effect of histological preparation on the tissue dimensions. Shrinkage of 20–25% of the plaque area is normally encountered during fixation. An ex vivo and a subsequent in vivo study on carotid atherosclerotic plaques revealed a strong correlation between MDCT and histology for the assessment of plaque area ($r^2 = 0.81$ and 0.73, respectively) (de Weert *et al.*, 2005; de Weert *et al.*, 2006). In addition, the

interobserver variability of plaque area measurements with MDCT was moderate with a coefficient of variation of 19% (de Weert *et al.*, 2006).

Two coronary in vivo studies compared the plaque volume assessed with MDCT and IVUS. One study found a strong correlation ($r = 0.8$) and an underestimation of the coronary plaque volume assessed with MDCT compared to IVUS (Achenbach *et al.*, 2004). The other study found a moderate correlation ($r = 0.55$) and an overestimation of coronary plaque area assessed with MDCT compared to IVUS (Moselewski *et al.*, 2004).

Plaque component quantification

The difference in density values between the major plaque components (lipid tissue, fibrous tissue and calcifications) is of great interest because this

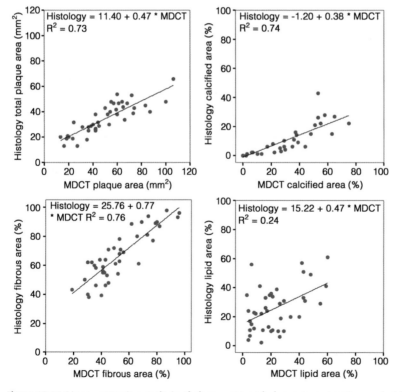

Figure 15.11 Linear regression analysis of plaque area and plaque component areas in MDCT images and histologic sections.

allows the plaque components to be quantified (Figure 15.10). An in vivo validation study, in which MDCT images of carotid arteries were compared with histological sections from the endarterectomy specimens, compared the areas of the major plaque components (Figure 15.11). As expected, MDCT overestimated the size of the calcifications but the correlation was good. In addition, the correlation for fibrous tissue was good, but was poor for lipid ($r^2 = 0.74$ and 0.24, respectively). An exploratory analysis revealed that the correlation between lipid areas on histological sections and in MDCT images improved with a decreasing amount of calcifications in the plaque (r^2 is 0.81 for noncalcified plaques) (de Weert *et al.*, 2006). Therefore, MDCT is capable of quantifying calcifications and fibrous tissue in atherosclerotic carotid plaque in good correlation with histology, and lipid can be adequately quantified in mildly calcified plaques.

The interobserver variability of area measurements of the different plaque components was moderate, with a coefficient of variation of 16%, 21% and 40% for calcified regions, fibrous regions and lipid regions, respectively (de Weert *et al.*, 2006).

Clinical applications

Risk prediction

The severity of stenosis in the carotid artery is a well-known predictor of cerebral infarction and is currently used as the main parameter in deciding whether the patient is advised to undergo carotid endarterectomy or stent placement. Plaque morphology is considered an additional independent predictor of cerebral infarction: plaques consisting of a necrotic lipid core covered by a thin fibrous cap (the unstable or vulnerable plaque) are prone to rupture (Fuster *et al.*, 1992a,b; Virmani *et al.*, 2002), leading to thromboembolic release of particles to the brain. CT of the plaque in the carotid bifurcation may provide clinicians with these additional independent predictors of (recurrent) stroke which may in the future compete with the severity of stenosis in treatment decisions.

Whether the presence of certain plaque features is a good reason for surgical intervention, has to be demonstrated in larger prospective studies, which will determine the significance of CT-assessed plaque features for stroke risk. Such studies will prove whether the concept of vulnerable plaque is applicable to carotid atherosclerosis. Even then, a randomized controlled trial will have to be performed to prove that surgical intervention is beneficial in patients with CT-assessed vulnerable plaques in the carotid artery. Which CT-assessed plaque features will be candidates for an improved risk assessment? To this end, a large prospective study is being conducted in which 800 patients with cerebrovascular symptoms undergo a CTA of the carotid arteries, and CT-derived parameters of the plaque will be related to future cerebrovascular events.

Lumen surface morphology

Several DSA studies have demonstrated that plaque ulcerations of a symptomatic carotid stenosis is a strong independent predictor of stroke (Eliasziw *et al.*, 1994; Rothwell *et al.*, 2000). Angiographic ulceration is associated with plaque rupture, intraplaque hemorrhage, a large lipid core and less fibrous tissue, all features of unstable vulnerable plaques (Lovett *et al.*, 2004). MDCT can assess luminal surface morphology with the same or better accuracy than DSA.

Lipid

Pathological studies have demonstrated that plaques with a high lipid volume are prone to rupture; additionally, the lipid content is highly thrombogenic after disruption (Davies *et al.*, 1994; Seeger *et al.*, 1995). Other studies have shown no significant difference in plaque morphology, with respect to lipid, between symptomatic and asymptomatic plaques. Duplex ultrasonography studies confirmed the hypothesis about the risk of lipid, by demonstrating that echolucent plaques which are supposed to correspond with lipid-rich plaques are associated with a higher risk for future ischemic cerebrovascular events (Polak *et al.*, 1998). These studies failed, however, in quantifying lipid or other plaque components. The important role of lipid is also strengthened by the success of ipid-lowering therapy in preventing acute atherosclerotic-related events. This success could be explained by the reduction of the lipid content of vulnerable plaques (Zhao *et al.*, 2001).

Calcifications

Coronary calcification is an independent predictor of coronary heart disease and stroke (Vliegenthart *et al.*, 2002; Vliegenthart *et al.*, 2005). Measures of carotid atherosclerosis, like intima-media thickness measured with B-mode ultrasound, are independent predictors of stroke (Hollander *et al.*, 2002). Whether carotid calcification assessed with MDCT is an independent predictor of stroke is currently under investigation in a large population-based study which includes over 2500 subjects.

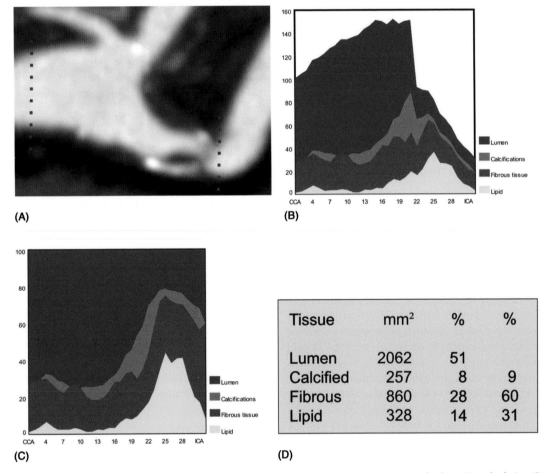

Figure 15.12 Sagittal MDCT image of the carotid bifurcation with an atheroscleric plaque (A). Absolute (B) and relative (C) area measurements of lumen, fibrous tissue, lipid tissue and calcifications in consecutive MDCT images. The x-axis represent the numbers of consecutive MDCT images. Volume measurements of the different plaque components (D).

Calcifications are one of the components of the atherosclerotic plaque and are related to the amount of plaque. Nevertheless, atherosclerotic plaque may almost totally consist of noncalcified components and these plaques are missed on noncontrast CT scans.

With CTA the total amount of plaque can be assessed and, subsequently, the relative contribution of calcium to the plaque. The percentage plaque area in carotid atherosclerosis assessed with CT is two-fold greater in asymptomatic versus symptomatic plaques (Shaalan *et al.*, 2004). This was not confirmed in a study in which microscopic plaque morphology from symptomatic and asymptomatic patients was compared (Fisher *et al.*, 2005). Another CT study demonstrated that calcified plaques (defined as plaques with a median density greater than 130 HU) were 21 times less likely to be symptomatic than noncalcified plaques (Nandalur *et al.*, 2005). In other words, the relative amount of noncalcified plaque components may be related to an increased risk of being symptomatic.

Plaque volume

In the early phase of atherosclerosis, preservation of a patent lumen is achieved by outward remodelling of the vessel wall. Therefore, significant atherosclerotic plaque is already present before moderate to severe luminal compromise is detected on DSA.

Since CT enables the visualization of the atherosclerotic plaque and the process of vascular remodeling, it can detect changes in atherosclerotic plaque volume which would have stayed unrecognized by luminal measurements only. The question arises whether the amount of plaque will be a better predictor of neurologic events than the severity of stenosis.

Natural history of atherosclerosis and pharmacological intervention

From manual or semiautomated measurements of plaque area in consecutive CT images in which

vessel thickening is present, it is possible to calculate the plaque volume and relative contribution of each plaque component (Figure 15.12). In addition, the spatial distribution of the plaque components can be depicted. These measures can be used in follow-up studies in which disease progression is evaluated. Moreover, they can be used as surrogate endpoints in clinical studies in which the effect of pharmacological intervention is studied.

REFERENCES

Achenbach, S., Moselewski, F., *et al.* (2004). Detection of calcified and noncalcified coronary atherosclerotic plaque by contrast-enhanced, submillimeter multidetector spiral computed tomography: a segment-based comparison with intravascular ultrasound. *Circulation*, **109**, 14–17.

Agatston, A. S., Janowitz, W. R., *et al.* (1990). Quantification of coronary artery calcium using ultrafast computed tomography. *Journal of American College of Cardiology*, **15**, 827–32.

Allison, M. A., Criqui, M. H., *et al.* (2004). Patterns and risk factors for systemic calcified atherosclerosis. *Arteriosclerosis, Thrombosis, and Vascular Biology*, **24**, 331–6.

Arad, Y., Spadaro, L. A., *et al.* (1998). Correlations between vascular calcification and atherosclerosis: a comparative electron beam CT study of the coronary and carotid arteries. *Journal of Computer Assisted Tomography*, **22**, 207–11.

Becker, C. R., Nikolaou, K., *et al.* (2003). Ex vivo coronary atherosclerotic plaque characterization with multidetector-row CT. *European Radiology*, **13**, 2094–8.

Cademartiri, F., Mollet, N. R., *et al.* (2005a). Influence of intracoronary attenuation on coronary plaque measurements using multislice computed tomography: observations in an ex vivo model of coronary computed tomography angiography. *European Radiology*, **15**, 1426–31.

Cademartiri, F., Runza, G., *et al.* (2005b). Influence of increasing convolution kernel filtering on plaque imaging with multislice CT using an ex-vivo model of Coronary Angiography Influenza dei filtri di convoluzione sulla misurazione dei valori di attenuazione della placca durante Angiografia Coronarica mediante TC multistrato. *La Radiologia Medica*, **110**, 234–40.

Cademartiri, F., van der Lugt, A., *et al.* (2002). Parameters affecting bolus geometry in CTA: a review. *Journal of Computer Assisted Tomography*, **26**, 598–607.

Caplan, L. R. (1991). Diagnosis and treatment of ischemic stroke. *Journal of the American Medical Association*, **266**, 2413–18.

Cumming, M. J. and Morrow, I. M. (1994). Carotid artery stenosis: a prospective comparison of CT angiography and conventional angiography. *AJR. American Journal of Roentgenology*, **163**, 517–23.

Davies, M. J., Woolf, N., *et al.* (1994). Lipid and cellular constituents of unstable human aortic plaques. *Basic Research in Cardiology*, **89** (Suppl. 1), 33–9.

de Monye, C., Cademartiri, F., *et al.* (2005). Sixteen-detector row CT angiography of carotid arteries: comparison of different volumes of contrast material with and without a bolus chaser. *Radiology*, **237**, 555–62.

de Monye, C., de Weert, T. T., *et al.* (2006). Optimization of CT angiography of the carotid artery with a 16-multi-detector-row CT scanner: craniocaudal scan direction reduces contrast material-related perivenous artifacts. *AJR. American Journal of Roentgenology*, **186**, 1737–45.

de Weert, T. T., Ouhlous, M., *et al.* (2005). In vitro characterization of atherosclerotic carotid plaque with multidetector computed tomography and histopathological correlation. *European Radiology*, **15**, 1906–14.

de Weert, T. T., Ouhlous, M., *et al.* (2006). In vivo characterization and quantification of atherosclerotic carotid plaque components with multidetector computed tomography and histopathological correlation. *Arteriosclerosis, Thrombosis and Vascular Biology*, in press.

Eliasziw, M., Streifler, J. Y., *et al.* (1994). Significance of plaque ulceration in symptomatic patients with high-grade carotid stenosis. North American Symptomatic Carotid Endarterectomy Trial. *Stroke*, **25**, 304–8.

Estes, J. M., Quist, W. C., *et al.* (1998). Noninvasive characterization of plaque morphology using helical computed tomography. *Journal of Cardiovascular Surgery*, **39**, 527–34.

Fisher, M., Paganini-Hill, A., *et al.* (2005). Carotid plaque pathology: thrombosis, ulceration, and stroke pathogenesis. *Stroke*, **36**, 253–7.

Fuster, V., Badimon, L., *et al.* (1992a). The pathogenesis of coronary artery disease and the acute coronary syndromes (1). *New England Journal of Medicine*, **326**, 242–50.

Fuster, V., Badimon, L., *et al.* (1992b). The pathogenesis of coronary artery disease and the acute coronary syndromes (2). *New England Journal of Medicine*, **326**, 310–18.

Heinz, E. R., Pizer, S. M., *et al.* (1984). Examination of the extracranial carotid bifurcation by thin-section dynamic CT: direct visualization of intimal atheroma in man (Part 1). *AJNR. American Journal of Neuroradiology*, **5**, 355–9.

Hoffmann, U., Kwait, D. C., *et al.* (2003). Vascular calcification in ex vivo carotid specimens: precision and accuracy of measurements with multi-detector row CT. *Radiology*, **229**, 375–81.

Hollander, M., Bots, M. L., *et al.* (2002). Carotid plaques increase the risk of stroke and subtypes of cerebral infarction in asymptomatic elderly: the Rotterdam study. *Circulation*, **105**, 2872–7.

Hong, C., Bae, K. T., *et al.* (2003). Coronary artery calcium: accuracy and reproducibility of measurements with multi-detector row CT–assessment of effects of different thresholds and quantification methods. *Radiology*, **227**, 795–801.

Koelemay, M. J., Nederkoorn, P. J., *et al.* (2004). Systematic review of computed tomographic angiography for assessment of carotid artery disease. *Stroke*, **35**, 2306–12.

Leber, A. W., Knez, A., *et al.* (2004). Accuracy of multi-detector spiral computed tomography in identifying and differentiating the composition of coronary atherosclerotic plaques: a comparative study with intracoronary ultrasound. *Journal of the American College of Cardiology*, **43**, 1241–7.

Link, J., Brossmann, J., *et al.* (1996). Spiral CT angiography and selective digital subtraction angiography of internal carotid artery stenosis. *AJNR. American Journal of Neuroradiology*, **17**, 89–94.

Lovett, J. K., Gallagher, P. J., *et al.* (2004). Histological correlates of carotid plaque surface morphology on lumen contrast imaging. *Circulation*, **110**, 2190–7.

Moselewski, F., Ropers, D., *et al.* (2004). Comparison of measurement of cross-sectional coronary atherosclerotic plaque and vessel areas by 16-slice multidetector computed tomography versus intravascular ultrasound. *American Journal of Cardiology*, **94**, 1294–7.

Naghavi, M., Libby, P., *et al.* (2003). From vulnerable plaque to vulnerable patient: a call for new definitions and risk assessment strategies: Part I. *Circulation*, **108**, 1664–72.

Nandalur, K. R., Baskurt, E., *et al.* (2005). Calcified carotid atherosclerotic plaque is associated less with ischemic symptoms than is noncalcified plaque on MDCT. *AJR. American Journal of Roentgenology*, **184**, 295–8.

Nikolaou, K., Becker, C. R., *et al.* (2004). Multidetector-row computed tomography and magnetic resonance imaging of atherosclerotic lesions in human ex vivo coronary arteries. *Atherosclerosis*, **174**, 243–52.

North American Symptomatic Carotid Endarterectomy Trial Collaborators (1991). Beneficial effect of carotid endarterectomy in symptomatic patients with high-grade carotid stenosis. North American Symptomatic Carotid Endarterectomy Trial Collaborators. *New England Journal of Medicine*, **325**, 445–53.

Oliver, T. B., Lammie, G. A., *et al.* (1999). Atherosclerotic plaque at the carotid bifurcation: CT angiographic appearance with histopathologic correlation. *AJNR. American Journal of Neuroradiology*, **20**, 897–901.

Polak, J. F., Shemanski, L., *et al.* (1998). Hypoechoic plaque at US of the carotid artery: an independent risk factor for incident stroke in adults aged 65 years or older. Cardiovascular Health Study. *Radiology*, **208**, 649–54.

Randomised trial of endarterectomy for recently symptomatic carotid stenosis: final results of the MRC European Carotid Surgery Trial (ECST). (1998). *Lancet*, **351**, 1379–87.

Randoux, B., Marro, B., *et al.* (2001). Carotid artery stenosis: prospective comparison of CT, three-dimensional gadolinium-enhanced MR, and conventional angiography. *Radiology*, **220**, 179–85.

Rothwell, P. M., Gibson, R., *et al.* (2000). Interrelation between plaque surface morphology and degree of stenosis on carotid angiograms and the risk of ischemic stroke in patients with symptomatic carotid stenosis. On behalf of the European Carotid Surgery Trialists' Collaborative Group. *Stroke*, **31**, 615–21.

Schroeder, S., Flohr, T., *et al.* (2001a). Accuracy of density measurements within plaques located in artificial coronary arteries by X-ray multislice CT: results of a phantom study. *Journal of Computer Assisted Tomography*, **25**, 900–6.

Schroeder, S., Kopp, A. F., *et al.* (2001b). Noninvasive detection and evaluation of atherosclerotic coronary plaques with multislice computed tomography. *Journal of the American College of Cardiology*, **37**, 1430–5.

Schroeder, S., Kuettner, A., *et al.* (2004). Reliability of differentiating human coronary plaque morphology using contrast-enhanced multislice spiral computed tomography: a comparison with histology. *Journal of Computer Assisted Tomography*, **28**, 449–54.

Seeger, J. M., Barratt, E., *et al.* (1995). The relationship between carotid plaque composition, plaque morphology, and neurologic symptoms. *Journal of Surgical Research*, **58**, 330–6.

Shaalan, W. E., Cheng, H., *et al.* (2004). Degree of carotid plaque calcification in relation to symptomatic outcome and plaque inflammation. *Journal of Vascular Surgery*, **40**, 262–9.

Stary, H. C. (2000). Natural history and histological classification of atherosclerotic lesions: an update. *Arteriosclerosis, Thrombosis, and Vascular Biology*, **20**, 1177–8.

Stary, H. C., Chandler, A. B., *et al.* (1994). A definition of initial, fatty streak, and intermediate lesions of atherosclerosis. A report from the Committee on Vascular Lesions of the Council on Arteriosclerosis, American Heart Association. *Circulation*, **89**, 2462–78.

Stary, H. C., Chandler, A. B., *et al.* (1995). A definition of advanced types of atherosclerotic lesions and a histological classification of atherosclerosis. A report from the Committee on Vascular Lesions of the Council on Arteriosclerosis, American Heart Association. *Circulation*, **92**, 1355–74.

Streifler, J. Y., Eliasziw, M., *et al.* (1994). Angiographic detection of carotid plaque ulceration. Comparison with surgical observations in a multicenter study. North American Symptomatic Carotid Endarterectomy Trial. *Stroke*, **25**, 1130–2.

Virmani, R., Burke, A. P., *et al.* (2002). Pathology of the unstable plaque. *Progress in Cardiovascular Disease*, **44**, 349–56.

Vliegenthart, R., Hollander, M., *et al.* (2002). Stroke is associated with coronary calcification as detected by electron-beam CT: the Rotterdam Coronary Calcification Study. *Stroke*, **33**, 462–5.

Vliegenthart, R., Oudkerk, M., *et al.* (2005). Coronary calcification improves cardiovascular risk prediction in the elderly. *Circulation*, **112**, 572–7.

Walker, L. J., Ismail, A., *et al.* (2002). Computed tomography angiography for the evaluation of carotid atherosclerotic plaque: correlation with histopathology of endarterectomy specimens. *Stroke*, **33**, 977–81.

Zhao, X. Q., Yuan, C., *et al.* (2001). Effects of prolonged intensive lipid-lowering therapy on the characteristics of carotid atherosclerotic plaques in vivo by MRI: a case-control study. *Arteriosclerosis, Thrombosis and Vascular Biology*, **21**, 1623–9.

16

Assessment of carotid plaque with conventional ultrasound

Stephen Meairs

University of Heidelberg, 68167 Mannheim, Germany

Introduction

Over three decades ago continuous-wave (CW) Doppler was introduced as the first ultrasound (US) investigation for evaluation of carotid stenosis. Since that time, the rapid development of noninvasive US techniques has resulted in a wide variety of clinical applications for assessment of carotid disease. This chapter will discuss the clinical merits and limitations of US techniques for evaluation of both early and advanced carotid disease. It will then address recent developments including carotid plaque perfusion and molecular imaging of carotid disease.

Ultrasound techniques for evaluation of carotid disease

Doppler sonography

US Doppler techniques are commonly used for examining the carotid arteries. Interpretation of Doppler signals is based on analysis of the audio signals and of the frequency spectrum. The Doppler effect is named after Christian Doppler, who described the effect of moving objects on the change in frequency of emitted light in 1842. This effect is familiar to anyone who has stood in one place and listened to a source of sound passing by. The rising pitch of the passing movement of sound rushes toward the listener and equally drops as the source leaves him behind. Similarly, the Doppler frequency shift, which is the difference between emitted and received US frequency, is proportional to the velocity of moving blood cells.

CW Doppler systems use two transducers, one of which emits while the other receives US continuously. This simple system is easily applicable for the detection of a broad range of flow velocity alterations including high blood flow velocities associated with severe stenosis. However, it provides only limited information about the topographic origin of the US-reflecting source. In contrast, pulsed waved (PW) Doppler systems, in which US is both emitted and received from a single piezoelectric crystal, provide a depth estimate of the insonated site. Although CW and PW Doppler are simple, inexpensive screening procedures for detection of stenoses and occlusions in the extracranial arteries, they have been largely replaced by more sophisticated US techniques offering real-time display of the vessel walls and lumen combined with color-coded visualization of blood flow.

Imaging techniques

A number of complementary ultrasonographic techniques are available for imaging of the carotid arteries.

B-mode scanning displays the morphologic features of normal and pathological vessels. Since the extracranial carotid arteries lie near the skin,

Carotid Disease: The Role of Imaging in Diagnosis and Management, ed. Jonathan Gillard, Martin Graves, Thomas Hatsukami and Chun Yuan. Published by Cambridge University Press. © Cambridge University Press 2007.

linear array transducers are commonly used at US frequencies of 7.0–12.0 MHz.

Duplex sonography combines integrated PW Doppler spectrum analysis and B-mode sonography. In addition to providing information about the presence and morphology of arterial lesions, the B-mode image serves as a guide for the placement of the PW Doppler sample volume. The common, internal and external carotid arteries (CCA, ICA, and ECA, respectively) are usually characterized by a relatively distinct Doppler frequency spectrum, which allows their identification upon insonation with a PW Doppler system. The emission frequency of the integrated PW Doppler system ranges between 4 and 7 MHz.

Color Doppler flow imaging (CDFI) preserves the advantages of duplex sonography and additionally visualizes color-coded blood flow patterns superimposed on the gray-scale B-mode image (Steinke *et al.*, 1990). Using a defined color scale, the direction and the average mean velocity of moving blood cells within the sample volume at a given point in time is encoded. Generation of color signals is based on the detection of frequency and phase shifts by means of a multigate transducer.

The technique of autocorrelation is used to obtain a real-time visualization of color-coded hemodynamics.

Power Doppler imaging (PDI) displays the amplitude of Doppler signals. Color and brightness of the signals are related to the number of blood cells producing the Doppler shift. PDI is more sensitive for detection of blood flow than CDFI. This is because PDI is less angle-dependent than CDFI, thus allowing better display of curving or tortuous vessels. By reliance upon Doppler amplitude, there is no aliasing. This improves display of vessel wall pathology in areas of turbulent flow. PDI is a valuable technique for displaying plaque surface structure (Steinke *et al.*, 1996) (Figure 16.1).

Real-time compound imaging enhances ultrasonographic visualization and characterization of carotid artery plaques (Jespersen *et al.*, 2000; Kofoed *et al.*, 2001). This technique acquires US beams, which are steered off-axis from the orthogonal beams used in conventional US. The number of frames and steering angles varies, depending on the transducer characteristics. Frames acquired from sufficiently different angles contain independent random speckle patterns, which are averaged

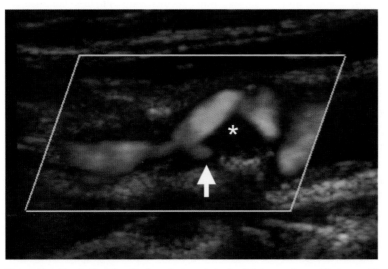

Figure 16.1 Power Doppler display of stenosis in the left internal carotid artery with deep ulceration (arrow). Duplex imaging allows simultaneous depiction of weakly echogenic plaque material, presumably lipid (*).

to reduce speckle and improve tissue differentiation. Real-time compound imaging improves
characterization of carotid plaque morphology
(Kern *et al.*, 2004).

B-mode flow imaging allows direct visualization
of blood reflectors without the limitations of
Doppler technology such as aliasing, signal drop-
out at orthogonal detection angles, and wall filter
limitations (Weskott, 2000; Henri and Tranquart,
2000). B-flow has been shown to be very effective in
visualizing hemodynamic flow and in detecting
stenotic lesions in the carotid artery (Umemura
and Yamada, 2001). Moreover, B-flow can provide a
detailed hemodynamic image of phenomena such
as bloodstream swirls. B-flow also visualizes bloodstream flow patterns at the site of wall ulcerations
or vascular tortuousness.

Three-dimensional (3D) ultrasound can be
used for both qualitative and quantitative analysis
of plaques in the carotid artery. Surface features
of carotid plaques, not readily appreciated in conventional two-dimensional (2D) B-mode scanning,
can be clearly demonstrated by 3D US. In some
cases, this may lead to a diagnosis not obtainable with other imaging techniques (Meairs *et al.*,
2000) (Figure 16.2). New developments in 3D US
image acquisition involve the use of position and
orientation measurement (POM) devices capable
of tracking scanheads in six degrees-of-freedom
(6-DOF) (Detmer *et al.*, 1994; Barry *et al.*, 1997).
This approach allows "freehand" scanning to
collect image data from different perspectives and
potentially offers the ability to maximize tissue
information that is not readily available from
one imaging plane alone. Methods for enhanced
reconstruction and visualization of 6-DOF US data
are now available (Meairs *et al.*, 2000).

Contrast harmonic imaging (CHI) is based on
the non-linear emission of harmonics by resonant
microbubbles pulsating in a US field. The emission
at twice the driving frequency, termed the second
harmonic, can be detected and separated from
the fundamental frequency. The advantage of
the harmonic over the fundamental frequency is
that contrast agent microbubbles resonate with

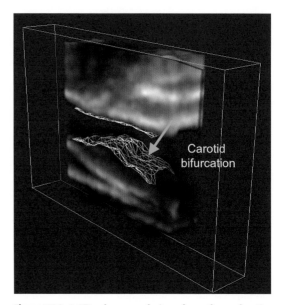

Figure 16.2 A 3D volume rendering of an atherosclerotic
plaque of the internal carotid artery using compound
reconstruction techniques for B-mode imaging. A grid on
the plaque surface demonstrates a surface defect (arrow)
corresponding to a traumatic plaque rupture.

harmonic frequencies, whereas adjacent tissues do
so very little. In this way, CHI may enhance the
signal-to-noise ratio and the ability of B-mode
scanners to differentiate bubbles in the tissue
vascular space from the echogenic surrounding
avascular tissue. This technique can be used to
visualize perfusion characteristics of carotid artery
plaques.

Monitoring early atherosclerosis with ultrasound

Decades of silent arterial wall alterations precede
cardiovascular clinical events, which then reflect
advanced atherosclerotic disease. The first morphological abnormalities of arterial walls can be
imaged by B-mode ultrasonography. This technique is one of the best methods for detection of
early stages of atherosclerotic disease, because it

is easily applicable, readily available, and demonstrates the wall structure with better resolution than magnetic resonance angiography or conventional angiography. Accordingly, US has been used in a number of studies to monitor the intima media thickness (IMT) of the carotid arteries, a measurement which has consequently been shown to be associated with cardiovascular risk factors and the incidence of cardiovascular disease.

IMT reflects not only early atherosclerosis, but also nonatherosclerotic intimal reactions such as intimal hyperplasia and intimal fibrocellular hypertrophy. This differentiation is important because epidemiological studies have shown that wall thickening as depicted by ultrasonographic measurements of IMT is different from atherosclerotic plaque regarding localization, risk factors and predictive value on cardiovascular events. As IMT is being increasingly used in clinical trials to serve as a surrogate endpoint for determining the success of interventions that lower risk factors provide for atherosclerosis, it is imperative that standardized methods be used to allow homogenous data collection and analysis.

Pignoli and coworkers were the first to identify a "double line" pattern of the carotid artery wall with B-mode US (Pignoli et al., 1986). They described the first echogenic line on the far wall to represent the lumen-intima interface and the second line to correspond to the media-adventitia interface. The distance between these two echogenic lines correlated highly with measurements of IMT in tissue specimens from CCAs. This initial report on measurement of IMT with B-mode US was later validated in vitro (Wong et al., 1993) and was shown to enable good intra- and interobserver reproducibility (Riley et al., 1992).

Since the focal location of sites of reactive intimal thickening and initial plaque development in the carotid arteries is related to geometric transitions, the selection of precise regions for measurement of IMT is important. Any single examination by US may not identify the site of maximal intimal thickening. Therefore, IMT examinations over a range of incident angles and axial locations are necessary. Several IMT sampling protocols have been introduced. The type of IMT sampling used, i.e. combined measurements at different sites, measurements only at the CCA, mean or maximum wall thickness, may largely depend on the research question and on the relative emphasis accorded to confirmed atherosclerotic lesions.

The recent Mannheim IMT consensus statement notes that although recent studies have shown that reduction of IMT values are significantly correlated with risk reduction and improvement of risk factor profiles in a large population, neither positive nor negative predictive values on ischemic risk reduction are known in individual subjects treated successfully for specific risk factors (Touboul et al., 2004). Thus, although IMT has been suggested to represent an important risk marker, it does not fulfill the characteristics of an accepted risk factor.

Assessment of advanced atherosclerotic disease

In the initial period of cerebrovascular ultrasonographic insonation the ophthalmic artery was used as an indirect test for detection of significant carotid artery stenosis (Maroon et al., 1969; Melis-Kisman and Mol, 1970). This periorbital technique provides quick information on the existence of collateral pathways. In the presence of severe stenosis or occlusion of the ICA retrograde blood supply from the ECA via the ophthalmic anastomosis can be easily detected with CW Doppler. However, with sufficient collateralization from the contralateral carotid or the vertebrobasilar systems, orthograde perfusion of the ophthalmic artery may occur. Accordingly, this indirect test fails to detect even hemodynamically significant ipsilateral carotid obstruction in up to 20% of patients. While detection of retrograde perfusion in the ophthalmic artery is a strong indicator of severe pathology within the ipsilateral extracranial carotid system, findings of normal perfusion of the ophthalmic branches cannot exclude severe carotid stenosis or occlusion.

Doppler sonography can be used to detect various degrees of carotid obstruction. According to the distribution of abnormal blood flow patterns within, proximal to, or distal to a narrowed arterial segment, this technique provides data on the extent, site, and degree of lesions of more than 40% lumen narrowing. Special transducers can be used to assess distal extracranial lesions of the ICA; e.g. carotid dissections (Meairs and Hennerici, 2000), fibromuscular dysplasia, or atypically located atherosclerosis.

Grading carotid artery stenosis with US

An international consensus meeting established criteria for the quantification of ICA stenosis (De Bray and Glatt, 1995). Recommendations for interpretation of Doppler shift velocities and residual area are summarized below.

- Mild stenosis (40–60%) is characterized by a local increase of peak and mean flow velocities. Systolic peak velocities range above 120 cm/s (4-MHz probe).
- Moderate stenosis (60–80%) shows a distortion of normal pulsatile flow in addition to a local increase of peak and mean frequencies. Typically, systolic flow decelerations are found in the poststenotic segment. The systolic peak velocity ranges from 120 to 240 cm/s.
- Severe stenosis (more than 80%) produces markedly increased peak flow velocities exceeding 240 cm/s and occasionally reaching over 600 cm/s. In addition, pre- and poststenotic blood flow velocity is significantly reduced compared with the contralateral unaffected carotid artery. Retrograde flow of the ophthalmic artery may occur.
- Subtotal stenosis (more than 95%) is characterized by variable, usually low peak flow velocities, which decrease once a stenosis becomes pseudo-occlusive. This condition is difficult to separate from complete occlusion and may be misdiagnosed.

- ICA occlusion usually shows a low velocity Doppler signal with predominant reversed signal component and absent diastolic flow at the presumed origin of the ICA (stump flow). Blood flow velocity in the CCA is reduced, and frequently retrograde perfusion of the ophthalmic artery occurs. In acute thrombotic occlusion, echolucent material fills the vascular lumen, which can hardly be differentiated on the gray-scale from blood flow in a patent ICA. The capacity of modern CDFI and PDI instruments to detect very slow blood flow velocities has markedly improved the sensitivity for the diagnosis of a subtotal ICA stenosis and pseudo-occlusion.

The combination of B-mode imaging and PW Doppler sonography in duplex instruments considerably improves the accuracy of the noninvasive diagnosis and grading of carotid stenosis. The degree of stenosis can be estimated from distinct parameters of the Doppler frequency spectrum. However, instead of Doppler shift frequencies, equivalent flow velocity values can be obtained after correction of the Doppler insonation angle according to the flow direction in the vessel segment. In CDFI three sources of information are available for the classification of carotid stenosis: the Doppler frequency spectrum, measurement of the residual vessel lumen and characteristic color flow patterns.

Doppler frequency spectrum

Assessment of the Doppler spectrum is important since it can often be recorded even when plaque calcification obscures adequate visualization of color flow patterns and of the residual vessel lumen. Parameters from the Doppler spectrum such as the peak systolic frequency or velocity (Taylor and Strandness, 1987) agree well with angiography for grading carotid stenosis.

Measurement of residual vessel lumen

Using sequential longitudinal and transverse sections, both CDFI and PDI allow reliable assessment of plaque configuration and relative obstruction by contrasting the intravascular surface. Assuming a concentric stenosis, the percentage area reduction in cross-sections is higher than the relative diameter. There is a good correlation between transverse lumen reduction on CDFI and diameter reduction on corresponding angiograms of carotid stenosis (Steinke *et al.*, 1992; Sitzer *et al.*, 1993). Measurement of local diameter and area reduction in carotid stenosis can be performed more reliably by PDI than by CDFI due to improved visualization of the residual stenotic lumen (Steinke *et al.*, 1996).

The volumetric potential of 3D US has important clinical implications in serial follow-up studies for observing the progression or regression of stenotic lesions and for evaluating the outcome of interventional procedures such as endarterectomy or stent placement (Yao *et al.*, 1998). Recent studies demonstrate that the volumetric change that must be observed to establish with 95% confidence that a plaque has undergone change is approximately 20–35% for plaques <100 mm^3 and approximately 10–20% for plaques >100 mm^3 (Landry *et al.*, 2004).

Color Doppler flow patterns

Color Doppler flow patterns can provide complementary information for establishing the degree of carotid artery stenosis. Low-grade stenosis (40–60%) is associated with a relatively long segment of decreased color saturation with absent or minimal poststenotic turbulence (Steinke *et al.*, 1990). In moderate obstructions (61–80%) the decreased color saturation is more circumscribed, while flow velocity remains high during diastole. Poststenotic flow is turbulent and flow reversal occurs frequently. High-grade stenosis (Figure 16.3) is characterized by a mosaic pattern indicating high flow velocity and mixed turbulence (Hallam *et al.*, 1989). A short segment of maximal color fading or aliasing with severe poststenotic turbulence and flow reversal provides further evidence for high-grade stenosis (Steinke *et al.*, 1990).

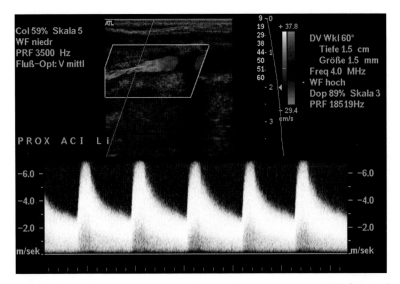

Figure 16.3 The Doppler spectrum identifies a high-grade stenosis of the left carotid artery with maximum peak velocity of >6 m/s causing left hemispheric stroke. CDFI demonstrates a mosaic pattern indicating high flow velocity and mixed turbulence.

Assessment of plaque morphology

US has been extensively used for study of carotid plaque morphology. High-resolution B-mode imaging alone, and in conjunction with color Doppler flow and PDI techniques, has been used to define parameters for identification of symptomatic or vulnerable plaques. These have included plaque echogenicity, plaque surface structure, plaque ulcerations, and plaque fibrous cap.

Carotid artery plaques of homogeneous, moderate intensity echogenicity consist mainly of fibrotic tissue (Hennerici et al., 1984). Such plaques rarely show ulceration, perhaps accounting for the lack of a significant correlation between homogeneous echogenicity and the occurrence of focal cerebral ischemia. Heterogeneous plaques represent matrix deposition, cholesterol accumulation, necrosis, calcification and intraplaque hemorrhage (Hennerici et al., 1984; Goes et al., 1990). Several studies have demonstrated that high-resolution B-mode scanning can characterize echomorphologic features of carotid plaques that correlate with histopathologic criteria (Comerota et al., 1990). Although echolucent areas within the plaque may represent thrombotic material or hemorrhage, lipid accumulation may produce similar echogenicity. Plaque calcification produces acoustic shadowing. Depending on the location of the plaque and on the extent of calcification, acoustic shadowing can be a major obstacle for visualization of plaque morphology.

Initial studies of plaque echogenicity with B-mode US reported an association between heterogeneous plaques and the occurrence of cerebrovascular events (Bluth et al., 1986; Langsfeld et al., 1989). Support for this association was provided by several investigations of endarterectomy specimens which suggested a correlation between intraplaque hemorrhage and transient ischemic attacks and stroke (Lusby et al., 1982; Imparato et al., 1983). Later studies, however, were unable to confirm these observations (Bassiouny et al., 1989; Leen et al., 1990). The issue on whether

differences in plaque echogenicity can distinguish between symptomatic and asymptomatic plaques continues to be a debatable subject. More recent ultrasonographic studies have renewed the notion that heterogeneous carotid plaques are more often associated with intraplaque hemorrhage and neurologic events, and conclude that evaluation of plaque morphology may be helpful in selecting patients for carotid endarterectomy (Golledge et al., 1997; Park et al., 1998). Others argue that lipid-rich plaques are more prone to rupture and suggest that an association between intraplaque hemorrhage and a high lipid content as revealed in B-mode US may support this theory (Gronholdt et al., 1997). However, these newer findings have been negated by other research groups finding little correlation between plaque morphology and histological specimens (Droste et al., 1997). One definitive study on the significance of heterogeneous plaque structure found no differences in volume of intraplaque hemorrhage, lipid core, necrotic core or plaque calcification in patients with highly stenotic carotid lesions undergoing endarterectomy, regardless of preoperative symptom status (Hatsukami et al., 1997). Other groups have also been unable to demonstrate that complicated plaques showing plaque rupture, thrombosis or intraplaque hemorrhage are associated with symptoms, and conclude that such plaques may occur at any time, irrespective of symptoms (Milei et al., 2003).

One significant problem in comparison of studies on the value of plaque echogenicity is standardization. Indeed, the use of image normalization procedures can have a profound effect on how plaques are classified (Nicolaides et al., 2005). Another important issue that may have been long overlooked in debates concerning the correlation of histological and US findings is the poor reproducibility of histological exams. Unfortunately, pathological correlation in studies of carotid plaque imaging cannot be reliably interpreted or compared because of incomparable and poorly reported histology methods (Lovett et al., 2005).

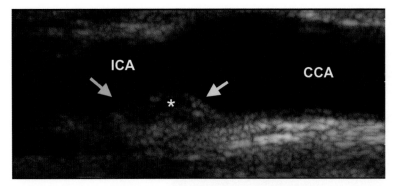

Figure 16.4 High-resolution B-mode scan (13 MHz dynamic range linear transducer) of heterogeneous plaque (arrows) of the internal carotid artery at the level of the carotid bifurcation. Common carotid artery (CCA) and internal carotid artery (ICA). The fibrous cap displays stronger echoes on the proximal plaque surface (yellow arrow) as on its more distal surface (green arrow) where fibrous cap thinning is evident. The plaque displays a relatively smooth plaque surface structure protruding into the lumen of the ICA. Beneath the plaque surface is an area of weaker echoes (*), corresponding to lipid accumulation.

Although a relatively good differentiation between smooth, irregular and ulcerative plaque surfaces was obtained for postmortem carotid artery specimens in early studies (Hennerici *et al.*, 1984), the in vivo accuracy as compared to findings at carotid endarterectomy has been considerably poorer (Widder *et al.*, 1990; Droste *et al.*, 1997). Commonly used parameters for identification of plaque ulceration have been surface defects showing a depth and length of ≥2 mm with a well-defined base in the recess. Using these criteria, B-mode imaging failed to provide a satisfactory diagnostic yield for ulcerative plaques with a sensitivity of only 47% (Comerota *et al.*, 1990). Although it is likely that the use of state-of-the-art US equipment applying new developments such as compound B-mode imaging, B-flow or pulse inversion CHI will considerably improve the identification of plaque ulceration, there are no reports that confirm this contention.

Erosions of the fibrous cap with inflammation and neoformation of early atherosclerotic lesions within, upon or immediately beneath fibrous caps are particularly suggestive of plaque instability (Bassiouny *et al.*, 1997). Plaques not associated with disruption usually have an intact fibrous cap of uniform thickness, well demarcated from the lesion and without focal erosion, inflammation or plaque neoformation. There has therefore been considerable interest in evaluation of the fibrous cap with B-mode US (Figure 16.4). One study comparing carotid endarterectomy specimens with preoperative carotid US results found that the best factors for characterization of carotid plaques were thinning and rupture of the fibrous cap (Lammie *et al.*, 2000). Likewise, determination of the mean fibrous cap thickness with a new US system based using automatic boundary detection has shown good discrimination between symptomatic and asymptomatic plaques (Devuyst *et al.*, 2005).

Plaque motion

Experimental work has suggested that analysis of plaque motion, i.e. translational plaque movements coincident with those of arterial walls, plaque rotations and local, plaque-specific deformations, may provide new insights into plaque modeling as well as into mechanisms of plaque rupture with subsequent embolism. Plaque surface movement may be attributable to deformations resulting from crack propagation of multiple local

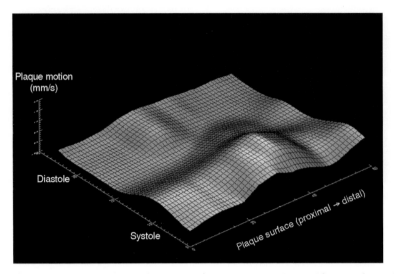

Figure 16.5 Grid of plaque surface motion from a symptomatic carotid artery plaque showing increased velocities at the center of the plaque during systole. A second phase of surface motion of smaller amplitude is seen in late diastole. Data acquisition was performed with an ECG-triggered, parallel motor system (slice thickness 0.2 mm). A nonparametric hierarchical motion estimation algorithm utilizing minimization of the sum-of-squared differences (SSD) of Laplacian-filtered pyramid images was used to compute the motion field.

internal tears in the plaque. Theoretically, identification of local variations in surface deformability might provide information on the relative vulnerability to plaque fissuring or rupture.

Four-dimensional (4D) ultrasonography has been used to acquire temporal 3D US data of carotid artery plaques (Meairs and Hennerici, 1999). This US data has been analyzed with motion detection algorithms to determine apparent velocity fields, also known as optical flow, of the plaque surface for characterization of plaque motion patterns in patients with symptomatic and asymptomatic carotid artery disease (Meairs and Hennerici, 1999). Asymptomatic plaques showed a homogenous orientation and magnitude of computed surface velocity vectors, coincident with arterial wall movement. Symptomatic plaques, however, demonstrated evidence for plaque deformation, irrespective of arterial wall movements (Figure 16.5). Further refinement of plaque motion analysis using radiofrequency signals (Horder et al., 1998) and new detection

algorithms (Golemati et al., 2003) may improve the clinical applicability of this promising approach for characterizing plaque vulnerability.

Echocontrast studies in evaluation of carotid stenosis

Commercially available contrast agents consist of microbubbles with average diameters of 3–6 μm in concentrations of about 10^8 microbubbles/milliliter. The microbubbles are normally stabilized against dissolution by surfactants, phospholipids, or a surface layer of partially denatured albumin. Current contrast agents can enhance the US signal by 10–30 dB, thus enabling the detection of flow in deeper and smaller vessels.

The first generation of US contrast agents consisted of air-filled microbubbles. Examples of such agents are Albunex®, which is produced by controlled sonication of a 5% human serum albumin solution, and Levovist®, which is a galactose-based agent stabilized by 0.01% palmitic acid.

Meairs, S., Beyer, J. and Hennerici, M. (2000). Reconstruction and visualization of irregularly sampled three- and four-dimensional ultrasound data for cerebrovascular applications. *Ultrasound in Medicine and Biology*, **26**, 263–72.

Meairs, S. and Hennerici, M. (1999). Four-dimensional ultrasonographic characterization of plaque surface motion in patients with symptomatic and asymptomatic carotid artery stenosis. *Stroke*, **30**, 1807–13.

Meairs, S. and Hennerici, M. (2000). Long-term follow-up of aneurysms developed during extracranial internal carotid artery dissection. *Neurology*, **54**, 2190.

Meairs, S., Timpe, L., Beyer, J. and Hennerici, M. (2000). Acute aphasia and hemiplegia during karate training. *Lancet*, **356**, 40.

Melis-Kisman, E. and Mol, J. M. F. (1970). L'applicationde l'effet Doppler à l'exploration cérébrovasculaire – Rapport préliminaire. *Revue Neurologique*, **122**, 470–2.

Milei, J., Parodi, J. C., Ferreira, M., *et al.* (2003). Atherosclerotic plaque rupture and intraplaque hemorrhage do not correlate with symptoms in carotid artery stenosis. *Journal of Vascular Surgery*, **38**, 1241–7.

Moreno, P. R., Purushothaman, K. R., Fuster, V., *et al.* (2004). Plaque neovascularization is increased in ruptured atherosclerotic lesions of human aorta: implications for plaque vulnerability. *Circulation*, **110**, 2032–8.

Nicolaides, A. N., Kakkos, S. K., Griffin, M., *et al.* (2005). Effect of image normalization on carotid plaque classification and the risk of ipsilateral hemispheric ischemic events: results from the asymptomatic carotid stenosis and risk of stroke study. *Vascular*, **13**, 211–21.

Park, A. E., McCarthy, W. J., Pearce, W. H., Matsumura, J. S. and Yao, J. S. (1998). Carotid plaque morphology correlates with presenting symptomatology. *Journal of Vascular Surgery*, **27**, 872–8.

Pignoli, P., Tremoli, E., Poli, A., Oreste, P. and Paoletti, R. (1986). Intimal plus medial thickness of the arterial wall: a direct measurement with ultrasound imaging. *Circulation*, **74**, 1399–406.

Riley, W. A., Barnes, R. W., Applegate, W. B., *et al.* (1992). Reproducibility of noninvasive ultrasonic measurement of carotid atherosclerosis. The Asymptomatic Carotid Artery Plaque Study. *Stroke*, **23**, 1062–8.

Rothwell, P. M., Gutnikov, S. A. and Warlow, C. P. (2003). Reanalysis of the final results of the European Carotid Surgery Trial. *Stroke*, **34**, 514–23.

Schumann, P. A., Christiansen, J. P., Quigley, R. M., *et al.* (2002). Targeted-microbubble binding selectively to GPIIb IIIa receptors of platelet thrombi. *Investigative Radiology*, **37**, 587–93.

Sitzer, M., Fuerst, G., Fischer, H., *et al.* (1993). Between-method correlations in quantifying internal carotid stenosis. *Stroke*, **24**, 1513–18.

Sitzer, M., Furst, G., Siebler, M. and Steinmetz, H. (1994). Usefulness of an intravenous contrast medium in the characterization of high-grade internal carotid stenosis with color Doppler-assisted duplex imaging. *Stroke*, **25**, 385–9.

Steinke, W., Hennerici, M., Rautenberg, W. and Mohr, J. P. (1992). Symptomatic and asymptomatic high-grade carotid stenoses in Doppler color-flow imaging. *Neurology*, **42**, 131–8.

Steinke, W., Kloetzsch, C. and Hennerici, M. (1990). Carotid artery disease assessed by color Doppler flow imaging: correlation with standard Doppler sonography and angiography. *American Journal of Neuroradiology*, **11**, 259–66.

Steinke, W., Meairs, S., Ries, S. and Hennerici, M. (1996). Sonographic assessment of carotid artery stenosis: comparison of power Doppler imaging and color Doppler flow imaging. *Stroke*, **27**, 91–4.

Strandness, D. E. and Eikelboom, B. C. (1998). Carotid artery stenosis–where do we go from here? *European Journal of Ultrasound*, **7** (Suppl. 3), S17–S26.

Taylor, D. C. and Strandness, D. E., Jr. (1987). Carotid artery duplex scanning. *Journal of Clinical Ultrasound*, **15**, 635–44.

Touboul, P. J., Hennerici, M. G., Meairs, S., *et al.* (2004). Mannheim Intima-Media Thickness Consensus on Behalf of the Advisory Board of the 3rd Watching the Risk Symposium 2004, 13th European Stroke Conference, Mannheim, Germany, May 14, 2004. *Cerebrovascular Diseases*, **18**, 346–9.

Umemura, A. and Yamada, K. (2001). B-mode flow imaging of the carotid artery. *Stroke*, **32**, 2055–7.

Van Liew, H. D. and Burkard, M. E. (1995). Bubbles in circulating blood: stabilization and simulations of cyclic changes of size and content. *Journal of Applied Physiology*, **79**, 1379–85.

Virmani, R., Kolodgie, F. D., Burke, A. P., *et al.* (2005). Atherosclerotic plaque progression and vulnerability to rupture: angiogenesis as a source of intraplaque hemorrhage. *Arteriosclerosis, Thrombosis, and Vascular Biology*, **25**, 2054–61.

Weissleder, R. and Mahmood, U. (2001). Molecular imaging. *Radiology*, **219**, 316–33.

Weller, G. E., Villanueva, F. S., Klibanov, A. L. and Wagner, W. R. (2002). Modulating targeted adhesion of an ultrasound contrast agent to dysfunctional endothelium. *Annals of Biomedical Engineering*, **30**, 1012–19.

Weskott, H. P. (2000). B-flow–a new method for detecting blood flow. *Ultraschall inder Medizin*, **21**, 59–65.

Widder, B., Paulat, K., Hackspacher, J., *et al.* (1990). Morphological characterization of carotid artery stenoses by ultrasound duplex scanning. *Ultrasound in Medicine and Biology*, **16**, 349–54.

Wong, M., Edelstein, J., Wollman, J. and Bond, M. G. (1993). Ultrasonic-pathological comparison of the human arterial wall. Verification of intima-media thickness. *Arteriosclerosis and Thrombosis*, **13**, 482–6.

Yao, J., van Sambeek, M. R., Dall'Agata, A., *et al.* (1998). Three-dimensional ultrasound study of carotid arteries before and after endarterectomy; analysis of stenotic lesions and surgical impact on the vessel. *Stroke*, **29**, 2026–31.

17

Assessment of carotid plaque with intravascular ultrasound

Gastón A. Rodriguez-Granillo and Patrick W. Serruys

Erasmus MC, Dr Molewaterplein 40, 3015 GD Rotterdam, The Netherlands

History

Intravascular ultrasound (IVUS) has a relatively short yet highly prolific history that started in the late 1980s. The vast majority of clinical IVUS has centered on the coronary arteries with very limited studies in the carotid territory. Although this book is mainly focused on carotid disease there are a number of successful coronary IVUS techniques, which could be applied to carotid data.

Early studies already demonstrated that the extension and severity of coronary atherosclerosis might be greatly underestimated with angiography, whereas highly accurate measurements could be obtained using IVUS (Glagov et al., 1987; McPherson et al., 1987; Gussenhoven et al., 1989). Later, plaque characterization by means of the visual assessment was attempted and correlation with histopathology offered questionable results (Gussenhoven et al., 1989a,b; Peters et al., 1994). Moving forward to the core of the past decade, interventional cardiologists sought to find an application of IVUS in the catheterization laboratory. As a result, several studies evaluated the potential of IVUS as an adjunctive tool for guiding percutaneous coronary interventions. IVUS has thereafter aided the evolution of angioplasty providing insights about the morphology of atherosclerotic plaque (Suzuki et al., 1999), the mechanisms involved in the restenotic process (Hoffmann et al., 1996; Shiran et al., 1998; de Feyter et al., 1999; Sheris et al., 2000), the assessment of lesion severity (Abizaid et al., 1998, 1999; Nishioka et al., 1999; Takagi et al., 1999) and complications (Sheris et al., 2000; Degertekin et al., 2003) and the guidance of percutaneous coronary interventions (Schiele et al., 1998; Fitzgerald et al., 2000; Frey et al., 2000; Mudra et al., 2001; Oemrawsingh et al., 2003).

More recently, IVUS has emerged as a highly accurate tool for the serial assessment of the natural history of coronary atherosclerosis and to evaluate the effect of different conventional and emerging drug therapies in the progression of atherosclerosis (Fang et al., 2002; Matsuzaki et al., 2002; Nissen et al., 2003; Nissen et al., 2004a,b; Tardif et al., 2004). Finally, the contemporary and future application of IVUS is linked to the study of different applications of the analysis of radiofrequency data, both for the improvement of plaque characterization (Nair et al., 2002; Kawasaki et al., 2005) and for the assessment of mechanical properties of plaques (de Korte et al., 1998, 2002). Overall, such insightful analysis of the radiofrequency data might potentially aid the detection of plaques with certain allegedly high-risk characteristics (Schaar et al., 2003; Rodriguez-Granillo et al., 2005a) and monitor their natural history in prospective natural history studies.

The technology

IVUS is a catheter-based diagnostic tool that provides a real-time, high-resolution, tomographic

Carotid Disease: The Role of Imaging in Diagnosis and Management, ed. Jonathan Gillard, Martin Graves, Thomas Hatsukami and Chun Yuan. Published by Cambridge University Press. © Cambridge University Press 2007.

view of coronary arteries. It thereby enables the assessment of morphology, severity and extension of coronary plaque. There are basically two types of commercially available IVUS imaging catheters: a single-element mechanically rotated transducer and a phased-array electronic system. Mechanical systems comprise a flexible cable with a single rotation transducer that revolves at 30 revolutions per second emitting and receiving ultrasound signals every 1° increment. Such catheters are covered with an echolucent outer sheath to prevent direct contact of the ultrasound element with the vessel wall. Phased-array catheters contain a 64-element annular array that enables a coordinated emission of the ultrasound signal.

Mechanical and phased-array catheters have relative advantages and disadvantages. Mechanical catheters have higher resolution but display specific artefacts such as nonuniform rotational distortion. In addition, far field imaging can be more problematic with mechanical catheters due to amplified attenuation and enhanced blood backscatter. On the other hand, phased-array catheters have lower resolution resulting in inferior near-field imaging and as they are not pulled back within a sheath, are more susceptible to nonuniform pull-back speed particularly in tortuous vessels.

Currently, the use of automated pullbacks has overcome the manual interrogation of the vessels, in particular since the former allows volumetric determination of direct (lumen and vessel) and indirect (e.g. plaque, neointima) measurements.

Safety

IVUS has been widely performed over the past two decades without significant or frequent adverse effects. In a recent large study that evaluated the long-term safety of IVUS, coronary spasm (easily reversed with intracoronary administration of nitrates) occurred in 1.9% of procedures and IVUS was not found to accelerate atherosclerosis (Guedes *et al.*, 2005).

Limitations of angiography

Quantitative angiographic measurements can be misleading since this technique only allows the evaluation of the profile of the lumen (Topol and Nissen, 1995). Compensatory expansive remodelled coronaries may present a significant increase in the burden of atherosclerotic plaque without evident changes in the degree of stenosis (Glagov *et al.*, 1987). Such phenomenon may impair the visual interpretation of this technique, yielding to significant interobserver variability and poor in vitro correlation (Grodin *et al.*, 1974). Coronary atherosclerosis is commonly a diffuse disease of the vessel wall, involving long segments of the coronaries, rarely sparing segments. The diffuse distribution of plaque has lead to misinterpretation of angiography, eventually having the appearance of small reference vessels with minimal disease (Topol and Nissen, 1995). Such masking of the true severity and extension of the disease has been clearly depicted by Mintz *et al.*, who showed that reference segments of treated lesions had a mean plaque burden of 51% (Mintz *et al.*, 1995).

Vessel foreshortening, irregular plaque distribution and irregular lumen geometry are all additional factors that further impair the accuracy of angiographic measurements.

Quantitative and qualitative IVUS

Contour detection at the leading edge of both the lumen and the media-adventitia interface (external elastic membrane, EEM) allows the assessment of two direct measurements (lumen and vessel area). From these contours, plaque volume $\sum_{n=1}^{n=m} (\text{Vessel}_{area} - \text{Lumen}_{area}) \cdot d$; where m refers to the total number of images, n to an individual image and d to distance between images and plaque burden (%) $\left(\frac{\text{Vessel}_{area} - \text{Lumen}_{area}}{\text{Vessel}_{area}} \right) \cdot 100$ can be estimated.

Several other area measurements can be obtained with IVUS, such as minimum and maximum lumen diameter, minimum and maximal plaque thickness, and lumen and plaque eccentricity (Mintz *et al.*, 2001). It is noteworthy that since the leading edge of the media is not well defined, IVUS measurements cannot determine the real (histological) plaque area delineated by the internal elastic membrane. Hence, the area enclosed within the EEM and lumen contours is solely a surrogate of the plaque area, comprising the media as well. However, the inclusion of the media into the plaque area does not affect the measurements, since it represents a negligible fraction of the "plaque plus media".

In addition to its precise quantitative measurements, IVUS has been used as a tool to characterize in vivo the composition of coronary plaques. Initially, this was attempted by means of the visual judgement of the images (Gussenhoven *et al.*, 1989a). Using this approach, plaques were qualitatively defined as soft (echolucent), fibrous (plaques with intermediate echogenicity between soft and highly echogenic plaques), mixed (plaques containing more than one acoustical subtype) or calcified (Mintz *et al.*, 2001).

It has been recognized that its value for identification of specific plaque components, particularly of lipid-rich plaques, is limited (Peters *et al.*, 1994). Nevertheless, IVUS remains a highly accurate tool regarding calcium detection (Tuzcu *et al.*, 1996). Dense calcium deposits reflect the entire ultrasound energy, thus causing a phenomenon called acoustic shadowing.

Coronary plaque characterization has currently evolved to a more automated approach, leading to more accurate results (Schartl *et al.*, 2001; de Winter *et al.*, 2003). More recently, spectral analysis of IVUS radiofrequency (RF) data has emerged as a promising tool to accurately and quantitatively assess the individual components of plaques (Nair *et al.*, 2002). Accurate characterization in vivo using IVUS RF data analysis has the potential to allow the assessment of the effects of pharmacological therapies on the coronary arteries, thereby enabling a better understanding of the disease and further development of new pharmacologic interventions (Rodriguez-Granillo *et al.*, 2005).

Progression-regression

Several angiographic studies have extensively explored the efficacy of lipid-lowering therapies to slow coronary plaque progression. A meta-analysis of such studies has concluded that the magnitude of the antiatherosclerotic effects is small compared with the effects of statins on the prevention of cardiovascular events (Balk *et al.*, 2004). Such clinical-angiographic discordance has been initially attributed to the aforementioned limitations of angiography, leading investigators to pursue the conductance of progression-regression studies with the aid of IVUS (Takagi *et al.*, 1997). Thereafter, several serial studies evaluated the impact of different medical strategies on the atherosclerotic burden over time with the aid of IVUS (Schartl *et al.*, 2001; Nissen *et al.*, 2004a; Okazaki *et al.*, 2004). However, results are still conflicting, showing no definitive differences in plaque volume over time thus reinforcing the discrepancies between the observed clinical benefit of medical therapies and the absence of a significant impact on plaque progression. Two major theories might explain such discrepancy. First, although IVUS provides accurate morphometric measurements, several factors such as intra- and interobserver variability, different position of the catheter, severely calcified vessels and artifacts can impair the reproducibility of serial measurements (Bekeredjian *et al.*, 1999; Blessing *et al.*, 1999; Gaster *et al.*, 2001). Secondly, it has been established that the histological composition of coronary plaques can precipitate atherothrombotic events regardless of the hemodynamical compromise of the lesion (Ambrose *et al.*, 1988; Davies *et al.*, 1993).

Whether the striking discordance between the clinical effects of validated antiatherosclerotic therapies and their effects on plaque volume is due to a significant change in plaque composition or to deficiencies in the methodology of IVUS studies remains unknown. Nevertheless, recent studies have shed some light by showing significant changes in plaque composition with no alteration in the plaque burden (Schartl *et al.*, 2001; Kawasaki *et al.*, 2005).

Vulnerable plaque

Major improvements in the management and diagnosis of patients with coronary artery disease have been accomplished. Still, a large number of victims who are apparently healthy die suddenly without prior symptoms (Kannel *et al.*, 1975; Falk *et al.*, 1995). Most of these events are related to plaque rupture (PR) and subsequent thrombotic occlusion at the site of nonflow-limiting atherosclerotic lesions in epicardial coronary arteries (Ambrose *et al.*, 1988; Little *et al.*, 1988). In addition, silent PR and its subsequent wound healing accelerate plaque growth and are a more frequent feature in arteries with less severe luminal narrowing (Burke *et al.*, 2001). These dire consequences of PR have brought about the development of several catheter-based techniques with the potential to detect in vivo vulnerability features of coronary atherosclerotic plaques (Asakura *et al.*, 2001; Regar *et al.*, 2002; Schaar *et al.*, 2004; Rodriguez-Granillo *et al.*, 2005a; in press).

The detection of ruptured plaques by IVUS has been recently reported by several investigators (Maehara *et al.*, 2002; Rioufol *et al.*, 2002; Hong *et al.*, 2004, 2005). In these studies, PR was found to be ubiquitous in culprit vessels of acute myocardial infarction patients (Rioufol, 2002; Hong *et al.*, 2004). Nevertheless, though less frequent, PR was also a common finding in nonculprit vessels and even in stable patients (Maehara *et al.*, 2002; Rioufol *et al.*, 2002). In addition, in agreement with angiographical findings, PR was nonuniformly distributed throughout the coronary tree, showing a clear clustering pattern involving particularly the proximal segments and sparing the distal segments and the left main coronary artery (Wang *et al.*, 2004; Hong *et al.*, 2005). Finally, the presence of PR has also been associated with high levels of C-reactive protein (Hong *et al.*, 2004).

Although these studies have provided valuable data regarding morphologic features of already ruptured plaques, it is important to stress that they do not provide evidence about the prospective detection of rupture-prone plaques.

Histological characteristics of thin-cap fibroatheroma (TCFA), the major predecessor of PR, have been extensively described (Falk *et al.*, 1995; Kolodgie *et al.*, 2001; Naghavi *et al.*, 2003). Indeed, an expert consensus document has established the major criteria for defining TCFA being: (1) the presence of a lipid-rich atheromatous core; (2) a thin fibrous cap with macrophage infiltration and decreased smooth muscle cell content; and (3) expansive remodeling (Schaar *et al.*, 2004).

IVUS RF data analysis: IVUS-VH and palpography

As aforementioned, plaque characterization through visual interpretation of gray-scale IVUS is suboptimal, especially when assessing heterogeneous, lipid-rich plaques (Peters *et al.*, 1994). Low echo-reflectance plaques are considered "soft" or lipid-rich. However, the accuracy of gray-scale IVUS for discriminating lipid from fibrous tissue is limited since in addition to large amounts of extracellular lipids (low echo-reflective areas), the lipid core contains cholesterol crystals, necrotic debris and microcalcifications (highly echoreflective areas) (Virmani *et al.*, 2000).

On the contrary, spectral analysis of IVUS RF data (IVUS-VH) has demonstrated its potential to provide an objective and accurate assessment of coronary plaque composition (Moore *et al.*, 1998; Nair *et al.*, 2002; Kawasaki *et al.*, 2005).

By means of the frequency domain analysis of the RF data, tissue maps that classify plaque into four major components were constructed (Nair *et al.*, 2002). In preliminary in vitro studies, four histological plaque components were correlated with a specific spectrum of the RF signal (Moore *et al.*, 1998; Nair *et al.*, 2002). These different plaque components were assigned color codes. Calcified, fibrous, fibrolipidic and necrotic core regions were

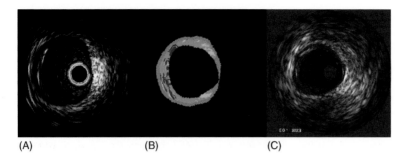

Figure 17.1 Matched cross-section of a left anterior coronary artery imaged by conventional (gray-scale) IVUS (A), IVUS-VH (B) and palpography (C). IVUS-VH color-coding labels calcified, fibrous, fibrolipidic and necrotic core regions as white, green, greenish-yellow and red, respectively. For palpography, the calculated local strain is also color-coded, from blue (for 0% strain) through yellow (for 2% strain) via red.

labelled white, green, greenish-yellow and red, respectively (Figure 17.1). IVUS RF data analysis may follow the progression of the disease not only with regards to its volume, but to its composition as well (Kawasaki *et al.*, 2005; Rodriguez-Granillo *et al.*, 2005b, in press). In addition, this novel IVUS application may potentially refine risk stratification strategies, and allow a more comprehensive pathophysiologic approach toward natural history studies. Recently, using this technique, we have identified in vivo a surrogate of TCFA (IVUS-derived TCFA, IDTCFA) as a more prevalent finding in acute coronary syndromes (ACS) than in stable angina patients. In addition, the distribution of IDTCFA lesions along the coronary vessels was clearly clustered (Rodriguez-Granillo *et al.*, 2005a).

Although the most accepted threshold to define a cap as "thin" has been set at 65 μm (Burke *et al.*, 1997), a number of important ex vivo studies have used higher (>200 μm) thresholds (Mann *et al.*, 1996; Felton *et al.*, 1997; Schaar *et al.*, 2003). It is well established that significant tissue shrinkage occurs during tissue fixation (Lee, 1984). Furthermore, postmortem contraction of arteries is an additional confounding factor (Fishbein and Siegel, 1996). Since the axial resolution of IVUS RF data is between 100 and 150 μm, we assumed that the absence of visible fibrous tissue overlying a necrotic core suggested a cap thickness of below

100–150 μm and used the absence of such tissue to define a thin fibrous cap (Nair and Vince, 2004).

The eccentric accumulation of a lipid-rich necrotic core within the vessel wall is usually separated from the lumen by a thin fibrous cap. This observation led to the hypothesis that vulnerable lesions might have mechanical properties that differ from those of chronic stable lesions. Indeed, both PR and increased inflammatory markers have been reported to occur more frequently in regions and patients with increased mechanical stress (Burleigh *et al.*, 1992; Loree *et al.*, 1992; Schaar *et al.*, 2004). The palpography rationale is that, at a defined pressure, soft tissue (lipid-rich) components will deform more than hard tissue components (fibrous-calcified) (de Korte *et al.*, 1998). Images have been obtained at different pressure levels and compared to determine the local tissue compression. The radial strain in the tissue is calculated by cross-correlation techniques on the RF signal and can be displayed as a color-coded image (Figure 17.1) (de Korte *et al.*, 1998). The sensitivity and specificity to detect vulnerable plaques has recently been assessed in postmortem human coronary arteries where vulnerable plaques were detected with a sensitivity of 88% and a specificity of 89% (Schaar *et al.*, 2003). In addition to ex vivo studies, this technique has also been tested in vivo, where palpography detected a high incidence of deformable plaques in ACS patients.

Coronary remodelling

Coronary artery remodelling was initially described by Glagov as a compensatory enlargement of the coronary arteries in response to an increase in plaque area (Glagov *et al.*, 1987). This concept has later evolved to a dynamic theory where vessels may also experience shrinkage in response to plaque growth (Pasterkamp *et al.*, 1995). Several studies have associated positive (expansive) remodelling to an increase in inflammatory marker levels, larger necrotic cores, pronounced medial thinning and worse clinical presentation (Pasterkamp *et al.*, 1998; Smits *et al.*, 1999; Burke *et al.*, 2002; Varnava *et al.*, 2002). IVUS has been utilized to assess the relationship between vascular remodelling and plaque composition (Mintz *et al.*, 1997; Tauth *et al.*, 1997; Sabate *et al.*, 1999; Fuessl *et al.*, 2001). More recently, we have shown a significantly larger necrotic core content in positively remodelled lesions, whereas the fibrotic burden of plaques was inversely correlated with the remodelling index (Rodriguez-Granillo *et al.*, 2005).

It is important though to stress that, ideally, the presence of coronary remodelling should be established by serial determinations (Hibi *et al.*, 2005).

Shear stress

Carotid and coronary studies have used MRI and IVUS to show that atherosclerosis has a tendency to arise more frequently in low-oscillatory shear stress regions such as in inner curvature of nonbranching segments and opposite to the flow-divider at bifurcations (Kimura *et al.*, 1996; Krams *et al.*, 1997; Jeremias *et al.*, 2000; Irace *et al.*, 2004). The pathophysiology of such a phenomenon can be explained by the fact that low-oscillatory shear stress induces a loss of the physiological flow-oriented alignment of the endothelial cells, thus causing an enhancement of the expression of adhesion molecules and a weakening of cell junctions, ultimately leading to an increase in permeability to lipids and macrophages (Berceli *et al.*, 1990; Kornet *et al.*, 1999; Kaazempur-Mofrad *et al.*, 2004; Slager *et al.*, 2005). Shear stress can be calculated by a combined approach using IVUS and angiography (Krams *et al.*, 1997). Indeed, the relation between shear stress and plaque vulnerability is currently the subject of intensive research efforts (Slager *et al.*, 2005).

Future directions

Since IVUS-virtual histology and palpography utilize the same source data (RF data analysis), information regarding both techniques might be obtained using the same pullback (Figure 17.1); potentially increasing the prognostic value of certain seemingly pejorative plaque characteristics assessed in prospective natural history studies. Another future avenue is the imaging of the vasa vasorum, which can now be achieved using micro bubble-contrast-enhanced IVUS, thus enabling the measurement of activity and inflammation within plaques (Carlier *et al.*, 2005).

As pictured along the chapter, IVUS has numerous applications that have supported the development and progress of interventional cardiology through the past decades. Toward the future, we foresee a pivotal role of IVUS for the detection of vulnerable plaque and the assessment of the effect of emergent medical strategies both related to plaque volume and composition. The utility of IVUS for carotid imaging has been less exploited and limited to the guidance of percutaneous coronary interventions (Clark *et al.*, 2004). This was driven by the excellent imaging quality provided by noninvasive B-mode carotid ultrasound.

However, the rising body of investigations using IVUS for the detection of vulnerable plaque might promote a more universal application of the

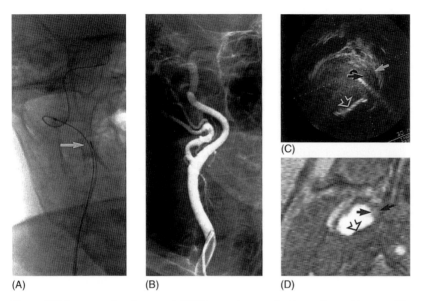

(A)   (B)   (D)

Figure 17.2 Intravascular ultrasound (IVUS) transducer at the internal carotid artery; (A): arrow indicates transducer location. Panel B shows a seemingly normal contrast angiography. IVUS (C) and corresponding MRA (D) cross-sections of the carotid bifurcation are shown. Wide eccentric plaque (between arrows) is seen similarly on both IVUS and magnetic resonance angiography. (Reproduced with permission from Rasanen, H. T. *et al.* (1999). *Stroke*, **30**, 827–33.)

technique potentially including imaging of mild carotid artery atherosclerosis (Rasanen *et al.*, 1999) (Figure 17.2).

REFERENCES

Abizaid, A., Mintz, G. S., Pichard, A. D., *et al.* (1998). Clinical, intravascular ultrasound, and quantitative angiographic determinants of the coronary flow reserve before and after percutaneous transluminal coronary angioplasty. *American Journal of Cardiology*, **82**, 423–8.

Abizaid, A. S., Mintz, G. S., Mehran, R., *et al.* (1999). Long-term follow-up after percutaneous transluminal coronary angioplasty was not performed based on intravascular ultrasound findings: importance of lumen dimensions. *Circulation*, **100**, 256–61.

Ambrose, J. A., Tannenbaum, M. A., Alexopoulos, D., *et al.* (1988). Angiographic progression of coronary artery disease and the development of myocardial infarction. *Journal of the American College of Cardiology*, **12**, 56–62.

Asakura, M., Ueda, Y., Yamaguchi, O., *et al.* (2001). Extensive development of vulnerable plaques as a pan-coronary process in patients with myocardial infarction: an angioscopic study. *Journal of the American College of Cardiology*, **37**, 1284–8.

Balk, E. M., Karas, R. H., Jordan, H. S., *et al.* (2004). Effects of statins on vascular structure and function: A systematic review. *American Journal of Medicine*, **117**, 775–90.

Bekeredjian, R., Hardt, S., Just, A., Hansen, A. and Kuecherer, H. (1999). Influence of catheter position and equipment-related factors on the accuracy of intravascular ultrasound measurements. *Journal of Invasive Cardiology*, **11**, 207–12.

Berceli, S. A., Warty, V. S., Sheppeck, R. A., *et al.* (1990). Hemodynamics and low density lipoprotein metabolism. Rates of low density lipoprotein incorporation and degradation along medial and lateral walls of the rabbit aorto-iliac bifurcation. *Arteriosclerosis*, **10**, 686–94.

Blessing, E., Hausmann, D., Sturm, M., *et al.* (1999). Intravascular ultrasound and stent implantation: intra-observer and interobserver variability. *American Heart Journal*, **137**, 368–71.

Burke, A. P., Farb, A., Malcom, G. T., *et al.* (1997). Coronary risk factors and plaque morphology in men with coronary disease who died suddenly. *New England Journal of Medicine*, **336**, 1276–82.

Burke, A. P., Kolodgie, F. D., Farb, A., *et al.* (2001). Healed plaque ruptures and sudden coronary death: evidence that subclinical rupture has a role in plaque progression. *Circulation*, **103**, 934–40.

Burke, A. P., Kolodgie, F. D., Farb, A., Weber, D. and Virmani, R. (2002). Morphological predictors of arterial remodeling in coronary atherosclerosis. *Circulation*, **105**, 297–303.

Burleigh, M. C., Briggs, A. D., Lendon, C. L., *et al.* (1992). Collagen types I and III, collagen content, GAGs and mechanical strength of human atherosclerotic plaque caps: span-wise variations. *Atherosclerosis*, **96**, 71–81.

Carlier, S., Kakadiaris, I. A., Dib, N., *et al.* (2005). Vasa vasorum imaging: a new window to the clinical detection of vulnerable atherosclerotic plaques. *Current Atherosclerosis Reports*, **7**, 164–9.

Clark, D. J., Lessio, S., O'Donoghue, M., Schainfeld, R. and Rosenfield, K. (2004). Safety and utility of intravascular ultrasound-guided carotid artery stenting. *Catheterization and Cardiovascular Intervention*, **63**, 355–62.

Davies, M. J., Richardson, P. D., Woolf, N., Katz, D. R. and Mann, J. (1993). Risk of thrombosis in human atherosclerotic plaques: role of extracellular lipid, macrophage, and smooth muscle cell content. *British Heart Journal*, **69**, 377–81.

de Feyter, P. J., Kay, P., Disco, C. and Serruys, P. W. (1999). Reference chart derived from post-stent-implantation intravascular ultrasound predictors of 6-month expected restenosis on quantitative coronary angiography. *Circulation*, **100**, 1777–83.

de Korte, C. L., van der Steen, A. F., Cespedes, E. I. and Pasterkamp, G. (1998). Intravascular ultrasound elastography in human arteries: initial experience in vitro. *Ultrasound in Medicine and Biology*, **24**, 401–8.

de Korte, C. L., Carlier, S. G., Mastik, F., *et al.* (2002). Morphological and mechanical information of coronary arteries obtained with intravascular elastography; feasibility study in vivo. *European Heart Journal*, **23**, 405–13.

de Winter, S. A. H. I., Hamers, R., de Feyter, P. J., *et al.* (2003). Computer assisted three-dimensional plaque characterization in ultracoronary ultrasound studies. *Computers in Cardiology*, **30**, 73–6.

Degertekin, M., Serruys, P. W., Tanabe, K., *et al.* (2003). Long-term follow-up of incomplete stent apposition in patients who received sirolimus-eluting stent for de novo coronary lesions: an intravascular ultrasound analysis. *Circulation*, **108**, 2747–50.

Falk, E., Shah, P. K. and Fuster, V. (1995). Coronary plaque disruption. *Circulation*, **92**, 657–71.

Fang, J. C., Kinlay, S., Beltrame, J., *et al.* (2002). Effect of vitamins C and E on progression of transplant-associated arteriosclerosis: a randomised trial. *Lancet*, **359**, 1108–13.

Felton, C. V., Crook, D., Davies, M. J. and Oliver, M. F. (1997). Relation of plaque lipid composition and morphology to the stability of human aortic plaques. *Arteriosclerosis, Thrombosis, and Vascular Biology*, **17**, 1337–45.

Fishbein, M. C. and Siegel, R. J. (1996). How big are coronary atherosclerotic plaques that rupture? *Circulation*, **94**, 2662–6.

Fitzgerald, P. J., Oshima, A., Hayase, M., *et al.* (2000). Final results of the Can Routine Ultrasound Influence Stent Expansion (CRUISE) study. *Circulation*, **102**, 523–30.

Frey, A. W., Hodgson, J. M., Muller, C., Bestehorn, H. P. and Roskamm, H. (2000). Ultrasound-guided strategy for provisional stenting with focal balloon combination catheter: results from the randomized Strategy for Intracoronary Ultrasound-guided PTCA and Stenting (SIPS) trial. *Circulation*, **102**, 2497–502.

Fuessl, R. T., Kranenberg, E., Kiausch, U., *et al.* (2001). Vascular remodeling in atherosclerotic coronary arteries is affected by plaque composition. *Coronary Artery Disease*, **12**, 91–7.

Gaster, A. L., Korsholm, L., Thayssen, P., Pedersen, K. E. and Haghfelt, T. H. (2001). Reproducibility of intravascular ultrasound and intracoronary Doppler measurements. *Catheterization and Cardiovascular Interventions*, **53**, 449–58.

Glagov, S., Weisenberg, E., Zarins, C. K., Stankunavicius, R. and Kolettis, G. J. (1987). Compensatory enlargement of human atherosclerotic coronary arteries. *New England Journal of Medicine*, **316**, 1371–5.

Grodin, C. M, Dyrda, I., Pasternac, A., *et al.* (1974). Discrepancies between cineangiographic and postmortem findings in patients with coronary artery disease and recent myocardial revascularization. *Circulation*, **49**, 703–9.

Guedes, A., Keller, P. F., L'Allier, P. L., *et al.* (2005). Long-term safety of intravascular ultrasound in nontransplant, nonintervened, atherosclerotic coronary arteries.

Journal of the American College of Cardiology, **45**, 559–64.

Gussenhoven, W. J., Essed, C. E., Frietman, P., *et al.* (1989). Intravascular echographic assessment of vessel wall characteristics: a correlation with histology. *International Journal of Cardiovascular Imaging*, **4**, 105–16.

Gussenhoven, E. J., Essed, C. E., Frietman, P., *et al.* (1989a). Intravascular ultrasonic imaging: histologic and echographic correlation. *European Journal of Vascular Surgery*, **3**, 571–6.

Gussenhoven, E. J., Essed, C. E., Lancee, C. T., *et al.* (1989b). Arterial wall characteristics determined by intravascular ultrasound imaging: an in vitro study. *Journal of the American College of Cardiology*, **14**, 947–52.

Hibi, K., Ward, M. R., Honda, Y., *et al.* (2005). Impact of different definitions on the interpretation of coronary remodeling determined by intravascular ultrasound. *Catheterization and Cardiovascular Intervention*, **65**, 233–9.

Hoffmann, R., Mintz, G. S., Dussaillant, G. R., *et al.* (1996). Patterns and mechanisms of in-stent restenosis. A serial intravascular ultrasound study. *Circulation*, **94**, 1247–54.

Hong, M. K., Mintz, G. S., Lee, C. W., *et al.* (2004). Comparison of coronary plaque rupture between stable angina and acute myocardial infarction: a three-vessel intravascular ultrasound study in 235 patients. *Circulation*, **110**, 928–33.

Hong, M. K., Mintz, G. S., Lee, C. W., *et al.* (2005). The site of plaque rupture in native coronary arteries: a three-vessel intravascular ultrasound analysis. *Journal of the American College of Cardiology*, **46**, 261–5.

Irace, C., Cortese, C., Fiaschi, E., *et al.* (2004). Wall shear stress is associated with intima-media thickness and carotid atherosclerosis in subjects at low coronary heart disease risk. *Stroke*, **35**, 464–8.

Jeremias, A., Huegel, H., Lee, D. P., *et al.* (2000). Spatial orientation of atherosclerotic plaque in non-branching coronary artery segments. *Atherosclerosis*, **152**, 209–15.

Kaazempur-Mofrad, M. R., Isasi, A. G., Younis, H. F., *et al.* (2004). Characterization of the atherosclerotic carotid bifurcation using MRI, finite element modeling, and histology. *Annals of Biomedical Engineering*, **32**, 932–46.

Kannel, W. B., Doyle, J. T., McNamara, P. M., Quickenton, P. and Gordon T. (1975). Precursors of sudden coronary death. Factors related to the incidence of sudden death. *Circulation*, **51**, 606–13.

Kawasaki, M., Sano, K., Okubo, M., *et al.* (2005). Volumetric quantitative analysis of tissue characteristics of coronary plaques after statin therapy using three-dimensional integrated backscatter intravascular ultrasound. *Journal of the American College of Cardiology*, **45**, 1946–53.

Kimura, B. J., Russo, R. J., Bhargava, V., *et al.* (1996). Atheroma morphology and distribution in proximal left anterior descending coronary artery: in vivo observations. *Journal of the American College of Cardiology*, **27**, 825–31.

Kolodgie, F. D., Burke, A. P., Farb, A., *et al.* (2001). The thin-cap fibroatheroma: a type of vulnerable plaque: the major precursor lesion to acute coronary syndromes. *Current Opinion in Cardiology*, **16**, 285–92.

Kornet, L., Hoeks, A. P., Lambregts, J. and Reneman, R. S. (1999). In the femoral artery bifurcation, differences in mean wall shear stress within subjects are associated with different intima-media thicknesses. *Arteriosclerosis, Thrombosis, and Vascular Biology*, **19**, 2933–9.

Krams, R., Wentzel, J. J., Oomen, J. A., *et al.* (1997). Evaluation of endothelial shear stress and 3D geometry as factors determining the development of atherosclerosis and remodeling in human coronary arteries in vivo. Combining 3D reconstruction from angiography and IVUS (ANGUS) with computational fluid dynamics. *Arteriosclerosis, Thrombosis, and Vascular Biology*, **17**, 2061–5.

Lee, R. M. K. W. (1984). A critical appraise of the effects of fixation, dehydration and embedding of cell volume. In *The Science of Biological Specimen Preparation for Microscopy and Microanalysis*, ed. J. P. Revel, T. Barnard and G. H. Haggis. IL: Chicago pp. 61–70.

Little, W. C., Constantinescu, M., Applegate, R. J., *et al.* (1988). Can coronary angiography predict the site of a subsequent myocardial infarction in patients with mild-to-moderate coronary artery disease? *Circulation*, **78**, 1157–66.

Loree, H. M., Kamm, R. D., Stringfellow, R. G. and Lee, R. T. (1992). Effects of fibrous cap thickness on peak circumferential stress in model atherosclerotic vessels. *Circulation Research*, **71**, 850–8.

Maehara, A., Mintz, G. S., Bui, A. B., *et al.* (2002). Morphologic and angiographic features of coronary plaque rupture detected by intravascular ultrasound. *Journal of the American College of Cardiology*, **40**, 904–10.

Mann, J. M. and Davies, M. J. (1996). Vulnerable plaque. Relation of characteristics to degree of stenosis in human coronary arteries. *Circulation*, **94**, 928–31.

Matsuzaki, M., Hiramori, K., Imaizumi, T., *et al.* (2002). Intravascular ultrasound evaluation of coronary plaque regression by low density lipoprotein-apheresis in familial hypercholesterolemia: the Low Density Lipoprotein-Apheresis Coronary Morphology and Reserve Trial (LACMART). *Journal of the American College of Cardiology*, **40**, 220–7.

McPherson, D. D., Hiratzka, L. F., Lamberth, W. C., *et al.* (1987). Delineation of the extent of coronary atherosclerosis by high-frequency epicardial echocardiography. *New England Journal of Medicine*, **316**, 304–9.

Mintz, G. S., Painter, J. A., Pichard, A. D., *et al.* (1995). Atherosclerosis in angiographically "normal" coronary artery reference segments: an intravascular ultrasound study with clinical correlations. *Journal of the American College of Cardiology*, **25**, 1479–85.

Mintz, G. S., Kent, K. M., Pichard, A. D., *et al.* (1997). Contribution of inadequate arterial remodeling to the development of focal coronary artery stenoses. An intravascular ultrasound study. *Circulation*, **95**, 1791–8.

Mintz, G. S., Nissen, S. E., Anderson, W. D., *et al.* (2001). American College of Cardiology Clinical Expert Consensus Document on Standards for Acquisition, Measurement and Reporting of Intravascular Ultrasound Studies (IVUS). A report of the American College of Cardiology Task Force on Clinical Expert Consensus Documents. *Journal of the American College of Cardiology*, **37**, 1478–92.

Moore, M. P., Spencer, T., Salter, D. M., *et al.* (1998). Characterisation of coronary atherosclerotic morphology by spectral analysis of radiofrequency signal: in vitro intravascular ultrasound study with histological and radiological validation. *Heart*, **79**, 459–67.

Mudra, H., di Mario, C., de Jaegere, P., *et al.* (2001). Randomized comparison of coronary stent implantation under ultrasound or angiographic guidance to reduce stent restenosis (OPTICUS Study). *Circulation*, **104**, 1343–9.

Naghavi, M., Libby, P., Falk, E., *et al.* (2003). From vulnerable plaque to vulnerable patient: a call for new definitions and risk assessment strategies: Part I. *Circulation*, **108**, 1664–72.

Nair, A. C. D. and Vince, D. G. (2004). Regularized Autoregressive Analysis of Intravascular Ultrasound Data: Improvement in Spatial Accuracy of Plaque Tissue Maps. *IEEE Transactions on Ultrasonics, Ferroelectrics, and Frequency Control*, **51**, 420–31.

Nair, A., Kuban, B. D., Tuzcu, E. M., *et al.* (2002). Coronary plaque classification with intravascular ultrasound radiofrequency data analysis. *Circulation*, **106**, 2200–6.

Nishioka, T., Amanullah, A. M., Luo, H., *et al.* (1999). Clinical validation of intravascular ultrasound imaging for assessment of coronary stenosis severity: comparison with stress myocardial perfusion imaging. *Journal of the American College of Cardiology*, **33**, 1870–8.

Nissen, S. E., Tsunoda, T., Tuzcu, E. M., *et al.* (2003). Effect of recombinant ApoA-I Milano on coronary atherosclerosis in patients with acute coronary syndromes: a randomized controlled trial. *Journal of the American Medical Association*, **290**, 2292–300.

Nissen, S. E., Tuzcu, E. M., Libby, P., *et al.* (2004a). Effect of antihypertensive agents on cardiovascular events in patients with coronary disease and normal blood pressure: the CAMELOT study: a randomized controlled trial. *Journal of the American Medical Association*, **292**, 2217–25.

Nissen, S. E., Tuzcu, E. M., Schoenhagen, P., *et al.* (2004b). Effect of intensive compared with moderate lipid-lowering therapy on progression of coronary atherosclerosis: a randomized controlled trial. *Journal of the American Medical Association*, **291**, 1071–80.

Oemrawsingh, P. V., Mintz, G. S., Schalij, M. J., *et al.* (2003). Intravascular ultrasound guidance improves angiographic and clinical outcome of stent implantation for long coronary artery stenoses: final results of a randomized comparison with angiographic guidance (TULIP Study). *Circulation*, **107**, 62–7.

Okazaki, S., Yokoyama, T., Miyauchi, K., *et al.* (2004). Early statin treatment in patients with acute coronary syndrome: demonstration of the beneficial effect on atherosclerotic lesions by serial volumetric intravascular ultrasound analysis during half a year after coronary event: the ESTABLISH Study. *Circulation*, **110**, 1061–8.

Pasterkamp, G., Wensing, P. J., Post, M. J., *et al.* (1995). Paradoxical arterial wall shrinkage may contribute to luminal narrowing of human atherosclerotic femoral arteries. *Circulation*, **91**, 1444–9.

Pasterkamp, G., Schoneveld, A. H., van der Wal, A. C., *et al.* (1998). Relation of arterial geometry to luminal narrowing and histologic markers for plaque vulnerability: the remodeling paradox. *Journal of the American College of Cardiology*, **32**, 655–62.

Peters, R. J., Kok, W. E., Havenith, M. G., *et al.* (1994). Histopathologic validation of intracoronary ultrasound imaging. *Journal of the American Society of Echocardiography*, **7**, 230–41.

Rasanen, H. T., Manninen, H. I., Vanninen, R. L., *et al.* (1999). Mild carotid artery atherosclerosis: assessment by 3-dimensional time-of-flight magnetic resonance angiography, with reference to intravascular ultrasound imaging and contrast angiography. *Stroke*, **30**, 827–33.

Regar, E. S. J., van der Giessen, W., van der Steen and Serruys, P. W. (2002). Real-time, in-vivo optical coherence tomography of human coronary arteries using a dedicated imaging wire. *American Journal of Cardiology*, **90**, 129H.

Rioufol, G., Finet, G., Ginon, I., *et al.* (2002). Multiple atherosclerotic plaque rupture in acute coronary syndrome: a three-vessel intravascular ultrasound study. *Circulation*, **106**, 804–8.

Rodriguez-Granillo, G. A., García-García, H., McFadden E., Valgimigli, M., *et al.* (2005a). In Vivo Intravascular Ultrasound-Derived Thin-Cap Fibroatheroma Detection Using Ultrasound Radio Frequency Data Analysis. *Journal of the American College of Cardiology*, **46**, 2038–42.

Rodriguez-Granillo, G. A., Serruys, P., McFadden, E., van Mieghem, C., *et al.* (2005b). First-in-man prospective evaluation of temporal changes in coronary plaque composition by in vivo ultrasound radio frequency data analysis: an integrated biomarker and imaging study (IBIS) substudy. *Eurointervention*, **1**, 282–8.

Rodriguez-Granillo, G. A., Serruys, P. W., Garcia-Garcia, H. M., *et al.* (2005). Coronary artery remodelling is related to plaque composition. *Heart*, **92**, 388–91.

Sabate, M., Kay, I. P., de Feyter, P. J., *et al.* (1999). Remodeling of atherosclerotic coronary arteries varies in relation to location and composition of plaque. *American Journal of Cardiology*, **84**, 135–40.

Schaar, J. A., De Korte, C. L., Mastik, F., *et al.* (2003). Characterizing vulnerable plaque features with intravascular elastography. *Circulation*, **108**, 2636–41.

Schaar, J. A., Muller, J. E., Falk, E., *et al.* (2004). Terminology for high-risk and vulnerable coronary artery plaques. Report of a meeting on the vulnerable plaque, June 17 and 18, 2003, Santorini, Greece. *European Heart Journal*, **25**, 1077–82.

Schaar, J. A., Regar, E., Mastik, F., *et al.* (2004). Incidence of high-strain patterns in human coronary arteries: assessment with three-dimensional intravascular palpography and correlation with clinical presentation. *Circulation*, **109**, 2716–19.

Schartl, M., Bocksch, W., Koschyk, D. H., *et al.* (2001). Use of intravascular ultrasound to compare effects of different strategies of lipid-lowering therapy on plaque volume and composition in patients with coronary artery disease. *Circulation*, **104**, 387–92.

Schiele, F., Meneveau, N., Vuillemenot, A., *et al.* (1998). Impact of intravascular ultrasound guidance in stent deployment on 6-month restenosis rate: a multicenter, randomized study comparing two strategies–with and without intravascular ultrasound guidance. RESIST Study Group. REStenosis after Ivus guided STenting. *Journal of the American College of Cardiology*, **32**, 320–8.

Sheris, S. J., Canos, M. R. and Weissman, N. J. (2000). Natural history of intravascular ultrasound-detected edge dissections from coronary stent deployment. *American Heart Journal*, **139**, 59–63.

Shiran, A., Mintz, G. S., Waksman, R., *et al.* (1998). Early lumen loss after treatment of in-stent restenosis: an intravascular ultrasound study. *Circulation*, **98**, 200–3.

Slager, C. J. W. J., Gijsen, F. J. H., Schuurbiers, J. C. H., *et al.* (2005). The role of shear stress in the generation of rupture-prone vulnerable plaques. *Nature Clinical Practice*, **2**, 401–7.

Smits, P. C., Pasterkamp, G., Quarles van Ufford, M. A., *et al.* (1999). Coronary artery disease: arterial remodelling and clinical presentation. *Heart*, **82**, 461–4.

Suzuki, T., Hosokawa, H., Katoh, O., *et al.* (1999). Effects of adjunctive balloon angioplasty after intravascular ultrasound-guided optimal directional coronary atherectomy: the result of Adjunctive Balloon Angioplasty After Coronary Atherectomy Study (ABACAS). *Journal of the American College of Cardiology*, **34**, 1028–35.

Takagi, T., Yoshida, K., Akasaka, T., *et al.* (1997). Intravascular ultrasound analysis of reduction in progression of coronary narrowing by treatment with pravastatin. *American Journal of Cardiology*, **79**, 1673–6.

Takagi, A., Tsurumi, Y., Ishii, Y., *et al.* (1999). Clinical potential of intravascular ultrasound for physiological assessment of coronary stenosis: relationship between quantitative ultrasound tomography and pressure-derived fractional flow reserve. *Circulation*, **100**, 250–5.

Tardif, J. C., Gregoire, J., L'Allier, P. L., *et al.* (2004). Effects of the acyl coenzyme A:cholesterol acyltransferase inhibitor avasimibe on human atherosclerotic lesions. *Circulation*, **110**, 3372–7.

Tauth, J., Pinnow, E., Sullebarger, J. T., *et al.* (1997). Predictors of coronary arterial remodeling patterns in patients with myocardial ischemia. *American Journal of Cardiology*, **80**, 1352–5.

Topol, E. J. and Nissen, S. E. (1995). Our preoccupation with coronary luminology. The dissociation between clinical and angiographic findings in ischemic heart disease. *Circulation*, **92**, 2333–42.

Tuzcu, E. M., Berkalp, B., De Franco, A. C., *et al.* (1996). The dilemma of diagnosing coronary calcification: angiography versus intravascular ultrasound.

Journal of the American College of Cardiology, **27**, 832–8.

Varnava, A. M., Mills, P. G. and Davies, M. J. (2002). Relationship between coronary artery remodeling and plaque vulnerability. *Circulation*, **105**, 939–43.

Virmani, R., Kolodgie, F. D., Burke, A. P., Farb, A. and Schwartz, S. M. (2000). Lessons from sudden coronary death: a comprehensive morphological classification scheme for atherosclerotic lesions. *Arteriosclerosis, Thrombosis, and Vascular Biology*, **20**, 1262–75.

Wang, J. C., Normand, S. L., Mauri, L. and Kuntz, R. E. (2004). Coronary artery spatial distribution of acute myocardial infarction occlusions. *Circulation*, **110**, 278–84.

18

Image postprocessing

William Kerwin, Dongxiang Xu and Fei Liu

University of Washington, Seattle WA, USA

Introduction

Atherosclerosis, the disease behind heart attacks and strokes, is characterized by build-up of plaque within the intimal layer of arteries. Clinical events occur due to *thrombosis*, in which a clot occludes the vessel at the lesion site and *embolization*, in which thrombotic materials from the site of a lesion are released into the blood stream and occlude distal vessels. To date, the primary clinical indicator for risk from atherosclerotic plaque has been stenosis, expressed as a percentage reduction in the lumen diameter of the vessel. Stenosis is typically assessed by angiography or duplex ultrasound.

However, stenosis provides an incomplete picture of risk. Arteries exhibiting only moderate stenosis account for a large percentage of strokes and heart attacks. Histological studies in various vascular beds have established that features of the atherosclerotic plaque itself dictate its clinical course in cases of moderate stenosis (Falk, 1992). Specific plaque features associated with clinical risk include a fibrous cap that is thin, ruptured, or ulcerated and a large lipid-rich necrotic core (Virmani *et al.*, 2000). Together these features define the "vulnerable plaque."

Given the significance of vulnerable plaque for patient prognosis, considerable interest exists in developing noninvasive means to measure plaque features and provide clinical indicators that augment stenosis. Research in recent years has shown that magnetic resonance imaging (MRI) is a powerful tool for identifying plaque features in the carotid artery. This has led to efforts to determine the image intensity characteristics associated with an array of plaque features (Hatsukami *et al.*, 2000; Yuan *et al.*, 2001; Mitsumori *et al.*, 2003; Chu *et al.*, 2004). Using these characteristics, manual outlining of plaque features has been shown to produce area measurements that strongly correlate with histological ground truth (Saam *et al.*, 2005).

The importance of plaque features suggests a role for image postprocessing techniques in optimally combining multicontrast MRI data and automatically identifying plaque regions. The purpose of this chapter is to present an overall framework for measuring the volumes of atherosclerotic plaque components in the carotid artery. The framework will be demonstrated with our software platform called the computer-aided system for cardiovascular disease evaluation (CASCADE). This system includes boundary detection, registration of multiple contrast weightings, and segmentation of internal plaque components. Among other uses, CASCADE is suitable for use in clinical trials to assess the effects of treatment on plaque composition.

Imaging vulnerable plaque

Vulnerable plaque

A section from a typical advanced atherosclerotic lesion surgically removed from a carotid artery is

Carotid Disease: The Role of Imaging in Diagnosis and Management, ed. Jonathan Gillard, Martin Graves, Thomas Hatsukami and Chun Yuan. Published by Cambridge University Press. © Cambridge University Press 2007.

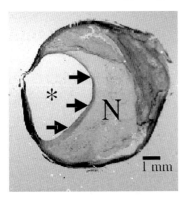

Figure 18.1 Histological specimen of an atherosclerotic plaque near the carotid bifurcation stained with Movat's pentachrome. A thin fibrous cap (arrows) separates the vessel lumen (*) from a large necrotic core (N).

shown in Figure 18.1. At the center is the lumen, which is the normal passageway for blood. Separating the lumen from the bulk of the lesion is an encapsulating fibrous layer (fibrous cap). Behind the cap lies the core of the lesion, which may include lipid-rich necrotic material, cholesterol crystals, calcification, intraplaque hemorrhage, loose matrix, and/or microvessels in various mixtures. A variety of cell types including smooth muscle cells and macrophages can be present. Various biological processes, most notably inflammation and angiogenesis, can also be occurring. Such lesions are thus characterized by great complexity, dynamic behavior, and variation across populations.

Retrospective histological evaluations of culprit lesions implicated in myocardial infarction and stroke have established which of these features are associated with clinical events. The most important feature is the status of the fibrous cap, which separates the highly thrombogenic core from the blood stream. Disruption of the fibrous cap precipitates a rapid sequence of events leading to thrombus formation (Davies and Thomas, 1985). Disrupted caps are typically thinned, previously ruptured, or eroded (Virmani *et al.*, 2000). In addition to the fibrous cap, other plaque features

can play a role in clinical events and sudden plaque progression. The most important internal feature is the necrotic core, which generally contains large deposits of lipid and may contain intraplaque hemorrhage. The strong association of large lipid-rich cores with clinical events is thought to arise from its weak structure and the extremely thrombogenic nature of the core (Davies *et al.*, 1993). Additionally, calcification within the plaque can be the source of thromboembolic events when they exist as calcific nodules protruding into the lumen, but calcification can also be associated with stable plaque (Virmani *et al.*, 2000). Loose matrix is an early phase of fibrous tissue thought to form as a result of injury, which may be a sign of ongoing disruptions (Wight and Merrilees, 2004). Ideally, loose matrix would be observed transforming into the denser collagen matrix of stable plaque.

Lesion indices

To evaluate the effects of plaque composition on outcome, noninvasive imaging techniques must be paired with algorithms to segment the plaque into its constituent components and quantify the relative amounts of each. We refer to the quantitative measurements as "lesion indices" and divide them into two categories. The first category consists of *morphological* indices, which quantify the size and shape of the vessel wall. Stenosis is an example of a morphological index. Additionally, measurements of the vessel wall itself are of interest, including maximal wall thickness, total wall volume, and the ratio of the wall area to the total vessel area (lumen plus wall). The fundamental challenge in obtaining these measurements is to identify the inner lumen boundary and outer wall boundary in medical images.

A second class of lesion indices consists of *compositional* indices. These quantify the amounts of plaque subcomponents within the diseased vessel wall. The calcium score provided by computed tomography (CT) is an example of a compositional index (Rumberger *et al.*, 1999).

The extent of high-density regions in CT images of vessel walls associates with the extent of calcification (Sutton-Tyrrell *et al.*, 2001), and can be used as a risk factor for heart attack and stroke (Vliegenthart *et al.*, 2002). Further techniques must be developed to assess the integrity of the fibrous cap and the size of the lipid core, both of which are thought to be more telling than the extent of calcification. The complete list of tissue types to be measured includes necrotic core, fibrous tissue, loose fibrous matrix, calcification, and intra-plaque hemorrhage. Quantifying these compo-nents requires the plaque to be divided up by tissue type and is thus equivalent to plaque segmentation. Once segmentation is complete, computing the indexes is simply a matter of computing volumes of different regions.

MRI of carotid plaque

The success of MRI in characterizing plaque composition derives from its excellent contrast between soft tissues, which provides anatomical and compositional detail. Contrast can also be changed by adjusting any of several imaging parameters. Multiple images with different contrast weightings can thus be combined for increased sensitivity to tissue differences. Various studies have concluded that accurate tissue characteriza-tion requires information combined from multiple MRI contrast weightings (Shinnar *et al.*, 1999; Yuan *et al.*, 2001; Clarke *et al.*, 2003; Mitsumori *et al.*, 2003; Chu *et al.*, 2004). Additionally, submillimeter pixel sizes and thin image slices (2 mm or less) are critical to differentiate distinct components that may occupy volumes smaller than 1 mm^3.

A standard in vivo carotid MRI protocol now includes T_1-weighted (T1W), T_2-weighted (T2W), proton-density-weighted (PDW), time-of-flight (TOF), and, possibly, contrast-enhanced T1W (CE-T1W) MRI (Yuan and Kerwin, 2004). To perform volumetric analysis of plaque composi-tion, stacks of axial images of the carotid artery are obtained. A dedicated carotid surface coil is employed to provide a longitudinal coverage of up

to 5 cm and maximal signal-to-noise ratio (Hayes *et al.*, 1996). Images are obtained at 10 or more locations, centered on the carotid bifurcation with a separation of 2 mm. This results in at least 2 cm coverage for all subjects. A representative set of images showing the different contrast weightings is shown in Figure 18.2.

Vessel wall morphology

The image processing challenge for measuring morphological indices of atherosclerotic plaque is one of boundary detection. In general, only a single contrast-weighting is required. The preferred imaging technique is double-inversion recovery T1W contrast, which has superior blood suppres-sion and provides sharp contrast between the plaque and lumen. The TOF weighting can, never-theless, be a valuable reference for differentiating juxtaluminal calcifications from the true lumen (Mitsumori *et al.*, 2003). Whereas both calcification and the lumen are dark on T1W images, the lumen is bright and calcification is dark on TOF. Fat suppression is also important for detecting the outer wall boundary of the vessel, which is typically abutted by fat.

Boundary detection

Boundary detection in medical imaging is typically performed using active contour methods, also known as "snakes" (Kass *et al.*, 1987). The basic active contour methodology seeks to identify a curve corresponding to edges in the image. Optimization of the curve is accomplished by minimizing an energy function that may depend on the image itself as well as the smoothness of the contour. A number of active contour approaches for specifically detecting vessel boundaries have been proposed (Han *et al.*, 2001, 2003).

We have found that excellent performance and flexibility for boundary detection in vessel wall imaging is afforded by B-spline snakes (Brigger *et al.*, 2000). In B-spline snakes, the boundary

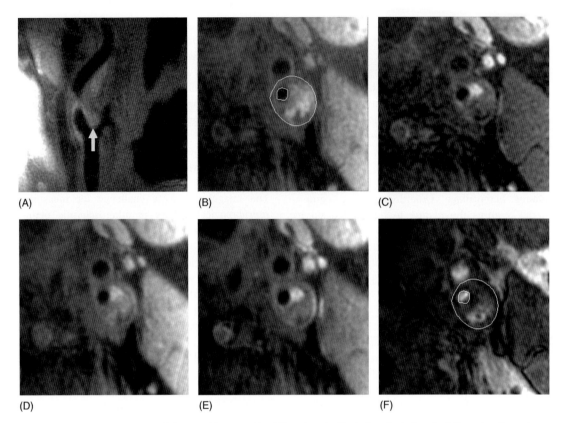

Figure 18.2 Multicontrast MRI of the carotid artery: (A) oblique longitudinal view depicting the bifurcation (arrow); (B) T1W; (C) T2W; (D) PDW; (E) CE-T1W; (F) TOF (contours in (B) and (F) indicate lumen and outer wall boundaries).

contour $C(u) = (c_x(u), c_y(u))$ is parameterized as a B-spline, such as

$$c_x(u) = \sum_{k=1}^{K} \xi_k \beta(u - k) \qquad (18.1)$$

$$c_y(u) = \sum_{k=1}^{K} \psi_k \beta(u - k), \qquad (18.2)$$

where $u \in [0, K)$, ξ_k and ψ_k are the spline coefficients, and cubic B-spline kernels are often used:

$$\beta(u) = \begin{cases} 2/3 + |u|^3/2 - u^2, & 0 \le |u| < 1 \\ (2 - |u|)^3/6, & 1 \le |u| < 2 \, . \\ 0, & 2 \le |u| \end{cases} \qquad (18.3)$$

The values of the spline coefficients are modified until an image-based energy functional is minimized. Our energy formulation is:

$$E = \frac{b}{l(C)} \int_0^K \left| \frac{dC(u)}{du} \right| n(u) \nabla I |_{C(u)} du, \qquad (18.4)$$

where $l(C)$ is the length of the contour, $n(u)$ is the inward-facing unit normal to the contour and the image gradient is computed at the corresponding point on the contour. Identifying a contour where the interior is brighter than the exterior is accomplished by setting $b = +1$ and a darker interior is found by setting $b = -1$. Scaling by the magnitude of the derivative of $C(u)$ prevents spline nodes from clustering in a region of high gradient and dividing by $l(C)$ weights all curves equally, regardless of length and avoids an infinitely expanding contour.

Such an approach has several advantages. First, the inherent smoothness of the spline means that no explicit smoothness term is required in the energy. Second, the node points of the spline, defined as $C(k)$ where k is an integer, can be manually moved if necessary for rapid manual correction of boundaries. Third, optimization can be formulated as simple gradient descent. The major challenge for the B-spline snake is to initialize it near the true boundary to ensure convergence.

Lumen detection

To find the lumen boundary, the B-spline snake is initialized by applying a region-based segmentation to each image around a user-defined point (mouse-click). Our method for segmenting an image into homogeneous regions is called the mean-shift algorithm (Fukunaga and Hostetler, 1975a). The mean-shift approach iteratively searches for clusters of pixels and has several distinct advantages for our application. First, it finds clusters with no prior knowledge of the number or locations of clusters. Second, it is relatively insensitive to the intensity range of the artery, which depends on the proximity of the artery to the surface coils and can differ by scanner manufacturer. Finally, the segmentation can be easily controlled by a single parameter that produces fine (many regions) to coarse (few regions) segmentation results.

As originally proposed, the mean shift algorithm iterates from an arbitrary starting point y_0 to a cluster center using:

$$y_{i+1} = \frac{\sum_{j=1}^{J} v_j h((\|y_i - v_j\|/r)^2)}{\sum_{j=1}^{J} h((\|y_i - v_j\|/r)^2)} \quad (18.5)$$

where h is a weighting function, r is the radius of the weighting function, and v_j is a vector of intensity values for the jth pixel. This equation

shifts the estimated cluster center to the weighted sample mean, centered at y_i, hence the name mean-shift.

Another interpretation (Comaniciu and Meer, 2002) shows that the mean shift algorithm performs gradient ascent on the estimated probability density function $f(y)$ using:

$$y_{i+1} = y_i + \frac{\hat{\nabla} f(y_i)}{\hat{f}(y_i)} \quad (18.6)$$

where $f(y)$ and its gradient are estimated using:

$$\hat{f}(y) = \beta \sum_{j=1}^{J} k((\|y - v_j\|/r)^2) \quad (18.7)$$

The parameter β is a constant that causes $f(y)$ to integrate to 1, but cancels out of the iterative formula (18.6). The function k, which weights each vector by its distance to y, makes (18.5) and (18.6) equivalent if

$$h(x) = -k'(x) \quad (18.8)$$

In our implementation, we use the above formulation to determine the mean shift, where we use the weighting function:

$$k(x) = \begin{cases} 1 - x & x < 1 \\ 0 & x \geq 1 \end{cases} \quad (18.9)$$

This is the Epanechnikov kernel for density estimation, which under asymptotic assumptions is optimal in the sense that it minimizes the mean square error of the density estimate (Comaniciu and Meer, 2002).

Once the cluster centers are identified, each pixel is assigned to a specific cluster using the k-nearest neighbor approach (Fukunaga and Hostetler, 1975b). Small regions are reassigned to neighboring regions by choosing the region with the closest mean intensity vector. Then, the boundaries of the segmented region are found, fed to the B-spline snake and the results displayed on the image (Figure 18.3). In our implementation of lumen detection, a slider bar is used to dynamically adjust the minimum region size. If the size of any region is lower than this threshold, the pixels within this region will be re-assigned to

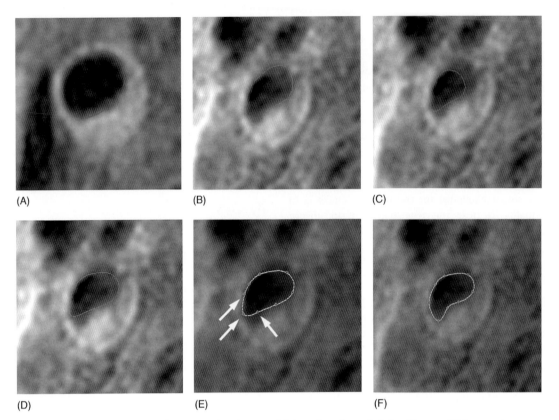

(A)   (B)   (C)

(D)   (E)   (F)

Figure 18.3 Lumen detection modes: (A) results of successful detection of a well-defined lumen; (B) incorrect detection due to flow artifact is adjusted (C–D) using the lumen size parameter to the correct answer in (D). Alternatively, the contour from (C) is placed into node adjustment mode (E) and three points (arrows) are adjusted to obtain the correct result in (F).

neighboring cluster centers so as to erase small noisy regions. The slider bar allows the user to rapidly step through alternative solutions.

Outer wall detection

Outer wall boundary detection proceeds in a manner similar to lumen detection (see Figure 18.4). An automated algorithm initializes a B-spline snake and is adjusted by interactive control of a single parameter. The B-spline snake itself can be further adjusted by moving of the node points. The methodology of the automated

algorithm is, however, significantly different from lumen detection. The outer boundary of the wall poses a more difficult challenge because unlike the lumen, it is not a uniform intensity and because it can be abutted by structures with similar intensities. As a result, the B-spline snake must contend with strong, false edges as well as poorly defined true edges.

To overcome the difficulties of outer wall detection, we use information from the prior, more proximal image to guide wall detection in the subsequent image. We refer to this approach as a "Markov model" because of its relationship

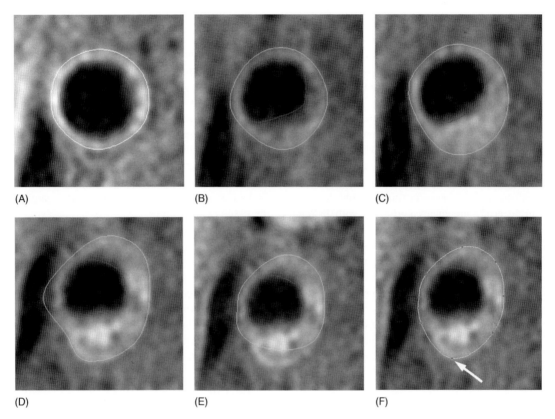

Figure 18.4 Wall detection modes: (A–C) successful outer wall boundary detection moving distally from the proximal common carotid artery (A); (D) erroneous boundary detection is corrected by (E) adjusting the thickness scaling factor and (F) moving one node point (arrow).

to Markov random processes, in which optimal prediction of a subsequent state depends only on the prior state. The information fed from the previous state is the wall thickness along eight equally-spaced radial lines emanating from the center of the lumen contour. These thicknesses are scaled by factors ranging from 0.5 to 1.5, added to the lumen contour in the subsequent image, and used to initialize the B-spline snake. The scaling factor yielding the lowest overall energy in the snake formulation (18.4) is used to generate the optimal outer wall contour. The user may also dynamically select the preferred scaling factor by adjusting a slider bar.

Morphological indices

From the lumen and wall boundaries, a number of morphological indices can be derived. These include the minimal lumen area, maximal wall area, total wall volume, and maximal wall thickness. To normalize for artery size, the lumen and wall areas can be divided by the total cross-sectional vessel area (i.e. lumen + wall). Investigations with manual boundary identification have shown that MRI produces measurements that are highly accurate, with in vivo and ex vivo measurements exhibiting correlation coefficients of 0.92 for wall volume, 0.91 for maximal wall area, and

0.90 for minimal lumen area (Luo *et al.*, 2003). Surprisingly, this same study showed that the correlations between these different morphological indices is quite low (less than 0.3), indicating that they provide unique characterizations of plaque burden. In further studies, these measurements were also shown to be highly reproducible across studies, with coefficients of variation as low as 5.8% for wall volume, 7.1% for maximal wall volume, and 4.1% for minimal lumen area (Saam *et al.*, 2006). A recent result further showed that measurements of mean wall thickness in the proximal common carotid artery are highly correlated with B-mode ultrasound measures of intima-media thickness (IMT), suggesting that MRI may provide a measure of overall cardiovascular risk similar to the established marker IMT (Underhill *et al.*, 2005).

The main advantages of the automated boundary detection procedures described here are that they permit these morphological indices of plaque burden to be extracted more rapidly and potentially with better reproducibility and inter-rater agreement. To test this assertion, we revisited six randomly selected subjects from a study previously used to assess measurement reproducibility. These subjects had a coefficient of variation for wall volume of 8.2% for manual boundary drawing, which was somewhat higher than the overall average of 5.8%. Two studies from these subjects were evaluated using the interactive boundary detection scheme described here, which resulted in a coefficient of variation of only 4.9%, significantly lower than that for manual drawing. To put this in perspective, a clinical trial aimed at detecting a 5% difference in wall volumes between treatment arms with 80% power would require 86 subjects per arm with a coefficient of variation 8.2%, but only 31 per arm with a coefficient of variation of 4.9%.

Plaque composition

The major benefit of MRI over other imaging modalities for carotid atherosclerosis is its ability to characterize plaque composition, not just morphology. The image processing challenge for measuring compositional indices is to segment the vessel wall into components. For this purpose, fusion of data from multiple contrast weightings is critical. This, in turn, introduces a further processing challenge because patient motion between successive acquisitions misaligns the images. Thus, a first step for compositional analysis is to register the multiple contrast weightings to eliminate patient shifts. Once this is completed, statistical models are used to classify regions by tissue type.

Registration

Registration of the remaining contrast weightings to the T1W image, with the wall boundaries already outlined, is accomplished in two steps. First, the vertical alignment of the different contrast weightings is established by finding the location within each stack of images where the common carotid artery bifurcates into the internal and external carotid arteries. This location is referred to as the zero point of the artery and more proximal locations within the common carotid artery are assigned negative location numbers. Distal locations in the internal carotid artery are assigned positive location numbers.

Once the vertical alignment is established, in-plane shifts by the patient are automatically eliminated. In developing an automated registration technique, we had to account for nonrigid deformations within the neck. Also, nearby structures can undergo true physiological changes, such as constriction of the adjacent jugular vein. Fortunately, for the small motions that occur within a single imaging session, the atherosclerotic carotid artery behaves more like a rigid body embedded in a deforming medium, simplifying the required motion correction. Additionally, we can take advantage of the known lumen and wall contours in the reference T1W images.

We therefore developed a registration algorithm for the carotid artery based on the active edge maps formulation (Kerwin and Yuan, 2001). In active edge maps, two images are registered by aligning edge information. Specifically, a set of edge points $X = \{x_1, \ldots, x_n\}$ is extracted from the reference image and the active edge map method seeks the transformation $T(x)$ that minimizes the registration energy:

$$E_{\text{reg}} = \sum_{i=1}^{n} E_{\text{image}}(T(x_i)) + E_{\text{internal}}(T) \qquad (18.10)$$

where E_{image} is an edge-based energy function determined by the target image, $T(x)$ maps the motion that has occurred between the reference and target images, and E_{internal} is an optional restriction on the form (e.g. smoothness) of the motion.

With this formulation, we take advantage of the points making up the lumen and outer wall contours as the set of edge points X, which ensures that only relevant carotid artery information will be utilized in registration. We then use:

$$E_{\text{image}} = -\sum_{m \in C} a(x)g(x - x_m) \qquad (18.11)$$

where g is a Gaussian function with width (σ) of two pixels, C is the set of points in the Canny edge map (Canny, 1986), and $a(x)$ equals 3 if x is in the lumen contour and 1 if it is in the wall contour. Use of a Gaussian kernel creates a continuous, differentiable image energy function for gradient-based optimization and extends the capture range of the registration algorithm so that the initial estimate of $T(x)$ is less critical. Use of the binary Canny edge map limits the influence of the surface coils, which produce stronger edges closer to the coils. The term $a(x)$ causes the lumen and wall contours to receive approximately equal weight despite the greater number of points in the wall contour.

For the motion, we assume $T(x)$ consists of simple in-plane shifts, which tends to be accurate for the carotid artery over the short imaging session and eliminates the need to define $E_{\text{internal}}(T)$. The range of possible shifts is restricted to ±2 mm in each direction. To overcome larger patient shifts,

we introduced a feature we call "smart drag" in which the user can move any image relative to the contours and upon releasing the image, the registration algorithm minimizes the energy within a 1 mm region surrounding that location. The registration procedure is illustrated in Figure 18.5.

Segmentation

In the next analysis step, homogeneous intensity regions within the artery wall are automatically detected, outlined and assigned a tissue type (necrotic core, calcification, fibrous tissue, or loose matrix) by the morphology-enhanced probabilistic plaque segmentation (MEPPS) algorithm (Liu *et al.*, 2006). It is a flexible, multicontrast plaque segmentation technique that is suitable for objectively testing various approaches for measuring plaque composition in vivo and to validate the method with histology.

In designing the MEPPS algorithm, we attempted to mimic the thought process used by the radiologist in manual review. First, manual review generally relies on relative intensities (e.g. hyper, hypo, or iso-intense) to describe image features. We therefore preprocess the images to establish a baseline iso-intensity (the median intensity in the region of interest) for each image and scale all pixel values relative to this baseline. Second, reviewers use morphological cues, such as local wall thickness, in addition to intensity when classifying regions. We therefore assign probability based on both intensity and morphology. Finally, reviewers intuitively use the most value-added contrast weightings in classifying regions, ignoring potentially confounding information from low-value weightings. We therefore sought to identify the most useful weightings for segmentation.

The core task of the MEPPS algorithm is to assign four probabilities to each pixel. These probabilities represent the likelihood that the pixel is necrotic core, calcification, loose matrix, or fibrous tissue. We base this probability on the pixel intensity in each contrast weighting – represented by the

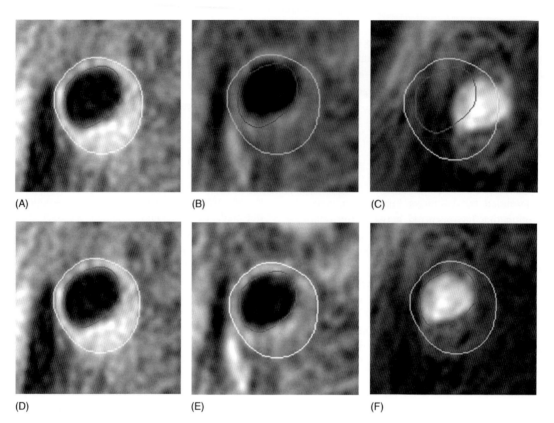

(A)   (B)   (C)

(D)   (E)   (F)

Figure 18.5 Registration: lumen and wall boundaries drawn on a T1W image (A) are slightly misaligned when mapped to the PDW image (B) and grossly misaligned with the TOF image (C). After Active Edge Map registration (D–F), all contours which agree are aligned with the image features.

vector $\mathbf{x}$ – and on two morphological factors: the local wall thickness t and the distance of the pixel from the lumen d. Thus, we determine the probability $\Pr(T_i|t,d,\mathbf{x})$, where T_i corresponds to one of the four tissue types (i.e. $i = 1,2,3,4$). The two distances t and d capture information about the local plaque morphology, typically used in manual review. For example, thin plaque regions are generally fibrous and loose matrix is most commonly seen adjacent to the lumen.

To estimate each probability, we can assume that the intensity of a given tissue does not vary with position in the plaque. For example, calcification has the same appearance whether it is adjacent to the lumen or deep within the plaque. Thus, $\mathbf{x}$ is conditionally independent of t and d, given T_i. This assumption allows us to cast the probability as a naïve-Bayesian network (Hecherman, 1995) and leads to the formula:

$$\Pr(T_i|t,d,\mathbf{x}) = \frac{p(t,d|T_i)p(\mathbf{x}|T_i)\Pr(T_i)}{\sum_{j=1}^{4}p(t,d|T_j)p(\mathbf{x}|T_j)\Pr(T_j)} \qquad (18.12)$$

The two conditionally independent probability density functions (PDFs) $p(\mathbf{x}|T_i)$ and $p(t,d|T_i)$, and the relative frequency of each of the four tissue types $\Pr(T_i)$ were estimated from a training set.

Once the probabilities for each pixel are determined, the final step is to classify each pixel as a given tissue. Although the pixels could be classified based on the highest probability alone, we utilize a competing contour formulation to define the final regions. This additional step provides two benefits. First, it provides the ability to easily edit the regions by modifying the contours, and second, it helps to eliminate isolated pixels and convoluted regions attributable to noise.

The contours delineating each tissue region are determined using the active region method (Paragios and Deriche, 2000). Each of four contours seeks one preassigned tissue. In order to produce reasonable boundaries, contours are moving under a smoothness constraint to maximize the total probability for the corresponding tissue within it. Based on Gibbs-Markov random field theory (Geman and Geman, 1984; Zhu and Yuille, 1996), using the level set method to represent each contour, the energy functional is designed as:

$$E(\Phi_i) = \sum_{i=1}^{4} \iint_{\Omega} -\log(\Pr(T_i))H(\Phi_i)dxdy$$

$$+ \lambda_1 \sum_{i=1}^{4} \iint_{\Omega} |\nabla H(\Phi_i)|dxdy \qquad (18.13)$$

$$+ \lambda_2 \iint_{\Omega} \left(\sum_{i=1}^{4} H(\Phi_i) - 1\right)^2 dxdy$$

where Φ_i is level set function and $H(\Phi)$ is the Heaviside function. The first item sums probability within the contours, the second one is a measure of total contour length and the third one constrains each pixel to belong to one, and only one contour. By using the level set method, topology changes of the curves are handled automatically, allowing individual contours to split and merge to form as many distinct regions as necessary.

Figure 18.6 shows the results of segmentation of an example based on probabilities. To visualize the pixel-wise probabilities in Figure 18.6, each pixel has been color coded to indicate the tissue with the highest probability. The intensity represents the difference between the highest and

Table 18.1. Correlations (R) of histology-guided measurements (total area per location) with manual segmentation and MEPPS

Tissue	Manual	MEPPS
Necrotic core	0.71	0.78
Calcification	0.76	0.83
Loose matrix	0.33	0.41
Fibrous tissue	0.78	0.82

Abbreviation: MEPPS = morphology-enhanced probabilistic plaque segmentation.

second highest probabilities, essentially providing a confidence metric in the classification. Also shown are the final contours delineating the tissue regions. The use of active contour methods to delineate the final regions has successfully overcome the presence of "holes" in the probability map that might otherwise have been misclassified.

Compositional indices

Measurements of plaque composition focus on computing the amounts of each component within the plaque. These compositional indices may characterize the total volume of each component or the total percentage of the wall volume attributable to the component. However, these measurements can be highly dependent on MRI coverage, for example, reducing the volume percentage if a large segment of relatively normal wall is included in the computation. A preferable technique may be to identify the maximal cross-sectional area of the component or its maximal area percentage.

The ability of MRI to measure compositional indices has been previously demonstrated by comparison with histological measurements. Correlation coefficients for histology versus MRI have been reported for necrotic cores ($r = 0.75$), calcification ($r = 0.74$), and loose matrix ($r = 0.70$) (Saam et al., 2005). These measurements are also highly reproducible from scan to scan, with

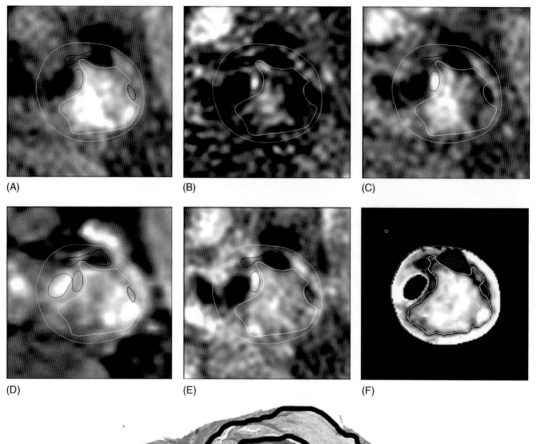

(A)   (B)   (C)

(D)   (E)   (F)

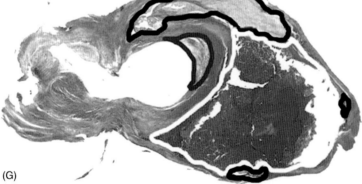

(G)

Figure 18.6 Segmentation results showing: (A)–(E) T1, T2, PD, TOF and CET1 MR images with manual, histology-confirmed drawings; (F) MEPPS segmentation; and (G) segmented histological image (yellow = necrotic core, purple = loose matrix, blue = calcification).

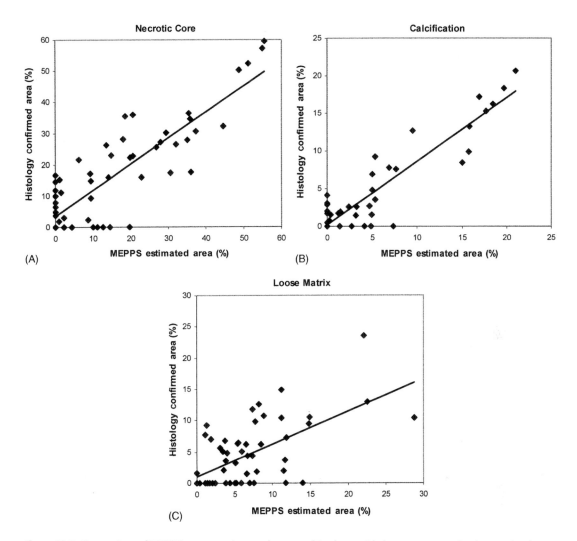

Figure 18.7 Comparison of MEPPS segmentation results versus histology-guided measurements for three main plaque tissues, with linear regression lines.

intraclass correlation coefficients of 0.99 reported for necrotic core and 0.90 for calcification (Saam *et al.*, 2006).

The ability of MEPPS to measure compositional indices was evaluated on 58 cross-sectional image sets (five contrast weightings per set) from 12 individuals undergoing carotid endarterectomy. Each set was independently segmented by MEPPS. The correlations (R) of histology guided measurements (total area per location) with manual segmentation and MEPPS are shown in Table 18.1. In addition, comparisons of the percentage areas from each location were made with histologically confirmed measurements and found to yield correlation coefficients of 0.86 for necrotic core, 0.93 for calcification, and 0.62 for loose matrix (Figure 18.7). These results suggest somewhat improved performance over previous manual

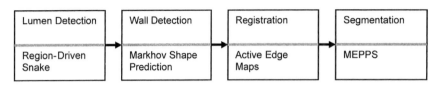

Figure 18.8 Process flow in automated plaque analysis with the computer-aided system for cardiovascular disease evaluation (CASCADE). Top boxes indicate general step to be accomplished; bottom boxes indicate method used by CASCADE.

evaluation results for necrotic core and calcification. The relatively poor performance for loose matrix is attributed to overestimation on the part of MEPPS. Retrospective evaluation showed that the algorithm was detecting regions with features identical to loose matrix, but attributed to flow artifacts by reviewers. Such regions can be easily deleted in manual editing for improved performance with minimal effort.

Conclusion

Together the image processing techniques presented in this chapter describe the process flow in Figure 18.8. The software platform we created to control these steps is the computer-aided system for cardiovascular disease evaluation (CASCADE; Xu *et al.*, 2004). With CASCADE, the user is guided through the interactive procedures to perform lumen detection via the region-driven snake, then wall detection using a Markov shape prediction, registration with active edge maps, and finally segmentation with MEPPS. Although alternative solutions to these procedures exist and future development should improve their effectiveness, the four principle processing steps of CASCADE remain.

This chapter focuses on the algorithms implemented in CASCADE to perform the four principal processing steps in carotid plaque characterization. Other researchers have proposed a number of alternative techniques for lumen and wall boundary detection (Han *et al.*, 2001, 2003; Adame *et al.*, 2004; Mansard *et al.*, 2004) and plaque segmentation (Clarke *et al.*, 2003; Adame *et al.*, 2004; Itskovitch *et al.*, 2004). These other techniques

perform equivalent tasks and could also be implemented within the CASCADE framework. Many of these, however, have not been used on in vivo data or have undergone very little validation.

CASCADE provides reliable, accurate, and quantitative information regarding plaque composition. This capability has enormous potential for assessing the response of carotid lesions to therapy. Treatment of atherosclerosis with drugs such as statins is thought to alter lesion composition (Zhao *et al.*, 2001). Thus, these techniques could be used in early phase clinical trials to determine whether lesion composition is responding as expected. Ultimately, we hope these measurements will correlate with clinical risk and provide clinicians with metrics other than stenosis for selecting the course of treatment. This goal requires long-term serial studies of large numbers of subjects. Such studies are currently underway.

For either application, CASCADE must be shown to provide both accurate and precise information regarding lesion morphology and composition. Validation efforts have shown that the morphological indices are highly reproducible and agree with corresponding ultrasound measurements. The compositional indices have been shown to predict histology measurements with high accuracy. The next challenge will be to maintain this performance in general use at multiple centers.

REFERENCES

Adame, I.M., van der Geest, R.J., Wasserman, B.A., *et al.* (2004). Automatic segmentation and plaque characterization in atherosclerotic carotid artery MR images. *Magma*, **16**, 227–34.

Brigger, P., Hoeg, J. and Unser, M. (2000). B-spline snakes: A flexible tool for parametric contour detection. *IEEE Transactions on Image Processing*, **9**, 1484–96.

Canny, J. (1986). A computational approach to edge detection. *IEEE Transactions on Pattern Analysis*, **8**, 679–98.

Chu, B., Kampschulte, A. and Ferguson, M. S., *et al.* (2004). Hemorrhage in the atherosclerotic carotid plaque: A high-resolution MRI study. *Stroke*, **35**, 1079–84.

Clarke, S. E., Hammond, R. R., Mitchell, J. R. and Rutt, B. K. (2003). Quantitative assessment of carotid plaque composition using multicontrast MRI and registered histology. *Magnetic Resonance in Medicine*, **50**, 1199–208.

Comaniciu, D. and Meer, P. (2002). Mean shift: a robust approach toward feature space analysis. *IEEE Transactions on Pattern Analysis and Machine Intelligence*, **24**, 603–19.

Davies, M. J. and Thomas, A. C. (1985). Plaque fissuring–the cause of acute myocardial infarction, sudden ischaemic death, and crescendo angina. *British Heart Journal*, **53**, 363–73.

Davies, M. J., Richardson, P. D., Woolf, N., Katz, D. R. and Mann, J. (1993). Risk of thrombosis in human atherosclerotic plaques: role of extracellular lipid, macrophage, and smooth muscle cell content. *British Heart Journal*, **69**, 377–81.

Falk, E. (1992). Why do plaques rupture? *Circulation*, **86**, III30–42.

Fukunaga, K. and Hostetler, L. D. (1975a). The estimation of the gradient of a density function, with applications in pattern recognition. *IEEE Transactions on Pattern Analysis and Machine Intelligence*, **21**, 32–40.

Fukunaga, K. and Hostetler, L. (1975b). k-nearest-neighbor bayes-risk estimation. *IEEE Transactions on Pattern Analysis and Machine Intelligence*, **21**, 285–93.

Geman, S. and Geman, D. (1984). Stochastic relaxation, Gibbs distributions, and the Bayesian restoration of images. *IEEE Transactions on Pattern Analysis*, **6**, 721–41.

Han, C., Hatsukami, T. S., Hwang, J. N. and Yuan, C. (2001). A fast minimal path active contour model. *IEEE Transactions on Image Processing*, **10**, 865–73.

Han, C., Kerwin, W. S., Hatsukami, T. S., Hwang, J. N. and Yuan, C. (2003). Detecting objects in image sequences using rule-based control in an active contour model.

IEEE Transactions on Biomedical Engineering, **50**, 705–10.

Hatsukami, T., Ross, R., Polissar, N. and Yuan, C. (2000). Visualization of fibrous cap thickness and rupture in human atherosclerotic carotid plaque in vivo with high resolution magnetic resonance imaging. *Circulation*, **102**, 959–64.

Hayes, C. E., Mathis, C. M. and Yuan, C. (1996). Surface coil phased arrays for high-resolution imaging of the carotid arteries. *Journal of Magnetic Resonance Imaging*, **6**, 109–12.

Hecherman, D. (1995). A tutorial on learning with Bayesian networks. Technical report, MSR-TR-95–06.

Itskovich, V. V., Samber, D. D., Mani, V., *et al.* (2004). Quantification of human atherosclerotic plaques using spatially enhanced cluster analysis of multi-contrast-weighted magnetic resonance images. *Magnetic Resonance in Medicine*, **52**, 515–23.

Kass, M., Witkin, A. and Terzopoulos, D. (1987). Snakes: active contour models. *International Journal of Computer Vision*, **1**, 321–31.

Kerwin, W. S. and Yuan, C. (2001). Active edge maps for medical image registration. *Proceedings of SPIE*, **4322**, 516–26.

Liu, F., Xu, D., Ferguson, M. S., *et al.* (2006). Automated in vivo Segmentation of Carotid Plaque MRI with Morphology-Enhanced Probability Maps. *Magnetic Resonance in Medicine*, in press.

Luo, Y., Polissar, N., Han, C., *et al.* (2003). Accuracy and uniqueness of three in vivo measurements of atherosclerotic carotid plaque morphology with black blood MRI. *Magnetic Resonance in Medicine*, **50**, 75–82.

Mansard, C. D., Canet Soulas, E. P., Anwander, A., *et al.* (2004). Quantification of multicontrast vascular MR images with nlsnake, an active contour model: in vitro validation and in vivo evaluation. *Magnetic Resonance in Medicine*, **51**, 370–9.

Mitsumori, L. M., Hatsukami, T. S., Ferguson, M. S., *et al.* (2003). In vivo accuracy of multisequence MR imaging for identifying unstable fibrous caps in advanced human carotid plaques. *Journal of Magnetic Resonance Imaging*, **17**, 410–20.

Paragios, N. and Deriche, R. (2000). Coupled geodesic active regions for image segmentation: a level set approach. *European Conference in Computer Vision*, 224–40.

Rumberger, J. A., Brundage, B. H., Rader, D. J. and Kondos, G. (1999). Electron beam computed tomographic coronary calcium scanning: a review and guidelines for use in asymptomatic persons. *Mayo Clinic Proceedings*, **74**, 538.

Saam, T., Ferguson, M.S., Yarnykh, V.L., *et al.* (2005). Quantitative evaluation of carotid plaque composition by *in vivo* MRI. *Arteriosclerosis, Thrombosis and Vascular Biology*, **25**, 234–9.

Saam, T., Kerwin, W.S., Chu, B., *et al.* (2006). Sample size calculation for clinical trials using magnetic resonance imaging for the quantitative assessment of carotid atherosclerosis. *Journal of Cardiovascular Magnetic Resonance*, in press.

Shinnar, M., Fallon, J.T., Wehrli, S., *et al.* (1999). The diagnostic accuracy of ex vivo MRI for human atherosclerotic plaque characterization. *Arteriosclerosis, Thrombosis and Vascular Biology*, **19**, 2756–61.

Sutton-Tyrrell, K., Kuller, L.H., Edmundowicz, D., *et al.* (2001). Usefulness of electron beam tomography to detect progression of coronary and aortic calcium in middle-aged women. *American Journal of Cardiology*, **87**, 560–4.

Underhill, H., Kerwin, W., Hatsukami, T. and Yuan, C. (2005). Is common carotid artery mean wall thickness by MRI comparable to intima-media thickness by B-Mode US? *Journal of Cardiovascular Magnetic Resonance*, **7**, 140–1.

Virmani, R., Kolodgie, F.D., Burke, A.P., Farb, A. and Schwartz, S.M. (2000). Lessons from sudden coronary death: a comprehensive morphological classification scheme for atherosclerotic lesions. *Arteriosclerosis, Thrombosis and Vascular Biology*, **20**, 1262–75.

Vliegenthart, R., Hollander, M., Breteler, M.M., *et al.* (2002). Stroke is associated with coronary calcification as detected by electron-beam CT: the Rotterdam Coronary Calcification Study. *Stroke*, **33**, 462–5.

Wight, T.N. and Merrilees, M.J. (2004). Proteoglycans in atherosclerosis and restenosis: key roles for versican. *Circulation Research*, **94**, 1158   –67.

Xu, D., Kerwin, W.S., Saam, T., Ferguson, M. and Yuan, C. (2004). CASCADE: Computer aided system for cardio-vascular disease evaluation. *International Society for Magnetic Resonance in Medicine*, abstract 1922.

Yuan, C. and Kerwin, W.S. (2004). MRI of atherosclerosis. *Journal of Magnetic Resonance Imaging*, **19**, 710–19.

Yuan, C., Mitsumori, L.M., Ferguson, M.S., *et al.* (2001). In vivo accuracy of multispectral magnetic resonance imaging for identifying lipid-rich necrotic cores and intraplaque hemorrhage in advanced human carotid plaques. *Circulation*, **104**, 2051–6.

Zhao, X.Q., Yuan, C., Hatsukami, T.S., *et al.* (2001). Effects of prolonged intensive lipid-lowering therapy on the characteristics of carotid atherosclerotic plaques in vivo by MRI: a case-control study. *Arteriosclerosis, Thrombosis and Vascular Biology*, **21**, 1623–9.

Zhu, S. and Yuille, A. (1996). Region competition: unifying snakes, region growing, and Bayesian/MDL for multi-band image segmentation. *IEEE Transactions on Pattern Analysis*, **18**, 884–900.

19

Nuclear imaging for the assessment of patients with carotid artery atherosclerosis

John R. Davies and Peter L. Weissberg

University of Cambridge Addenbrooke's Hospital, Hills Rd, Cambridge, CB2 2QQ, UK

Introduction

Atherosclerosis affecting the carotid arteries is an important cause of thromboembolic stroke and thus, its identification in patients at risk of stroke is desirable. Over the past three decades many attempts have been made to utilize nuclear imaging technology to identify atherosclerotic lesions in the carotid arteries. Early studies focused on providing the clinician with noninvasive alternatives for angiography such as ultrasound, computerized tomography (CT) and magnetic resonance (MR). The ability to identify lesions in large vessels such as the carotid artery, meant that developing nuclear imaging techniques as a means of simply confirming the presence of atherosclerosis was no longer justified. However, interest in developing novel nuclear imaging techniques has resurfaced following the realization that, much like coronary disease and myocardial infarction, thromboembolic stroke caused by carotid atheroma occurs as a result of plaque rupture. It is now widely accepted that the risk of plaque rupture is dictated by particular pathological processes at the cellular and molecular level, the identification of which nuclear imaging is ideally suited.

This chapter begins by outlining the basic principles that underpin nuclear imaging. This is followed by an overview of the cellular and molecular pathways that predispose to plaque inflammation, rupture, and thrombosis. The chapter then concentrates on methods for targeting these pathways by way of nuclear imaging. As well as detailing the relevant human studies, this section also outlines the most promising techniques that have so far only been tested in experimental models. The chapter concludes with a summary of the progress so far and a brief look into the future.

The basic principles of nuclear imaging as applied to imaging of the atherosclerotic plaque

Imaging with radionuclide tracer compounds is a multistage process. It begins with production of the radionuclide and its conjugation with a tracer compound. This is followed by administration of the tracer compound to the patient and its subsequent detection by techniques such as single photon emission computed tomography (SPECT) and positron emission tomography (PET). Both SPECT and PET rely on the detection of photons emitting as a result of radioactive decay of the radionuclide tagged tracer compound. In SPECT, imaging detectors are used to sense single gamma photons that are emitted from the radionuclide tag. The casing which houses the detector crystals also contains collimators which ensure

Carotid Disease: The Role of Imaging in Diagnosis and Management, ed. Jonathan Gillard, Martin Graves, Thomas Hatsukami and Chun Yuan. Published by Cambridge University Press. © Cambridge University Press 2007.

that each crystal can only detect photons that are travelling along a certain path. This ensures that the origin of emitted photons can be pinpointed and images that detail the distribution of the tracer compound can be faithfully constructed by the computer software. The distance between adjacent collimators dictates the spatial resolution of the machine. The smaller the distance the higher the spatial resolution, but the lower the detection sensitivity due to higher numbers of photons that fail to reach the detectors. In practice the spatial resolution of most human SPECT scanners is between 1 and 2 cm. PET imaging relies on the detection of paired photons that are emitted from the tracer compound at 180° to one another. These photons are the product of the energy released when positrons, ejected from the nucleus of the radionuclide, annihilate with adjacent electrons. A ring of scintillation crystals housed in the casing of the PET machine detects the emitted photon pairs which hit detectors on opposite sides of the detection ring within nanoseconds of one another. This allows the PET scanner to detect the line along which the photons originated from without the need for collimation, which means that a higher spatial resolution can be achieved without compromising detection sensitivity. A whole body human PET scanner typically has a spatial resolution of between 4 and 6 mm.

In both SPECT and PET the detected photon emission is corrected to account for errors due to attenuation, scatter, random decay events and dead time, following which 2D and 3D topographical images can be reconstructed.

The small size of most atherosclerotic lesions and their anatomical proximity to other structures places exacting demands on nuclear imaging systems. However, in contrast to coronary arteries, the carotid vessels are larger and are not subject to excessive motion, making them a much easier imaging target for nuclear techniques. Ideally, tracers for atheroma imaging should bind specifically to plaque constituents and should be rapidly cleared from the circulation to allow for sufficient contrast between the plaque and the blood pool.

Uptake in adjacent tissues should also be minimal. If a tracer satisfies these criteria then the problems created by low spatial resolution (often referred to as partial volume effects) can be easily overcome. However, the resulting image will not have sufficient detail to identify the exact anatomical location of tracer uptake. To overcome this, sequential anatomical imaging, most notably by CT, is now increasingly being used.

The biology of plaque inflammation, rupture and thrombosis

Advanced atherosclerotic lesions comprise a lipid-rich core covered by a smooth muscle cell and matrix-rich fibrous cap. The vulnerable plaque, whether it be present in carotid, coronary or peripheral arteries is typified by an abundance of inflammatory cells and their protein products (Davies, 1996; Libby et al., 1997; Golledge et al., 2000), all of which provide potential targets for radionuclide tracers. Macrophages play a central role in the destabilization of atherosclerotic lesions. Circulating monocytes are recruited to atheromatous lesions in response to the expression of adhesion molecules and chemotactic proteins such as monocyte chemotactic protein-1 (MCP-1) (Rosenfeld, 2002). Once recruited, they differentiate into macrophages and ingest oxidized lipoproteins thereby generating foam cells (Vainio and Ikonen, 2003). Foam cells and newly recruited macrophages secrete a host of proinflammatory cytokines as well as enzymes such as matrix metalloproteinases (MMP) that break down the connective tissue of the fibrous cap resulting in structural changes that reduce its ability to resist the mechanical forces imposed by the flowing blood (Libby et al., 1996). In addition, foam cells present in the vulnerable plaque frequently exhibit endoplasmic reticular (ER) stress which is associated with phosphatidyl serine (PS) expression on the cell surface, which in turn, contributes to foam cell apoptosis (Tabas, 2004). Extensive upregulation of caspases is seen in atherosclerotic lesions (Chen *et al.*, 2004) and overt apoptosis of macrophages is commonly observed in fibrous caps at the site of plaque rupture with apoptosis further augmenting surface PS expression (Kolodgie *et al.*, 2000). Foam cell apoptosis leads to the build-up of extracellular cholesterol as well as the release of inflammatory cytokines and prothrombotic proteins such as interleukins, tumor necrosis factor-alpha and tissue factor. The inflammatory milieu that results from macrophage activation, foam cell formation and apoptosis reduces the mechanical strength of the plaque. MMPs catalyze the breakdown of matrix proteins thus thinning the protective fibrous cap. The build up of extracellular cholesterol leads to an expansion of the lipid core. Thus the forces that are required to breach the fibrous cap and tear it away from the underlying lipid core are dangerously reduced. When plaque rupture occurs, the highly thrombogenic lipid core comes into contact with the circulating blood, which activates platelets and the intrinsic and extrinsic coagulation cascade pathways. The extent to which the thrombus blocks the vessel lumen and impedes blow flow depends predominantly on the size of the thrombogenic stimulus, which in turn depends on the size of the lipid core and the degree to which it is exposed to the circulating blood following plaque rupture.

Radionuclide tracers have been developed that can identify some of the important pathways associated with plaque instability and thrombosis including macrophage recruitment, foam cell formation, matrix breakdown enzymes, macrophage metabolism, apoptosis, fibrin deposition and platelet activation (Figure 19.1). Table 19.1 provides a summary of some of the studies that have been carried out.

Imaging of lipoprotein phagocytosis and foam cell generation

Vulnerable lesions are characterized by high levels of low density lipoprotein (LDL) accumulation, oxidation and phagocytosis by plaque macrophages and foam cells. Lipid metabolism therefore provides a suitable target for identifying high-risk plaques.

Oxidized LDL (oxLDL) particles have been successfully radiolabelled allowing investigators to identify lipid accumulation within macrophages and foam cells present in atheromatous plaques (Iuliano *et al.*, 1996). Lees *et al.* used ^{99m}Tc-oxLDL to successfully image symptomatic human carotid lesions in vivo (Lees *et al.*, 1988). They found that uptake of ^{99m}Tc-oxLDL by carotid plaques was significantly higher compared with normal carotids ($p = 0.02$). Uptake of ^{99m}Tc-oxLDL above that of the normal carotid artery was observed in 10 out of 11 carotid plaques (91%, confidence limits 58.7–99.8). No correlation between the degree of stenosis and the target to background uptake ratio was seen.

Given that the clinical utility of radiolabelled autologous oxLDL is likely to be limited because of its time-consuming preparation process, several groups have synthesized and tested antibody tracers that bind to epitopes on the oxidized LDL molecule. The majority of studies performed thus far have used radiolabelled malondialdehyde-2 (MDA-2), a prototype murine monoclonal antibody that binds to the malondialdehyde epitope on the oxLDL molecule. Experiments in hypercholesterolaemic apolipoprotein E null (apoE−/−) mice and Wantanabe heritable hyperlipidaemic (WHHL) rabbits have shown that lipid-rich lesions accumulated approximately 20 times more ^{125}I-MDA2 than normal arterial tissue (Tsimikas *et al.*, 1999). Immunohistochemistry confirmed co-localization of ^{125}I-MDA2 uptake with macrophage foam cells. In an ex vivo autoradiography study, ^{125}I-MDA2 has been shown to have the capability to track changes in macrophage foam cell density following dietary manipulation (Tsimikas *et al.*, 2000). Immunohistology revealed that decreased uptake of ^{125}I-MDA2 following dietary plaque regression did not correlate with a decrease in plaque size but was associated with a decrease in macrophage foam cell number, an increase in VSMCs and a higher collagen content (Torzewski *et al.*, 2004). These results suggest that MDA-2 could be used as

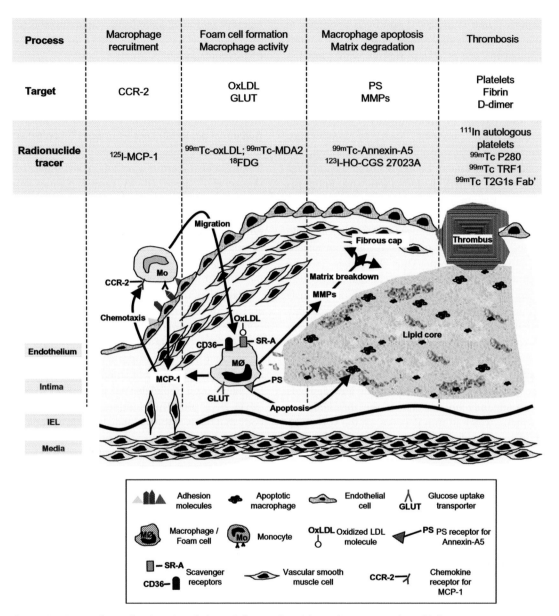

Process	Macrophage recruitment	Foam cell formation Macrophage activity	Macrophage apoptosis Matrix degradation	Thrombosis
Target	CCR-2	OxLDL GLUT	PS MMPs	Platelets Fibrin D-dimer
Radionuclide tracer	^{125}I-MCP-1	^{99m}Tc-oxLDL; ^{99m}Tc-MDA2 ^{18}FDG	^{99m}Tc-Annexin-A5 ^{123}I-HO-CGS 27023A	^{111}In autologous platelets ^{99m}Tc P280 ^{99m}Tc TRF1 ^{99m}Tc T2G1s Fab'

Figure 19.1 Targets for nuclear imaging of plaque inflammation. Schematic representation of inflammatory cells, molecules and processes that present potential targets for the identification of vulnerable plaques. CCR-2, chemokine receptor 2; CD36, cluster differentiation 36; GLUT, glucose uptake transporter; IEL, internal elastic lamina; MCP-1, monocyte chemotactic protein-1; MMP, matrix metalloproteinase; OxLDL, oxidized low density lipoprotein; PS, phosphatidyl serine; SR-A, scavenger receptor-A.

Table 19.1. Overview of radiolabelled tracers for imaging of atheroscelorosis

Target mechanism	Target cell/molecule	Tracer	Human studies	Animal studies	Ex vivo histological correlation	In vivo imaging attempted	Notes	Reference
Macrophage chemotaxis	CCR-2	^{125}I-MCP-1	✗	✓	✓	✗	Excellent correlation with macrophage number. Fast plasma clearance	Ohtsuki et al., 2001
LDL phagocytosis and foam cell generation	oxLDL	^{99m}Tc-oxLDL	✓	✓	✓	✓	Rapid plasma clearance c.f. native LDL tracers	Lees et al., 1988
		^{125}I-MDA2	✗	✓	✓	✓	Also capable of tracking changes in foam cell number	Tsimikas et al., 2000
		^{125}I-IK17	✓	✓	✓	✗	In vitro staining of human plaques -IK17 localizes to lipid core	Shaw et al., 2001
MMP activity	MMP	^{123}I-HO-CGS 27023A	✗	✓	✓	✓	Significant increase in uptake in lesioned carotid c.f. sham and control. Rapid plasma clearance	Kopka et al., 2004
		^{111}In-MMP inhibitor	✗	✓	✓	✓		Kolodgie et al., 2001
Apoptosis	PS	^{99m}Tc-Annexin-A5	✓	✓	✓	✓	Co-localization with apoptotic macrophages. Uptake in humans correlates with vulnerable histological features	Kolodgie et al., 2003; Kietselaer et al., 2004
Macrophage activity	GLUT	^{18}FDG	✓	✓	✓	✓	PET tracer. Good correlation between tracer uptake and macrophage number. Uptake in humans unstable > stable plaque	Rudd et al., 2002; Davies et al., 2005; Dunphy et al., 2005

Target mechanism	Target cell/molecule	Tracer	Human studies	Animal studies	Ex vivo histological correlation	In vivo imaging attempted	Notes	Reference
Coagulation	Fibrin	^{99m}Tc T2G1s Fab'	×	✓	N/A	✓	Uptake ratio lesion:control = 2:1 *in vivo* and 4:1 *ex vivo*	Cerqueira *et al.*, 1992
	D-dimer	^{99m}Tc TRF1	✓	✓	N/A	✓	Uptake seen in only 5/8 patients. No histological correlate	Ciavolella *et al.*, 1999
Platelets	Autologous platelets	^{111}In autologous platelets	✓	×	N/A	✓	Inconsistent results between studies – may be due to inconsistent use of antiplatelet agents	Minar *et al.*, 1989; Moriwaki *et al.*, 1995
	GPIIb/IIIa	^{99m}Tc P748	×	✓	N/A	✓		Vallabhajosula, 1996
		^{99m}Tc P280	✓	×	N/A	✓	Uptake in 11/18 patients. No histological correlate	Vallabhajosula *et al.*, 1996
		^{99m}Tc DMP-444	×	✓	✓	✓	Tracer uptake correlated with platelet number/ thrombus weight	Mitchel *et al.*, 2000

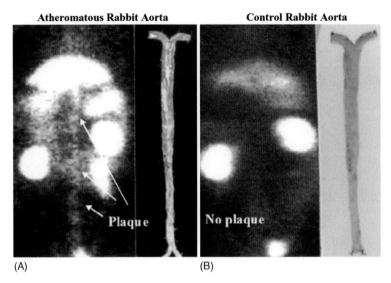

Figure 19.2 *In vivo* gamma camera images of experimental aortic atheroma following injection of ^{99m}Tc-MDA2. (A) Watanabe heritable hyperlipidaemic (WHHL) rabbit injected with 5 mCi of ^{99m}Tc-MDA2 showing selective uptake in the aorta (arrows). (B) A control normocholesterolemic, nonatherosclerotic New Zealand White rabbit shows no aortic uptake. Interestingly, there is significantly more liver, spleen, and gut uptake of ^{99m}Tc-MDA2 in the WHHL rabbit, where increased oxidation-specific epitopes are known to exist. Reproduced with permission from Tsimikas *et al.* (1999). *Journal of Nuclear Cardiology*, **6**, 41–53.

a marker of plaque stability. Preliminary studies carried out on WHHL rabbits following intravenous injection of ^{99m}Tc-MDA2 (Tsimikas *et al.*, 1999) have confirmed the feasibility of in vivo gamma imaging of aortic plaque (Figure 19.2). However, a visible signal was only seen in 4 out of 7 WHHL rabbits and no quantification of the in vivo images was attempted. Therefore, the in-vivo imaging capability of this technique remains in doubt.

In an attempt to increase tracer affinity and specificity and thus increase uptake into the plaque, genetically engineered antibodies against human oxLDL have been synthesized. Their small molecular size should enable higher lesion to blood ratios which should allow more effective in-vivo imaging. In vitro and ex vivo experiments carried out in experimental animal models and on excised human carotid atheroma have given promising results (Shaw *et al.*, 2001). This approach to imaging of lipid uptake appears to hold promise but we await in vivo studies in patients with carotid atherosclerosis to determine its utility.

Imaging macrophage stress and apoptosis in atherosclerotic plaque

Apoptotic cells express PS on their cell surface and, therefore, nuclear imaging of PS expression may identify vulnerable plaques at risk of rupture (Kolodgie *et al.*, 2003). This expectation may be confounded by the likelihood of PS expression on other constituents of the plaque such as platelets in overlying thrombus, and on red blood cell membrane remnants in the necrotic core of the lesions. However, given that thrombus and intraplaque hemorrhage are both associated with plaque vulnerability, this may not present a problem in clinical practice.

Annexin-A5 has a high affinity for the aberrantly expressed PS on the cell surface. Accordingly, ^{99m}Tc-labeled annexin-A5 has been used for noninvasive imaging of experimental atherosclerotic lesions in rabbits induced by de-endothelialization of the infradiaphragmatic aorta followed by 12 weeks of a high fat, high cholesterol diet (Kolodgie et al., 2003). All animals received radiolabelled annexin-A5 intravenously, and the abdominal aortic atherosclerotic lesions could be observed 2–3 hours later. Ex vivo images clearly showed uptake of radiotracer corresponding to the lesion distribution within the excised aorta and to tracer uptake seen on the in vivo images. There was no radiotracer uptake in areas without visible atherosclerotic lesions. A control annexin-A5 mutant that is incapable of binding to PS did not accumulate in the lesions. Similarly, there was no localization of ^{99m}Tc-annexin-A5 in control rabbits without atherosclerotic lesions. Annexin-A5 uptake in atherosclerotic lesions was approximately 10-fold greater than in the nonatherosclerotic aortic wall. The mean percent-injected dose per gram annexin-A5 uptake in the specimens with lesions correlated with the histologic severity of atherosclerotic lesions; the radiotracer uptake demonstrated that annexin accumulation predominantly occurred in AHA type IV lesions with only minimal uptake in type II and III lesions. There was a direct relationship of annexin-A5 uptake with macrophage burden ($r = 0.47$, $p = 0.04$) and the magnitude of histologically-verified apoptosis. No association was observed between smooth muscle cell burden and radiotracer uptake ($r = 0.08$, $p = 0.73$). The results of this study confirm the ability of annexin-A5 to image apoptosis within the atherosclerotic plaque, paving the way for human studies.

^{99m}Tc-annexin-A5 has subsequently been used to image atheroma in four patients with carotid vascular disease (Kietselaer et al., 2004), two of whom had suffered a recent transient ischemic attack (TIA). Tc^{99m}-annexin-A5 uptake was seen in the cervical region in the two patients with recent TIA. No uptake was discernible in the other two patients who had both suffered a TIA more than 6 months prior to imaging and who were also being treated with high-dose statins (Figure 19.3). All patients underwent carotid endarterectomy after imaging. The positive Tc^{99m}-annexin-A5 uptake correlated with plaque macrophage content whereas both patients with negative annexin scans had smooth muscle cell-rich lesions. One of the two patients with recent TIA had a severe stenosis in the contralateral carotid, but without annexin-A5 uptake. Whilst these studies suggest that annexin-A5 has promise as an atheroma-imaging agent, it is too early to speculate on its clinical utility. In addition, a lack of anatomical detail on the emission scans makes it difficult to be sure that the uptake is indeed related to atherosclerotic plaque.

Imaging of plaque macrophage activity with fluorine-18 labelled deoxyglucose PET

Deoxyglucose competes with glucose for uptake into metabolically active cells where it accumulates in proportion to metabolic activity. When labelled with fluorine-18, its accumulation can be imaged and, more importantly, quantified by PET. Fluorine-18 labelled deoxyglucose (FDG) PET has been used extensively to estimate myocardial glucose utilization (Phelps et al., 1978) and is becoming the imaging method of choice for identifying tumors (Strauss and Conti, 1991). The recognition that FDG-PET might have a role in imaging inflammation led to its use in diagnosing and following patients with systemic vasculitides (Bleeker-Rovers et al., 2003; Meller et al., 2003). In one study of 20 patients with suspected vasculitis, FDG-PET was reported to have 100% positive predictive value and 82% negative predictive value for the diagnosis of vasculitis (Bleeker-Rovers et al., 2003). It has been particularly useful in diagnosing and monitoring the response to treatment in Takayasu's arteritis (Andrews et al., 2004; Webb et al., 2004). Thus, FDG-PET clearly has the capacity to measure vascular inflammation.

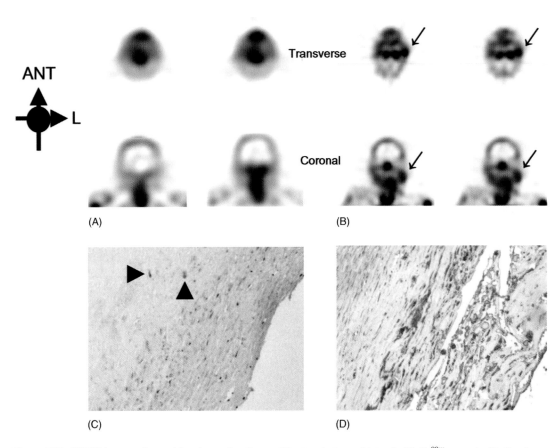

Figure 19.3 SPECT images of unstable atherosclerotic carotid artery lesions obtained with Tc^{99m}-annexin-A5. Panel A shows transverse and coronal views obtained by SPECT in Patient I, who had a left-sided TIA 3 days before imaging. Patient I had significant stenoses of both carotid arteries; however, the uptake of Tc^{99m}-annexin-A5 is evident only in the culprit lesion (see arrows). Histopathology of an endarterectomy specimen from patient I (B, antiannexin-A5 antibody) shows substantial infiltration of macrophages into the neointima, with extensive binding of annexin-A5 (brown staining). In contrast, SPECT images of patient II (C), who had had a right-sided TIA 3 months before imaging, do not show annexin-A5 uptake in the carotid region on both sides. Doppler ultrasonography revealed a clinically significant obstructive lesion on the affected side. Histopathological analysis of an endarterectomy specimen from patient II (D) shows a lesion rich in smooth-muscle cells, with negligible binding of annexin-A5. ANT, anterior; L, left. Reproduced with permission from Kietselaer *et al.* (2004). *New England Journal of Medicine*, **350**, 1472–3.

The first studies to show that FDG-PET might have a role in imaging atherosclerosis were performed in cholesterol-fed rabbits. Vallabhajosula *et al.* showed that sufficient FDG was taken up by macrophage-rich atherosclerotic lesions in the aortic arch to be imaged in a conventional human PET scanner (Vallabhajosula *et al.*, 1996).

The same group showed that FDG uptake appeared to be related to macrophage content of the plaque. Using a similar model, Lederman *et al.* showed that a positron-sensitive fibreoptic probe placed in contact with the arterial intima could detect high FDG uptake in atherosclerotic segments of the iliac artery (Lederman *et al.*, 2001). These studies coincided with reports that approximately 50% of patients undergoing FDG-PET for cancer were found, incidentally, also to have high FDG uptake into large arteries (Yun *et al.*, 2001), assumed to be due to atherosclerosis. Compared with those with no vascular uptake, the patients with high vascular FDG uptake had more risk factors for atherosclerosis (Yun *et al.*, 2002). These studies strongly suggested that atherosclerotic plaques could be imaged by FDG-PET. Indeed, it is now recognized that atherosclerotic FDG uptake may be misinterpreted as representing the presence of tumor in oncological scans (Hanif *et al.*, 2004).

The first clinical study of FDG-PET imaging of human atherosclerosis was published recently (Rudd *et al.*, 2002). In this study Rudd *et al.* used autoradiography to demonstrate that when human atherosclerotic plaques were incubated ex vivo with tritiated deoxyglucose ($[^3H]DG$), it was taken up by plaque macrophages, and not by surrounding vascular smooth muscle cells. They subsequently undertook FDG-PET scans on eight patients who had experienced a recent TIA and in whom there was angiographic evidence of internal carotid artery stenosis. FDG-PET images were co-registered with CT angiograms to ensure that any PET "hot spots" coincided with identified stenotic plaques. They demonstrated FDG accumulation into all eight symptomatic plaques with significantly less FDG uptake into six contralateral asymptomatic plaques (difference in mean FDG uptake rate of 2.1×10^{-5} sec^{-1}, $p = 0.005$) and no discernible uptake into normal arteries (Figure 19.4).

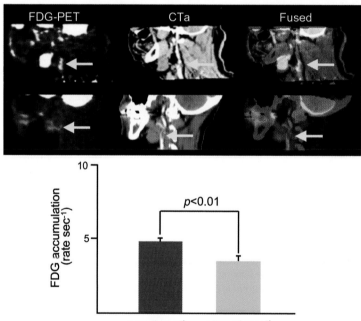

Figure 19.4 PET images from patients with unstable carotid disease following administration of FDG. (A) FDG-PET (left column), CT angiography (middle column) and fused (right column) images from patient with symptomatic carotid stenosis (top row) and contralateral asymptomatic carotid stenosis (bottom row). The yellow arrows highlight areas of FDG uptake corresponding to stenotic carotid plaque. (B) A graph showing FDG accumulation rate in symptomatic versus asymptomatic carotid plaques. Note that FDG uptake into symptomatic plaque was significantly higher. Modified from original figure reproduced with permission from Rudd *et al.* (2002). *Circulation*, **105**, 2708–11.

These studies provide proof of principal that FDG-PET can image atherosclerotic plaque inflammation and suggest that it can also quantify plaque inflammatory cell activity. If confirmed, these observations suggest that FDG-PET could be used to identify potentially unstable plaques and to monitor effects of drug therapy on plaque inflammation. Confirmation that FDG-PET can quantify plaque macrophages has come from a recent study in atherosclerotic rabbits which demonstrated a close correlation between FDG uptake and plaque macrophage content ($r = 0.81$, $p < 0.0001$) (Ogawa *et al.*, 2004). If FDG-PET is able to identify only those plaques that are most actively inflamed, then it follows that not all plaques should take up significant amounts of FDG. It is becoming clear that this is indeed the case. Three studies have been published recently in which patients with suspected cancer were imaged by both CT and FDG-PET (Tatsumi *et al.*, 2003; Ben Haim *et al.*, 2004; Dunphy *et al.*, 2005). CT measures calcium which is an almost universal component of atherosclerosis, such that the presence or absence of calcium in the vessel wall is taken to include or exclude the presence of atherosclerosis (Budoff *et al.*, 1998). All studies demonstrated substantial disparity between CT positive and PET positive plaques. However, these findings are not inconsistent with current understanding of plaque cell biology which would predict that calcification is a consequence of cell death induced by inflammation. Thus FDG uptake indicates current inflammation and therefore potential instability, whilst CT calcification identifies past inflammation and, therefore, relative stability (Weissberg, 2004).

These studies all suggest that FDG-PET may have an important role to play in identifying vulnerable plaques. However, this approach has a number of important limitations that must be overcome if it is to be of wider clinical use. FDG-PET provides little or no anatomical resolution and so must be combined and co-registered with another imaging modality to ensure that the PET signal arises from an atherosclerotic plaque and not an adjacent metabolically active structure, such as a lymph node. This will no doubt be facilitated by the wider availability of combined PET/CT scanners. However, any co-registered imaging modality that relies on angiographic principles will be no better at identifying nonstenotic lesions than conventional angiography. Co-registration with high resolution MRI, which can characterize nonstenotic as well as stenotic lesions, offers promise for imaging large arteries, such as the carotid. It also has the advantage of not adding to radiation exposure. Our group has recently completed a study in which both FDG-PET and MRI were carried out on a cohort of patients ($n = 12$) with symptomatic carotid disease due to undergo carotid endarterectomy (Davies *et al.*, 2005). Surprisingly, we found that five out of 12 plaques targeted for endarterectomy had the same degree of FDG uptake as normal vessel walls. In addition, nonstenotic plaques with high FDG uptake were identified in three out of these five patients (Figure 19.5). This study reinforces the advantages of combining FDG-PET with MRI and suggests that this technique may provide a method of selecting appropriate lesions for surgical or percutaneous intervention in patients at risk of stroke.

Other targets for nuclear imaging of plaque inflammation

Unlike the tracers described above, the ones outlined below have not been tested in vivo in patients with carotid atherosclerosis. They have been included in this chapter because they are potential tracers for carotid imaging in the future.

Imaging of monocyte recruitment

MCP-1 labelled with iodine-125 (^{125}I) has been shown to accumulate selectively in lipid-rich, macrophage-rich regions of experimental atherosclerosis in rabbits where the radiotracer uptake is closely correlated with the severity of lesions (Ohtsuki *et al.*, 2001). The ratio of radioactivity in plaque to normal vessel was 6:1.

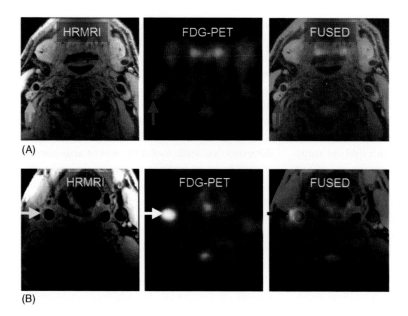

Figure 19.5 Combined PET and MRI imaging to identify FDG uptake in nonstenotic plaque. High-resolution MRI and FDG-PET scans taken from a patient who had suffered a recent right carotid territory stroke. (A) Transaxial images taken at the level of the proximal right internal carotid (RIC) artery. There is a large atherosclerotic plaque in the RIC artery causing severe luminal stenosis (green arrow). Despite its size, only low FDG uptake is demonstrated (blue and red arrows). (B) Axial images taken at the level of the proximal common carotid arteries (CCA). The yellow arrow highlights a nonstenotic plaque in the wall of the right CCA. The white arrow points to an area of high FDG uptake, the location of which is confirmed on the fused scan as the right CCA (black arrow). Reproduced with permission from Davies *et al.* (2005). *Stroke*, **36**, 2642–7.

Furthermore, there was a strong correlation between percent injected dose per gram accumulation of ^{125}I-MCP-1 in the atherosclerotic lesions and quantitative estimates of the number of macrophages per unit area ($r = 0.85$, $p < 0.0001$). Encouragingly, plasma clearance of the tracer was also rapid with a clearance half-life of 10 minutes, suggesting that external imaging of inflamed plaques with MCP-1 tracers may be possible.

At present no in vivo imaging studies using the above tracer compounds have been published. Therefore, it remains uncertain as to whether this approach to noninvasive external imaging of macrophage recruitment is achievable in vivo in man. However, the importance of macrophage recruitment with regards to plaque instability

justifies the ongoing efforts of investigators in this field.

Imaging of plaque matrix metalloproteinases (MMP)

In unstable plaques there is excessive secretion of MMP enzymes that break down the connective tissue matrix of the plaque. When activated by oxLDL and proinflammatory cytokines, macrophages secrete inactive MMP, including interstitial collagenases (MMP-1), gelatinase B (MMP-9), and stromolysins (MMP-3), which are activated *in situ* by plasmin (Lendon *et al.*, 1991; Galis *et al.*, 1994). Immunohistochemistry shows that MMP production is predominantly in the vicinity of macrophages in human coronary atherosclerotic lesions (Narula *et al.*, 2003). Kopka *et al.* have successfully synthesized a number of synthetic radiolabelled MMP inhibitors, that bind to the active zinc(II) ion on a broad spectrum of MMPs (Kopka *et al.*, 2004). They studied a ^{123}I-labelled molecule (HO-CGS 27023A) in apoE−/− mice that had undergone carotid artery ligation followed by a high cholesterol diet to induce rapid development of atherosclerosis (Schafers *et al.*, 2004). They showed that following injection of ^{123}I-HO-CGS 27023A, uptake into lesioned carotid arteries was significantly higher than into normal arterial tissue from the contralateral carotid artery and carotid arteries from the sham and control mice (Figure 19.6). In addition, predosing mice with unlabelled ligand prevented uptake, indicating a high level of specific binding. Clearance of the tracer from the circulation was rapid allowing for clear plaque identification on gamma images. Ex vivo gamma counting of arteries from the lesioned mice confirmed uptake into the artery that was not found in the contralateral artery. Micro-autoradiography of the imaged lesions using ^{125}I-HO-CGS 27023A confirmed co-localization of tracer distribution and MMP-9 immunostaining.

A similar broad-spectrum MMP inhibitor radiolabelled with indium-111 has been used to image atherosclerotic lesions in NZW rabbits induced by balloon de-endothelialization of the abdominal aorta and dietary manipulation (Kolodgie *et al.*, 2001). Following intravenous injection of the tracer, gamma camera imaging revealed significantly higher aortic tracer uptake in those on a high cholesterol diet than those where the diet was interrupted with normal chow (0.033 ± 0.019% injected dose/gram; lesion-to-non-lesion ratio 11:1). In turn, images confirmed that the animals on the interrupted diet regime had higher concentrations of tracer uptake than the control animals who were maintained on a cholesterol-free diet (0.015 ± 0.005% injected dose/gram, $p=0.01$). Threshold analysis of histological sections showed a significantly higher level of immunostaining for MMP in the plaque

segments that demonstrated high tracer uptake relative to those with low uptake.

These preliminary observations suggest that MMP might prove to be a suitable target for in vivo imaging of atherosclerosis. Recent reports of ^{11}C and ^{18}F labelling of MMP inhibitors also raise the possibility of PET imaging studies (Zheng *et al.*, 2002). The superior spatial resolution and tracer detection sensitivity of PET would allow more sophisticated quantification and would enable investigators to make use of combined PET/CT machines to provide anatomical co-registration.

Targeting of atherosclerosis-related thrombus

Vulnerable plaques provide a highly thrombogenic substrate and have often gone through both symptomatic and asymptomatic episodes of rupture, thrombosis and repair (Davies and Thomas, 1984). This phenomenon provides an opportunity to detect such plaques with radiotracers targeted to the various components that make up thrombus. Imaging approaches have targeted the two main thrombotic mechanisms, fibrin formation and platelet activation.

Imaging of fibrin and its related molecules

Radiolabelled fibrinogen has proven to be a poor candidate for thrombus imaging based on its slow accumulation into arterial thrombi. A small pilot study to assess the potential of radio-iodinated fibrinogen failed to image symptomatic plaques in four patients with angiographically proven carotid disease (Mettinger *et al.*, 1978). Most studies designed to detect fibrin and its breakdown products have centered on the use of radiolabelled antibodies. Cerqueira *et al.* used a canine model of acute arterial thrombosis to test the ability of a monoclonal antibody fragment, T2G1s Fab′, to bind specifically to fibrin to allow in vivo detection (Cerqueira *et al.*, 1992). Carotid and femoral thrombi were induced by means of temporary

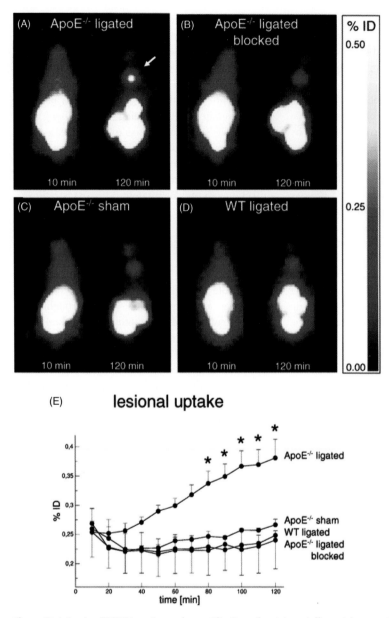

Figure 19.6 In vivo SPECT imaging and quantification of matrix metalloproteinase activity in experimental carotid lesions using the tracer [123I]HO-CGS 27023A. Representative planar images taken 10 minutes (left) and 120 minutes (right) after injection in apolipoprotein E-deficient mice (A–C) and wild-type mice (D) 4 weeks after carotid ligation. (A) Unblocked; (B) after predosing with 6 mmol/L CGS27023A; (C) sham-operated; (D) wild-type; (E) and (F) quantitative uptake of the radioligand in the carotid lesion and tissues over time is expressed as % ID. *P<0.05 between unblocked and predosed lesional uptake. The signal in the abdominal cavity is nonspecific and probably reflects metabolism of the original compound, because there is no inhibition after predosing in all experiments. Reproduced with permission from Schafers *et al.* (2004). *Circulation,* **109**, 2554–9.

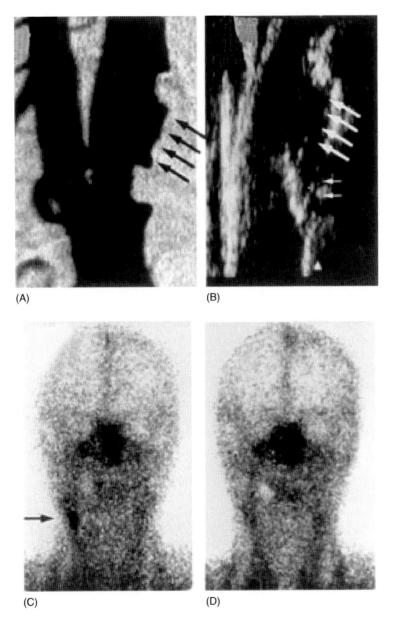

(A)   (B)

(C)   (D)

Figure 19.7 In vivo gamma camera imaging of platelet accumulation in a symptomatic patient with carotid atherosclerosis. Carotid angiogram (A); B-mode ultrasound (B); gamma camera imaging following injection of ^{111}In-labelled platelets (C); and ^{99m}Tc-labelled human serum albumin (D) in a 58-year-old man who suffered from transient ischemic attacks with left hemiparesis. Large arrows in (A) and (B) indicate obviously ulcerated lesions in the right internal carotid artery. Small arrows in (B) point to the carotid bifurcation. Arrow in (C) highlights a pathological, positive platelet accumulation in the right carotid artery. No tracer uptake can be seen in the "control" images following injection of ^{99m}Tc-labelled human serum albumin (D). Modified with permission from original figure by Moriwaki et al. (1995). *Arteriosclerosis, Thrombosis and Vascular Biology*, **15**, 2234–40.

luminal occlusion, crush injury and thrombin injection. Sham-operated carotid arteries served as controls. ^{99m}Tc-T2G1s Fab′ was injected following temporary occlusion and a series of planar gamma images was obtained. Plasma clearance of the tracer was adequate with a half-life of 2 hours. Ex vivo quantification revealed a thrombus to blood ratio of 4:2. Visual analysis of the in vivo images showed uptake by 2 hours in all carotid thrombi. In vivo thrombus to contralateral carotid ratio was 2:2 at 2 hours post injection. The same tracer however, had a sensitivity of only 50% for the detection of chronic arterial thrombi in patients with left ventricular thrombus, aortic aneurysms, and peripheral arterial grafts (Stratton et al., 1994). Given that chronic thrombus buried within atheromatous lesions is likely to be less accessible to tracers injected systemically, this result suggests that T2G1s Fab′ is an unlikely candidate for the detection of anything but recent plaque disruption.

A series of studies have been carried out using monoclonal antibodies directed against D-dimers of cross-linked fibrin. Preliminary data were obtained from a rabbit model of arterial and venous thrombosis which confirmed the ability to image the uptake of ^{131}I labelled antibody fragments (Scopinaro et al., 1992). An in vitro human study of TRF1, a novel D-dimer monoclonal antibody fragment, revealed significantly higher binding to atheromatous vessels compared with normal vessels, both of which were obtained during bypass surgery (Greco et al., 1993). Indirect immunofluorescence confirmed TRF1 uptake within the plaque wall. The same group has also carried out an in vivo imaging study using a ^{99m}Tc labelled antibody fragment (Ciavolella et al., 1999). Eight patients with carotid atheroma awaiting endarterectomy were enrolled. Following antibody injection, a dynamic gamma imaging protocol was employed up to 3 hours following injection. At 6 hours postinjection, carotid endarterectomy was performed. Atherosclerotic lesions were detected on scintigraphic images in five of eight patients at 3 hours postinjection. This correlated with those

lesions with higher vessel to blood ratios detected on analysis of the endarterectomy specimens. No ex vivo immunohistochemical evaluation was carried out to confirm the localization of the tracer within the plaque. However, no surface thrombus was evident on macroscopic examination and therefore the authors concluded that, given the presence of fibrin within atherosclerotic plaques and previous in vitro findings, the in vivo uptake was most likely to correspond to fibrin deposition deep in the substance of the plaque. The origin of fibrin deposited in plaque is still unclear as is its significance in relation to plaque instability. It is not clear whether fibrin accumulates within the plaque as a result of plaque rupture, due to hemorrhage from fragile capillaries that form beneath the fibrous cap or due to a passage across the intact endothelium over a period of months or years. This uncertainty makes it difficult to assess the clinical value of this imaging method at present.

Platelet imaging

Thrombi associated with disruption of the plaque surface are composed mainly of platelets, and therefore platelet scintigraphy is theoretically more likely to succeed in terms of acute thrombus imaging than labelling fibrin. Scintigraphic platelet imaging can be achieved in a number of ways, including radiolabelling of autologous platelets, use of monoclonal antibodies against surface receptors and intracellular targets, and binding of synthetic peptides to molecules on the platelet cell membrane.

Human atheroma imaging studies utilizing radiolabelled autologous platelets have produced inconsistent results (Isaka et al., 1986; Minar et al., 1989; Moriwaki et al., 1995, 2000). However, this could be due to important design differences. In a study of 60 patients, 38 of whom had carotid circulation cerebrovascular events, Moriwaki et al. (1995) showed that ^{111}In-labeled platelet accumulation correlated with overall plaque burden and plaque ulceration as detected by careful B-mode ultrasound examination (Figure 19.7). In contrast, Minar *et al.* (1989) in a similar study found no correlation between radiotracer uptake and ultrasound parameters. However, in the former study, images were taken 48 hours following tracer administration and antiplatelet medications were stopped 3 weeks prior to imaging. In the latter study, antiplatelet medications were continued and images were taken 24–26 hours after injection. Therefore, in the first study there is likely to have been higher platelet activity and more time for the accumulation of the ^{111}In-labeled tracer. Nevertheless, the need to image 48 hours after tracer injection in patients not receiving antiplatelet therapy would seriously limit the applicability of this technique to patients with suspected acute vascular events. ^{111}In-platelet scintigraphy has been used to study the effects of antiplatelet agents (Isaka *et al.*, 1986; Moriwaki *et al.*, 2000). Isaka *et al.* investigated the effects of aspirin and ticlopidine (an ADP receptor antagonist) in patients with suspected ischemic cerebrovascular disease (Isaka *et al.*, 1986). They found that tracer accumulation diminished in carotid lesions following treatment with aspirin, but not after ticlopidine. However, there was no control arm and the study was unblinded. Moriwaki *et al.* performed a similar study on the effect of a novel antiplatelet agent, E5510 (Moriwaki *et al.*, 2000). They enrolled patients with carotid or aortic atheroma in which there was high tracer uptake at baseline. The study cohort was split into two, with one half taking the study drug and the other half not. E5510 resulted in a 50% reduction in tracer uptake, whilst there was no significant change in patients in whom the agent was withheld. These two studies demonstrate the potential of noninvasive nuclear imaging to assess the effects of both established and novel pharmacological agents.

Platelet activation in response to exposure of subendothelial tissues following plaque rupture leads to an upregulation of GPIIb/IIIa receptors on the cell surface. Rapid uptake of ^{99m}Tc-P748, a synthetic peptide ligand to the GPIIb/IIIa receptor, has allowed effective imaging of carotid artery thrombus induced in dogs by crush injury (Vallabhajosula, 1996). A similar tracer, ^{99m}Tc-P280, has been injected into nine patients with carotid atherosclerosis who subsequently underwent SPECT imaging of the neck. Uptake was demonstrated in 11 of 18 carotid arteries, but to our knowledge no histological correlation was carried out to assess the sensitivity and specificity of the tracer for labelling platelets (Vallabhajosula *et al.*, 1996). Further studies are clearly needed to address this issue.

Summary

Over the last 30 years, many attempts have been made to image the atherosclerotic plaque using radionuclide-tagged tracer molecules. However, the number of successful in vivo human studies has been few, highlighting the challenging nature of plaque imaging. However, the last decade has seen an upsurge in the number of reported studies, in response to the need for cellular and molecular imaging of the atherosclerotic plaque. Current clinical practice still relies heavily on the use of X-ray angiography to guide both diagnosis and the selection of lesions for interventional treatment, despite the fact that it cannot identify potentially unstable plaques. Nuclear imaging is capable of identifying many of the molecular processes that contribute to plaque rupture and therefore provides one potential solution to the challenge of identifying unstable plaques prior to rupture. However, there is a need to find suitable tracers that can infiltrate the plaque in high enough concentrations to enable in vivo imaging by way of an external detection system, whether that be SPECT or PET. Most atherosclerotic plaques are small in size and lie adjacent to the vessel lumen that often contains a significant concentration of tracer. Therefore advances in detector technology are needed to enable detection of small quantities of tracer and to improve the spatial resolution of SPECT and PET machines.

Given that nuclear imaging provides very little in the way of anatomical information, it is advantageous to combine it with an anatomical imaging modality such as CT or MRI. For this reason, the use of combined PET/CT scanners has become more widespread and research into combining PET with MRI is currently underway.

In terms of functional imaging of human carotid atherosclerosis, 99mTc-annexin-A5-SPECT and FDG-PET currently hold the most promise. FDG-PET has been successfully combined with both CT and MRI to produce high quality images that provide the necessary anatomical and functional data to enable plaque inflammation to be accurately localized within the vascular tree. 99mTc-annexin-A5-SPECT has yet to be combined with anatomical imaging modalities but there is no reason why this should not be possible. It is also likely that in the near future annexin-A5 will be conjugated with a positron-emitting radionuclide to allow PET imaging of apoptosis within the carotid plaque. In addition there are several tracers in preclinical assessment, such as those that identify plaque MMPs and the monocyte chemoattractant, MCP-1. These tracers have the necessary pharmacokinetic profile to improve on what has been achieved with FDG and 99mTc-annexin-A5 imaging.

Before nuclear imaging can become an everyday tool in the clinical management of patients with carotid disease, further studies are necessary, both to optimize currently available techniques and to develop novel tracers with improved pharmacokinetics. In addition, prospective outcome studies involving larger patient numbers need to be carried out to confirm a correlation between high tracer uptake and increased clinical risk. Despite the need for further studies, what is clear is that the current reliance on X-ray angiography is far from ideal and that every effort should be made to find newer technologies to enable clinicians to lower the significant morbidity and mortality caused by carotid atherosclerosis.

Acknowledgements

We would like to acknowledge the hard work carried out by the other members of the team at Cambridge University, not least Dr. Tim Fryer, Dr. David Izquierdo, Dr. John Clark, Dr. Jonathan Gillard, and Dr. Liz Warburton. We would also like to thank The British Heart Foundation who has provided generous funding for our scientific program.

REFERENCES

Andrews, J., Al Nahhas, A., Pennell, D. J., *et al.* (2004). Non-invasive imaging in the diagnosis and management of Takayasu's arteritis. *Annals of the Rheumatic Diseases*, **63**, 995–1000.

Ben Haim, S., Kupzov, E., Tamir, A. and Israel, O. (2004). Evaluation of 18F-FDG uptake and arterial wall calcifications using 18F-FDG PET/CT. *Journal of Nuclear Medicine*, **45**, 1816–21.

Bleeker-Rovers, C. P., Bredie, S. J., van der Meer, J. W., Corstens, F. H. and Oyen, W. J. (2003). F-18-fluorodeoxyglucose positron emission tomography in diagnosis and follow-up of patients with different types of vasculitis. *Netherlands Journal of Medicine*, **61**, 323–9.

Budoff, M. J., Shavelle, D. M., Lamont, D. H., *et al.* (1998). Usefulness of electron beam computed tomography scanning for distinguishing ischemic from nonischemic cardiomyopathy. *Journal of the American College of Cardiology*, **32**, 1173–8.

Cerqueira, M. D., Stratton, J. R., Vracko, R., Schaible, T. F. and Ritchie, J. L. (1992). Noninvasive arterial thrombus imaging with 99mTc monoclonal antifibrin antibody. *Circulation*, **85**, 298–304.

Chen, J., Mehta, J. L., Haider, N., *et al.* (2004). Role of caspases in Ox-LDL-induced apoptotic cascade in human coronary artery endothelial cells. *Circulation Research*, **94**, 370–6.

Ciavolella, M., Tavolaro, R., Taurino, M., *et al.* (1999). Immunoscintigraphy of atherosclerotic uncomplicated lesions in vivo with a monoclonal antibody against D-dimers of insoluble fibrin. *Atherosclerosis*, **143**, 171–5.

Davies, M. J. (1996). Stability and instability: two faces of coronary atherosclerosis. The Paul Dudley White Lecture 1995. *Circulation*, **94**, 2013–20.

Davies, J. R., Rudd, J. H., Fryer, T. D., *et al.* (2005). Identification of culprit lesions after transient ischemic attack by combined 18F fluorodeoxyglucose positron-emission tomography and high-resolution magnetic resonance imaging. *Stroke*, **36**, 2642–7.

Davies, M. J. and Thomas, A. (1984). Thrombosis and acute coronary-artery lesions in sudden cardiac ischemic death. *New England Journal of Medicine*, **310**, 1137–40.

Dunphy, M. P., Freiman, A., Larson, S. M. and Strauss, H. W. (2005). Association of vascular 18F-FDG uptake with vascular calcification. *Journal of Nuclear Medicine*, **46**, 1278–84.

Galis, Z. S., Sukhova, G. K., Lark, M. W. and Libby, P. (1994). Increased expression of matrix metalloproteinases and matrix degrading activity in vulnerable regions of human atherosclerotic plaques. *Journal of Clinical Investment*, **94**, 2493–503.

Golledge, J., Greenhalgh, R. M. and Davies, A. H. (2000). The symptomatic carotid plaque. *Stroke*, **31**, 774–81.

Greco, C., Di Loreto, M., Ciavolella, M., *et al.* (1993). Immunodetection of human atherosclerotic plaque with 125I-labeled monoclonal antifibrin antibodies. *Atherosclerosis*, **100**, 133–9.

Hanif, M. Z., Ghesani, M., Shah, A. A. and Kasai, T. (2004). F-18 fluorodeoxyglucose uptake in atherosclerotic plaque in the mediastinum mimicking malignancy: another potential for error. *Clinical Nuclear Medicine*, **29**, 93–5.

Isaka, Y., Kimura, K., Etani, H., *et al.* (1986). Effect of aspirin and ticlopidine on platelet deposition in carotid atherosclerosis: assessment by indium-111 platelet scintigraphy. *Stroke*, **17**, 1215–20.

Iuliano, L., Signore, A., Vallabajosula, S., *et al.* (1996). Preparation and biodistribution of 99m technetium labelled oxidized LDL in man. *Atherosclerosis*, **126**, 131–41.

Kietselaer, B. L., Reutelingsperger, C. P., Heidendal, G. A., *et al.* (2004). Noninvasive detection of plaque instability with use of radiolabeled annexin A5 in patients with carotid-artery atherosclerosis. *New England Journal of Medicine*, **350**, 1472–3.

Kolodgie, F. D., Edwards, S., Petrov, A., *et al.* (2001). Non-invasive detection of matrix metalloproteinase upregulation in experimental atherosclerotic lesions and its abrogation by dietary modification. *Circulation*, **104**, 694, abstract.

Kolodgie, F. D., Narula, J., Burke, A. P., *et al.* (2000). Localization of apoptotic macrophages at the site of plaque rupture in sudden coronary death. *American Journal of Pathology*, **157**, 1259–68.

Kolodgie, F. D., Petrov, A., Virmani, R., *et al.* (2003). Targeting of apoptotic macrophages and experimental atheroma with radiolabeled annexin V: a technique with potential for noninvasive imaging of vulnerable plaque. *Circulation*, **108**, 3134–9.

Kopka, K., Breyholz, H. J., Wagner, S., *et al.* (2004). Synthesis and preliminary biological evaluation of new radioiodinated MMP inhibitors for imaging MMP activity in vivo. *Nuclear Medicine and Biology*, **31**, 257–67.

Lederman, R. J., Raylman, R. R., Fisher, S. J., *et al.* (2001). Detection of atherosclerosis using a novel positron-sensitive probe and 18-fluorodeoxyglucose (FDG). *Nuclear Medicine Communications*, **22**, 747–53.

Lees, A. M., Lees, R. S., Schoen, F. J., *et al.* (1988). Imaging human atherosclerosis with 99mTc-labeled low density lipoproteins. *Arteriosclerosis*, **8**, 461–70.

Lendon, C. L., Davies, M. J., Born, G. V. and Richardson, P. D. (1991). Atherosclerotic plaque caps are locally weakened when macrophages density is increased. *Atherosclerosis*, **87**, 87–90.

Libby, P., Geng, Y. J. and Aikawa, M., *et al.* (1996). Macrophages and atherosclerotic plaque stability. *Current Opinion Lipidology*, **7**, 330–5.

Libby, P., Geng, Y. J., Sukhova, G. K., Simon, D. I. and Lee, R. T. (1997). Molecular determinants of atherosclerotic plaque vulnerability. *Annals of the New York Academy of Sciences*, **811**, 134–42.

Meller, J., Strutz, F., Siefker, U., *et al.* (2003). Early diagnosis and follow-up of aortitis with (18)F FDG PET and MRI. *European Journal of Nuclear Medicine and Molecular Imaging*, **30**, 730–6.

Mettinger, K. L., Larsson, S., Ericson, K. and Casseborn, S. (1978). Detection of atherosclerotic plaques in carotid arteries by the use of 123I-fibrinogen. *Lancet*, **1**, 242–4.

Minar, E., Ehringer, H., Dudczak, R., *et al.* (1989). Indium-111-labeled platelet scintigraphy in carotid atherosclerosis. *Stroke*, **20**, 27–33.

Mitchel, J., Waters, D., Lai, T., *et al.* (2000). Identification of coronary thrombus with a IIb/IIIa platelet inhibitor radiopharmaceutical, technetium-99m DMP-444: A canine model. *Circulation*, **101**, 1643–6.

Moriwaki, H., Matsumoto, M., Handa, N., *et al.* (1995). Functional and anatomic evaluation of carotid atherothrombosis. A combined study of indium 111 platelet scintigraphy and B-mode ultrasonography. *Arteriosclerosis, Thrombosis, and Vascular Biology*, **15**, 2234–40.

Moriwaki, H., Matsumoto, M., Handa, N., *et al.* (2000). Effect of E5510, a novel antiplatelet agent, on platelet deposition in atherothrombotic lesions: evaluation by 111In platelet scintigraphy. *Nuclear Medicine Communications*, **21**, 1051–8.

Narula, J., Virmani, R. and Zaret, B. (2003). Radionuclide imaging of atherosclerotic lesions. In *Atlas of Nuclear Cardiology*, ed. E. Braunwald, V. Dilsizian and J. Narula. Current Medicine, Philadelphia, pp. 217–35.

Ogawa, M., Ishino, S., Mukai, T., *et al.* (2004). (18)F-FDG accumulation in atherosclerotic plaques: immunohistochemical and PET imaging study. *Journal of Nuclear Medicine*, **45**, 1245–50.

Ohtsuki, K., Hayase, M., Akashi, K., Kopiwoda, S. and Strauss, H. W. (2001). Detection of monocyte chemoattractant protein-1 receptor expression in experimental atherosclerotic lesions: an autoradiographic study. *Circulation*, **104**, 203–8.

Phelps, M. E., Hoffman, E. J., Selin, C., *et al.* (1978). Investigation of 18F 2-fluoro-2-deoxyglucose for the measure of myocardial glucose metabolism. *Journal of Nuclear Medicine*, **19**, 1311–19.

Rosenfeld, M. E. (2002). Leukocyte recruitment into developing atherosclerotic lesions: the complex interaction between multiple molecules keeps getting more complex. *Arteriosclerosis, Thrombosis, and Vascular Biology*, **22**, 361–3.

Rudd, J. H. F., Warburton, E. A., Fryer, T. D., *et al.* (2002). Imaging Atherosclerotic Plaque Inflammation With 18F-Fluorodeoxyglucose Positron Emission Tomography. *Circulation*, **105**, 2708–11.

Schafers, M., Riemann, B., Kopka, K., *et al.* (2004). Scintigraphic imaging of matrix metalloproteinase activity in the arterial wall in vivo. *Circulation*, **109**, 2554–9.

Scopinaro, F., Di Loreto, M., Banci, M., *et al.* (1992). Anti D dimer monoclonal antibodies: a possible scintigraphic agent for immunodetection of thrombi. *Nuclear Medicine Communications*, **13**, 723–9.

Shaw, P. X., Horkko, S., Tsimikas, S., *et al.* (2001). Human-derived anti-oxidized LDL autoantibody blocks uptake of oxidized LDL by macrophages and localizes to atherosclerotic lesions in vivo. *Arteriosclerosis, Thrombosis, and Vascular Biology*, **21**, 1333–9.

Stratton, J. R., Cerqueira, M. D., Dewhurst, T. A. and Kohler, T. R. (1994). Imaging arterial thrombosis: comparison of technetium-99m-labeled monoclonal antifibrin antibodies and indium-111-platelets. *Journal of Nuclear Medicine*, **35**, 1731–7.

Strauss, L. G. and Conti, P. S. (1991). The applications of PET in clinical oncology. *Journal of Nuclear Medicine*, **32**, 623–48.

Tabas, I. (2004). Apoptosis and plaque destabilization in atherosclerosis: the role of macrophage apoptosis induced by cholesterol. *Cell Death Differentiation*, **11** (Suppl. 1), S12–S16.

Tatsumi, M., Cohade, C., Nakamoto, Y. and Wahl, R. L. (2003). Fluorodeoxyglucose uptake in the aortic wall at PET/CT: possible finding for active atherosclerosis. *Radiology*, **229**, 831–7.

Torzewski, M., Shaw, P. X., Han, K. R., *et al.* (2004). Reduced in vivo aortic uptake of radiolabeled oxidation-specific antibodies reflects changes in plaque composition consistent with plaque stabilization. *Arteriosclerosis, Thrombosis, and Vascular Biology*, **24**, 2307–12.

Tsimikas, S., Palinski, W., Halpern, S. E., *et al.* (1999). Radiolabeled MDA2, an oxidation-specific, monoclonal antibody, identifies native atherosclerotic lesions in vivo. *Journal of Nuclear Cardiology*, **6**, 41–53.

Tsimikas, S., Shortal, B. P., Witztum, J. L. and Palinski, W. (2000). In vivo uptake of radiolabeled MDA2, an oxidation-specific monoclonal antibody, provides an accurate measure of atherosclerotic lesions rich in oxidized LDL and is highly sensitive to their regression. *Arteriosclerosis, Thrombosis, and Vascular Biology*, **20**, 689–97.

Vainio, S. and Ikonen, E. (2003). Macrophage cholesterol transport: a critical player in foam cell formation. *Annals of Medicine*, **35**, 146–55.

Vallabhajosula, S. (1996). Technetium-99m-P748, Platelet specific techtide for imaging arterial thrombus: preclinical studies in a canine model of intra-arterial thrombus. *Journal of Nuclear Medicine*, **37** (Suppl.), 152, abstract.

Vallabhajosula, S., Machac, K. and Knesaurek, J. (1996). Imaging atherosclerotic macrophage density by positron emission tomography using F-18 flurodeoxyglucose (FDG). *Journal of Nuclear Medicine*, **37**, 38, abstract.

Vallabhajosula, S., Weiberger, J., Machac, J., *et al.* (1996). Technetium-99m P280, activated platelet specific techtide™: phase II clinical studies in patients with carotid atherosclerosis. *Journal of Nuclear Medicine*, **37** (Suppl.), 272, abstract.

Webb, M., Chambers, A., Al Nahhas, A., *et al.* (2004). The role of 18F-FDG PET in characterising disease activity in Takayasu arteritis. *European Journal of Nuclear Medicine Molecular Imaging*, **31**, 627–34.

Weissberg, P. L. (2004). Noninvasive imaging of atherosclerosis: the biology behind the pictures. *Journal of Nuclear Medicine*, **45**, 1794–5.

Yun, M., Jang, S., Cucchiara, A., Newberg, A. B. and Alavi, A. (2002). 18F FDG uptake in the large arteries: a correlation study with the atherogenic risk factors. *Seminars in Nuclear Medicine*, **32**, 70–6.

Yun, M., Yeh, D., Araujo, L. I., *et al.* (2001). F-18 FDG uptake in the large arteries: a new observation. *Clinical Nuclear Medicine*, **26**, 314–19.

Zheng, Q. H., Fei, X., Liu, X., *et al.* (2002). Synthesis and preliminary biological evaluation of MMP inhibitor radiotracers 11C methyl-halo-CGS 27023A analogs, new potential PET breast cancer imaging agents. *Nuclear Medicine and Biology*, **29**, 761–70.

20

USPIO – enhanced magnetic resonance imaging of carotid atheroma

Simon P. S. Howarth, Tjun Tang, Martin J. Graves, Rikin Trivedi, Jamie Harle and Jonathan H. Gillard

University of Cambridge, Cambridge CB2 ZQQ, UK

Background

It is well described that vulnerable atheroma has a thin fibrous cap overlying a large, necrotic lipid core often with associated inflammation (Stary, 1994; Stary et al., 1994; Stary et al., 1995; Stary, 2000a,b; Stary, 2001). Over half of the ischemic strokes in the developed world are thought to be due to rupture of extracranial plaque and a significant proportion of this plaque can be found either at the carotid bifurcation or just above the bifurcation in the internal carotid artery (Pasterkamp et al., 1998; Kiechl and Willeit, 1999; Ono et al., 2001; Zhang et al., 2001; Gaigalaite, 2002; Hollander et al., 2002). Plaque rupture involves the mechanical failure of the fibrous cap, thereby exposing the blood to the necrotic lipid core. This endothelial disruption leads to platelet aggregation and the formation of a luminal thrombus which can then either totally occlude the lumen or, more commonly, throw off emboli to the distal intracranial vasculature. Plaques also develop in this manner with organization of the thrombus eventually leading to the seeding of a new fibrous cap from systemic endothelial progenitor cells (Pulvirenti et al., 2000; Littlewood and Bennett, 2003; Stoneman and Bennett, 2004) and an increase in the overall level of stenosis. Histologically this can be demonstrated with many plaque specimens showing evidence of multiple fibrous caps within the substance of the plaque (Figure 20.1).

Fibrous caps are thought to thin and weaken due to a number of mechanisms including direct mechanical fatigue (Tang et al., 2001; Stehbens, 2002; Wu et al., 2003; Tang et al., 2004), apoptotic cell death with the fibrous cap (Littlewood and Bennett, 2003) and weakening of the extracellular collagen matrix by enzymes such as matrix metalloproteinases (Browatzki et al., 2005; Chen et al., 2005; Kong et al., 2005; May et al., 2005; Newby, 2005; Solini et al., 2005), secreted by activated macrophages amongst other immune cells. This inflammatory process is thought to be crucial in the development of vulnerable plaque and may indeed be the key to its future definition.

Conventional clinical risk assessment of patients is based upon the findings of the North American symptomatic carotid endarterectomy trial (NASCET) and European carotid surgery trial (ECST) and is based solely on luminal stenosis (Rothwell and Warlow, 1999; Henderson et al., 2000; Bond et al., 2002; Cunningham et al., 2002; Naylor et al., 2003; Rothwell et al., 2003a,b). These trials showed a benefit from carotid endarterectomy in symptomatic patients who have a stenosis of 70% or more. More recently the asymptomatic carotid surgery trial (ACST) (Halliday et al., 1995; Robless et al., 1998; Naylor, 2004; Rothwell and Goldstein, 2004) has likewise

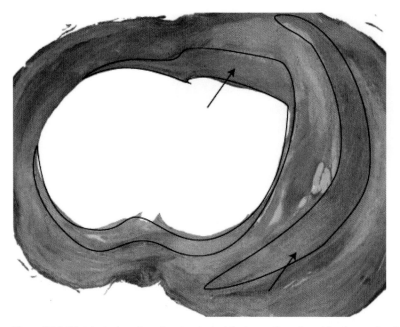

Figure 20.1 Histological section showing typical features of a vulnerable plaque showing multiple fibrous caps (arrow heads).

reported a benefit of endarterectomy in totally asymptomatic carotid stenosis of 70% or more. None of these trials were able to answer the question as to whether patients with 50–69% stenosis would also benefit from intervention.

Although important, methods used to measure luminal stenosis, namely conventional X-ray angiography, Doppler ultrasound, computerized tomography angiography and contrast-enhanced magnetic resonance angiography, do not give any information about the plaque components or their relative proportions. Further, the process of arterial remodelling may underestimate the atheroma burden present in a particular patient and therefore their risk of stroke. Cross-sectional, high-resolution magnetic resonance imaging (MRI) and, to a certain extent, intravascular ultrasound (IVUS) have allowed this deficiency to be overcome but in vivo imaging of inflammation has until recently been impossible. IVUS is, of course, highly invasive whereas MRI provides an ideal platform

for the noninvasive in vivo assessment of plaque biology.

Ultrasmall paramagnetic iron oxide (USPIO)-enhanced MRI imaging is a promising noninvasive method to identify high-risk atheromatous plaques, of which inflammation plays a significant role as previously discussed. Lesions at risk for rupture usually show accumulation of macrophages (Ross, 1999) either at the shoulders of the plaque or in the necrotic lipid core.

USPIO

Super-paramagnetic iron oxide (SPIO) agents consist of microcrystalline magnetite cores coated with dextrans or siloxanes with typical diameters of 5–200 nm. After injection they accumulate in the reticuloendothelial system (RES) of the liver (Kupffer cells) and the spleen. Iron oxide particles function as contrast-enhancing agents by creating a large dipolar magnetic field gradient that acts on

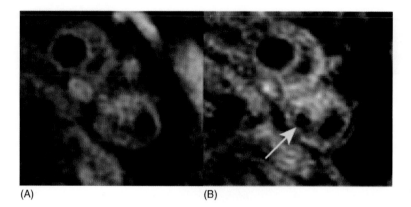

(A)   (B)

Figure 20.2 Pre (A) and postUSPIO (B) MR imaging of a symptomatic carotid plaque. Focal USPIO uptake can be seen at 24 hours (yellow arrow head).

the water molecules that diffuse close to the particles (Bulte *et al.*, 1999, 2002). SPIO particles have a very large T_2/T_1 ratio so that although they increase both T_1 and T_2 relaxation, in general the T_2 effects dominate to the extent that negative contrast is observed in both T_1-weighted and T_2-weighted imaging. The predominant T_2 effects create an area of hypointensity on conventional spin-echo MR sequences that is enhanced further by compaction, for example within cells (Figure 20.2). The intracellular compaction also appears to reduce the T_1 effect considerably (Bulte *et al.*, 2001; Billotey *et al.*, 2003). Gradient echo MR sequences appear to be even more sensitive than spin-echo sequences for detecting the contrast agent, by virtue of the inherent T_2^* sensitivity of these sequences (Bulte *et al.*, 1992; Bulte *et al.*, 1995; Bulte *et al.*, 1998; Bulte *et al.*, 1999; Billotey *et al.*, 2003; Foster-Gareau *et al.*, 2003). The degree of magnetic susceptibility effect (blooming) can be controlled by specifying data acquisition parameters that have more or less T_2 and T_2^* dependence. It should therefore be noted that the extent of signal drop is not directly proportional to SPIO concentration, since the blooming effect may extend some distance depending upon the imaging parameters.

USPIO agents, typically with a mean diameter less than 50 nm, have a different biodistribution. They do not accumulate in the RES so rapidly which results in a longer plasma half-life. This feature together with the fact that the T_2/T_1 ratio decreases with decreasing particle size, has led to some USPIO agents being proposed as potential blood pool agents for magnetic resonance angiography (MRA), e.g. code 7228 (*Ferumoxytol*, Advanced Magnetics Inc, Cambridge, MA). In addition USPIO particles with a mean diameter of less than 10 nm will accumulate in lymph nodes by, for example, direct transcapillary passage through endothelial venules where they are readily phagocytosed by monocyte-derived macrophages. This has led to at least one USPIO agent, ferumoxtran-10 (*Sinerem*, Laboratoire Guerbet, Paris; *Combidex*, Advanced Magnetics, Cambridge, MA), being used for the detection of metastatic disease in lymph nodes. Metastatic nodes demonstrate less uptake of this agent allowing differentiation of normal-sized metastatic nodes from uninvolved normal nodes that appear hypointense. Since macrophage accumulation in the vessel wall is a marker of vulnerability it has been thought that USPIOs may also accumulate within atherosclerotic lesions. Studies in hyperlipidemic rabbits (Corot *et al.*, 2003; Corot *et al.*, 2004; Crowe, 2005) have revealed that USPIO particles are taken up by macrophage-laden aortic plaques as intracellular inclusions and reveal areas of focal signal loss on T_2^*-weighted

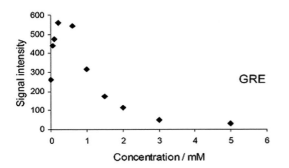

Figure 20.3 Graph to show relationship between USPIO concentration and signal intensity on standard GRE imaging at 1.5 T. It can clearly be seen that low concentrations of USPIO result in a signal enhancement, whereas higher concentrations lead to signal loss (via its T_2^* effect). (Graph courtesy of Dr. L. Crowe, Brompton Hospital, London, UK.)

MRI within the vessel wall when compared with precontrast images. Indeed it was as part of a study investigating the use of Sinerem for the staging of lymph node metastases that focal signal loss was first incidentally noted in segments of arterial wall in vivo that was attributed to USPIO uptake in atherosclerotic plaques (Schmitz et al., 2001).

The signal intensity changes with increasing concentration of Sinerem are shown in Figure 20.3. The figure shows an increase in signal intensity at low concentrations due to the predominately T_1 shortening effects of the Sinerem followed by a signal decrease with increasing concentration as T_2/T_2^* effects start to dominate (Crowe, 2005). Whilst conventional imaging sequences use relatively long TE gradient echo or spin echo sequences resulting in Sinerem uptake being depicted as areas of hypointensity, the use of imaging sequences with ultrashort echo times (uTE) can reduce the T_2^* influence and provide images where the Sinerem signal can be seen to increase.

Clinical studies

Sinerem has been used in the evaluation of human carotid atheroma (Schmitz et al., 2002; Kooi et al., 2003; Schmitz, 2003; Trivedi et al., 2003; Trivedi

et al., 2004a,b) in which areas of focal signal loss on in vivo MR images have been shown to correspond to accumulation of iron particles in ex vivo specimens. USPIOs are thought to accumulate predominantly in macrophages in ruptured and rupture-prone human atherosclerotic lesions.

Kooi first showed that USPIO uptake induces significant signal decreases in the in vivo T_2^*w MR images obtained using an electrocardiogram (ECG)-triggered gradient echo sequence with a TE of 20 ms, acquired 24 hours after intravenous administration of USPIO (Kooi et al., 2003). Moreover clustering of iron oxide particles in tissue may lead to additional T_2^* shortening and the "blooming effect" (Chambon et al., 1993). This signal decrease was found to be attenuated in images acquired after 72 hours. This suggested that there is an active process of accumulation and excretion of USPIO particles.

Trivedi et al. went on to investigate in more detail the in vivo temporal relationship of signal intensity reduction on MRI after USPIO administration in symptomatic patients scheduled for carotid endarterectomy (Trivedi et al., 2004a). An ECG-triggered quadruple inversion recovery (QIR) prepared (Yarnykh and Yuan, 2002) spiral sequence was used. The QIR preparation suppresses the high luminal signal both pre- and post-Sinerem administration, whilst the spiral acquisition provides a highly time-efficient method for data collection. Two acquisitions with effective echo times of 5.6 ms and 15.0 ms were acquired. Eight consecutive patients with severe internal carotid artery stenosis underwent multisequence MR imaging of the carotid bifurcation before and 24, 36, 48, and 72 hours after USPIO administration. There was a distinct temporal variation in the size of the area showing signal intensity loss between images from any one patient. The earliest discernible signal loss was evident by 24 hours becoming more visually obvious at 36 hours after infusion and remaining so at 48 hours after infusion (Figure 20.4). The area of signal loss began to decrease after 48 hours but was still visible on images taken 96 hours after infusion.

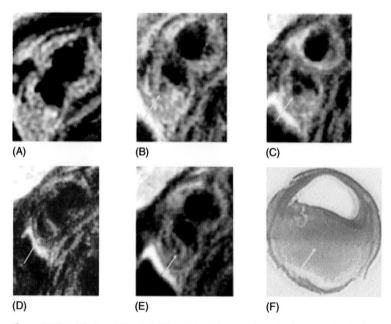

(A)   (B)   (C)

(D)   (E)   (F)

Figure 20.4 Axial short TE spiral T_2^*-weighted images through the same level of the internal carotid artery of a patient before infusion (A) and at 24 hours (B); 36 hours (C); 48 hours (D); and 96 hours (E) after infusion of Sinerem, and the matched histological section obtained 8 days after infusion, stained with elastin van Gieson to demonstrate plaque morphology (F). (A), The fibrous cap is visualized as showing no signal loss on the preinfusion image. (B), An area of signal loss is evident in subendothelial region (arrow). (C) and (D), The area of signal loss has increased in size (arrow). (E), The size of the area of signal loss has decreased but is still visible. (F), The excised plaque shows typical features of the "vulnerable" plaque, a thin fibrous cap (arrowhead) overlying a large lipid core (arrow).

The area of signal intensity loss localized to the fibrous cap region on histological co-registration and localization suggesting that it is the macrophages that are taking up the USPIO. This was confirmed with double staining techniques using Perls (an iron stain) and anti-CD 68 (for macrophages) (Figure 20.5). Transmission electron microscopy was utilized to visualize the USPIO particles within the phagolysosomes of the macrophages (Figure 20.6). This temporal change in the resultant signal intensity reduction on MRI suggests an optimal time window for the detection of macrophages on postinfusion imaging.

This study was later validated with a larger cohort of 30 patients whereby over 90% of symptomatic patients who were also scheduled for carotid endarterectomy showed USPIO enhancement. Qualitative MR analysis was highly sensitive (92.5) and moderately specific (64%) for detection of USPIO particles in atheromatous plaque. In addition there was good agreement between MR imaging and histology.

Howarth *et al.* also used USPIO to compare patients with symptomatic and asymptomatic carotid stenosis. They reported that USPIO appeared to show a dual contrast effect with signal enhancement being seen in plaques with little inflammation and large fibrous caps. Although seen best on T_1-weighted imaging, the effect was also seen on T_2^*-weighted imaging (GRE spiral) (Figure 20.7). They concluded that this phenomenon may be due to the signal enhancement seen on

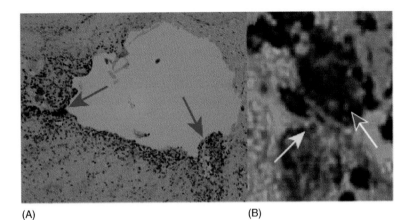

(A)   (B)

Figure 20.5 Double stained symptomatic plaque using Perls stain (for iron) and CD68 (macrophages). Inset shows USPIO particles in CD68-positive macrophages.

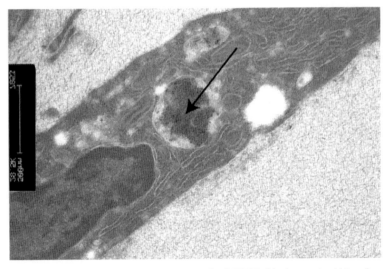

Figure 20.6 Transmission electron micrograph of USPIO (black arrow) within a human monocyte macrophage (image courtesy of Dr. Jeremy Skepper and Dr. Karin Muller, Multi Imaging Centre, University of Cambridge, UK).

gradient echo imaging at low concentrations of USPIO (Figure 20.3).

Symptomatic patients had more focal areas of signal drop than asymptomatics, thus suggesting that their plaques had large inflammatory infiltrates. Asymptomatic plaques showed significantly more enhancement in both T_1-weighted and T_2^*-weighted images than symptomatic plaque

suggesting more stability as a result of thicker fibrous caps. However some asymptomatic plaques also showed focal areas of signal drop, suggesting an occult macrophage burden. It is perhaps this group that would benefit most from this technique, allowing identification of inflammation within otherwise morphologically ''stable'' plaques.

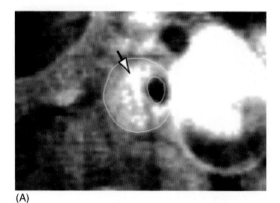

(A)

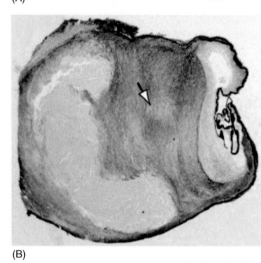

(B)

Figure 20.7 Post-USPIO imaging of an asymptomatic carotid plaque with corresponding histology. Note the signal enhancement associated with the thick fibrous cap (arrowheads).

The conclusion was that, if validated by larger studies, USPIO particles may prove a useful dual contrast medium able to enhance the risk stratification of patients with carotid stenosis thus improving patient selection for intervention.

The contralateral side of symptomatic patients given USPIO were also analyzed. It was found that 95% patients showed bilateral USPIO uptake (Figure 20.8) suggesting an inflammatory burden within their carotid atheroma bilaterally. Only one

patient with USPIO signal decrease on the symptomatic side showed no signal decrease on the asymptomatic side. This finding highlights the truly systemic nature of vulnerable atheroma and that patients showing inflammatory activity on one side may be more likely to have it contralaterally than truly asymptomatic patients. Thus patients who have a symptomatic carotid stenosis and who are found to have contralateral disease should be closely followed up with a low threshold for intervention.

Methods of analysis

T$_2$*-weighted imaging

The region of interest approach

As previously discussed, although T$_2$*-weighted imaging does allow the visualisation of the effect of USPIO particles, there has been much debate in the literature as how best to quantify this and whether the degree of signal loss is in any way proportional to the inflammatory load within the plaque. Trivedi *et al.* used manually delineated regions of interest and calculated the normalized signal change between pre- and post-USPIO images. The signal was normalized to the signal in the adjacent sternocleidomastoid muscle and any ROIs drawn that showed an actual normalized signal drop were taken to indicate USPIO uptake. This showed only a moderate correlation with macrophages staining positively for USPIO on Perls staining (Pearson's product moment 0.6).

Although useful, this technique has an inherent problem of bias and observer error leading to some question as to its usefulness in quantification of inflammatory burden.

The quadrant approach and its statistical challenges

A more recent approach has been to arbitrarily divide the vessel wall in each slice into quadrants

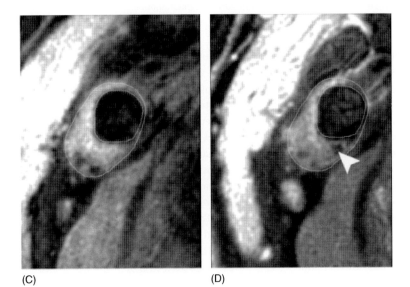

(A)

(B)

(C)

(D)

Figure 20.8 Pre-(left) and post-USPIO (right) imaging showing USPIO uptake in both the symptomatic plaque (A) and the contralateral asymptomatic plaque (B) in the same patient.

by constructing perpendiculars to the horizontal axis across the image (Figure 20.9) This technique has the advantage that data points come from the whole vessel and every section has plaque rather than the rather biased population of ROIs. Thus, a quadrant showing signal loss, once normalized to adjacent muscle, is taken to mean USPIO uptake in that quadrant. Whilst eliminating operator bias, this technique has a number of problems associated with it. First, small focal areas of signal loss may be lost in a quadrant when regions of signal enhancement are found around it, limiting the

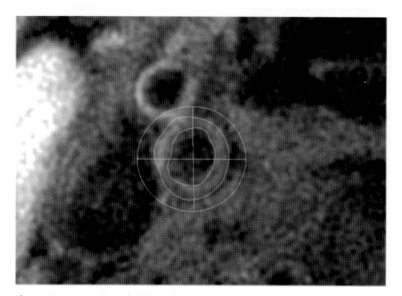

Figure 20.9 Screenshot of CMR Tools (London) showing method of quadrant segmentation.

spatial resolution of the analysis. Second, any statistical analysis needs to consider the quadrants as populations and compare one population with another (for example, quadrants from symptomatic patients against quadrants from asymptomatic patients). In order for parametric statistics to be useful, a number of assumptions are made as a matter of course. A simple two-tailed t-test assumes that the quadrants are normally distributed and that each quadrant represents a totally independent observation. In taking only 10 symptomatic cases, it is clear that the signal change in the quadrants appears to be very close to a normal distribution (Figure 20.10). However, the assumption that each quadrant represents a completely independent observation is obviously over simplistic.

One quadrant is likely to depend on another to some extent not only within the slice but also between the slices (Figure 20.11). Data will therefore be clustered and simple parametric statistics will therefore falter since the number of degrees of freedom for a simple t-test will be related to the number of quadrants rather than

the number of patients and therefore the overall test statistic will be calculated to be artificially high. Thus any *p*-value will be artificially low.

In an attempt to tackle these problems, a complex repeated measures mixed model was used to model true variances in quadrant data from ten symptomatic individuals. Patient group (symptomatic or asymptomatic) was fitted as a fixed effect, and patient as a random effect. Slice and quadrant were used to define the within-patient correlation. The best fitting correlation structure was selected using the Akaike Information Criterion. Estimates of signal change within each group were calculated with appropriate 95% confidence intervals adjusting for the correlation between measurements made on the same subject. An estimate of the difference between groups with appropriate 95% confidence interval was also calculated, together with a *p*-value testing the hypothesis of no difference between groups. Model assumptions regarding homogeneity of variance were verified by inspection of residual plots. Distributional assumptions regarding normality were verified by assessment of normal probability

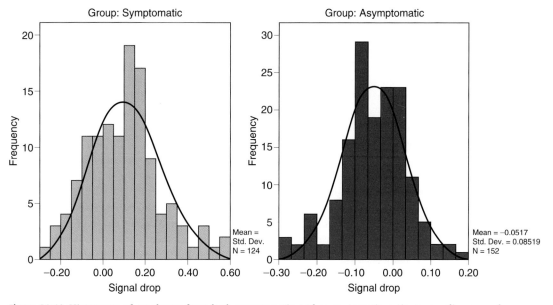

Figure 20.10 Histograms of quadrants from both symptomatic and asymptomatic patients revealing normal distributions.

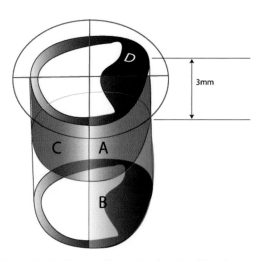

Figure 20.11 Diagram illustrating that signal loss in quadrant A is not independent and will depend to a certain extent on quadrants B, C and D, in other words, within slice and between slice correlation. Thus, individual quadrants cannot be deemed to be completely independent observations statistically.

plots. The analysis was carried out using PROC MIXED in SAS for Windows version 8.2.

This repeated measures mixed model shows promise in the analysis of USPIO enhanced T_2^*-weighted imaging and may well aid in detailed analysis of signal loss secondary to USPIO uptake.

T_2^* quantification

Although T_2^*-weighted imaging allows visualization of USPIO uptake, the need to normalize the signal in quadrants to the adjacent muscle is problematic. It makes assumptions that the signal in the muscle should not change following USPIO infusion and that any change in muscle signal will be related to varying sensitivity of the surface coil across the field of view between the two imaging sessions, 36 hours apart. This is clearly an inaccurate assumption and the need to normalize the signal to the adjacent muscle is a potential source of significant error and variability. Further, the signal response at the muscle ROI may very well be different to the signal response at the carotid wall quadrant and the two may not be directly comparable.

An accurate and reliable quantitative assessment of in vivo inflammatory atheroma burden is crucial for studies designed to look at the efficacies of new pharmacological interventions currently aimed at the stabilization of vulnerable plaque target inflammatory activity. One potential solution is to measure the carotid wall T_2^* before and after administration of USPIO particles as an index of macrophage quantification. It should be noted that T_2^* relaxometry for quantitative imaging is strongly hampered by large-scale field inhomogeneities, which lead to signal losses and an overestimation of the relaxation rate R_2^* ($1/T_2^*$). This is of course a potentially major problem in USPIO-enhanced imaging although a number of methods to ameliorate the problem have been reported in the literature. These techniques include increasing the spatial resolution, altering the slice-selection gradient or using a tailored radiofrequency pulse. A further technique is to use 3D high-resolution static magnetic field (B_0) maps to recover the signal loss in images acquired by a 2D multiecho sequence. Dahnke *et al.* have reported a method utilizing a combination of these techniques (Dahnke and Schaeffter, 2005). Their corrected T_2^* maps show reduced influence of the local field variation and demonstrate a better spatial distribution of the agent.

Light from the dark spot?

As has already been discussed, conventional USPIO-enhanced MR sequences have relied on the T_2^* susceptibility effect of iron oxide to visualize a hypointensity in the post-USPIO imaging that was not present in the pre-USPIO imaging. There are, of course, a number of problems using such a "negative" contrast agent. First, species other than iron oxide can result in low signal on T_2^*-weighted imaging, the most obvious example of which is calcium. Large calcified deposits

particularly in the shoulders of the plaque or the lipid core can produce large areas of signal loss. It is primarily for this reason that pre-USPIO imaging needs to be performed. Unfortunately it is very difficult to accurately match pre- and 36 hours postimaging locations. Therefore when estimating signal reductions from pre- to post-USPIO imaging, it is inevitable that slightly different volumes of tissue will be considered and therefore this will produce an inherent error in the signal difference calculation.

If it were possible to demonstrate USPIO particle uptake as hyperintense rather than hypointense, it may be possible to do away with preimaging and therefore the inherent error that this inevitably causes. Recently three different approaches have been adopted to make this seemly impossible task a reality; uTE, inversion recovery on-resonance water suppression (IRON) imaging and Gradient echo acquisition for superparamagnetic particles with positive contrast (GRASP).

Ultra-short TE imaging

Crowe *et al.* (2005) have shown that if an imaging sequence with an extremely short echo time (TE), i.e. 80 μs, is used then the T_2/T_2^* effects can be substantially reduced and the USPIO signal made hyperintense due to the T_1 shortening effects of the agent. This effect can be further enhanced by acquiring two images, one with a relatively "long" TE, i.e. XX ms and the other with the "ultra-short" TE and performing a subtraction image. This technique was assessed in a rabbit model of atherosclerosis (Figure 20.12). uTE imaging should not render calcified deposits high signal as previously discussed and therefore potentially eliminate the necessity for pre-USPIO imaging.

IRON imaging

IRON imaging (Stuber, 2005) uses a completely different principle to that of uTE imaging but the goal is the same; positive contrast where previously there was only the possibility of negative contrast.

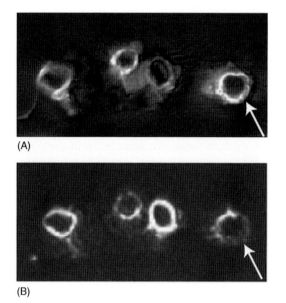

(A)

(B)

Figure 20.12 Ultra short echo time (UTE) imaging of ex vivo hyperlipidemic rabbit aorta following administration of different concentrations of USPIO. UTE imaging (B) is compared with GRE imaging (A). USPIO uptake can easily be seen (white arrows) (image courtesy of Dr. L. Crowe, Brompton Hospital, London, UK).

IRON is an imaging methodology that enables the signal-enhanced visualization of nondiamagnetic materials. Using a spectrally selective saturation prepulse, the signal originating from on-resonant protons can be suppressed. However, this saturation pulse does not affect off-resonant protons in close proximity to nondiamagnetic particles such as USPIO. Therefore, signal enhancement adjacent to these particles can be generated while the on-resonant background appears signal-attenuated. Changing the bandwidth of the saturation pulse can change the size of the area of enhancement. Fat saturation is obtained by adding preceding dual-inversion prepulses and timing the read out for the point at which the on-resonance spins cross zero magnetization. In this case the signal enhancement is created in tissue adjacent to the USPIO so this type of imaging may well not be useful for accurate spatial localization of the USPIO effect but rather confirmation that it is actually present at all.

A similar technique has been proposed by Cunningham *et al.* who also used a spectrally selective RF pulse to excite and refocus the off-resonance water surrounding USPIO-labelled cells both in an animal model in vivo and in a phantom (Cunningham *et al.*, 2002). Thus only the fluid and tissue adjacent to the cells were visible in the image. They also found that there was a significant linear correlation ($r = 0.87$, $p < 0.005$) between the estimated number of cells and signal observed, opening up the possibility that this technique may be useful for quantification of USPIO uptake.

GRASP imaging

Mani *et al.* have recently published the technique of GRASP imaging to obtain positive contrast with USPIO uptake (Mani *et al.*, 2006). GRASP images off-resonant spins in a similar fashion to the IRON sequence. In a conventional gradient echo acquisition, after an excitation pulse, the slice selection gradient dephases the spins. To rephase the excited spins, normally the full 100% rephasing gradient is used to compensate for the slice selection area. This is indicated by the magnetic moment of zero at the completion of the rephasing gradient pulse. If the amplitude of this rephasing gradient is decreased (for example, to 25%), it creates a gradient imbalance that will effectively reduce the signal under normal circumstances. However, in locations where a negative local gradient (caused by a super paramagnetic material) is present, the gradient balance is restored and a bright signal can be seen. Locations where a dipole field is not present will appear dark, thus providing positive contrast in regions where super paramagnetic material is present with respect to the background.

The GRASP sequence generated positive signal enhancement in the phantoms containing iron. For all rephasing values ≤30%, positive contrast was observed. This sequence has yet to be tested in vivo but shows promise as a useful tool for localizing USPIO uptake particularly in tissue with significant intrinsic T_2^* effects.

The future for USPIO

Although showing great promise for the noninvasive assessment of carotid atheroma, it is likely that the future for USPIO compounds will lie with more targeted agents. Work on agents of this sort thus far in humans has been limited to fibrin-targeted gadolinium-based imaging. However, molecular targeting of contrast agents to either membrane-bound receptors or free proteins will eventually allow "in vivo microscopy" at an exquisite resolution with the use of high-field clinical systems. Such potential targets could include Interleukin (IL)-1 receptors, matrix metalloproteinase (MMP)-7, MMP-9 and tumor necrosis factor (TNF) alpha to name but a few. Receptors involved in the apoptotic pathway in vascular smooth muscle cells (VSMCs) are also under scrutiny as potential targets although, as yet, no useable agents have come forth from this research.

Macrophage markers, well known in histological circles such as MAC387 and CD68 could well be used as targeted moieties for specific USPIOs to further aid localization of USPIOs to these cells and lastly, USPIO-tagged HDL may well be a possibility in the future.

As novel sequences are developed and more clinical work is done, a consensus may finally be reached in the literature as to how best quantify USPIO uptake in inflammatory atheroma and how this may change over time and following pharmaceutical intervention. It is quite clear that USPIO-enhanced MR imaging will have a major role to play in the development of atheroma-stabilizing drugs of the future and may have a place in the risk stratification of asymptomatic atheroma and medium stenotic atheroma and selection for subsequent intervention.

Acknowledgement

Dr. Sam Miller for statistical support in preparation of this chapter.

REFERENCES

Billotey, C., Wilhelm, C., Devaud, M., *et al.* (2003). Cell internalization of anionic maghemite nanoparticles: Quantitative effect on magnetic resonance imaging. *Magnetic Resonance in Medicine*, **49**, 646–54.

Bond, R., Narayan, S. K., Rothwell, P. M. and Warlow, C. P. (2002). Clinical and radiographic risk factors for operative stroke and death in the European carotid surgery trial. *European Journal of Vascular and Endovascular Surgery*, **23**, 108–16.

Browatzki, M., Larsen, D., Pfeiffer, C. A., *et al.* (2005). Angiotensin II stimulates matrix metalloproteinase secretion in human vascular smooth muscle cells via nuclear factor-kappaB and activator protein 1 in a redox-sensitive manner. *Journal of Vascular Research*, **42**, 415–23.

Bulte, J. W., Brooks, R. A., Moskowitz, B. M., Bryant, L. H., Jr. and Frank, J. A. (1998). T_1 and T_2 relaxometry of monocrystalline iron oxide nanoparticles (MION-46L): theory and experiment. *Academic Radiology*, **5** (Suppl. 1), S137–40; discussion S145–6.

Bulte, J. W., Brooks, R. A., Moskowitz, B. M., Bryant, L. H., Jr. and Frank, J. A. (1999). Relaxometry and magnetometry of the MR contrast agent MION-46L. *Magnetic Resonance in Medicine*, **42**, 379–84.

Bulte, J. W., De Jonge, M. W., Kamman, R. L., *et al.* (1992). Dextran-magnetite particles: contrast-enhanced MRI of blood-brain barrier disruption in a rat model. *Magnetic Resonance in Medicine*, **23**, 215–23.

Bulte, J. W., Douglas, T., Mann, S., *et al.* (1995). Initial assessment of magnetoferritin biokinetics and proton relaxation enhancement in rats. *Academic Radiology*, **2**, 871–8.

Bulte, J. W., Douglas, T., Witwer, B., *et al.* (2001). Magneto-dendrimers allow endosomal magnetic labeling and in vivo tracking of stem cells. *Nature Biotechnology*, **19**, 1141–7.

Bulte, J. W., Duncan, I. D. and Frank, J. A. (2002). In vivo magnetic resonance tracking of magnetically labeled cells after transplantation. *Journal of Cerebral Blood Flow and Metabolism*, **22**, 899–907.

Chambon, C., Clement, O., Le Blanche, A., Schouman-Claeys, E. and Frija, G. (1993). Superparamagnetic iron oxides as positive MR contrast agents: in vitro and in vivo evidence. *Magnetic Resonance in Imaging*, **11**, 509–19.

Chen, F., Eriksson, P., Hansson, G. K., *et al.* (2005). Expression of matrix metalloproteinase 9 and its regulators in the unstable coronary atherosclerotic plaque. *International Journal of Molecular Medicine*, **15**, 57–65.

Corot, C., Petry, K. G., Trivedi, R., *et al.* (2004). Macrophage imaging in central nervous system and in carotid atherosclerotic plaque using ultrasmall superparamagnetic iron oxide in magnetic resonance imaging. *Investigative Radiology*, **39**, 619–25.

Corot, C., Violas, X., Robert, P., Gagneur, G. and Port, M. (2003). Comparison of different types of blood pool agents (P792, MS325, USPIO) in a rabbit MR angiography-like protocol. *Investigative Radiology*, **38**, 311–19.

Crowe, L. (2005). Ex vivo MR imaging of atherosclerotic rabbit aorta labelled with USPIO – Enhancement of iron loaded regions in UTE imaging. *Proceedings of the International Society of Magnetic Resonance in Medicine*, **13**, 115.

Cunningham, E. J., Bond, R., Mehta, Z., *et al.* (2002). Long-term durability of carotid endarterectomy for symptomatic stenosis and risk factors for late postoperative stroke. *Stroke*, **33**, 2658–63.

Dahnke, H. and Schaeffter, T. (2005). Limits of detection of SPIO at 3.0 T using T2 relaxometry. *Magnetic Resonance in Medicine*, **53**, 1202–6.

Foster-Gareau, P., Heyn, C., Alejski, A. and Rutt, B. K. (2003). Imaging single mammalian cells with a 1.5 T clinical MRI scanner. *Magnetic Resonance in Medicine*, **49**, 968–71.

Gaigalaite, V. (2002). Atherosclerosis-related stroke: risk factors, location, outcome. *Medicina (Kaunas)*, **38**, 617–23.

Halliday, A. W., Thomas, D. J. and Mansfield, A. O. (1995). The asymptomatic carotid surgery trial (ACST). *International Angiology*, **14**, 18–20.

Henderson, R. D., Eliasziw, M., Fox, A. J., Rothwell, P. M. and Barnett, H. J. (2000). Angiographically defined collateral circulation and risk of stroke in patients with severe carotid artery stenosis. North American Symptomatic Carotid Endarterectomy Trial (NASCET) Group. *Stroke*, **31**, 128–32.

Hollander, M., Bots, M. L., Del Sol, A. I., *et al.* (2002). Carotid plaques increase the risk of stroke and subtypes

of cerebral infarction in asymptomatic elderly: the Rotterdam study. *Circulation*, **105**, 2872–7.

Kiechl, S. and Willeit, J. (1999). The natural course of atherosclerosis. Part II: vascular remodeling. Bruneck Study Group. *Arteriosclerosis, Thrombosis and Vascular Biology*, **19**, 1491–8.

Kong, Y. Z., Huang, X. R., Ouyang, X., *et al.* (2005). Evidence for vascular macrophage migration inhibitory factor in destabilization of human atherosclerotic plaques. *Cardiovascular Research*, **65**, 272–82.

Kooi, M. E., Cappendijk, V. C., Cleutjens, K. B., *et al.* (2003). Accumulation of ultrasmall superparamagnetic particles of iron oxide in human atherosclerotic plaques can be detected by in vivo magnetic resonance imaging. *Circulation*, **107**, 2453–8.

Littlewood, T. D. and Bennett, M. R. (2003). Apoptotic cell death in atherosclerosis. *Current Opinion in Lipidology*, **14**, 469–75.

Mani, V., Briley-Saebo, K. C., Itskovich, V. V., Samber, D. D. and Fayad, Z. A. (2006). Gradient echo acquisition for superparamagnetic particles with positive contrast (GRASP): sequence characterization in membrane and glass superparamagnetic iron oxide phantoms at 1.5T and 3T. *Magnetic Resonance in Medicine*, **55**, 126–35.

May, A. E., Schmidt, R., Bulbul, B. O., *et al.* (2005). Plasminogen and matrix metalloproteinase activation by enzymatically modified low density lipoproteins in monocytes and smooth muscle cells. *Thrombosis and Haemostasis*, **93**, 710–15.

Naylor, A. R. (2004). The Asymptomatic Carotid Surgery Trial: bigger study, better evidence. *British Journal of Surgery*, **91**, 787–9.

Naylor, A. R., Rothwell, P. M. and Bell, P. R. (2003). Overview of the principal results and secondary analyses from the European and North American randomised trials of endarterectomy for symptomatic carotid stenosis. *European Journal of Vascular and Endovascular Surgery*, **26**, 115–29.

Newby, A. C. (2005). Dual role of matrix metalloproteinases (matrixins) in intimal thickening and atherosclerotic plaque rupture. *Physiological Reviews*, **85**, 1–31.

Ono, K., Watanabe, S., Daimon, Y., *et al.* (2001). Diagnosis of carotid artery atheroma by magnetic resonance imaging. *Japanese Circulation Journal*, **65**, 139–44.

Pasterkamp, G., Schoneveld, A. H., Hillen, B., *et al.* (1998). Is plaque formation in the common carotid artery representative for plaque formation and luminal stenosis in other atherosclerotic peripheral arteries? A post mortem study. *Atherosclerosis*, **137**, 205–10.

Pulvirenti, T. J., Yin, J. L. and Chaufour, X. (2000). P2X (purinergic) receptor redistribution in rabbit aorta following injury to endothelial cells and cholesterol feeding. *Journal of Neurocytology*, **29**, 623–31.

Robless, P., Emson, M., Thomas, D., Mansfield, A. and Halliday, A. (1998). Are we detecting and operating on high risk patients in the asymptomatic carotid surgery trial? The Asymptomatic Carotid Surgery Trial Collaborators. *European Journal of Vascular and Endovascular Surgery*, **16**, 59–64.

Ross, R. (1999). Atherosclerosis is an inflammatory disease. *American Heart Journal*, **138**, S419–20.

Rothwell, P. M. and Warlow, C. P. (1999). Prediction of benefit from carotid endarterectomy in individual patients: a risk-modelling study. European Carotid Surgery Trialists' Collaborative Group. *Lancet*, **353**, 2105–10.

Rothwell, P. M., Eliasziw, M., Gutnikov, S. A., *et al.* (2003a). Analysis of pooled data from the randomised controlled trials of endarterectomy for symptomatic carotid stenosis. *Lancet*, **361**, 107–16.

Rothwell, P. M., Gutnikov, S. A. and Warlow, C. P. (2003b). Reanalysis of the final results of the European Carotid Surgery Trial. *Stroke*, **34**, 514–23.

Rothwell, P. M. and Goldstein, L. B. (2004). Carotid endarterectomy for asymptomatic carotid stenosis: asymptomatic carotid surgery trial. *Stroke*, **35**, 2425–7.

Schmitz, S. A. (2003). Iron-oxide-enhanced MR imaging of inflammatory atherosclerotic lesions: overview of experimental and initial clinical results. *Rofo*, **175**, 469–76.

Schmitz, S. A., Taupitz, M., Wagner, S., *et al.* (2002). Iron-oxide-enhanced magnetic resonance imaging of atherosclerotic plaques: postmortem analysis of accuracy, inter-observer agreement, and pitfalls. *Investigation Radiology*, **37**, 405–11.

Schmitz, S. A., Taupitz, M., Wagner, S., *et al.* (2001). Magnetic resonance imaging of atherosclerotic plaques using superparamagnetic iron oxide particles. *Journal of Magnetic Resonance Imaging*, **14**, 355–61.

Solini, A., Santini, E. and Ferrannini, E. (2005). Enhanced angiotensin II-mediated effects in fibroblasts of patients with familial hypercholesterolemia. *Journal of Hypertension*, **23**, 367–74.

Stary, H. C. (1994). Changes in components and structure of atherosclerotic lesions developing from childhood to middle age in coronary arteries. *Basic Research in Cardiology*, **89** (Suppl. 1), 17–32.

Stary, H. C. (2000a). Lipid and macrophage accumulations in arteries of children and the development of atherosclerosis. *American Journal of Clinical Nutrition*, **72**, 1297S–1306S.

Stary, H. C. (2000b). Natural history and histological classification of atherosclerotic lesions: an update. *Arteriosclerosis, Thrombosis and Vascular Biology*, **20**, 1177–8.

Stary, H. C. (2001). The development of calcium deposits in atherosclerotic lesions and their persistence after lipid regression. *American Journal of Cardiology*, **88**, 16E–19E.

Stary, H. C., Chandler, A. B., Dinsmore, R. E., *et al.* (1995). A definition of advanced types of atherosclerotic lesions and a histological classification of atherosclerosis. A report from the Committee on Vascular Lesions of the Council on Arteriosclerosis, American Heart Association. *Circulation*, **92**, 1355–74.

Stary, H. C., Chandler, A. B., Glagov, S., *et al.* (1994). A definition of initial, fatty streak, and intermediate lesions of atherosclerosis. A report from the Committee on Vascular Lesions of the Council on Arteriosclerosis, American Heart Association. *Arteriosclerosis and Thrombosis*, **14**, 840–56.

Stehbens, W. E. (2002). The fatigue hypothesis of plaque rupture and atherosclerosis. *Medical Hypotheses*, **58**, 359–60.

Stoneman, V. E. and Bennett, M. R. (2004). Role of apoptosis in atherosclerosis and its therapeutic implications. *Clinical Science (London)*, **107**, 343–54.

Stuber, M. (2005). Shedding light on the dark spot with IRON – a method that generates positive contrast in the presence of superparamagnetic nanoparticles. *Proceedings of the International Society of Magnetic Resonance in Medicine*, **13**, 2608.

Tang, D., Yang, C., Kobayashi, S. and Ku, D. N. (2001). Steady flow and wall compression in stenotic arteries: a three-dimensional thick-wall model with fluid-wall interactions. *Journal of Biomechanical Engineering*, **123**, 548–57.

Tang, D., Yang, C., Zheng, J., *et al.* (2004). 3D MRI-based multicomponent FSI models for atherosclerotic plaques. *Annals of Biomedical Engineering*, **32**, 947–60.

Trivedi, R., U-King-Im, J. and Gillard, J. (2003). Accumulation of ultrasmall superparamagnetic particles of iron oxide in human atherosclerotic plaque. *Circulation*, **108**, e140; author reply e140.

Trivedi, R. A., Im, U. K., Graves, M. J., *et al.* (2004a). In vivo detection of macrophages in human carotid atheroma: temporal dependence of ultrasmall superparamagnetic particles of iron oxide-enhanced MRI. *Stroke*, **35**, 1631–5.

Trivedi, R. A., Im, U. K., Graves, M. J., Kirkpatrick, P. J. and Gillard, J. H. (2004b). Noninvasive imaging of carotid plaque inflammation. *Neurology*, **63**, 187–8.

Wu, H. C., Chen, S. Y., Shroff, S. G. and Carroll, J. D. (2003). Stress analysis using anatomically realistic coronary tree. *Medical Physics*, **30**, 2927–36.

Yarnykh, V. L. and Yuan, C. (2002). T1-insensitive flow suppression using quadruple inversion-recovery. *Magnetic Resonance in Medicine*, **48**, 899–905.

Zhang, S., Hatsukami, T. S., Polissar, N. L., Han, C. and Yuan, C. (2001). Comparison of carotid vessel wall area measurements using three different contrast-weighted black blood MR imaging techniques. *Magnetic Resonance in Medicine*, **19**, 795–802.

21

Gadolinium-enhanced plaque imaging

William Kerwin

University of Washington, Seattle WA, USA

Introduction

The use of magnetic resonance imaging (MRI) for evaluation of atherosclerotic plaque has mostly focused on morphological aspects of the disease. The ability of MRI to provide high resolution depictions of the vessel lumen, outer wall boundary and plaque substructures is well established (Yuan and Kerwin, 2004). Such information, however, tells only part of the story of the plaque. Microscopic processes, such as infiltration of macrophages, can have profound effects on disease progression. Fortunately, MRI offers the ability to assess such processes through the use of injected contrast agents.

The development of contrast agents for MRI is a rapidly expanding area, with most agents utilizing gadolinium and its ability to shorten MR relaxation times T_1 and T_2. In T_1-weighted images, regions with accumulation of the agent are characteristically brighter and in T_2-weighted images, high concentration regions appear darker. Chelates of gadolinium including Gd-DTPA are currently available for clinical use and were initially approved for applications in detecting lesions of the central nervous system. Experimental uses under investigation include magnetic resonance angiography (MRA) and MRI of atherosclerosis. Techniques exist in these areas for first pass imaging in which the agent is restricted to the blood stream, late phase enhancement in which the agent has diffused into the extracellular space of the tissue, and dynamic imaging in which the transfer from the blood stream to the tissue is observed over time.

This chapter reviews the state of the art in contrast-enhanced MRI of atherosclerosis. It begins with an overview of clinically available and developmental contrast agents. Next, late-phase enhancement characteristics and their association with specific plaque components are discussed. The remainder of the chapter will discuss the challenges and quantitative advantages of dynamic contrast-enhanced imaging of plaque.

Contrast agents used in plaque imaging

Gadolinium-based agents

The majority of plaque imaging experiments in humans have utilized small molecular weight gadolinium agents such as Gd-DTPA (Magnevist, Berlex), and Gd-DTPA-BMA (Omniscan, GE Healthcare). These agents exhibit similar longitudinal relaxivities (R_1) of approximately 4 mMol^{-1}sec^{-1}, producing an effective T_1 given by:

$$\left(\frac{1}{T_1}\right)_{\text{effective}} = \left(\frac{1}{T_1}\right)_{\text{intrinsic}} + MR_1 \tag{21.1}$$

where M is the concentration of the agent in mMol (Lauffer, 1996). These agents are characterized by rapid distribution into the extracellular space, relatively rapid clearance by the kidneys, and a well-established understanding

Carotid Disease: The Role of Imaging in Diagnosis and Management, ed. Jonathan Gillard, Martin Graves, Thomas Hatsukami and Chun Yuan. Published by Cambridge University Press. © Cambridge University Press 2007.

of their pharmacokinetics. Given the large body of research involving these agents, they will be the focus of subsequent sections of this chapter. Nevertheless, a number of promising new agents are emerging for plaque imaging and must be mentioned here, with the caveat that most are far from being approved for clinical use.

One focus of the new agents is the burgeoning area of contrast-enhanced MRA. Although the ability of commonly available contrast agents to generate high blood signal in time-of-flight imaging has shown great promise for MRA, the rapid distribution of the agents into the extravascular space limits the lumen contrast improvement. Several agents are nearing clinical availability for MRA based on maintaining the agents within the blood pool.

One of these agents is MS-325 (Epix Medical, Cambridge, MA), which binds to albumin with an 80–96% bound fraction in human plasma and exhibits a six- to ten-fold higher relaxivity effect than Gd-DTPA (Lauffer et al., 1998). The intravascular confinement of albumin prevents bound MS-325 from diffusing into the extravascular space. In combination with the higher relaxivity effects, this makes MS-325 an excellent agent for MRA in both first-pass and steady-state acquisitions (Grist et al., 1998). Confinement to the blood pool also enables MS-325 to potentially gauge tissue blood volume (Krause et al., 2003). Measuring permeability of the agent into the extravascular space is also conceivable, but the different pharmacokinetics of bound and unbound forms complicates the analysis (Turetschek et al., 2001).

Another blood pool agent is P792 (Guerbet SA, Paris), which is a macromolecular gadolinium chelate that is predominately restricted to the blood stream by its large size. Experiments suggest that P792 may have larger maximal effects on relaxivity than MS-325 in MRA experiments (Corot et al., 2003). P792 has also been shown to be useful in kinetic modeling of dynamic contrast-enhanced (DCE) MRI, where the slow transfer of the large molecule reduces the need for rapid imaging (Pradel et al., 2003).

Finally, a new agent with an apparent affinity for plaque is gadofluorine (Schering AG), which is a gadolinium-based agent with a perfluorinated side chain (Barkhausen et al., 2003). The effect of the hydrophobic side chain is to induce the molecules to aggregate in solution, forming large micelles with multiple gadolinium atoms. In the blood stream, the micelles remain in the plasma for long durations making gadofluorine a potential blood pool agent. Additionally, the hydrophobic side chain is lipophilic which may explain the observed affinity of the agent for plaque. In rabbits, gadofluorine was found to remain within plaques several days after administration, a sufficient time for its elimination from the blood pool. MRI showed distinct enhancement of such plaque regions with a strong association with regions staining with Sudan red (i.e. lipids) in subsequent histological analysis (Barkhausen et al., 2003).

Molecular imaging agents

The next generation of contrast agents promises to usher in a new era of contrast-enhanced MRI wherein specific tissue receptors, interaction with cell types, and different pharmacokinetic behavior are employed in tailoring agents to specific diseases (Weinmann et al., 2003). Detection of the vulnerable atherosclerotic plaque is one of the foremost targets of these disease-specific agents.

Flacke et al. (2001) described a method for generating nanoparticles with greater than 50 000 gadolinium atoms per nanoparticle and high avidity for fibrin. These ligand-targeted nanoparticles were shown to form a thin layer over the surface of clots in scanning electron micrographs which resulted in high enhancement of clots in vitro and in dogs. Winter et al. (2003a) demonstrated a nearly two-fold increased reduction in relaxivity for a similar fibrin-targeted agent based on a different gadolinium formulation. These agents may one day be used for early detection of clot material – a potential sign of vulnerable plaque – within entire vascular beds.

Another target of molecular contrast agents in the investigation of atherosclerosis is factors influencing angiogenesis. Angiogenesis is significant because the resulting neovasculature may contribute to plaque progression through intraplaque hemorrhage and to plaque disruption through inflammatory processes. Winter *et al.* (2003b) proposed such an agent with roughly 90 000 gadolinium atoms per particle that targeted the $\alpha_v\beta_3$-integrin, which is expressed in the vascular wall and is associated with angiogenesis. In cholesterol-fed rabbits, the aorta wall showed greater enhancement with this agent than in rabbits fed a control diet. Histological analysis confirmed a significant expansion of the adventitial vasa vasorum of the cholesterol-fed rabbits compared to the controls.

USPIOs

A major alternative to gadolinium-based agents are ultrasmall particles of superparamagnetic iron oxides (USPIOs). USPIOs (e.g. Sinerem®, Guerbet SA, Paris) suspended in solution and injected into patients at low concentrations result in positive contrast on T_1-weighted images (Chambon *et al.*, 1993). Their relaxation effects have the ability to enhance blood in MRA with results similar to those obtained with P792 (Corot *et al.*, 2003). Of greater value is the propensity of macrophages to phagocytose the USPIOs leading to a macrophage-specific agent (Schmitz *et al.*, 2001). Allowing for sufficient time for macrophage uptake – usually at least 24 hours – T_2*-weighted images show significant signal reduction due to susceptibility effects of the USPIOs (Ruehm *et al.*, 2001). In experiments with human carotid endarterectomy subjects, Kooi *et al.* (2003) showed that macrophages within plaques were positive for iron in histological and electron microscopy evaluations of endarterectomy specimens. In MRI of corresponding locations, significant signal reductions were observed.

Delayed plaque enhancement with gadolinium

The observation of enhancing regions in plaque after injection of a gadolinium contrast agent was first reported in animals by Lin *et al.* (1997) and in humans by Aoki *et al.* (1999). The dominant feature noted was a bright rim attributed to growth of the vaso vasorum in the adventitia (Figure 21.1a). Others noted patchy enhancement within the plaque itself (Figure 21.1b) (Wasserman *et al.*, 2002; Yuan *et al.*, 2002). This led investigators including Weiss *et al.* (2001), Yuan *et al.* (2002) and Wasserman *et al.* (2002), to consider whether CE-MRI provides unique information regarding plaque composition and vulnerability.

Imaging techniques

CE-MRI of atherosclerosis using gadolinium agents requires special considerations in the method of image acquisition. Most importantly, the proximity of the large vessel lumen, with its high concentration can lead to difficulties in interpretation of the images if care is not taken to suppress the blood signal. Typically, two options are available, spatial saturation bands and double inversion recovery (DIR). Both techniques rely on dephasing of the net magnetization of the blood outside of the image plane and subsequent inflow of the dephased blood. The DIR technique generally provides better suppression of the blood signal because suppression is applied over a broader area and more time is allowed for inflow of suppressed blood. In CE-MRI, this advantage becomes even greater as the rapid recovery from spatial saturation due to T_1 shortening further undermines that technique.

One problem that arises in DIR imaging is that the timing of the inversion must be carefully set relative to the T_1 of the blood for optimal suppression. However, the T_1 of the blood depends on the unknown concentration of the contrast agent. To overcome this issue, Yarnykh and Yuan (2002) proposed the quadruple inversion recovery (QIR)

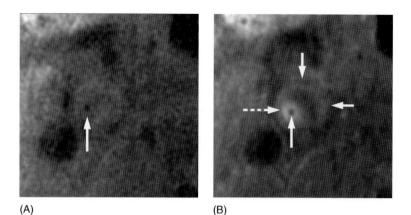

(A)   (B)

Figure 21.1 Pre-CE (A) and post-CE (B) cross-sectional MR images of a severely diseased carotid artery. The long arrows point to the narrowed lumen. The short arrows delineate the enhanced adventitia after injection with contrast. The enhancement surrounding the lumen (dotted arrow) is attributed to the presence of loose proteoglycan matrix.

technique, which adds a second double inversion recovery pulse set to the sequence. This leads to perfect suppression for two values of T_1 and nearly perfect suppression over a wide range of T_1 values.

Enhancement of the adventitial vasa vasorum

The observation of enhancement along the adventitial boundary of the plaque (Aoki *et al.*, 1999) and its probable association with neovasculature is of great interest because angiogenesis is thought to have a role in plaque formation. Specifically, these vessels are thought to provide a pathway for leukocyte infiltration and inflammatory activation (O'Brien *et al.*, 1996; deBoer *et al.*, 1999). Therefore, they may be indicators of vulnerable plaque.

A unique opportunity allowed us to assess the possible link between adventitial enhancement and neovasculature histologically. A subject with severe atherosclerosis was scheduled for resection of the right carotid artery for a symptomatic high-grade recurrent stenosis. One week prior to surgery, an MRI examination with a gadolinium contrast agent (Omniscan, GE Healthcare, Little Chalfont) revealed significant postcontrast enhancement along the adventitial boundary of the vessel (Figure 21.1). Following surgery, the

resected artery was fixed, sectioned at 1 mm intervals, and stained with Mallory's trichrome. Histology sections were then matched to the MR images using the shape and size of the lumen and wall. Finally, the large vessels of the adventitia (≥ 0.02 mm diameter) were counted within each section. The inclusion of the adventitia in the resected artery permitted this histological analysis.

To compare the histological results with MRI enhancement, the average intensity of the carotid outer rim was measured on pre- and postcontrast DIR T_1-weighted images. Ten axial locations separated by 2 mm were available and the average percent change in outer rim intensity was computed for each. Comparison to the corresponding number of vessels in histology (Figure 21.2) revealed a strong correlation ($r = 0.70$, $p < 0.03$). The clinical relevance of the adventitial enhancement requires further investigation.

Tissue specific characteristics

Of potentially greater interest is the delayed enhancement of structures within the plaque, especially near the lumen surface, where plaque disruption occurs. Utilizing the DIR and QIR

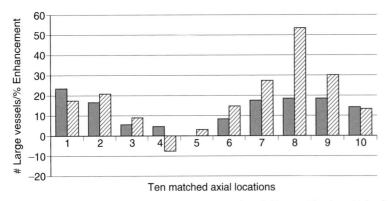

Figure 21.2 Association of large adventitial neovessels (solid bars) with adventitial enhancement (striped bars) in a carotid endarterectomy specimen.

techniques, several researchers have uncovered tantalizing links between enhancement and plaque characteristics. Yuan *et al.* (2002) and Wasserman *et al.* (2002) both found higher enhancement associated with fibrous tissue, suggesting that contrast enhanced (CE) MRI might be valuable for assessing the status of the fibrous cap, a key component of plaque stability. Yuan *et al.* also found the highest enhancement associated with areas of dense neovasculature, which are thought to contribute to plaque destabilization (McCarthy *et al.*, 1999; Moulton *et al.*, 2003). Weiss *et al.* (2001) found an association between high enhancement and serum markers of inflammation, suggesting CE MRI might be valuable for evaluating plaque inflammation. Inflammation plays a critical role in plaque initiation, progression, and disruption and represents an emerging target in the treatment of atherosclerosis.

To further explore the links between enhancement and tissue types, 18 patients scheduled for endarterectomy were enrolled in an MRI study. The protocol was identical to that used in the study by Yuan *et al.*, 2002. After acquiring pre- and post-contrast images at a total of 76 locations within these subjects, an expert reviewer placed matched regions of interest (ROIs) on both sets of images corresponding to uniform-appearing structures within the plaques. For each matched set of ROIs, the percent enhancement was computed.

Following carotid endarterectomy, the specimens were formalin fixed, decalcified, and embedded in paraffin. Sections (10 mm thick) corresponding to the image locations were identified after staining with Hematoxylin & Eosin and Mallory's Trichrome. The sections were then independently evaluated by a reviewer who was unaware of the imaging results and categorized the tissue types into five histopathological classifications (Stary *et al.*, 1995; Virmani *et al.*, 2000): Necrotic core, Calcification, Matrix, Neovasculature I (one to four microvessels per 200× field measuring under 0.02 mm in diameter), and Neovasculature II (five or more microvessels under 0.02 mm in diameter per 200× field or any number of microvessels measuring greater than 0.02 mm).

Comparison between histology and MRI enhancement was performed on a quadrant basis ($n = 198$). Each location was divided into four quadrants and for each quadrant, the percent enhancement of any ROI within the quadrant was recorded. Also, for each quadrant the set of tissues present in histology was recorded. This facilitated the search for a link between a specific level of enhancement and the presence of certain tissue types in the vicinity.

Table 21.1 summarizes the signal enhancement in MRI quadrants with and without specified histological features. Only neovasculature II showed

Table 21.1. Association of tissues with delayed enhancement

| Tissue type | Percent enhancement | | p-value |
	Present	Absent	
Matrix	79 ± 54	57 ± 52	0.07
Necrotic Core	55 ± 48	79 ± 57	0.19
Calcification	69 ± 55	66 ± 54	0.51
Neovasculature I	54 ± 42	79 ± 54	0.43
Neovasculature II	109 ± 52	51 ± 46	0.002

a statistically significant association with hyper-enhancement. Specifically, when neovasculature II was present, the mean percent increase was 109%±52% versus 51%±46% when it was absent ($p = 0.002$). The 109% average enhancement associated with neovasculature II was also the highest of all tissue components evaluated. Although marginal in terms of statistical significance, the presence of loose matrix was also associated with a higher level of enhancement (79% vs. 57%) and a necrotic core was associated with a lower level of enhancement (55% vs. 79%). Because inflammatory cells such as macrophages are associated with neovasculature and loose matrix (deBoer *et al.*, 1999; Virmani *et al.*, 2000), these findings suggest areas of strong enhancement may also be indicative of inflammation.

Effect of contrast enhancement on measurements of plaque composition

The association of enhancement with particular plaque features has provided the most utility in the quantitative assessment of plaque composition. Cai *et al.* (2005) recently showed that the propensity for fibrous tissue to enhance, while necrotic tissue does not can be used to accurately identify the fibrous cap and necrotic core regions of the plaque. Specifically, the fibrous cap was outlined as the highly enhancing region between the dark necrotic core and the lumen. Measurements of the cap area, length, and maximum thickness were

shown to correlate with equivalent measurements from histology with correlation coefficients of 0.80, 0.73, and 0.78, respectively. Furthermore, the percentage area of minimal enhancement correlated with histological measurements of necrotic core percentage with R equal to 0.87.

Dynamic imaging of plaque enhancement

Although late phase enhancement has been shown to provide additional information for characterizing plaque composition, the major contributions of CE MRI were expected to be in quantification and identification of inflammation. Because quantitative measurements of late phase enhancement are dependent on factors such as dose, scanner parameters, and timing, researchers turn to DCE MRI for quantitative studies. In DCE MRI, the time course of enhancement assists in characterizing tissue by showing not just *what* enhances but also *how* it enhances. For example, both neovasculature and loose matrix have strong enhancement in late phase images; these two tissues can be distinguished in dynamic images because loose matrix should enhance more slowly because it relies on diffusion of the contrast agent from the blood, rather than direct connection to the vascular system. Quantitative characterizations are then possible via kinetic modeling of contrast agent uptake.

Imaging techniques

Quantitative DCE MRI utilizes multiple image acquisitions over the course of contrast agent injection. It requires a sequence that provides rapid imaging to capture the changing enhancement patterns as the agent distributes through the vascular system and into the tissues. Additionally, the sequence must not suppress the blood signal, which then serves as an indicator of agent concentration in the blood. A typical imaging technique is a 2D spoiled gradient-recalled echo (SPGR) T_1-weighted sequence with

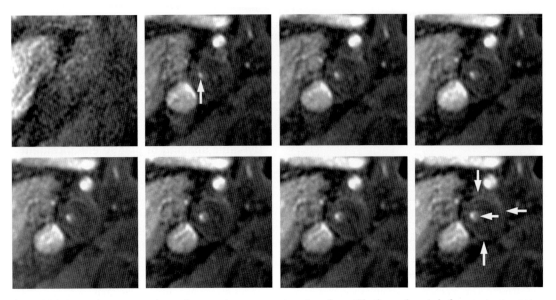

Figure 21.3 Dynamic contrast enhanced magnetic resonance imaging of carotid atherosclerosis before contrast agent arrival (top left) and at 15-second intervals following bolus arrival. The lumen is marked by an arrow in frame 2. Dynamic enhancement is apparent in a region of loose matrix surrounding the lumen and in the adventitia (short and long arrows, respectively, in final frame).

parameters: TR = 100 ms, TE = 3.5 ms, flip = 60°, thickness = 3 mm, gap = 1 mm, field-of-view = 16 × 12 cm, matrix = 256 × 144. Blood saturation bands are placed above and below each block of image locations to induce a T_1 recovery for measurement of signal increases due to contrast agent concentration in the blood. Each acquisition is repeated 10 or more times, with a repetition interval on the order of 15 sec. Coincident with the second image in the sequence, a standard dose (0.1 mmol/kg) of a gadolinium-based contrast agent is injected at a rate of 2 ml/sec via power injector. Examples of the resulting sequence of images are depicted in Figure 21.3.

Image processing

One challenge in DCE MRI is that quantitative kinetic modeling of enhancement requires exact registration of the images in the sequence. However, patient motion during imaging occurs.

Even small shifts on the order of 1 mm can have dramatic consequences since the pixel size is well under 1 mm and the entire vessel is often less than 1 cm in diameter.

To combat patient motion in DCE MRI of atherosclerosis, the Kalman Filtering Registration and Smoothing (KFRS) algorithm was proposed (Kerwin *et al.*, 2002). This technique is essentially an estimation theoretic approach to the problem, modeling enhancement and motion stochastically and seeking the linear minimum mean square error (LMMSE) estimate of the true sequence of images. The stochastic model assumes that the change in signal intensity of a given image pixel is dictated by a random process with known statistics. Furthermore, image noise and patient shifts are assumed to be dictated by known random processes. Given this model, a Kalman filter efficiently predicts the sequence of images given all prior images. These predictions are used in a maximum-likelihood registration procedure.

Finally, a Kalman smoother efficiently produces optimal estimates given all images in the sequence, not just prior ones.

Kinetic modeling

Once the sequence of DCE MRI images has been acquired and registered, it must be mathematically analyzed to glean the biologically relevant information from the time course of enhancement. The biological information accessible in this way consists of various measurements related to tissue permeability and blood supply. The measurements are extracted by fitting a prior model of the contrast agent kinetics to the observed brightness variations. Ideally, measurements are taken over time of blood plasma concentration $C_p(t)$ and tissue concentration $C_t(t)$ of the agent. In DCE MRI, the change in signal intensity is sometimes used in lieu of concentration or, for greater accuracy, the change in longitudinal relaxation rate ΔR_1 is used (Tofts, 1997).

One common approach is a two-compartment model of contrast agent kinetics, such as that illustrated in Figure 21.4. The total tissue concentration is given by:

$$C_t = v_p C_p + v_e C_e \qquad (21.2)$$

where C_e is the concentration in the extravascular extracellular space (EES), and v_p and v_e are the respective partial volumes of plasma and EES. The change in EES concentration over time is dictated by

$$\dot{C}_e = k_{ep}(C_p - C_e) \qquad (21.3)$$

where k_{ep} is the transfer rate of contrast agent between plasma and EES. Further complexity can be introduced to the model by assuming different exchange rates from plasma to EES and from EES back to plasma.

Unfortunately, even if matching transfer rates are assumed, parameter estimates for the two-compartment model can be unstable, an issue of "global identifiability" (Audoly et al., 2001). For example, if $C_t(t)$ is similar in shape to $C_p(t)$, this can be accounted for by setting $v_p = C_t/C_p$, by making k_{ep} very large and setting $v_e = C_t/C_p$, or any combination of these. Small changes in the observed data can thus lead to large changes in the estimated parameters. Therefore, care must be taken to ensure this model is applied in situations with high signal-to-noise ratios, where model instabilities have less impact, or in situations where unstable solutions are unlikely. Otherwise, further simplification of the model is warranted.

One simplification employed by Patlak (1983) assumes that the movement of contrast agent from the tissue back to the plasma is negligible. The result is a linear model of contrast agent dynamics that depends only on v_p and the term $K^{trans} = v_e k_{ep}$ according to

$$\frac{C_t(t)}{C_p(t)} = v_p + K^{trans} \frac{\int_0^t C_p(\tau)d\tau}{C_p(t)} \qquad (21.4)$$

This model will be valid if the transfer rate from EES to plasma is slow compared to the time span of the observations.

For situations where this is not true, an alternative assumption employed by Tofts and Kermode (1991) is that v_p is negligible. This leads to the general differential equation governing contrast agent uptake:

$$\dot{C}_t = k^{trans}\left(C_p - \frac{C_t}{v_e}\right) \qquad (21.5)$$

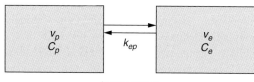

Image Voxel

Figure 21.4 Two-compartment model of contrast agent exchange: the total concentration in a volume of tissue is determined by a partial volume of plasma v_p, a partial volume of extravascular extracellular space v_e and their respective concentrations C_p and C_e. Dynamic interchange of contrast agent is determined by the rate constant k_{ep}.

The physiological definition of K^{trans} relates to blood flow, capillary surface area, and permeability, making it a good indicator of blood supply (Tofts *et al.*, 1999). The solution to this differential equation is:

$$C_t(t) = K^{trans} \int_0^t C_p(\tau) e^{\{-k_{ep}(t-\tau)\}} d\tau \qquad (21.6)$$

If $C_p(t)$ is known, the parameters k_{ep}, K^{trans}, and $v_e = K^{trans}/k_{ep}$ can be extracted. Typically, the blood concentration is periodically sampled and fitted with a multiexponential curve to approximate $C_p(t)$ (Tofts, 1997).

Results of kinetic modeling in carotid atherosclerosis

Figure 21.5 illustrates the application of the Patlak kinetic model to an advanced atherosclerotic plaque. The color-coded values of v_p are shown to be high in the lumen (as expected since the lumen is 100% blood). Surrounding the lumen, a region of high K^{trans} was found to be associated with proteoglycan-rich fibrous matrix. Elevated K^{trans} in the outer rim of the wall is also seen,

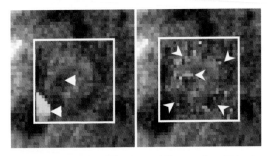

Figure 21.5 Pixel-level kinetic modeling results within the boxed region of the dynamic images of Figure 21.3. Increasing values of v_p (left) and K^{trans} (right) are shown as red, then yellow pixels. Uncolored regions have values near zero. Note the high v_p values in the lumen of the carotid artery and jugular vein (arrows) and the high values of K^{trans} surrounding the lumen and adventitial boundary (arrow heads).

a feature common to virtually all diseased arteries studied.

In histological studies, average values of v_p have been shown to correlate strongly with total neovasculature content (Kerwin *et al.*, 2003) and average values of K^{trans} have been shown to correlate with total macrophage content (Kerwin *et al.*, 2006). In Figure 21.6, we show the results of a study in which the average values of K^{trans} were computed for 26 arteries. The values were compared between subjects with quantities of seven plaque components that were either above or below the median. Significance was assessed by a *t*-test. Imaging was conducted within 1 week prior to surgery and plaque composition was quantified by histological analysis of the surgical specimen. This investigation showed strongly elevated K^{trans} in subjects with higher levels of macrophages and neovasculature and reduced values for subjects with large necrotic cores or heavily calcified plaques. The association of macrophages and neovasculature with K^{trans} is particularly important because both features are associated with an active inflammatory process within the plaque (O'Brien *et al.*, 1996; deBoer *et al.*, 1999).

Diffusion modeling

Carotid atherosclerosis also offers an alternative interpretation of contrast agent dynamics. In the standard kinetic models described above, contrast agent delivery to a voxel is assumed to arise from vasculature within that voxel. The models, however, become invalid when the bulk of the contrast agent arrives via diffusion over some considerable difference. Although most biological tissues are compatible with the former model, the juxtaluminal layer of large arteries likely follows a diffusion model.

From a theoretical standpoint, uptake of the contrast agent from the lumen may be described as a passive diffusion process dictated by $\partial C/\partial t = D \, \partial^2 C/\partial x^2$, where C is concentration, t is time, x is distance from the lumen surface, and D is the

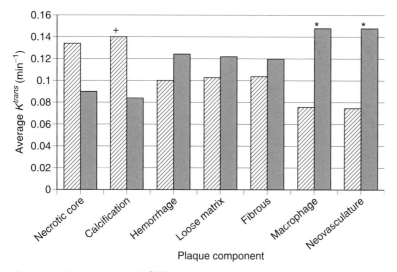

Figure 21.6 Average value of K^{trans} for subjects with plaques that had percentages of the indicated component higher (solid bars) versus lower (striped bars) than the group median (+: $p < 0.05$; *: $p < 0.01$).

diffusion coefficient in cm^2/sec. If concentration in the lumen is assumed to obey a single exponential decay and change in signal intensity is assumed to be proportional to concentration within the plaque, an effective diffusion coefficient D_{eff} that best describes enhancement of the entire juxtaluminal region can be found. The parameter D_{eff} reflects the rate at which the contrast agent penetrates into the plaque from the lumen.

The concept of diffusion modeling is illustrated in Figure 21.7, assuming a constant concentration within the vessel lumen. As time progresses, concentration within the tissue increases, as does the depth of penetration. Plotting concentration versus time at different depths shows a range of possible curve behaviors.

To test this concept in vivo, we analyzed the images of Figure 21.3. The juxtaluminal region was divided into three bands averaging 1, 2, and 3 pixels from the lumen surface. The average changes in signal intensity within each band were then simultaneously fit with a *single* diffusion equation to obtain D_{eff} for the entire region (Figure 21.8). Although the data are noisy, they exhibit a

reasonably good fit to the three parametric curves shown. The quality of this fit is quite remarkable considering all three curves are derived from a single diffusion parameter.

The histopathological significance of D_{eff} remains to be tested. We expect that the increased permeability and breakdown of the fibrous matrix associated with inflammation will lead to an elevated value of D_{eff}, and hence identify fibrous caps that are likely inflamed and/or may become disrupted. Whether this type of modeling can be reliably and reproducibly performed in vivo is also untested.

Conclusion

The ability of DCE MRI to extract quantitative physiological parameters is an exciting development in plaque imaging. Kinetic modeling of the entire plaque distills plaque characteristics to a single quantity, akin to measuring stenosis. In combination with stenosis, this information could lead to clinical decisions being made on the paired data. Of course, large scale studies are needed to

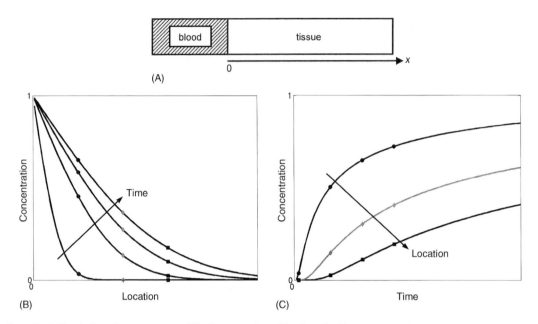

Figure 21.7 Simulation of contrast agent diffusion assuming a blood pool with constant, unit concentration is in contact with a uniform tissue (A). Curves are shown of concentration versus location x at successive times after contrast agent arrival (B) and of concentration versus time at different spatial locations (C). The circles, squares, and diamonds are corresponding points of the two plots.

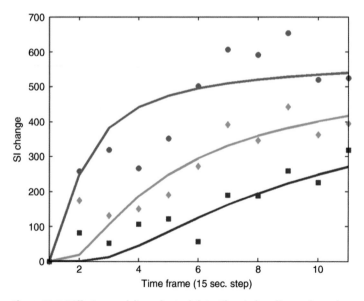

Figure 21.8 Diffusion modeling of actual data. The circles, diamonds, and squares are measurements of signal intensity (SI) change at depths of 1, 2, and 3 pixels. The curves are fit to these data points based on the diffusion model and a single diffusion parameter.

assess the clinical relevance of the contrast enhancement data.

At present, the most sought after feature to detect by CE MRI is inflammation, characterized by macrophage infiltration into the vessel wall and plaque. Additionally, inflammation is commonly associated with neovasculature which provides nutrition to the inflammatory cells, is induced by vascular growth factors expressed by the cells (Chen *et al.*, 1999), and provides a pathway for further inflammatory infiltration (deBoer, 1999) The interest in inflammation stems from the fact that inflammatory cells contribute to both plaque initiation and destabilization (Libby, 2002). Inflammation is a natural target for CE MRI because the increased blood supply and permeability associated with inflammation provides a significant pathway for agent entry and because macrophages are established targets of tissue-specific agents. Potential future targets of contrast agents in atherosclerosis are many and varied, with fibrous matrix molecules such as proteoglycan an attractive option, given their implications for cap stability.

The prospect of developing contrast agents that highlight specific features of atherosclerotic plaque such as macrophages, neovasculature or fibrin is certainly an exciting development in imaging of atherosclerosis. These tools provide the potential for visualizing the plaque features associated with rupture and clinical events. MRI with targeted contrast agents may one day be used to assess the stability of individual plaques based on their enhancement characteristics. Alternatively, the ability to image enhancement over broad regions suggests that agents specific to plaque features could be used in screening exams to assess overall plaque burden. To date, however, results with targeted agents are preliminary and such applications will require extensive efficacy and safety studies, likely making their wide-scale use a decade or more away.

In the nearer term, the mainstays of CE MRI of plaque will be currently approved chelates of gadolinium, USPIOs, and blood pool agents

nearing approval. A disadvantage of USPIOs is the need to wait a day or more after injection for macrophage uptake, which means pre- and post-contrast images must be obtained on separate days. This imposition may limit their applicability, although their strong association with macrophages makes them a powerful tool within certain applications. Basic gadolinium agents, on the other hand, result in nearly instantaneous enhancement allowing pre- and postcontrast images to be acquired within the same session. Over time, a shift away from small molecular weight agents and toward blood pool agents is expected, owing to the better performance in MRA and dynamic applications.

Although standard gadolinium agents produce nonspecific enhancement, they still provide considerable useful information for gauging atherosclerotic plaque. Contrast-enhanced T_1-weighted images can serve as additional weightings in a comprehensive multicontrast evaluation of plaque composition. Wasserman *et al.* showed that in such a role, contrast-enhanced images provide similar information to T_2-weighted images with higher contrast-to-noise ratios (Wasserman *et al.*, 2002). The further facilitation of MRA by contrast agents presents an opportunity for combined angiographic and contrast-enhanced plaque assessment of diseased vessels.

In terms of clinical and preclinical applications of CE MRI of atherosclerosis, the first use is likely to emerge in drug development. For example, the effectiveness of pharmaceutical agents targeting plaque inflammation could be judged based on their measured effects on contrast enhancement characteristics. Ultimately, the hope is to develop techniques based on CE MRI that provide a risk assessment for individual plaques. This information could then be used by the clinician in deciding the course of treatment.

The material presented in this chapter was based largely on experience in the human carotid artery. While the carotid represents a clinically important vessel, the ultimate hope is to extend these techniques for use on plaques in other vessels.

Currently such applications are difficult because other clinically significant vessels, most notably the coronary arteries, are smaller, less superficially located, or undergoing greater motion than the carotid arteries. Although imaging of plaque in the aorta and coronary arteries has been demonstrated, further technological advances are needed to make it clinically feasible. In the near term, the clinical benefit of this technique for vessels other than the carotid artery is most likely to come from therapies shown to have positive effects in carotid plaque that have a similar effect throughout the vascular system.

REFERENCES

Aoki, S., Aoki, K., Ohsawa, S., *et al.* (1999). Dynamic MR imaging of the carotid wall. *Journal of Magnetic Resonance Imaging*, **9**, 420–7.

Audoly, S., Bellu, G., D'Angio, L., Saccomani, M. P. and Cobelli, C. (2001). Global identifiability of nonlinear models of biological systems. *IEEE Transactions in Biomedical Engineering*, **48**, 55–65.

Barkhausen, J., Ebert, W., Heyer, C., Debatin, J. F. and Weinmann, H. J. (2003). Detection of atherosclerotic plaque with gadofluorine-enhanced magnetic resonance imaging. *Circulation*, **108**, 605–9.

Cai, J., Hatsukami, T. S., Ferguson, M. S., *et al.* (2005). In vivo quantitative measurement of intact fibrous cap and lipid rich necrotic core size in atherosclerotic carotid plaque: a comparison of high resolution contrast enhanced MRI and histology. *Circulation*, **112**, 3437–44.

Chambon, C., Clement, O., Le Blanche, A., Schouman-Claeys, E. and Frija, G. (1993). Superparamagnetic iron oxides as positive MR contrast agents: in vitro and in vivo evidence. *Magnetic Resonance Imaging*, **11**, 509–19.

Chen, Y. X., Nakashima, Y., Tanaka, K., *et al.* (1999). Immunohistochemical expression of vascular endothelial growth factor/vascular permeability factor in atherosclerotic intimas of human coronary arteries. *Arteriosclerosis, Thrombosis and Vascular Biology*, **19**, 131–9.

Corot, C., Violas, X., Robert, P., Gagneur, G. and Port, M. (2003). Comparison of different types of blood pool agents (P792, MS325, USPIO) in a rabbit MR angiography-like protocol. *Investigative Radiology*, **38**, 311–19.

deBoer, O. J., van der Wal, A. C., Teeling, P. and Becker, A. E. (1999). Leucocyte recruitment in rupture prone regions of lipid-rich plaques: a prominent role for neovascularization? *Cardiovascular Research*, **41**, 443–9.

Flacke, S., Fischer, S., Scott, M. J., *et al.* (2001). Novel MRI contrast agent for molecular imaging of fibrin: implications for detecting vulnerable plaques. *Circulation*, **104**, 1280–5.

Grist, T. M., Korosec, F. R., Peters, D. C., *et al.* (1998). Steady-state and dynamic MR angiography with MS-325: initial experience in humans. *Radiology*, **207**, 539–44.

Kerwin, W. S., Cai, J. and Yuan, C. (2002). Noise and motion correction in dynamic contrast-enhanced MRI for analysis of atherosclerotic lesions. *Magnetic Resonance in Medicine*, **47**, 1211–17.

Kerwin, W., Hooker, A., Spilker, M., *et al.* (2003). Quantitative magnetic resonance imaging analysis of neovasculature volume in carotid atherosclerotic plaque. *Circulation*, **107**, 851–6.

Kerwin, W., O'Brien, K., Ferguson, M., Hatsukami, T. and Yuan, C. (2006). Inflammation in carotid atherosclerotic plaque is associated with elevated neovasculature and permeability: a dynamic contrast-enhanced MRI study. *Radiology*, in press.

Kooi, M. E., Cappendijk, V. C., Cleutjens, K. B., *et al.* (2003). Accumulation of ultrasmall superparamagnetic particles of iron oxide in human atherosclerotic plaques can be detected by in vivo magnetic resonance imaging. *Circulation*, **107**, 2453–8.

Krause, M. H., Kwong, K. K. and Xiong, J. (2003). MRI of blood volume with MS 325 in experimental choroidal melanoma. *Magnetic Resonance Imaging*, **21**, 725–32.

Lauffer, R. B. (1996). MRI contrast agents: basic principles. In *Clinical Magnetic Resonance Imaging*, ed. R. Edelman, J. Hesselink and M. Zlatkin, Philadelphia, PA: W. B. Saunders Co., pp. 177–91.

Lauffer, R. B., Parmelee, D. J., Dunham, S. U., *et al.* (1998). MS-325: albumin-targeted contrast agent for MR angiography. *Radiology*, **207**, 529–38.

Libby, P. (2002). Inflammation in atherosclerosis. *Nature*, **420**, 868–74.

Lin, W., Abendschein, D. R. and Haacke, E. M. (1997). Contrast-enhanced magnetic resonance angiography of carotid arterial wall in pigs. *Journal of Magnetic Resonance Imaging*, **7**, 183–90.

McCarthy, M. J., Loftus, I. M., Thompson, M. M., *et al.* (1999). Angiogenesis and the atherosclerotic carotid plaque: an association between symptomatology and plaque morphology. *Journal of Vascular Surgery*, **30**, 261–8.

Moulton, K. S., Vakili, K. and Zurakowski, D. (2003). Inhibition of plaque neovascularization reduces macrophage accumulation and progression of advanced atherosclerosis. *Proceedings of the National Academy of Sciences of the United States of America*, **100**, 4736–41.

O'Brien, K. D., McDonald, T. O., Chait, A., Allen, M. D. and Alpers, C. E. (1996). Neovascular expression of E-selectin, intercellular adhesion molecule-1, and vascular cell adhesion molecule-1 in human atherosclerosis and their relation to intimal leukocyte content. *Circulation*, **93**, 672–82.

Patlak, C. S. (1983). Graphical evaluation of blood-to-brain transfer constants from multiple-time uptake data. *Journal of Cerebral Blood Flow and Metabolism*, **3**, 1–7.

Pradel, C., Siauve, N., Bruneteau, G., *et al.* (2003). Reduced capillary perfusion and permeability in human tumour xenografts treated with the vegf signalling inhibitor zd4190: an in vivo assessment using dynamic MR imaging and macromolecular contrast media. *Magnetic Resonance Imaging*, **21**, 845–51.

Ruehm, S. G., Corot, C., Vogt, P., Kolb, S. and Debatin, J. F. (2001). Magnetic resonance imaging of atherosclerotic plaque with ultrasmall superparamagnetic particles of iron oxide in hyperlipidemic rabbits. *Circulation*, **103**, 415–22.

Schmitz, S. A., Taupitz, T., Wagner, S., *et al.* (2001). Magnetic resonance imaging of atherosclerotic plaques using superparamagnetic iron oxide particles. *Journal of Magnetic Resonance Imaging*, **14**, 355–61.

Stary, H. C., Chandler, A. B., Dinsmore, R. E., *et al.* (1995). A definition of advanced types of atherosclerotic lesions and a histological classification of atherosclerosis. A report from the committee on vascular lesions of the council on arteriosclerosis, American Heart Association. *Circulation*, **92**, 1355–74.

Tofts, P. S. and Kermode, A. G. (1991). Measurement of the blood-brain barrier permeability and leakage space using dynamic MR imaging. 1. Fundamental concepts. *Magnetic Resonance in Medicine*, **17**, 357–67.

Tofts, P. S. (1997). Modeling tracer kinetics in dynamic Gd-DTPA MR imaging. *Journal of Magnetic Resonance Imaging*, **7**, 91–101.

Tofts, P. S., Brix, G., Buckley, D. L., *et al.* (1999). Estimating kinetic parameters from dynamic contrast-enhanced T1-weighted MRI of a diffusable tracer: standardized quantities and symbols. *Journal of Magnetic Resonance Imaging*, **10**, 223–32.

Turetschek, K., Floyd, E., Helbich, T., *et al.* (2001). MRI assessment of microvascular characteristics in experimental breast tumors using a new blood pool contrast agent (MS-325) with correlations to histopathology. *Journal of Magnetic Resonance Imaging*, **14**, 237–42.

Virmani, R., Kolodgie, F. D., Burke, A. P., Farb, A. and Schwartz, S. M. (2000). Lessons from sudden coronary death: a comprehensive morphological classification scheme for atherosclerotic lesions. *Arteriosclerosis, Thrombosis and Vascular Biology*, **20**, 1262–75.

Wasserman, B. A., Smith, W. I., Trout, H. H., *et al.* (2002). Carotid artery atherosclerosis: in vivo morphologic characterization with gadolinium-enhanced double-oblique MR imaging initial results. *Radiology*, **223**, 566–73.

Weinmann, H. J., Ebert, W., Misselwitz, B. and Schmitt-Willich, H. (2003). Tissue-specific MR contrast agents. *European Journal of Radiology*, **46**, 33–44.

Weiss, C. R., Arai, A. E., Bui, M. N., *et al.* (2001). Arterial wall MRI characteristics are associated with elevated serum markers of inflammation in humans. *Journal of Magnetic Resonance Imaging*, **14**, 698–704.

Winter, P. M., Caruthers, S. D., Yu, X., *et al.* (2003a). Improved molecular imaging contrast agent for detection of human thrombus. *Magnetic Resonance in Medicine*, **50**, 411–16.

Winter, P. M., Morawski, A. M., Caruthers, S. D., *et al.* (2003b). Molecular imaging of angiogenesis in early-stage atherosclerosis with alpha(v)beta3-integrin-targeted nanoparticles. *Circulation*, **108**, 2270–4.

Yarnykh, V. L. and Yuan, C. (2002). T1-insensitive flow suppression using quadruple inversion-recovery. *Magnetic Resonance in Medicine*, **48**, 899–905.

Yuan, C., Kerwin, W. S., Ferguson, M. S., *et al.* (2002). Contrast enhanced high resolution MRI for atherosclerotic carotid artery tissue characterization. *Journal of Magnetic Resonance Imaging*, **15**, 62–7.

Yuan, C. and Kerwin, W. S. (2004). MRI of atherosclerosis. *Journal of Magnetic Resonance Imaging*, **19**, 710–19.

22

Carotid magnetic resonance direct thrombus imaging

Alan Moody

Sunnybrook Health Sciences Centre, Toronto ON, Canada

Atherosclerosis is the basis of the majority of carotid artery disease which, via occlusive/stenotic disease and subsequent thromboembolic events, results in end organ (brain) damage. The ability to identify atherosclerotic carotid disease, characterize those patients with disease likely to cause end organ damage and then treat this disease as noninvasively as possible underlies many research questions into carotid disease at the present time. An improved understanding of the biological processes and interactions within atherosclerotic plaque enables a more rational and targeted approach to answering some of these questions. This is the case when designing new imaging techniques that attempt to specifically identify markers of high risk.

Over the last few years there has been a rapid expansion in our knowledge of the vascular biology of vessel wall disease. The American Heart Association (AHA) has defined a progression from minimal, nonthreatening, vessel wall disease to disease that is increasingly recognized as responsible for causing the terminal events leading to asymptomatic and symptomatic thromboembolic disease with subsequent end organ damage (Stary et al., 1995). The AHA classification defines type V disease as due to fibrous thickening not thought to be responsible for thromboembolic disease. Conversion of this to type VI disease however identifies high-risk atherosclerotic plaque. The three histological markers that define this stage

are: surface erosions; thrombus and intraplaque hemorrhage.

In recent years there have been a number of modifications to the classical concept of atherosclerotic disease that have significant implications for our understanding of this disease and the opportunities for its treatment. Until recently the measurement of vessel stenosis has been at the heart of patient risk stratification. Vessel wall disease causing significant ($>50\%$) stenosis appears a useful marker of disease severity as evidenced by a number of carotid endarterectomy trials (ECAS, 1991; Barnett et al., 1998) though its discriminatory power to accurately identify which severe lesions are really high risk remains poor. A number of years ago Glagov pointed out that the early stages of disease result in remodeling of the vessel wall such that the lumen is preserved despite the increasing extent of atherosclerotic disease (Glagov et al., 1987). This situation can exist with even quite severe disease such that the reliance on measuring stenosis to assess disease can give a false sense of security. This observation was further supported by studies correlating preevent angiographic data with postevent postmortem data. In the coronary arteries Ambrose has shown fatal culprit lesion stenosis is commonly nonsevere when imaged just prior to a fatal coronary event (Ambrose et al., 1988). Analysis of large endarterectomy trials shows that while severe stenosis is related to a higher event rate, this group only

Carotid Disease: The Role of Imaging in Diagnosis and Management, ed. Jonathan Gillard, Martin Graves, Thomas Hatsukami and Chun Yuan. Published by Cambridge University Press. © Cambridge University Press 2007.

makes up a proportion of patients with some degree of carotid vessel wall disease. From these trials it can be seen that a significant number of those suffering stroke are patients previously identified as having nonsevere (<70%) stenoses. What has become clear therefore from these results is that measuring lesser degrees of stenosis can now no longer be relied upon to exclude high risk vessel wall disease, and in order to overcome this limitation the diagnostic target should now be considered the vessel wall itself.

Removing the simple quantitative measure of vessel wall stenosis leaves a diagnostic vacuum as there is at present no simple or accurate replacement. In light of this, there have been increasing attempts to define qualitative and quantitative characteristics of vessel wall disease that will prospectively identify at risk and high risk disease while still asymptomatic. As a result, understanding the processes that result in plaque progression, plaque disruption and subsequent symptom generation is becoming increasingly important.

An element of the atheromatous plaque now becoming appreciated as potentially important in progression and rupture is intraplaque hemorrhage (IPH) (Virmani *et al.*, 2005). Hemorrhage may be of different ages and result in layers of thrombi reflecting a repetitive, often asymptomatic process (Burke *et al.*, 2001). This reflects the fact that while it is known that IPH is often associated with symptomatic events, commonly the hemorrhage is of insufficient severity, or located distant from the luminal surface or other plaque components that would lead to amplification of the effect of IPH, such that surface plaque disruption does not occur. The volume increase caused by IPH is known to be a cause of rapid increase in luminal stenosis and may, by resorption of hemorrhage, also account for a reduction in stenosis. It is now becoming clear however that beyond these mechanical effects of plaque expansion, hemorrhage into the substance of the plaque may have a far more fundamental role in the pathobiology of plaque progression.

The discovery that lipid accumulation within pulmonary artery atherosclerosis, associated with pulmonary hypertension (Arbustini *et al.*, 2002), is at least in part due to the accumulation of cholesterol from red blood cell membranes secondary to intraplaque hemorrhage, provides another explanation as to how and why cholesterol accumulates within plaque, and again emphasizes the importance of IPH. Furthermore, the same process has subsequently been confirmed to exist in systemic atherosclerosis (Kolodgie *et al.*, 2003). The cholesterol level within the erythrocyte membrane is greater than any other cell by up to one and a half to two times. The level of cholesterol also directly reflects the plasma cholesterol level and has been found in hypercholesterolemic patients to be up to seven times normal. Introduction of red blood cells into the plaque substance can therefore result in the accumulation of large quantities of free cholesterol especially in patients with raised circulating cholesterol. This therefore acts as a ready source of cholesterol for the plaque lipid pool that will steadily increase with repeated episodes of intraplaque hemorrhage. The environment of the plaque also seems to play a significant role in the way in which intraplaque erythrocytes and therefore cholesterol is handled; nondiseased vessel wall will tend to remove these components completely with no residual lipid pool, in contradistinction to already diseased vessel wall containing macrophages which accumulate red blood cells and initiate the extraction of cholesterol (Wartman and Laipply, 1949).

Inflammation is now accepted as a major process in the progression of atherosclerosis and now represents a therapeutic target (Choudhury *et al.*, 2005). The accumulation of extracellular lipid is driven by macrophages within the plaque which release phagocytosed oxidized low-density lipoprotein (LDL) upon cell death adding to the lipid core. Release of proteolytic enzymes from macrophages and monocytes has also been suggested as a means by which the plaque surface can become destabilized with eventual plaque rupture. Recent evidence indicates that the presence of red blood cells within the plaque could also interfere with macrophage/monocyte activity causing macrophage activation. Excessive erythrophagocytosis following repeat microhemorrhages eventually leads to phagoparesis which in turn reduces the clearance of apoptotic bodies within the plaque (Tabas, 2005; Schrijvers et al., 2005). The presence of these residual apoptotic bodies is a strong stimulus for escalating inflammation which in turn can trigger plaque softening and rupture. The contents of the red blood cell can also have a profound effect on the atherosclerotic process. Red blood cell derived heme is a reactive oxygen species which causes the oxidation of LDL and the expression of adhesion molecules such as vascular cell adhesion molecule (VCAM) and intercellular adhesion molecule (ICAM) (Morita, 2005).

IPH therefore appears to be a significant event within the plaque that can drive different aspects of plaque progression, many of which result in increased risk of plaque rupture. Chronically the lipid core size may gradually increase with accumulation of erythrocyte derived free cholesterol. With increase in size of the core the risk of plaque instability increases (Felton et al., 1997). More acutely IPH may lead to a sudden increase in size of plaque following a large volume increase due to intraplaque hemorrhage. The presence of red blood cells within the plaque may also cause an acceleration of the inflammatory process and has the potential to trigger surface rupture via disturbance of apoptosis. Not only are the whole red blood cells themselves or their membranes a stimulus for plaque progression and inflammation, but breakdown products of hemoglobin such as heme or methemoglobin, have also been known to stimulate inflammation and cause endothelial activation (Liu and Spolarics, 2003), thus generating a stimulus for carotid plaque activation even in the absence of surface disruption.

IPH commonly occurs by disruption of the surface fibrous cap allowing communication between the lumen and the intraplaque contents. However, histopathological studies have shown that not all cases of IPH are necessarily accompanied by surface disruption (Burke et al., 2002). This therefore poses the question as to the mechanism of IPH in these patients. Micro computerized tomography (CT) studies have elegantly shown the network of vessels that develop within the adventitia and media, and eventually intima of vessels with atherosclerotic plaque. These microvessels are not normal in their morphology and tend to be fragile and leak readily especially near to the luminal surface (Virmani et al., 2005). The formation of these vessels is under the control of growth factors acting upon the vasa vasorum as well as on local and bone marrow derived endothelial progenitor cells to bring about neo-angiogenesis (Garin et al., 2005; Khurana et al., 2005). Furthermore the control of vessel proliferation also appears to play a significant role in the translation of the beneficial effects of known antiatheroma drugs such as statins (Wilson et al., 2002).

An obvious mechanism by which neovessels may contribute to both acute and chronic phases of plaque progression is by bleeding into the plaque, producing IPH. Micro CT studies have examined the distribution of the new vessels with respect to luminal stenosis (Barger and Beeuwkes, 1990) and shown that these vessels are centered on the stenosis itself. However the origin of the vasa vasorum vessels is proximal to the stenosis; this results in a potential mechanism by which microvessel rupture may be induced especially in high-grade stenoses. The gradient across the stenotic section of the vessel goes from high pressure in the prestenotic region to low pressure poststenosis. In addition the turbulence that results within the poststenotic region leads to a significant decrease in luminal pressure brought about by the Bernoulli effect. This is in contrast to the pressure within the plaque microvessels, which are supplied by prestenotic vessels, and therefore exposed to the prestenotic high intravascular pressure. Therefore, there is a theoretical pressure difference between the intraplaque microvessels and the intraluminal blood pressure overlying the distal plaque. In addition to the generally abnormal morphology of the neo-microvessels which makes them prone to rupture, physiological stress that is communicated via elevation in systemic blood pressure (i.e. diurnal, seasonal and climate variation; physical exercise) will also be directly transmitted to the atherosclerotic plaque microcirculation which may be sufficient, especially in tightly stenotic disease, to cause micro-vessel rupture and IPH. This in turn may provide the trigger for plaque rupture. Even if insufficient to cause plaque rupture the hemorrhage will contribute to fuelling plaque progression.

In support of this hypothesis one would expect that plaques that have undergone rupture would have a greater density of neovessels compared with those without rupture. This has been confirmed by McCarthy et al. by looking at the endarterectomy specimens in patients with and without symptoms (McCarthy et al., 1999). They found a greater proportion of vessels in the plaques of symptomatic patients and these vessels were larger and more irregular in shape. Furthermore the increased density of vessels was also associated with more IPH, increased plaque rupture and the frequency of pre- and perioperative emboli, linking the presence of these vessels with the production of symptoms. A further study by Moreno also has not only confirmed this finding in aortic atheroma but has localized the site of increased vessel formation which is commonly in the base of the plaque (Moreno et al., 2004). Their study further showed that vessel density was positively associated with lipid-rich plaques and those with plaque inflammation and IPH. There is now therefore both theoretical and experimental evidence that plaque neovessels are significantly involved in intraplaque hemorrhage and both are closely associated with plaque rupture.

IPH is by definition a marker of complicated plaque and therefore readily identifies the plaque and if the patient is at increased risk of a vascular event. The identification of the culprit lesion in symptomatic patients may be important. First it confirms the diagnosis, and second may identify the specific lesion that has caused symptoms.

This may be particularly important in guiding therapeutic interventions. As already stated the culprit lesion can often be accompanied by a number of other asymptomatic stenotic lesions not responsible for producing symptoms which could therefore make lesion identification difficult if a means were not available to better characterize plaque. Identification of asymptomatic complicated disease could also have significant implications. Knowing that this type of lesion poses greater risk to the patient its recognition, while asymptomatic, affords a window of opportunity during which time therapeutic interventions can be undertaken. This concept has been further extended in the last few years as it has been appreciated that the onset of symptomatic disease may have a significant delay (3–4 days) subsequent to plaque rupture. Within the coronary arteries angiographic data days before acute myocardial infarction has shown the presence of culprit coronary lesions but producing no acute symptoms (Ojio et al., 2000). Analysis of thrombectomy specimens of patients suffering acute myocardial infarction has also shown heterogeneous aging of thrombus with over half the patients demonstrating thrombi which were days or weeks old (Rittersma et al., 2005). Similarly in the carotid circulation recent articles have emphasized that a definitive stroke is most likely to occur in the first few days following a warning transient ischemic attack (TIA) (Johnston et al., 2000; Lovett et al., 2003; Gladstone et al., 2004). This again supports the model of an initial plaque event that is then followed after an interval by an accelerated process resulting in a significant thromboembolic event. While acute thromboembolism is likely to represent the final stages of plaque rupture these data support the theory that plaque disruption is followed by successive thrombotic events measured in days and weeks. This presymptomatic period may represent a significant opportunity for detection and treatment; thus the presence of hemorrhage or thrombus may be a useful marker to identify "the vulnerable and already-disturbed plaque" described by Rittersma.

While the complete natural history of the development, progression and disruption of the atherosclerotic plaque remains to be fully elucidated, intraplaque hemorrhage appears to be a significant event that may not only identify a culprit lesion retrospectively, but may, because of the repetitive nature of the disease, also act as a marker of future events thus providing a means of identifying high-risk patients prior to symptom development. From the above it also appears that this event may not only be an important step in acute plaque events, but also by stimulating inflammation and contributing to the lipid core it also plays a significant role in driving the major substrates of the intraplaque environment. Repetitive intraplaque hemorrhage should therefore not only be regarded as an abortive attempt at plaque rupture but a significant contribution to the cumulative atherosclerotic process. Visualization of IPH could therefore provide a means of detecting the "fuelling" of the disease process and act as a significant marker of plaque pathophysiology whatever stage (acute, subacute, chronic) the vessel is imaged.

In order to investigate and exploit this pathophysiological marker a means of detecting, quantifying and following its behavior over time is required. This should be noninvasive, repeatable and have no effect on the disease process itself. This would ideally be an imaging technique and magnetic resonance imaging (MRI) has been successfully applied to the specific identification of blood products that allow the identification of thrombosis. As blood undergoes thrombosis hemoglobin within red blood cells captured within the thrombus undergoes a predictable maturation. Initially oxyhemoglobin is reduced to deoxyhemoglobin and then oxidation causes the production of methemoglobin. This is brought about by the conversion of Fe^{++} to Fe^{+++}. This results in a highly paramagnetic species because of five unpaired electrons. When present within tissues undergoing MRI this paramagnetism brings about significant T_1 shortening, similar in effect to the presence of gadolinium contrast agent. On the appropriate T_1-weighted sequence therefore this will result in the production of high signal. The possibility therefore exists that methemoglobin can be used as an endogenous contrast agent and in the appropriate setting the high signal generated could be used as a marker for the presence of methemoglobin and thus thrombus.

Proof of concept that methemoglobin could be used as an endogenous T_1 shortening contrast agent was demonstrated in vitro simply by generating methemoglobin of various concentrations. The resultant alteration of T_1 can be shown to be directly related to the methemoglobin concentration (Moody et al., 2000). Application of this technique was initially applied in a clinical setting in which a large volume thrombus was generated in vivo: venous thromboembolic disease. Applying T_1-weighted MRI to patients suspected of suffering deep vein thrombosis or pulmonary embolism, the identification of high signal within the deep veins of the legs or the arteries of the lungs was shown to accurately identify intravascular thrombus (Moody, 1997; Moody et al., 1997; Fraser et al., 2002). This work therefore supported the utility of methemoglobin to provide useful in vivo intravascular contrast in the clinical setting.

At the same time as intravascular methemoglobin was under investigation there was increasing interest in using MRI to directly image atherosclerotic disease within the vessel wall. Toussaint et al. provided early in vivo evidence of the power of MRI to differentiate plaque components including the lipid core, fibrous cap and intraplaque hemorrhage (Toussaint et al., 1996). Because of the known association of T_2-weighted images with the presence of diseased tissue, early efforts focused on the T_2 appearances of plaque and the identification of hemorrhage within the plaque using T_1-weighted imaging was generally ignored (Toussaint et al., 1995). Size of lipid core and cap thickness represented the main targets of MR imaging. Underappreciation of the presence of IPH in these early studies may in part have been related to the type of sequences used. Many investigators have concentrated on the application of spin echo techniques which appear to generate less methemoglobin-related high signal on T_1-weighted images and seem less sensitive to IPH (Taber *et al.*, 1996). Cappendijk *et al.* have shown that gradient echo techniques are significantly more sensitive to IPH than spin echo methods which may account for the increased difficulty detecting IPH with this latter technique (Cappendijk *et al.*, 2004).

Ideally imaging will not only act as a surrogate of histopathology, enabling accurate disease assessment without the need to depend on surgical specimens extracted from patients usually with severe disease, but also provide information relating to present and future disease activity. A reliable marker will allow the survey of any patient whether symptomatic or asymptomatic, with severe or mild disease. In order to reach this point, imaging characteristics need to be correlated with relevant clinical parameters such as signs, symptoms, end organ damage and patient outcome. Exploiting the already proven ability of MRI to generate high signal from methemoglobin, the possibility exists to specifically target hemorrhage within plaque using this technique. The possible utility of such an approach in an acute clinical setting has been demonstrated in patients suffering acute stroke. By concentrating on the single characteristic of IPH despite the difficulty of performing MRI in the acute phase of this patient population it was shown that IPH was commonly present in the proximal internal carotid artery ipsilateral to the side of cerebral infarction, and often independent of the degree of carotid stenosis (Moody *et al.*, 1999).

A great advantage the study of carotid disease has over other vascular beds is the ability to make direct correlation of histology with imaging appearances as patients undergo carotid endarterectomy. The relationship of intraplaque hemorrhage and MRI high signal in the carotid artery can therefore be studied more accurately by the study of endarterectomy specimens in patients suffering cerebral ischemia. Using targeted high resolution multiparametric MRI, Yuan has shown that it is possible to identify the lipid core and IPH with high

accuracy in 18 patients undergoing carotid endarterectomy (Yuan *et al.*, 2001). Further application of this multiparametric technique also provides a means of aging the IPH (Chu *et al.*, 2004). A further study of 63 patients undergoing endarterectomy confirmed that the presence of high signal using a single image acquisition with a heavily T_1-weighted fat-suppressed gradient echo sequence had a high positive predictive value (93%) for intraplaque hemorrhage. While this was a selected group, symptomatic with high-grade stenotic disease, it provided evidence that a simple low resolution technique could accurately identify complicated plaque and is potentially applicable to large populations (Moody *et al.*, 2003).

Using this technique on 120 patients routinely attending for imaging of their carotid vessels Murphy showed IPH on the side ipsilateral to symptoms of cerebral ischemia in 60% (Murphy *et al.*, 2003). The technique also had the advantage of imaging the contralateral carotid artery thus providing an estimate of the asymptomatic IPH rate in this selected high-risk group. This was found to be 36% providing evidence from a large population that IPH may occur silently and is not directly correlated to symptom production.

These techniques provide a means by which the natural history of different components of plaque contents can be followed, specifically IPH. A question that needs addressing is the influence of IPH on the progression of disease. The newly appreciated concept of red blood cells fueling the lipid core was tested by Takaya *et al.* by assessing plaque size progression (Takaya *et al.*, 2005). They found that the increase in vessel wall volume and necrotic core volume was significantly higher in patients with IPH over an 18-month period. This same group was also found to have more new hemorrhages within the plaque when compared with controls (no IPH at baseline).

Trials investigating the effect of IPH on symptom production and end organ damage are at present scarce. Preliminary data from Daniels *et al.* in a clinical follow-up study of 38 patients over 2 years demonstrated a 13% occurrence rate of cerebral ischemia in patients with previous cerebral ischemic events (Daniels *et al.*, 2005). All of those patients with recurrence had previously detected carotid high signal with MRI. Similarly Yamada followed 40 patients (Yamada *et al.*, 2005) for a median of 6 months and also found a recurrence rate of 12.5%, again only in those patients with IPH at initial presentation. These data therefore support the hypothesis that repetitive IPH results in further acute events within the plaque resulting in thromboembolism and end organ effects. Altaf *et al.* has further investigated the relationship of carotid IPH

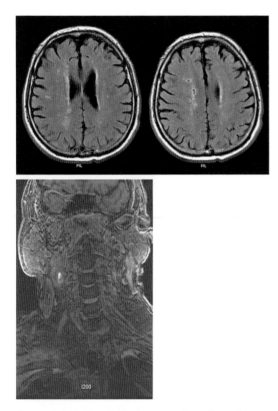

Figure 22.1 FLAIR axial images (top) show deep white matter ischemic lesions more on the right than the left. The low resolution coronal MR direct thrombus image (below) demonstrates high signal intensity in keeping with complicated plaque within the right carotid artery.

and end organ disease. Preliminary results from a study investigating the occurrence of high-intensity transient signals (HITS) detected by transcranial Doppler has shown that the rate of HITS generation is higher in patients with IPH (Altaf *et al.*, 2005). Furthermore, analysis of the MRI appearances of the brain in patients with and without IPH also demonstrated a significant increase in the number of white matter lesions ipsilateral to carotid IPH (Altaf *et al.*, 2006) (Figure 22.1). These findings along with evidence of plaque progression therefore lend significant support to the theoretical importance of IPH in the natural history of atherosclerotic plaque pathophysiology and the production of end organ damage.

The development of a simple and quick technique to identify complicated plaque irrespective of the degree of stenosis could provide a useful means of rapidly assessing an individual's vascular risk. Similarly large cohorts of patients can be surveyed for the presence of advanced disease without the need for prolonged high resolution imaging. This will therefore allow the study of populations who may or may not be at risk of advanced atherosclerotic disease. Until now much of our knowledge has relied on surgical resection specimens such as endarterectomy which have a tendency to select advanced disease thus not providing a reflection of the full spectrum of disease. Bitar has applied this rapid screening technique to investigating the effect of gender on carotid disease of patients presenting with cerebral ischemic symptoms (Bitar *et al.*, 2005a). In a cohort of 86 symptomatic patients (55 male, 31 female) there was a significant difference between the two gender groups with women having a far lower prevalence of IPH compared to men. When further analyzed the prevalence of IPH was found to increase with age, and women demonstrated IPH up to 15 years later than men. This suggests a difference in the vascular biology between the genders and is in keeping with the data correlating proliferation of the vasa vasorum and gender presented by Virmani *et al.* (2005) (Figure 22.2). Delay in the onset of IPH

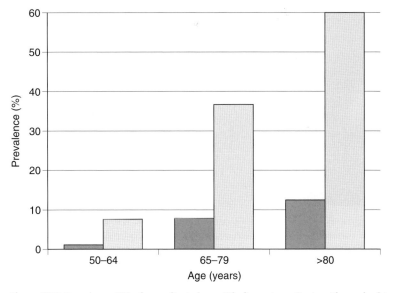

Figure 22.2 Prevalence (%) of complicated carotid plaque in patients with cerebral ischemic symptoms defined by age group and gender.

potentially accounts for some of the differences in the symptomatic presentation of cardiovascular disease in women. These techniques can therefore provide useful insights into pathobiology encouraging novel lines of investigation.

While low resolution, but high-contrast images may be of use in screening patients for the presence or absence of complicated plaque, investigation of the site and pathobiology of the atherosclerotic process requires high-resolution techniques. These can therefore provide intraplaque localization of disease that can be related to other elements of the disease process. High resolution in the literature has usually referred to images that are at least of 500 micron in-plane resolution. Through-plane resolution, i.e. slice thickness, has usually been greater in the order of 2–3 mm. Direct comparison with histology which utilizes slices of tissue in the order of a few microns is therefore still not possible. Attempts to resolve structures such as the thinned fibrous cap, which measures in the order of 65 microns in the coronary artery and in the order of 200 microns in the carotid artery,

with in vivo MRI is not achievable using these techniques (Wasserman *et al.*, 2005). Coverage of the diseased area with sufficient slices can also be problematic. A means of extending this coverage, providing an increased number of thinner slices is provided by 3D techniques which also allow multiplanar reconstruction of the volume data in any chosen plane. Using such techniques Bitar has shown that up to 40 500 micron thick slices with 500 micron in-plane resolution (i.e. 500 micron isotropic voxels) can be achieved which provides sufficient resolution so that each slice can be divided into up to 16 segments resulting in 640 data points per patient (Bitar *et al.*, 2005b). Comparing a lower resolution technique with that of this higher resolution method for the detection of IPH, sensitivity, specificity and positive predictive values all improved (68% → 83%; 89% → 99%; 69% → 96%) as did the interobserver agreement (0.58 → 0.85). The added spatial resolution allows the more precise localization of IPH which appears to be more commonly found in isolation, deep within the plaque closer to the adventitial rather

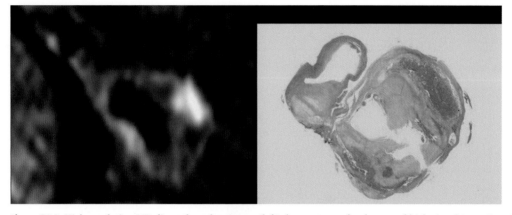

Figure 22.3 High-resolution MR direct thrombus image (left) demonstrates focal areas of high signal intensity within the wall of the internal carotid artery that correlate with areas of intraplaque hemorrhage on histology (right).

than the luminal surface (Bitar *et al.*, personal communications, 2005) (Figure 22.3). The latter is therefore supportive of the model described by Kolodgie *et al.* suggesting IPH derives, at least in part, from deep adventitial neovessels (Kolodgie *et al.*, 2003).

IPH is an important element of atherosclerotic plaque pathobiology. Its presence is a ready marker of plaque disruption, either from the luminal surface or due to neovessel rupture. Whatever the source, it is abnormal and indicates a significant step toward the development of symptomatic disease. In light of this, noninvasive identification of IPH provides a means of studying disease processes within populations as well as individual patient. Groups of patients suffering common diseases or identified with risk factors for atherosclerosis can therefore undergo cross-sectional and longitudinal study combining routine imaging of the carotid lumen (i.e. degree of stenosis) and end organ damage (brain ischemic changes) with imaging of vessel wall complicated disease as represented by IPH. Instead of waiting for patients to present with symptoms the opportunity exists to study the silent effects of atherosclerotic disease, locally in the vessel and within the end organ at a previously unrecognized stage, providing insights into the pathobiology of systemic disease on the vasculature.

REFERENCES

Altaf, N., Daniels, L., Beech, A., *et al.* (2005). Magnetic resonance direct thrombus imaging of the carotid plaque is associated with increased thromboembolization. *13th annual meeting of the International Society for Magnetic Resonance in Medicine.* Miami, Florida.

Altaf, N., Daniels, L., Morgan, P. S., *et al.* (2006). Cerebral white matter hyperintense lesions are associated with unstable carotid plaques. *European Journal of Vascular and Endovascular Surgery*, **31**, 8–13.

Ambrose, J. A., Tannenbaum, M. A., Alexopoulos, D., *et al.* (1988). Angiographic progression of coronary artery disease and the development of myocardial infarction. *Journal of the American College of Cardiology*, **12**, 56–62.

Arbustini, E., Morbini, P., D'armini, A. M., *et al.* (2002). Plaque composition in plexogenic and thromboembolic pulmonary hypertension: the critical role of thrombotic material in pultaceous core formation. *Heart*, **88**, 177–82.

Barger, A. C. and Beeuwkes, R., 3rd. (1990). Rupture of coronary vasa vasorum as a trigger of acute myocardial infarction. *American Journal of Cardiology*, **66**, 41G–43G.

Barnett, H. J., Taylor, D. W., Eliasziw, M., *et al.* (1998). Benefit of carotid endarterectomy in patients with symptomatic moderate or severe stenosis. North American Symptomatic Carotid Endarterectomy Trial Collaborators. *New England Journal of Medicine*, **339**, 1415–25.

Bitar, R., Leung, G., Kiss, A., *et al.* (2005a). Prevalence of intraplaque hemorrhage in vasculopathic patients with asymptomatic carotid stenosis. *2005 American Heart Association Scientific Sessions.* Dallas, Texas.

Bitar, R., Moody, A. R., Leung, G., *et al.* (2005b). 3D high-resolution Magnetic Resonance Direct Thrombus Imaging (hiresMRDTI) and 3D conventional MRDTI (convMRDTI): a radiological-histological comparative study. *Radiological Society of North America Meeting.* Chicago, Illinois.

Burke, A. P., Kolodgie, F. D., Farb, A., Weber, D. and Virmani, R. (2002). Morphological predictors of arterial remodeling in coronary atherosclerosis. *Circulation,* **105**, 297–303.

Burke, A. P., Kolodgie, F. D., Farb, A., *et al.* (2001). Healed plaque ruptures and sudden coronary death: evidence that subclinical rupture has a role in plaque progression. *Circulation,* **103**, 934–40.

Cappendijk, V. C., Cleutjens, K. B., Heeneman, S., *et al.* (2004). In vivo detection of hemorrhage in human atherosclerotic plaques with magnetic resonance imaging. *Journal of Magnetic Resonance Imaging,* **20**, 105–10.

Choudhury, R. P., Lee, J. M. and Greaves, D. R. (2005). Mechanisms of disease: macrophage-derived foam cells emerging as therapeutic targets in atherosclerosis. *Nature Clinical Practice. Cardiovascular Medicine,* **2**, 309–15.

Chu, B., Kampschulte, A., Ferguson, M. S., *et al.* (2004). Hemorrhage in the atherosclerotic carotid plaque: a high-resolution MRI study. *Stroke,* **35**, 1079–84.

Daniels, L., Altaf, N., Morgan, P., *et al.* (2005). Natural history of complicated carotid plaque detected by MRI in symptomatic moderate carotid artery stenosis. *The 14th European Stroke Conference.* Bologna, Italy.

ECAS (1991). MRC European Carotid Surgery Trial: interim results for symptomatic patients with severe (70–99%) or with mild (0–29%) carotid stenosis. European Carotid Surgery Trialists' Collaborative Group. *Lancet,* **337**, 1235–43.

Felton, C. V., Crook, D., Davies, M. J. and Oliver, M. F. (1997). Relation of plaque lipid composition and morphology to the stability of human aortic plaques. *Arteriosclerosis, Thrombosis and Vascular Biology,* **17**, 1337–45.

Fraser, D. G., Moody, A. R., Morgan, P. S., Martel, A. L. and Davidson, I. (2002). Diagnosis of lower-limb deep venous thrombosis: a prospective blinded study of magnetic resonance direct thrombus imaging. *Annals of Internal Medicine,* **136**, 89–98.

Garin, G., Mathews, M. and Berk, B. C. (2005). Tissue-resident bone marrow-derived progenitor cells: key players in hypoxia-induced angiogenesis. *Circulation Research,* **97**, 955–7.

Gladstone, D. J., Kapral, M. K., Fang, J., Laupacis, A. and Tu, J. V. (2004). Management and outcomes of transient ischemic attacks in Ontario. *Canadian Medical Association Journal,* **170**, 1099–104.

Glagov, S., Weisenberg, E., Zarins, C. K., Stankunavicius, R. and Kolettis, G. J. (1987). Compensatory enlargement of human atherosclerotic coronary arteries. *New England Journal of Medicine,* **316**, 1371–5.

Johnston, S. C., Gress, D. R., Browner, W. S. and Sidney, S. (2000). Short-term prognosis after emergency department diagnosis of TIA. *Journal of the American Medical Association,* **284**, 2901–6.

Khurana, R., Simons, M., Martin, J. F. and Zachary, I. C. (2005). Role of angiogenesis in cardiovascular disease: a critical appraisal. *Circulation,* **112**, 1813–24.

Kolodgie, F. D., Gold, H. K., Burke, A. P., *et al.* (2003). Intraplaque hemorrhage and progression of coronary atheroma. *New England Journal of Medicine,* **349**, 2316–25.

Liu, X. and Spolarics, Z. (2003). Methemoglobin is a potent activator of endothelial cells by stimulating IL-6 and IL-8 production and E-selectin membrane expression. *American Journal of Physiology. Cell Physiology,* **285**, C1036–46.

Lovett, J. K., Dennis, M. S., Sandercock, P. A., *et al.* (2003). Very early risk of stroke after a first transient ischemic attack. *Stroke,* **34**, e138–40.

McCarthy, M. J., Loftus, I. M., Thompson, M. M., *et al.* (1999). Angiogenesis and the atherosclerotic carotid plaque: an association between symptomatology and plaque morphology. *Journal of Vascular Surgery,* **30**, 261–8.

Moody, A. R. (1997). Direct imaging of deep-vein thrombosis with magnetic resonance imaging. *Lancet,* **350**, 1073.

Moody, A. R., Allder, S., Lennox, G., Gladman, J. and Fentem, P. (1999). Direct magnetic resonance imaging of carotid artery thrombus in acute stroke. *Lancet,* **353**, 122–3.

Moody, A. R., Liddicoat, A. and Krarup, K. (1997). Magnetic resonance pulmonary angiography and direct imaging of embolus for the detection of pulmonary emboli. *Investigative Radiology,* **32**, 431–40.

Moody, A. R., Morgan, P., Fraser, D. and Hunt, B. J. (2000). Methaemoglobin T1 high signal: its generation and application to MR thrombus imaging. *World Congress of the International Union of Angiology*. Ghent, Belgium.

Moody, A. R., Murphy, R. E., Morgan, P. S., *et al.* (2003). Characterization of complicated carotid plaque with magnetic resonance direct thrombus imaging in patients with cerebral ischemia. *Circulation*, **107**, 3047–52.

Moreno, P. R., Purushothaman, K. R., Fuster, V., *et al.* (2004). Plaque neovascularization is increased in ruptured atherosclerotic lesions of human aorta: implications for plaque vulnerability. *Circulation*, **110**, 2032–8.

Morita, T. (2005). Heme oxygenase and atherosclerosis. *Arteriosclerosis, Thrombosis and Vascular Biology*, **25**, 1786–95.

Murphy, R. E., Moody, A. R., Morgan, P. S., *et al.* (2003). Prevalence of complicated carotid atheroma as detected by magnetic resonance direct thrombus imaging in patients with suspected carotid artery stenosis and previous acute cerebral ischemia. *Circulation*, **107**, 3053–8.

Ojio, S., Takatsu, H., Tanaka, T., *et al.* (2000). Considerable time from the onset of plaque rupture and/or thrombi until the onset of acute myocardial infarction in humans: coronary angiographic findings within 1 week before the onset of infarction. *Circulation*, **102**, 2063–9.

Rittersma, S. Z., Van Der Wal, A. C., Koch, K. T., *et al.* (2005). Plaque instability frequently occurs days or weeks before occlusive coronary thrombosis: a pathological thrombectomy study in primary percutaneous coronary intervention. *Circulation*, **111**, 1160–5.

Schrijvers, D. M., De Meyer, G. R., Kockx, M. M., Herman, A. G. and Martinet, W. (2005). Phagocytosis of apoptotic cells by macrophages is impaired in atherosclerosis. *Arteriosclerosis, Thrombosis and Vascular Biology*, **25**, 1256–61.

Stary, H. C., Chandler, A. B., Dinsmore, R. E., *et al.* (1995). A definition of advanced types of atherosclerotic lesions and a histological classification of atherosclerosis. A report from the Committee on Vascular Lesions of the Council on Arteriosclerosis, American Heart Association. *Arteriosclerosis, Thrombosis and Vascular Biology*, **15**, 1512–31.

Tabas, I. (2005). Consequences and therapeutic implications of macrophage apoptosis in atherosclerosis: the importance of lesion stage and phagocytic efficiency. *Arteriosclerosis, Thrombosis and Vascular Biology*, **25**, 2255–64.

Taber, K. H., Hayman, L. A., Herrick, R. C. and Kirkpatrick, J. B. (1996). Importance of clot structure in gradient-echo magnetic resonance imaging of hematoma. *Journal of Magnetic Resonance Imaging*, **6**, 878–83.

Takaya, N., Yuan, C., Chu, B., *et al.* (2005). Presence of intraplaque hemorrhage stimulates progression of carotid atherosclerotic plaques: a high-resolution magnetic resonance imaging study. *Circulation*, **111**, 2768–75.

Toussaint, J. F., Lamuraglia, G. M., Southern, J. F., Fuster, V. and Kantor, H. L. (1996). Magnetic resonance images lipid, fibrous, calcified, hemorrhagic, and thrombotic components of human atherosclerosis in vivo. *Circulation*, **94**, 932–8.

Toussaint, J. F., Southern, J. F., Fuster, V. and Kantor, H. L. (1995). T2-weighted contrast for NMR characterization of human atherosclerosis. *Arteriosclerosis, Thrombosis and Vascular Biology*, **15**, 1533–42.

Virmani, R., Kolodgie, F. D., Burke, A. P., *et al.* (2005). Atherosclerotic plaque progression and vulnerability to rupture: angiogenesis as a source of intraplaque hemorrhage. *Arteriosclerosis, Thrombosis and Vascular Biology*, **25**, 2054–61.

Wartman, W. B. and Laipply, T. C. (1949). The fate of blood injected into the arterial wall. *American Journal of Pathology*, **25**, 383–8.

Wasserman, B. A., Wityk, R. J., Trout, H. H., 3rd and Virmani, R. (2005). Low-grade carotid stenosis: looking beyond the lumen with MRI. *Stroke*, **36**, 2504–13.

Wilson, S. H., Herrmann, J., Lerman, L. O., *et al.* (2002). Simvastatin preserves the structure of coronary adventitial vasa vasorum in experimental hypercholesterolemia independent of lipid lowering. *Circulation*, **105**, 415–18.

Yamada, N., Higashi, M., Otsubo, R., *et al.* (2005). Characterization of carotid plaque by using an inversion-recovery based T1-weighted imaging in correlation with ipsilateral ischemic events. *13th annual meeting of the International Society for Magnetic Resonance in Medicine*. Miami, Florida.

Yuan, C., Mitsumori, L. M., Ferguson, M. S., *et al.* (2001). In vivo accuracy of multispectral magnetic resonance imaging for identifying lipid-rich necrotic cores and intraplaque hemorrhage in advanced human carotid plaques. *Circulation*, **104**, 2051–6.

23

The proximal carotid arteries – image-based computational modelling

Yun Xu and N. B. Wood

Imperial College London, South Kensington Campus,
London SW7 2AZ, UK

Introduction

The carotid bifurcation is a site of particular interest for arterial disease studies, since it is a focal site where atherosclerosis is common, particularly affecting the carotid sinus, at the origin of the internal carotids. Moreover, as the atherosclerotic plaque forms, it may become vulnerable to rupture, releasing emboli and promoting the formation of thrombus more distally, leading to stroke.

The long-standing hypothesis that hemodynamic forces correlate with the initiation and progression of atherosclerosis has been the driver for numerous computational and experimental studies of the carotid arteries over the years. Research on the combination of magnetic resonance imaging (MRI) and computational fluid dynamics (CFD) began almost a decade ago, leading to subsequent publications on studies of large artery hemodynamics under physiologically realistic anatomical and flow conditions (Milner *et al.*, 1998; Taylor *et al.*, 1999; Long *et al.*, 2000a,b; Wood *et al.*, 2001). The use of conventional and 3D ultrasound imaging to acquire in vivo geometrical information for CFD analysis has not been widely adopted although some attempts have been made (Gill *et al.*, 2000; Augst *et al.*, 2003; Barratt *et al.*, 2004; Glor *et al.*, 2005). Computerised tomography (CT) imaging has also been used for reconstruction of subject-specific models of coronary stenoses and abdominal aortic aneurysms (Raghavan *et al.*, 2000; Achenbach *et al.*, 2001; Leung *et al.*, 2005), but this technique is limited by the associated ionizing radiation.

CFD allows the simulation of complete flow fields within a specified domain, in space and time, via the numerical solution of the equations of motion. With the continuing advances in computer technology, and high-resolution imaging and image processing techniques, the combination of in vivo imaging and CFD now allows patient-specific flow simulations and opens the way to patho-physiological and clinical utility (Taylor *et al.*, 1999; Steinman *et al.*, 2002; Zhao *et al.*, 2002; Lee *et al.*, 2004).

Image-based computer modelling is able to simulate parameters that cannot be measured, or derived directly from imaging measurements, with acceptable resolution (e.g. Wood *et al.*, 2001). Research on the development of atherosclerosis (DeBakey *et al.*, 1985; Ku *et al.*, 1985; Giddens *et al.*, 1993; Malek *et al.*, 1999) has supported early suggestions (Fry, 1968; Caro *et al.*, 1969) that arterial wall shear stress was an important determinant of the observed patterns of arterial disease. Moreover, related research showed that endothelial shear stress is a signalling parameter for blood flow, both in short-term control of hemodynamics

Carotid Disease: The Role of Imaging in Diagnosis and Management, ed. Jonathan Gillard, Martin Graves, Thomas Hatsukami and Chun Yuan. Published by Cambridge University Press. © Cambridge University Press 2007.

and longer-term responses of the arterial system to blood flow variations (Davies, 1995; Wootton and Ku, 1999; Levick, 2003). The induced responses generally involve gene expression (Resnick and Gimbrone, 1995; Davies *et al.*, 1999; Malek *et al.*, 1999), giving additional potential importance to these methods. Therefore, research has focused on the computation of the spatial and temporal distributions of wall shear stress (Friedman and Fry, 1993) and related parameters (He and Ku, 1996; Steinman *et al.*, 2002; Glor *et al.*, 2003a; Thomas *et al.*, 2003). Flow regimes have been identified as "athero-prone" or "athero-protective", depending on flow structure and the associated wall shear stress patterns, giving rise to up-regulation and down-regulation of specific ranges of genes (Dai *et al.*, 2004; Passerini *et al.*, 2004).

Further recent applications include fluid-structure interaction: the modelling of arterial wall mechanics coupled with the flow field, particularly involving atherosclerotic plaques or stenoses (Bathe and Kamm, 1999; Tang *et al.*, 2001; Lee and Xu, 2002; Lee *et al.*, 2004). Here a principal aim is to determine stress distributions in the plaques with a view to predicting rupture, an initiating factor in stroke or coronary events (Richardson *et al.*, 1989; Richardson, 2002). Again, in vivo image-based modelling allows patient-specific studies, opening the way to related clinical decision support. Key problems associated with analysis of carotid plaque are the adequacy of resolution of in vivo images to determine the plaque structure, and the complexity and variability of the mechanical properties of postoperative or postmortem samples, between subjects and with time (Holzapfel *et al.*, 2004). A further question relates to the transition from laminar to turbulent flow in the poststenotic zones of the more severe stenoses (Wood and Xu, 2003).

Another application of patient-specific image-based modelling is clinical decision support via "virtual surgery", i.e. the predictive simulation of alternative vascular surgical interventions for optimizing treatment. Taylor *et al.* (1999) at Stanford have developed an interactive system whereby surgeons are able to simulate alternative femoral graft geometries. It is hoped that the work on carotid plaque will lead to clinical diagnosis and decision support, e.g. for plaque rupture prediction or providing additional information on the effects of drug therapy.

In drug studies it has been found that anti-hypertensive therapy may not only affect arterial wall thickness (Mayet *et al.*, 1995), but that different agents can have different morphological, and hence fluid dynamic outcomes (Stanton *et al.*, 2001; Ariff *et al.*, 2002); this could be potentially important in future clinical research. The mass transfer of substances between the flowing blood and the artery wall, including large molecules like albumin and lipids, and small molecules such as oxygen and nitric oxide has important potential applications (Rappitsch and Perktold, 1996; Ma *et al.*, 1997; Stangeby and Ethier, 2002; Tarbell, 2003) and the substances modelled could include drugs at their sites of action (pharmacokinetics and pharmacogenomics).

In this chapter we will concentrate our discussion on computational simulation based on MR and ultrasound imaging. Our examples will relate to the exploration of flow structure and wall shear stress distributions, and the latter's relationship with arterial disease patterns.

Imaging

The motion of a fluid is highly sensitive to the shape and dynamics of the boundaries that surround the fluid domain. Hence, an accurate description of 3D vessel geometry is essential for accurate modelling of blood flow using CFD, and magnetic resonance angiography (MRA) has been the most popular technique for obtaining this information in vivo. However, for superficial vessels such as the carotid and femoral arteries, extravascular 3D ultrasound can be a cost-effective alternative to MRA. Regardless of which imaging technique is used, the rationale remains the same: to construct a 3D volume of interest from a series of 2D cross-sectional slices.

Time-of-flight (TOF) angiography has been the most widely used method of MRA, performed with the gradient echo sequence enhanced by flow compensation. The sequence is versatile and robust, and has been applied to virtually every part of the body (Dumoulin and Hart, 1986; Dumoulin *et al.*, 1987). "Black-blood" MRI allows both the vessel lumen and outer wall to be imaged at relatively high resolution, providing information for both the lumen shape and wall thickness, required for wall stress analysis. A more recently introduced sequence, SSFP ("steady-state free precession"), gives high resolution of both lumen and vascular structures (Hargreaves *et al.*, 2003).

For 3D ultrasound imaging, the system usually consists of a standard 2D ultrasound scanner and an electromagnetic position and orientation measurement (EPOM) device (Barratt *et al.*, 2001). The EPOM sensor is mounted on the scan-probe and tracks its position and orientation. An image and the corresponding position/orientation are captured simultaneously when an R-wave trigger is detected and a set of nonparallel transverse slices with their position and orientation are recorded and stored on a computer for off-line analysis.

The resulting 2D transverse images are often segmented manually or semiautomatically to delineate the lumen contours. This may take a number of steps including preprocessing, edge detection and smoothing. Numerous image processing algorithms have been developed to accomplish these tasks (e.g. Kass *et al.*, 1988; Ji *et al.*, 1994; Long *et al.*, 1998). A key issue is to obtain a continuous and smooth contour whilst preserving as much original geometry as possible. By stacking the segmented lumen contours a 3D object can be constructed. Smoothing of the image data is required in order to minimize imaging artefacts, random errors due to subject movement, and beat-to-beat variation during the scan. More recently, fully 3D segmentation techniques have been developed (e.g. Antiga and Steinman, 2004), which may find increasing application in the future.

CFD modelling

Governing equations

The Navier-Stokes (N-S) equations of fluid motion for a homogeneous medium, derived by the nineteenth century mathematicians M. Navier in France and Sir G. G. Stokes in England, are exact for laminar flows of simple fluids. They express Newton's law of the conservation of momentum in the fluid, and are combined with the equation of continuity. The equations may be expressed in various forms, such as in partial differential Cartesian coordinate form or integro-differential form. They are written below as vectorial statements, in incompressible form, for an arbitrary fluid volume V:

$$\rho \frac{\partial}{\partial t} \int_V dV + \rho \int_S (U - U_S) \cdot n dS = 0 \qquad (23.1)$$

$$\rho \frac{\partial}{\partial t} \int_V U dV + \rho \int_S U(U - U_S) \cdot n dS$$
$$= \int_S [-p + \mu \nabla U + \mu (\nabla U)^T] \cdot n dS \qquad (23.2)$$

U is the instantaneous fluid velocity at time t, p is the instantaneous static pressure relative to a datum level, n is the unit vector orthogonal to and directed outward from a surface S of the volume, and ρ and μ are, respectively, the fluid density and viscosity. The former is constant under the incompressible assumption and the second is constant for a Newtonian fluid. The surface S here moves locally at velocity U_S. The superscript "T" represents the transpose of the quantity expressed in matrix form (we deal with a set of numerical values of the terms in the equation for each cell of a computational mesh). The equations cannot be solved analytically, except under a restricted range of approximations (Schlichting, 1979; Wood, 1999). Therefore, for most flows of practical interest, we use numerical solution methods, which have become more important as computers have become faster and able to store large amounts of data.

The form of equations (23.1) and (23.2) is appropriate for "finite volume" numerical analysis, used in many CFD codes, where V is the volume of a cell of the mesh on which the computation is carried out. If the boundaries are rigid, the velocity of the boundary $U_S = 0$. Alternatives to finite volume codes are finite difference, where a differential form of the N-S equations is used, and finite element codes, developed from structural analysis methods.

Boundary conditions

The solution of the N-S equations, whether analytical or numerical, requires a solution domain, the cardiovascular region of interest, and conditions on its boundary, including the "no-slip" condition at the blood-endothelium boundary, imposed by the frictional action of the fluid viscosity, and the impervious and rigid wall conditions, meaning all velocity components are zero at the wall. These are complemented by velocities and/or pressures at the inlet and outlet(s) to the domain. The flow solution is specific to the geometry of the domain (fixed or moving) and the boundary conditions. Therefore, it depends both on the local geometry and the geometry and cardiovascular characteristics of the regions contiguous with the domain of interest.

The required velocity distribution may be obtained from magnetic resonance velocity imaging (e.g. phase contrast [PC] and echo planar imaging [EPI]), which exploits the fact that motion through magnetic field gradients results in a phase shift in the net transverse magnetization of moving material compared with that of stationary material imaged at the same physical location. If the pressure level is unimportant, as in the rigid wall cases, the distal pressure may be set to zero at each time step, so that pressure in the domain represents a relative pressure floating in time. The pressure distribution at each time-step will be correctly determined, but if the absolute pressure distribution is required, as with fluid/wall coupling, it must be related to the time-varying absolute pressure (Zhao et al., 2002). If it is not feasible or practicable to measure the required velocity profiles via MR, the flow waveforms may be measured with Doppler ultrasound and the time-varying velocity profiles may be derived using Womersley's approximate analytical solution (Holdsworth et al., 1999; Nichols and O'Rourke, 2005).

Computational mesh

Having made a "virtual" reconstruction of the imaged domain, the numerical solution requires a grid on which the solution variables are calculated. Generally, the grids are said to be "structured" (hexahedral cells) or "unstructured" (including tetrahedral cells); both may be divided into blocks to fit different parts of the domain. Unstructured meshes can more readily fit into a complex geometry, but mesh refinement at boundaries may require special measures.

Resolution and accuracy of the numerical solution

Whilst the N-S equations are exact for laminar flows in simple fluids, the resolution and accuracy of the solution depends on the algebraic discretization method, the size and form of the mesh cells, and the time step for unsteady flows. Since numerical solutions require iterative methods, finding the number of iterations required for adequate convergence is a further criterion (e.g. Hirsch, 1988; Ferziger and Peric, 1996). Moreover, for complex flows, experimental confirmation of some aspect of the solution may be required, such as the reattachment point or zone of a separated flow, particularly if laminar-turbulent transition is involved (Bluestein et al., 1997; Mittal et al., 2001).

Parameters simulated

The computed solution comprises numerical values of flow field parameters on the computational mesh, at the nodes or on the faces of the cells. The principal parameters are the fluid velocity vectors, which may be resolved into orthogonal coordinate directions, and the "static" pressure (pressure experienced by walls lying parallel with the flow). The wall shear stress (WSS) is of particular interest in artery studies (e.g. Glor *et al.*, 2003a). The best method of interrogating a 3D, time-varying solution is via a graphical display, of which numerous commercial packages are available.

Examples

We have constructed CFD models of the carotid artery bifurcations for over 20 normal subjects as well as hypertensive patients based on either MRI or extravascular 3D ultrasound images, and selected examples of these are given in Figure 23.1. A comparative study was performed on the reconstructions from black-blood MRI and extra-vascular 3D ultrasound of carotid bifurcations (Glor *et al.*, 2003b). Overall, extravascular 3D ultrasound proved to be able to generate 3D in vivo carotid geometries suitable for CFD simulations, comparable to those reconstructed from

MRI. Despite some limitations, extravascular 3D ultrasound has potential to become a relatively inexpensive, fast and accurate alternative to MRI for CFD-based hemodynamics studies of super-ficial arteries.

Because of the importance of accurate representation of 3D vessel geometry to subsequent CFD analysis, it is necessary to assess the reproduci-bility of image-based reconstruction procedures. We have carried out a series of reproducibility studies for each imaging modality adopted, and an example of these for extravascular 3D ultra-sound-based carotid reconstruction is given here (Augst, 2003). The volunteer was imaged twice within a few weeks and analyzed using the methods described earlier. Doppler ultrasound flow measurements were also made which were used as boundary conditions for flow simulations. Figure 23.2 shows the comparison of vessel cross-sectional areas between the two scans, while Figure 23.3 shows the comparison of measured flow waves in each of the carotid arteries as well as predicted wall shear stress. It is clear that the difference in lumen cross-sectional areas is rather small, but the measured flow waves in the internal and external carotid arteries are notice-ably different. All these have an effect on computed velocity profiles and shear stress, and results shown in Figure 23.3 indicate that patterns of WSS and oscillatory shear index (OSI) are similar between models constructed from the initial and follow-up scans although quantitative differ-ences exist.

The methods described here were designed to be applicable to serial investigations and clinical use. One such example is the study on the effect of antihypertensive drugs on carotid hemo-dynamics. In this study, a number of hyper-tensive subjects were scanned before and after treatment with different antihypertensive thera-pies. Their carotid bifurcations were recon-structed and flow simulations were carried out to determine a variety of shear stress derived parameters. Shown in Figure 23.4 are the com-puted patterns of WSS and OSI before and

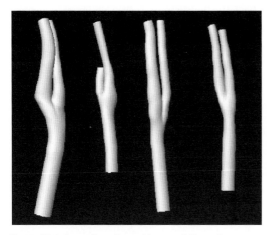

Figure 23.1 Examples of carotid artery bifurcation reconstructed from 3D ultrasound images.

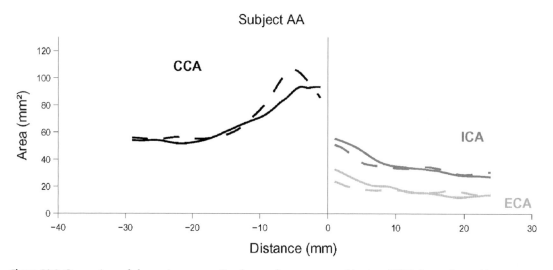

Figure 23.2 Comparison of change in cross-sectional area of common carotid artery (CCA), internal carotid artery (ICA) and external carotid artery (ECA) along the scan direction for first (solid) and second scan (dashed) for subject AA.

after treatment. It can be observed that there is a great similarity between initial and posttreatment results for this subject. The areas of high OSI and low WSS can be found in similar locations, but values for OSI appear to be lower and WSS levels slightly higher in the after treatment set.

The examples presented here are for rigid wall models where arterial wall compliance is not considered. Modelling of coupled fluid/wall interactions requires solutions of the equations of motion for both the flow and the wall, and has become a specific topic in computational mechanics in recent years. A practical problem in coupled fluid/wall modelling of blood flows is the difficulty in acquiring subject-specific data about the arterial wall thickness and mechanical properties. The effects of wall compliance on carotid hemodynamics have been investigated by Zhao *et al.* (2002) who observed a general reduction in the magnitude of WSS, but the global characteristics of the flow and stress patterns remained unchanged.

There are a number of practical limitations associated with subject-specific carotid flow simulations based on in vivo images. The most obvious one is the significant amount of computational effort required to carry out the simulation as well as efforts involved in converting image data into an appropriate CFD input file. The latter consists of a well-designed computational mesh generated for the specific carotid geometry reconstructed from a set of anatomical images and the necessary CFD boundary conditions. This process usually requires the input from an experienced operator even with the help of specialized software.

Standardized imaging protocols with high-quality images will certainly help to reduce the manpower needed for model reconstruction and preparation, and to minimize operator dependence of the reconstruction process. With further advancement in computer hardware and CFD software, patient-specific flow analysis based on noninvasively acquired images is likely to play an increasing role as a diagnostic,

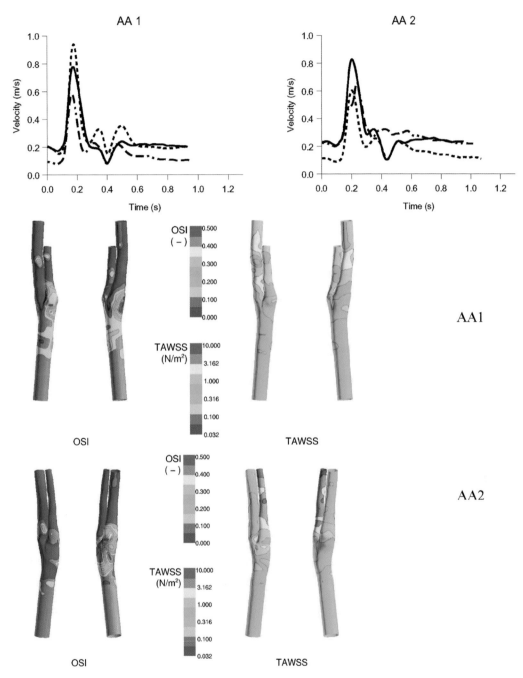

Figure 23.3 Comparison of measured centerline velocities in each vessel (CCA: solid line, ECA: dashed line, ICA: chain-dotted line) and computed oscillatory shear index (OSI) and TAWSS (time-averaged wall shear stress) for subject AA (AA1: first scan, AA2: second scan).

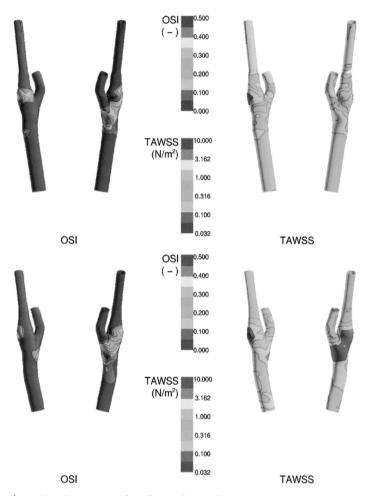

Figure 23.4 Comparison of oscillatory shear index (OSI) and TAWSS (time-averaged wall shear stress) for a hypertensive subject before (top) and after treatment (bottom).

predictive and surgical planning tool for vascular diseases.

Acknowledgements

The following people have contributed to the data used here: Drs. B. Ariff, A. D. Augst, D. C. Barratt, Professors A. D. Hughes and S. A. Thom.

REFERENCES

Achenbach, S., Giesler, T., Ropers, D., *et al.* (2001). Detection of coronary artery stenoses by contrast-enhanced, retrospectively electrocardiographically-gated, multislice spiral computed tomography. *Circulation*, **103**, 2535–8.

Antiga, L. and Steinman, D. A. (2004). Robust and objective decomposition and mapping of bifurcating vessels. *IEEE Transactions on Medical Imaging*, **23**, 704–13.

Ariff, B., Stanton, A., Barratt, D.C., *et al.* (2002). Comparison of the effects of antihypertensive treatment with angiotensin II blockade and beta-blockade on carotid wall structure and haemodynamics: protocol and baseline demographics. *Journal of the Renin-Angiotensin-Aldosterone System*, **3**, 116–22.

Augst, A. (2003). Haemodynamics in human carotid artery bifurcations: A combined CFD and 3D ultrasound study [PhD]. Imperial College London, University of London.

Barratt, D.C., Davies, A.H., Hughes, A.D., Thom, S.A. and Humphries, K.N. (2001). Optimisation and evaluation of an electromagnetic tracking device for high accuracy three-dimensional imaging of the carotid arteries. *Ultrasound in Medicine and Biology*, **27**, 957–68.

Barratt, D.C., Ariff, B.B., Humphries, K.N., *et al.* (2004). Reconstruction and quantification of the carotid artery bifurcation from 3-D ultrasound images. *IEEE Transactions in Medical Imaging*, **23**, 567–83.

Bathe, M. and Kamm, R.D. (1999). A fluid-structure interaction finite element analysis of pulsatile blood flow through a compliant stenotic artery. *Journal of Biomechanical Engineering*, **121**, 361–9.

Bluestein, D., Niu, L., Schoephoerster, R.T. and Dewanjee, M.K. (1997). Fluid mechanics of arterial stenosis: relationship to the development of mural thrombus. *Annals of Biomedical Engineering*, **25**, 344–56.

Caro, C.G., FitzGerald, J.M. and Schroter, R.C. (1969). Arterial wall shear and early atheroma in man. *Nature*, **223**, 1159–61.

Dai, G., Kaazempur-Mofrad, M.R., Natarajan, S., *et al.* (2004). Distinct endothelial phenotypes evoked by arterial waveforms derived from atherosclerosis-susceptible and -resistant regions of human vasculature. *Proceedings of the National Academy of Sciences*, **101**, 14871–6.

Davies, P.F. (1995). Flow-mediated endothelial mechanotransduction. *Physiological Reviews*, **75**, 519–60.

Davies, P.F., Polacek, D.C., Handen, J.S., Helmke, B.P. and DePaola, N. (1999). A spatial approach to transcriptional profiling: mechanotransduction and the focal origin of atherosclerosis. *Trends in Biotechnology*, **17**, 347–51.

DeBakey, M.E., Lawrie, G.M. and Glaeser, D.H. (1985). Patterns of atherosclerosis and their surgical significance. *Annals of Surgery*, **201**, 115–31.

Dumoulin, C.L. and Hart, H.R. (1986). Magnetic resonance angiography. *Radiology*, **161**, 717–20.

Dumoulin, C.L., Souza, S.P. and Hart, H.R. (1987). Rapid scan magnetic resonance angiography. *Magnetic Resonance in Medicine*, **5**, 238–45.

Ferziger, J.H. and Peric, M. (1996). *Computational Methods for Fluid Dynamics*. Berlin: Springer-Verlag.

Friedman, M.H. and Fry, D.L. (1993). Arterial permeability dynamics and vascular disease. *Atherosclerosis*, **104**, 189–94.

Fry, D.L. (1968). Acute endothelial damage associated with increased blood velocity gradients. *Circulation Research*, **22**, 165–97.

Giddens, D.P., Zarins, C.K. and Glagov, S. (1993). The role of fluid mechanics in the localization and detection of atherosclerosis. *Journal of Biomechanical Engineering*, **115**, 588–94.

Gill, J.D., Ladak, H.M., Steinman, D.A. and Fenster, A. (2000). Accuracy and variability assessment of a semiautomatic technique for segmentation of the carotid arteries from three-dimensional ultrasound images. *Medical Physics*, **27**, 1333–42.

Glor, F.P., Long, Q. and Hughes, A.D. (2003a). Reproducibility study of magnetic resonance image-based computational fluid dynamics prediction of carotid bifurcation flow. *Annals of Biomedical Engineering*, **31**, 142–1.

Glor, F.P., Ariff, B., Crowe, L., *et al.* (2003b). Carotid geometry reconstruction: a comparison between MRI and Ultrasound. *Medical Physics*, **30**, 3251–61.

Glor, F.P., Ariff, B., Hughes, A.D., *et al.* (2005). Operator dependence of 3-D ultrasound-based computational fluid dynamics for the carotid bifurcation. *IEEE Transactions in Medical Imaging*, **24**, 451–6.

Hargreaves, B.A., Vasanawala, S.S., Nayak, K.S., Hu, B.S. and Nishimura, G.G. (2003). Fat-suppressed steady-state free precession imaging using phase detection. *Magnetic Resonance in Medicine*, **50**, 210–13.

He, X. and Ku, D.N. (1996). Pulsatile flow in the human left coronary artery bifurcation: average conditions. *Journal of Biomechanical Engineering*, **118**, 74–82.

Hirsch, C. (1988). *Numerical Computation of Internal and External Flows*. New York, NY: Wiley.

Holdsworth, D.W., Norley, C.J.D., Frayne, R., Steinman, D.A. and Rutt, B.K. (1999). Characterization of common carotid artery blood-flow waveforms in normal human subjects. *Physiological Measurement*, **20**, 219–40.

Holzapfel, G., Sommer, G. and Regitnig, P. (2004). Anisotropic mechanical properties of tissue components in human atherosclerotic plaques. *Journal of Biomechanical Engineering*, **126**, 657–65.

Ji, T.L., Sundareshan, M.K. and Roehrig, H. (1994). Adaptive image contrast enhancement based on human visual properties. *IEEE Transactions in Medical Imaging*, **13**, 573–86.

Kass, M., Witkin, A. and Terzopoulos, D. (1988). Snake: active contour models. *International Journal of Computerized Vision*, **1**, 321–31.

Ku, D.N., Giddens, D.P., Zarins, C.Z. and Glagov, S. (1985). Pulsatile flow and atherosclerosis in the human carotid bifurcation. *Arteriosclerosis*, **5**, 293–302.

Lee, K.W. and Xu, X.Y. (2002). Modelling of flow and wall behaviour in a mildly stenosed tube. *Medical Engineering and Physics*, **24**, 575–86.

Lee, K.W., Wood, N.B. and Xu, X.Y. (2004). Ultrasound image-based computer model of a common carotid artery with a plaque. *Medical Engineering and Physics*, **26**, 823–40.

Levick, J.R. (2003). *An Introduction to Cardiovascular Physiology*, 4th edn. London, UK: Arnold, pp. 144–6.

Leung, J.H., Wright, A.R., Cheshire, N., *et al.* (2005). The effect of thrombus on wall stress in an abdominal aortic aneurysm model. In ed. H. Rodrigues, M., Cerraziola, M., Doblaré, J. Ambrósio and M. Viceconti, *Proceedings II of the International Conference of Computational Bioengineering*; Sept. 2005, Lisbon, Portugal: IST Press, pp. 413–20.

Long, Q., Xu, X.Y., Collins, M.W., Griffith, T.M. and Bourne, M. (1998). The combination of magnetic resonance angiography and computational fluid dynamics: a critical review. *Critical Reviews in Biomedical Engineering*, **26**, 227–76.

Long, Q., Xu, X.Y., Ariff, B., *et al.* (2000a). Reconstruction of blood flow patterns in a human carotid bifurcation: a combined CFD and MRI study. *Journal of Magnetic Resonance Imaging*, **11**, 299–311.

Long, Q., Xu, X.Y., Bourne, M. and Griffith, T.M. (2000b). Numerical study of blood flow in an anatomically realistic aorto-iliac bifurcation generated from MRI data. *Magnetic Resonance Medicine*, **43**, 565–76.

Ma, P., Li, X. and Ku, D.N. (1997). Convective mass transfer at the human carotid bifurcation. *Journal of Biomechanics*, **30**, 565–71.

Malek, A.M., Alper, S.L. and Izumo, S. (1999). Hemodynamic shear stress and its role in atherosclerosis. *Journal of the American Medical Association*, **282**, 2035–42.

Mayet, J., Stanton, A.V., Sinclair, A.-M., *et al.* (1995). The effects of antihypertensive therapy on carotid vascular structure in man. *Cardiovascular Research*, **30**, 147–52.

Milner, J.S., Moore, J.A., Rutt, B.K. and Steinman, D.A. (1998). Hemodynamics of human carotid artery bifurcations: Computational studies in models reconstructed from magnetic resonance imaging of normal subjects. *Journal of Vascular Surgery*, **28**, 143–56.

Mittal, R., Simmons, S.P. and Udaykumar, H.S. (2001). Application of large-eddy simulation to the study of pulsatile flow in a modeled arterial stenosis. *Journal of Biomechanical Engineering*, **123**, 325–32.

Nichols, W.W. and O'Rourke, M.F. (2005). *McDonald's Blood Flow in Arteries: Theoretical, Experimental and Clinical Principles*, 5th edn. London, UK: Hodder Arnold.

Passerini, A.G., Polacek, D.C. and Shi, C. *et al.* (2004). Coexisting proinflammatory and antioxidative endothelial transcription profiles in a disturbed flow region of the adult porcine aorta. *Proceedings of the National Academy of Sciences*, **101**, 2482–7.

Raghavan, M.L., Vorp, D.A., Federle, M.P., Makaroun, M.S. and Webster, M.W. (2000). Wall stress distribution on three-dimensionally reconstructed models of human abdominal aortic aneurysm. *Journal of Vascular Surgery*, **31**, 760–9.

Rappitsch, G. and Perktold, K. (1996). Pulsatile albumin transport in large arteries: a numerical study. *Journal of Biomechanical Engineering*, **118**, 511–19.

Resnick, N. and Gimbrone, M.A. (1995). Hemodynamic forces are complex regulators of endothelial gene expression. *Journal of the Federation of American Societies for Experimental Biology*, **9**, 874–82.

Richardson, P.D., Davies, M.J. and Born, G.V. (1989). Influence of plaque configuration and stress distribution on fissuring of coronary atherosclerotic plaques. *Lancet*, **2**, 941–4.

Richardson, P.D. (2002). Biomechanics of plaque rupture: Progress, problems and new frontiers. *Annals of Biomedical Engineering*, **30**, 524–36.

Schlichting, H. (1979). *Boundary Layer Theory*, 7th edn. New York, NY: McGraw-Hill.

Stangeby, D.K. and Ethier, C.R. (2002). Computational analysis of coupled blood-wall arterial LDL transport. *Journal of Biomechanical Engineering*, **124**, 1–8.

Stanton, A.V., Chapman, J.N., Mayet, J., *et al.* (2001). Effects of blood pressure lowering with amlodipine or lisinopril on vascular structure of the common carotid artery. *Clinical Science (Lond.)*, **101**, 455–64.

Steinman, D. A., Thomas, J. B., Ladak, H. M., *et al.* (2002). Reconstruction of carotid bifurcation hemodynamics and wall thickness using computational fluid dynamics and MRI. *Magnetic Resonance in Medicine*, **47**, 149–59.

Tang, D. L., Yang, C., Kobayashi, S. and Ku, D. N. (2001). Steady flow and wall compression in stenotic arteries: A three-dimensional thick-wall model with fluid-wall interactions. *Journal of Biomechanical Engineering*, **123**, 548–57.

Tarbell, J. M. (2003). Mass transport in arteries and the localization of atherosclerosis. *Annual Review of Biomedical Engineering*, **5**, 79–118.

Taylor, C. A., Draney, M. T. and Ku, J. P. (1999). Predictive medicine: computational techniques in therapeutic decision-making. *Computer Aided Surgery*, **4**, 231–47.

Thomas, J. B., Milner, J. S., Rutt, B. K. and Steinman, D. A. (2003). Reproducibility of image-based computational fluid dynamics models of the human carotid bifurcation. *Annals of Biomedical Engineering*, **31**, 132–41.

Wood, N. B. (1999). Aspects of fluid dynamics applied to the larger arteries. *Journal of Theoretical Biology*, **199**, 137–61.

Wood, N. B., Weston, S. J., Kilner, P. J., Gosman, A. D. and Firmin, D. N. (2001). Combined MR imaging and CFD simulation of flow in the human descending aorta. *Journal of Magnetic Resonance Imaging*, **13**, 699–713.

Wood, N. B. and Xu, X. Y. (2003). Turbulence in stenoses: survey and early numerical results. In *Recent Advances in Fluid Dynamics: Proceedings of the Fourth International Conference on Fluid Mechanics*; July 28–31. Dalian, China: © 2003 Tsinghua University Press & Springer-Verlag.

Wood, N. B., Exarchou, I., Xu, X. Y., *et al.* (2005). Progress with the study of retinal hemodynamics in normotensive and hypertensive patients. In *Proceedings of the ASME 2005 Summer Bioengineering Conference*; June 2005. Vail CO, USA. Abstract 68962.

Wootton, D. M. and Ku, D. N. (1999). Fluid mechanics of vascular systems, diseases, and thrombosis. *Annual Review of Biomedical Engineering*, **1**, 299–329.

Zhao, S. Z., Ariff, B. and Long, Q. (2002). Inter-individual variations in wall shear stress and mechanical stress distributions at the carotid artery bifurcation of healthy humans. *Journal of Biomechanics*, **35**, 1367–77.

24

Mechanical image analysis using finite element method[1]

Dalin Tang[1], Chun Yang[1,2] and Chun Yuan[3]

[1]Worcester Polytechnic Institute, Worcester, MA, USA
[2]Beijing Normal University, Beijing, China
[3]University of Washington, Seattle, WA 98195, USA

Introduction and general modeling considerations

Development in medical image technology has led to impressive progress in image-based computational modeling which adds a new dimension (mechanical analysis) to atherosclerotic plaque image analysis. While current patient screening and diagnosis are mainly based on 2D images and experiences from radiologists and physicians, plaque progression and rupture are believed to be related to plaque morphology, mechanical forces, vessel remodeling, blood conditions (cholesterol, sugar, etc.), chemical environment, and lumen surface conditions (inflammation) (Fuster *et al.*, 1990; Fuster, 1998; Suri and Laxminarayan, 2003). The mechanisms governing plaque progression and causing plaque rupture are not fully understood. The motivations of using computational models to perform mechanical image analysis are based on the following:

(i) mechanical forces play an essential role in plaque progression and rupture. Plaque itself would not rupture if no forces were acting on it. Both mechanical forces and plaque structure are key factors in the progression and rupture process and should be examined together;

(ii) fluid-structure interaction (FSI) plays an essential role in plaque mechanical analysis. Plaque structure, flow environment and material properties are the three elements for FSI models. By analyzing plaques using FSI models, the plaque is placed in a more realistic environment, and more accurate assessment and predictions are possible;

(iii) 3D multicomponent computational models based on 3D geometry reconstructed from magnetic resonance imaging (MRI) data will advance the current screening and diagnosis techniques;

(iv) a computational plaque vulnerability index, if one can be identified and validated, will be very useful for plaque assessment and monitoring.

The controlling factors affecting mechanical forces in the plaque are classified into three groups (see Table 24.1) so that we can better understand different computational models with their associated assumptions and limitations. In the following, Section 2 provides a brief review of image-based finite-element (FE) models in the literature; Sections 3–4 cover some basic results from 3D multi-component models with fluid-structure interactions; Sections 5–6 are discussions and concluding remarks.

Carotid Disease: The Role of Imaging in Diagnosis and Management, ed. Jonathan Gillard, Martin Graves, Thomas Hatsukami and Chun Yuan. Published by Cambridge University Press. © Cambridge University Press 2007.

Table 24.1. Controlling factors for plaque computational mechanical models

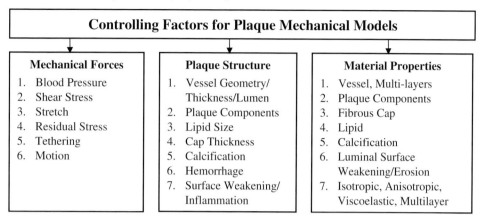

Controlling Factors for Plaque Mechanical Models		
Mechanical Forces	**Plaque Structure**	**Material Properties**
1. Blood Pressure	1. Vessel Geometry/ Thickness/Lumen	1. Vessel, Multi-layers
2. Shear Stress	2. Plaque Components	2. Plaque Components
3. Stretch	3. Lipid Size	3. Fibrous Cap
4. Residual Stress	4. Cap Thickness	4. Lipid
5. Tethering	5. Calcification	5. Calcification
6. Motion	6. Hemorrhage	6. Luminal Surface Weakening/Erosion
	7. Surface Weakening/ Inflammation	7. Isotropic, Anisotropic, Viscoelastic, Multilayer

Review of image-based computational models for atherosclerotic plaques

2D structure-only plaque models

2D structure-only models were used by several authors to investigate stress/strain distributions in atherosclerotic plaques. To test the hypothesis that plaque rupture occurs at sites of high circumferential stress in the diseased vessel, Cheng *et al.* introduced a finite element model to calculate the stress distributions in 24 coronary artery lesions based on histological specimens (Cheng *et al.*, 1993). Linear orthotropic elastic models were used for all plaque components (lipid, calcification, plaque fibrous tissue and artery). A mean intra-luminal pressure of 110 mmHg was imposed in the lumen. The FE model was solved by HKS ABAQUS 4.9. Their results indicated that the maximum circumferential stress in plaques that ruptured was significantly higher than maximum stress in stable specimens (4091 ± 1199 vs. 1444 ± 485 mm Hg, $p < 0.0001$). However, plaque rupture may not always occur at the region of highest stress, suggesting that local variations in plaque material properties contribute to plaque rupture.

Loree *et al.* used the same linear orthotropic model to investigate effects of fibrous cap and lipid pool on peak circumferential stress in atherosclerotic vessels (Loree *et al.*, 1992). They concluded that subintimal plaque structural features such as thickness of the fibrous cap are more important factors in the distribution of stress in the plaque than stenosis severity. To find out the impact of calcification on atherosclerotic plaque stability, Huang *et al.* studied 20 human coronary lesions (10 ruptured and 10 stable) derived from post-mortem coronary arteries (Huang *et al.*, 2001). All materials were assumed to be isotropic, incompressible, and hyperelastic. The nonlinear Mooney-Rivlin model was used. A commercial finite element package ADINA (ADINA R & D, Water Town, MA) was used to solve the 2D structural models. Their results indicated that maximum stress was not correlated with percentage of calcification, but it was positively correlated with the percentage of lipid ($p = 0.024$). In a more recent paper, Williamson *et al.* study sensitivity of wall stresses in diseased arteries to material properties (Williamson *et al.*, 2003). Both linear orthotropic models and nonlinear isotropic models were used and the material parameter values used can be found in Williamson *et al.*, 2003, Tables 3 and 4. Their results show that the stresses within the arterial wall, fibrous plaque, calcified plaque, and lipid pool have low sensitivities for variation in the elastic modulus. Even a ±50% variation in elastic modulus leads to less than a 10% change in stress at the site of rupture. It should be noted that some of the conclusions from 2D models may need to be modified when 3D models are used and the plaque component size becomes large enough to affect stress/strain distributions (see Section 3).

3D structure-only plaque models

Few 3D structure-only papers for atherosclerotic plaque mechanical analysis can be found in the current literature. Holzapfel *et al.* introduced a multilayer anisotropic 3D model with eight distinct arterial components associated with specific mechanical responses (Holzapfel *et al.*, 2002). A human external iliac artery was excised within 24 hours after death. A straight segment of the artery (20.0 mm) with an eccentric stenosis was scanned by means of high-resolution MRI (resolution $0.3 \times 0.3 \times 1.0$ mm^3). Mechanical tests were conducted to provide a fundamental basis for the formulation of large strain constitutive laws (see Table 1 of their paper). The 3D finite-element material model was solved by ABAQUS V5.8 to analyze the balloon-artery interaction during balloon expansion and stent deployment. The multilayer anisotropic model was compared with some simplified models (neglecting axial *in situ* pre-stretch, assuming plane strain states, and isotropic material responses), and maximum stress deviations of up to 600% were found. Their findings suggest that model simplifications need to be carefully justified. Computational predictions may be different from different models and should be interpreted with extreme caution.

3D fluid-only MRI-based models

In a series of papers, Long *et al.* combined computational fluid dynamics (CFD) modeling and MRI techniques together to perform patient-specific flow analysis based on in vivo MRI images from real patients (Long *et al.*, 1997, 2000, 2003). Their results showed that geometry of the carotid bifurcation was highly complex, involving helical curvature and out-of-plane branching. These geometrical features resulted in patterns of flow and wall shear stress significantly different from those found in simplified planar carotid bifurcation models. Comparisons between the predicted flow patterns and MR measurement demonstrated good quantitative agreement. Adding artery wall thickness to investigate its correlation with flow wall shear stress, Steinman *et al.* introduced a novel approach for noninvasively reconstructing artery wall thickness and local hemodynamics at the human carotid bifurcation (Steinman *et al.*, 2002). 3D models of the lumen and wall boundaries, from which wall thickness can be measured, were reconstructed from black blood MR. Phase contrast (PC) MRI was used to measure time-varying inlet/outlet flow rates which are used as boundary conditions (BC) for the subject-specific CFD model. Their results show good agreement between simulated and measured velocities, and demonstrate a correspondence between wall thickening and low and oscillating shear at the carotid bulb. However, a quantitative general relationship between WSS and wall thickness was not found. The paper by Steinman (Steinman, 2002) provides an excellent review and serves as a good reference for image-based CFD modeling.

3D CFD models with fluid-structure interactions

Zhao *et al.* introduced MRI-based FSI models to quantify flow shear stress and wall stress patterns in normal subjects in a clinical setting, and to define regions of low wall shear stress and high mechanical stress (Zhao *et al.*, 2002). Their fluid and solid models were solved iteratively by CFX4 (fluid) and ABAQUS (solid, shell model with linear elasticity). Their results revealed that some regions of the artery wall are exposed simultaneously to low wall shear stress and high mechanical stress and that these regions correspond to areas where atherosclerotic plaque develops. Younis *et al.* used FSI models with full 3D nonlinear hyperelastic model to investigate interindividual variations in flow dynamics and wall mechanics at the carotid artery bifurcation, and its effects on atherogenesis, in three healthy humans (Younis *et al.*, 2004). Kaazempur-Mofrad *et al.* used MRI-based FSI models to study the correlations between fluid dynamic parameters and histological markers of atherosclerosis (Kaazempur-Mofrad *et al.*, 2004). Four patients with atherosclerotic plaques were imaged using MRI and ultrasound, and subsequently underwent carotid endarterectomy. For each patient, a geometric model and a numerical mesh were constructed from MRI data (without plaque components), and velocity boundary conditions established. The model was solved by ADINA. Correlations attempted between the various fluid dynamic variables and the biological markers were interesting but inconclusive. Tendencies of maximum wall shear stress temporal gradient and average wall shear stress to correlate negatively with macrophages and lipid, and positively with collagen and smooth muscle cells, as well as tendencies of oscillatory shear index to correlate positively with macrophages and lipid and negatively with collagen and smooth muscle cells, were observed. While fluid-structure interactions are included in the above models, investigations were mainly focused on flow behaviors. Plaque components were not included in those FSI models.

MRI-based multi-component models with fluid-structure interactions

Image acquisition and 3D geometry reconstruction

Patients were recruited using an established recruitment protocol approved by University of Washington Institutional Review Board with informed consent obtained. MRI was conducted on a 3T Philips Achieva (Philips Medical Systems, Best) whole body scanner. A carotid-phased array coil was used for all scans. Multicontrast images of carotid atherosclerosis were generated to characterize plaque tissue composition, luminal and vessel wall morphology and inflammation (Yuan *et al.*, 1998, 2001a,b, 2002; Yuan and Kerwin, 2004). A computer package computer-aided system for cardiovascular disease evaluation (CASCADE) developed by the Vascular Imaging Laboratory at the University of Washington was used to perform image analysis and segmentation (Kerwin *et al.*, 2003). CASCADE allows for all contrast weightings to be simultaneously displayed, indexed relative to the carotid bifurcation, and analyzed serially along the length of the carotid artery. CASCADE automated analysis tools are able to accurately identify specific plaque features, including the lumen, wall boundary, necrotic core, calcifications, and other components. Upon completion of a review, an extensive report is generated and segmented contour lines for different plaque components for each slice are stored as digital files for 3D geometry reconstruction (Figure 24.1).

Geometry reconstruction and mesh generation were done using ADINA. All the segmented 2D slices were read into ADINA input file, point by point. For in vivo data, the geometry was reduced by 10% before read into ADINA so that the actual in vivo shape could be recovered with initial stress/strain conditions when initial axial prestretch and pressurization were applied. Geometry from ex vivo images does not need the reduction step, but axial prestretch and initial pressurization are needed to obtain initial stress/strain distributions in the plaque structure. 3D surfaces, volumes and computational meshes were made under ADINA computing environment. Intensive interactions and additional programming from the operator/researcher were needed due to the complexity of plaque morphology and components. Figure 24.1 shows 16 MRI slices (selected from a set of 24 slices) of a human carotid plaque sample,

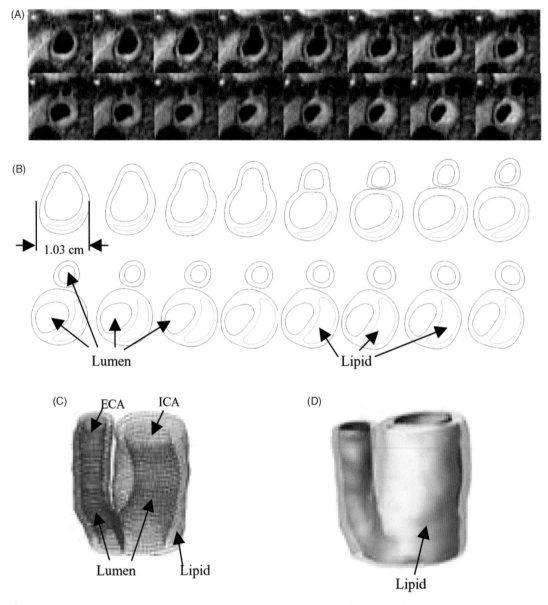

Figure 24.1 In vivo 3D magnetic resonance imaging (MRI) of a human carotid plaque and 3D reconstruction. (A) 16 MRI (T_1-weighted) slices (S0-S15) selected from a 24-slice set, slice spacing: 0.5 mm. Each image shown here is cut from the whole-neck image; (B) segmented contour plots using CASCADE showing plaque components; (C) reconstructed geometry with contour lines; and (D) 3D geometry showing lipid core and lumen.

(A)

(B)

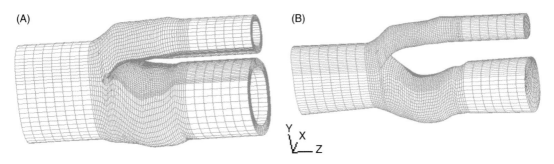

Figure 24.2 (A) Finite element mesh for the solid domain; (B) finite element mesh for the fluid domain.

the segmented component contour plots, and the reconstructed 3D geometry. Finite element meshes for fluid and solid domains are given in Figure 24.2. Fifty-six fluid volumes and 654 wall volumes were created to deal with the complex geometry and plaque components in the vessel wall. The diameter of the vessel is about 10 mm (outer diameter including vessel wall). Some smoothing (third-order spline) was applied to correct numerical and MRI artifacts, as well as overly unsmooth spots that affect the convergence of the model. The vessel was extended uniformly at both ends by 3 cm and 6 cm, respectively, so that it became long enough for our simulations. Geometries of other plaque samples were constructed using the same procedures.

The solid and fluid models

Both the artery wall and the components in the plaque were assumed to be hyperelastic, isotropic, incompressible and homogeneous. For the fluid model, the flow was assumed to be laminar, Newtonian, viscous and incompressible. The incompressible Navier-Stokes equations with arbitrary Lagrangian-Eulerian formulation were used as the governing equations which are suitable for problems with fluid-structure interactions and frequent mesh adjustments. Flow velocity at the flow-vessel interface was set to zero for steady flow and set to move with vessel wall (no-slip condition) for unsteady flow. Putting these together, we have

(summation convention is used) (Tang *et al.*, 2004c):

$$\rho\big(\partial\mathbf{u}/\partial t + ((\mathbf{u} - \mathbf{u_g}) \cdot \nabla)\mathbf{u}\big) = -\nabla_p + \mu\nabla^2\mathbf{u},$$
(equation of motion for fluid)

(24.1)

$$\nabla \cdot \mathbf{u} = 0, \qquad \text{(equation of continuity)} \quad (24.2)$$

$$\mathbf{u}|_\Gamma = \partial\mathbf{x}/\partial t, \partial\mathbf{u}/\partial n|_{\text{inlet,outlet}} = 0, \quad \text{(BC for velocity)}$$
(24.3)

$$p|_{\text{inlet}} = p_{\text{in}}(\mathbf{t}), p|_{\text{outlet}} = p_{\text{out}}(\mathbf{t}),$$
(pressure conditions)
(24.4)

$$\rho v_{i,tt} = \sigma_{ij,j}, \ i,j = 1,2,3; \ \text{sum over j},$$
(equation of motion for solids)
(24.5)

$$\varepsilon_{ij} = \big(v_{ij} + v_{j,i}\big)/2, \ i,j = 1,2,3$$
(strain-displacement relation)
(24.6)

$$\sigma_{ij} \cdot n_j|_{\text{out\_wall}} = 0, \quad \text{(natural equilibrium BC)}$$
(24.7)

$$\sigma^r_{ij} \cdot n_j|_{\text{interface}} = \sigma^s_{ij} \cdot n_j|_{\text{interface}},$$
(natural traction equilibrium BC)
(24.8)

where $\mathbf{u}$ and p are fluid velocity and pressure, $\mathbf{u_g}$ is mesh velocity, Γ stands for vessel inner boundary, $f_{\bullet,j}$ stands for derivative of f with respect to the jth variable, σ is stress tensor (superscripts indicate different materials), ε is strain tensor, $\mathbf{v}$ is solid displacement vector. The 3D nonlinear modified

Mooney-Rivlin model was used to describe the material properties of the vessel wall and plaque components (Bathe, 1996, 2002). The strain energy function is given by:

$$W = c_1(I_1 - 3) + c_2(I_2 - 3) + D_1[\exp(D_2(I_1 - 3)) - 1], \quad (24.9)$$

$$I_1 = \sum Cii, \ I_2 = \tfrac{1}{2}[I_1^2 - C_{ij}C_{ij}], \quad (24.10)$$

where I_1 and I_2 are the first and second strain invariants, $\mathbf{C} = [C_{ij}] = \mathbf{X}^T\mathbf{X}$ is the right Cauchy-Green deformation tensor, $\mathbf{X} = [X_{ij}] = [\partial x_i/\partial a_j]$, (x_i) is current position, (a_i) is original position (Bathe, 1996, 2002), c_i and D_i are material parameters chosen to match experimental measurements (Tang *et al.*, 2004a,b). The parameter values and stress-stretch curves used for the baseline multi-component model, together with pressure conditions, are given in Figure. 24.3.

The fully coupled FSI models were solved by ADINA. The artery was stretched axially and pressurized gradually to specified conditions. Mesh analysis was performed until differences between solutions from two consecutive meshes were negligible (less than 1% in L_2-norm). It takes

three periods to obtain periodic solutions. More details of the computational models and solution methods can be found from Tang *et al.* (2004a,b, 2005c) and Bathe (1996, 2002).

Solutions from the model based on in vivo MRI images

Simulations were conducted using the plaque sample given in Figure 24.1. The stenosis severity for this sample plaque is about 65% (by area). Flow velocity, pressure and plaque stress/strain distributions on different cut-surfaces were examined for critical patterns that may be related to plaque progression and rupture. Figure. 24.4 gives maximum principal stress and strain distributions (Stress-P_1 and Strain-P_1), flow velocity and pressure on a sagittal cut showing the bifurcation. Maximum Stress-P_1 value is located on a healthy part of the vessel where vessel wall is thin (Figure 24.4[a]). Figure 24.4(b) shows a maximum Strain-P_1 on a healthy location with large curvature. Flow velocity is higher at the stenosis narrowing of internal carotid artery,

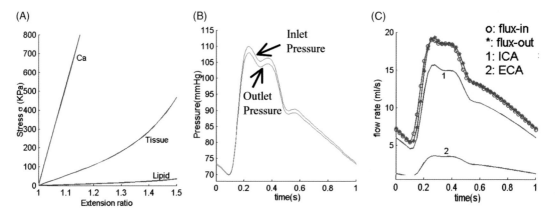

Figure 24.3 Material curves and pressure conditions for the multicomponent plaque model. (A) Stress-stretch curves derived from the modified Mooney-Rivlin model. The parameters are ($c_2 = 0$ for all materials): vessel and fibrous tissue: $c_1 = 368000$, $D_1 = 144000$, $D_2 = 2.0$; lipid: $c_1 = 20000$, $D_1 = 20000$, $D_2 = 1.5$; Ca: $c_1 = 3680000$; $D_1 = 1440000$, $D_2 = 2.0$, unit: dyn/cm^2; (B) pressure conditions specified at the inlet (common carotid artery) and outlets (internal carotid artery [ICA] and external carotid artery [ECA] C); (C) flow rate corresponding to the pressure conditions.

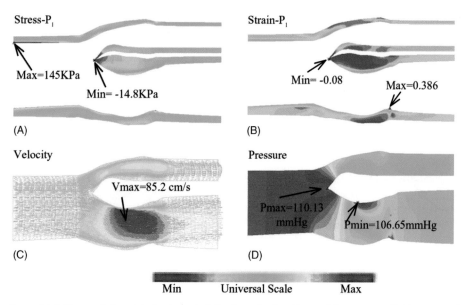

Figure 24.4 Flow and stress/strain characteristics from the baseline multicomponent fluid structure interaction (FSI) model. (A) maximum principal stress plot showing the location of maximum Stress-P_1 at a healthy site; (B) maximum principal strain plot showing the location of maximum Strain-P_1; (C) flow velocity has maximum in the stenotic region; and (D) pressure plot showing a minimum at the stenosis origin.

with a pressure minimum at the origin of the stenosis (Figures 24.4[c]−[d]).

The bifurcation section is good showing the flow features. However, it does not show the location and position of the lipid pool very well. Figure 24.5 presents other cut-surfaces showing lipid pool position and cap thickness which are more closely related to critical stress/strain behaviors. Figures 24.5(a)−(b) are from the plaque sample without modification. Maximum Stress-P_1 is observed again on the healthy side of the vessel where curvature is larger. To find out when the maximum stress would appear at the plaque cap, the plaque sample was modified so that the cap thickness became ½ and ¼ of original cap thickness. Maximum Stress-P_1 was found at the thin cap of the plaque on the y-cut surface with ¼ original cap thickness (Figure 24.5[c]). Figures 24.5(d)−(e) show Stress-P_1 plots on slice-17 with the original and ¼ cap thickness respectively. Maximum Stress-P_1

appeared at a location with large curvature in (d), and moved to the thin cap in (e).

Higher pressure and stenosis severity

Effects of other controlling factors can be investigated using parameter evaluation techniques, i.e. perform simulations with adjusted conditions and seek critical flow and stress/strain behaviors. Maximum Stress-P_1 value increased 68% when prescribed inlet pressure changed from 70 to 110 mmHg to 90−150 mmHg (see Figure 24.5[f]). Figure 24.5(g) shows that maximum Stress-P_1 increased from 142 KPa to 186 KPa when stenosis severity increased from 65% to 78% (by area). It is worth noting that stress level would be lower for more severe stenosis if plaque cap was not thin enough or the lipid pool was not present (Tang *et al.*, 2001, 2005b).

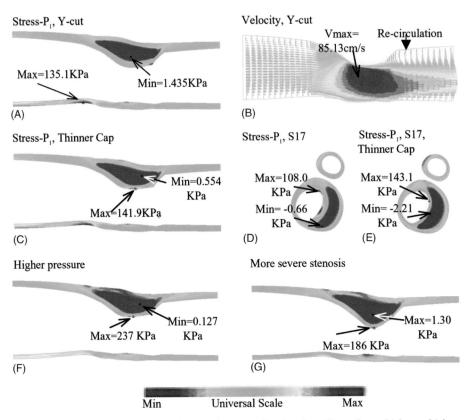

Figure 24.5 Plots from various cut surfaces and case studies showing effects of cap thickness, high pressure and stenosis severity on stress distributions. (A) Stress-P_1 on a Y-cut surface showing the location of maximum Stress-P_1 at a healthy site with large curvature; (B) velocity plot showing maximum velocity and flow recirculation; (C) maximum of Stress-P_1 occurs at thin cap of the lipid pool when cap thickness is reduced to ¼ of original thickness; (D) Stress-P_1 plot on slice 17 showing maximum at a site with large curvature; (E) Stress-P_1 plot on slice 17 with ¼ cap thickness showing maximum at the cap; (F) 36% pressure increase leads to 67% stress increase; and (G) with a large lipid pool and thin cap, more severe stenosis leads to higher stress in the plaque. Maximum stress from a 78% (by area) stenosis is 31% higher than that from the 65% stenosis as shown by (C).

Finite element models using other plaque samples

Effects of modeling assumptions: 2D and 3D models, axial stretch, fluid-structure interactions

As it can be seen clearly from the previous Figure, flow velocity and pressure are truly 3D. It has also been demonstrated that axial stretch and fluid structure interactions play important roles in

plaque stress/strain analysis (Tang *et al.*, 2001, 2004a). A 2D plaque model using only one cross-sectional slice will not be able to include 3D flow behavior, axial stretch and 3D fluid-structure interactions. These factors lead to considerable differences between computational results from 2D and 3D models. However, 2D models can still be used as a good starting point to get some initial data and insight because it is computationally inexpensive and easier to implement.

Local stress behaviors under pulsating pressure conditions

A plaque (plaque sample #2) with a large calcification and a lipid pool was chosen for this study (Tang *et al.*, 2005b). The 3D plaque geometry was reconstructed from 36 2D slices (resolution: 0.2 × 0.23 × 0.5 mm³). Inlet pressure was specified to be 90–150 mmHg with wave front similar to that given by Figure 24.3. Six sites were selected to track stress behaviors under pulsating pressure (Figure. 24.6). Figure 24.6(e) shows that the thin cap location (P4) has much greater (>400%) stress variation than other locations.

Effects of material parameters

Starting from the baseline model for plaque #2, material parameters for vessel, calcification and lipid-rich core were varied (changing material parameters for one tissue type while holding the other two unchanged) incrementally within a specified range and Stress-P_1 values from three selected sites are plotted in Figure 24.7. Stress-P_1 at the lipid cap increased by about 50% with a 50% vessel stiffness decrease, decreased 6% with 100% calcification stiffness increase, and increased by 22% with 50% lipid core stiffness decrease. Changes at the other two locations are much less noticeable.

Plaque structure, lipid core cap thickness, cap erosion

Plaque structure and component size are important factors. If we change the calcification

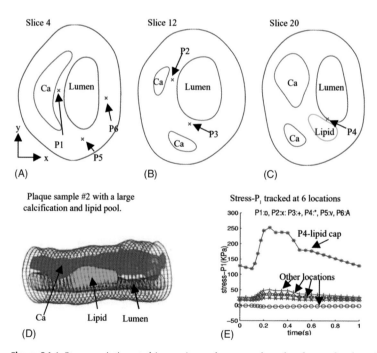

Figure 24.6 Stress variation at thin cap is much greater than that from other locations. (A)–(C) Normal and critical sites are selected to track stress/strain variations. P1: from calcification (Ca) cap; P2: from a thicker Ca cap; P3: from a thicker Ca cap; P4: from a thin lipid core cap (most vulnerable site); P5: normal point to observe stress-xx; P6: normal point to observe stress-yy. (D) Plaque sample #2 with a large calcification and a lipid pool. (E) Stress-P_1 tracked at six locations.

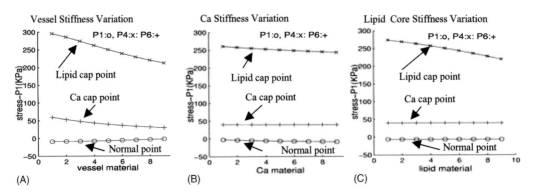

Figure 24.7 Material properties of vessel and plaque components have different levels of effects on stress distributions as shown by plots of Stress-P1 at three selected sites with different material parameters. Plaque sample #2 is used. Point selection was shown in Figure 24.6. Pin = 150 mmHg, Pout = 126 mmHg, axial-stretch = 10%. For each material, nine cases were computed with Case 1 being the softest and Case 9 being the stiffest. (A) Vessel: $c_1 = 60\,000–124\,000$; $D_1 = 20\,000–52\,000$; $D_2 = 1.6–2.4$; calcium (Ca) and lipid: baseline values; (B) Ca: $c_1 = 600\,000–1\,240\,000$; $D_1 = 200\,000–520\,000$; $D_2 = 1.6–2.4$; vessel and lipid: baseline values; (C) Lipid: $c_1 = 3\,400–6\,600$; $D_1 = 3\,400–6\,600$; $D_2 = 1.1–1.9$; vessel and Ca: baseline values.

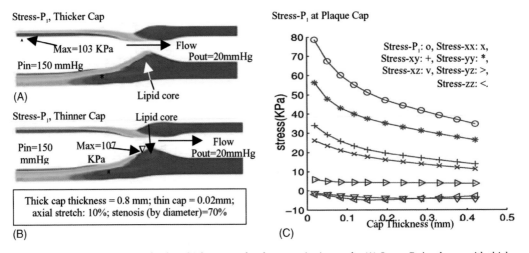

Figure 24.8 Thinner plaque cap leads to higher stress level: a quantitative study. (A) Stress-P_1 in plaque with thicker cap; (B) maximum of Stress-P_1 appears at the plaque cap when the cap is made thin enough; (C) Stress-P_1 at the plaque cap increases almost exponentially when cap thickness decreases.

or the lipid pool to normal tissue in plaque #2, stress/strain distributions will be very different. This is different from results obtained from 2D models (see 2D structure-only plaque models). It is

known that lipid core and its cap thickness have considerable effect on stress distributions and extreme stress locations. We choose plaque sample #3 for this case study (Figures 24.8–24.9).

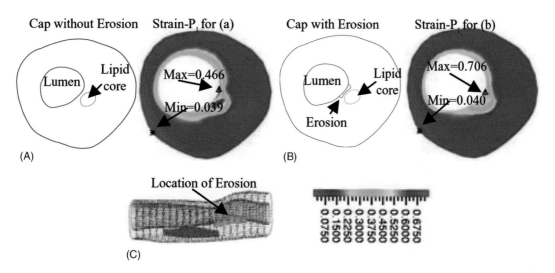

Figure 24.9 Plaque cap erosion/weakening causes large strain increase. Maximal principal stress showed very little change (Figure not shown). However, maximum of Strain-P_1 (maximal principal strain) increased about 50% when half of the cap was made 50% softer.

Figure 24.8(a)−(b) shows band plots of Stress-P_1 on a sagittal cut of the vessel with cap thickness 0.8 mm and 0.02 mm, respectively. Maximal Stress-P_1 appeared at the thin (healthy) side when cap thickness was 0.8 mm and moved to the cap site when the cap was adjusted thinner (Figures 24.8[a]−[b]). Figure 24.8(c) presents stress values tracked at the middle of the cap for 11 cases with cap thickness adjusted incrementally from 0.42 mm to 0.02 mm. Stress-P_1 values increased about 100% corresponding to the cap thickness variations. Other stress components showed similar patterns.

Cap erosion and inflammation weaken vessel surface (plaque cap) and may lead to large strain variations. Using plaque sample #3, we made half (in cap thickness) of plaque cap softer to represent cap erosion (stiffness was reduced by 50%). For the plaque with cap erosion, maximal stress value changed less than 1% (Figure not shown), Figure 24.9(b) shows that maximum Strain-P_1 increased by about 50% due to the cap weakening.

Critical site selection method and computational plaque vulnerability index (CPVI)

When the computational models are solved and results are obtained, it is still extremely challenging to identify critical indicators from the huge 3D time-dependent data set to make accurate plaque assessment due to complexity of plaque structure and stress/strain behaviors. One popular hypothesis is that maximal stress may be related to possible plaque rupture and may be used for plaque vulnerability assessment. Our results indicate that maximal stress often appears at the healthy part of the vessel where vessel wall is thinner than the diseased plaque side or where the vessel has a large curvature, and that local maximum stress values at critical sites may be a better indicator (Figures 24.4, 24.5, 24.10). A critical site-tracking method was proposed to identify critical sites and stress/strain conditions which are more closely related to plaque

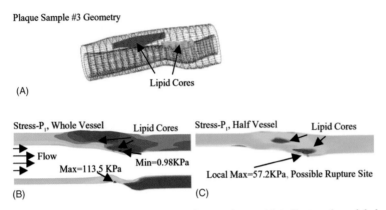

Figure 24.10 Local stress/strain extreme values are better risk indicators than global maximal stress/strain values. (A) Plaque sample #3 geometry; (B) Stress-P_1 plot for the whole sagittal slice showing maximum on the healthy side of the vessel; (C) Stress-P_1 plot for the upper half diseased vessel showing a local maximum stress at the plaque cap and a minimum in the lipid pool.

rupture risk, therefore, may provide more accurate assessment (Tang *et al.*, 2005a). Stress/strain conditions and locations which may be related to plaque rupture are called "critical stress/strain conditions" and "critical sites". Critical sites include locations of very thin cap, weakened cap sites, and other sites of special interest. Initial results were obtained from 34 MRI 2D slices from 14 autopsy patients (human coronary plaques). 2D models were used to calculate critical stress/strain values at selected critical sites (Figure 24.11, site selection). Following the American Heart Association's (AHA) classifications (Stary *et al.*, 1992, 1994, 1995), histopathological analysis was performed to the histological sections and a histopathological plaque vulnerability index (HPVI) was assigned to each section (Figure 24.11). Definition of HPVI is given in Table 24.2 (Tang *et al.*, 2005a). CPVI was determined to each 2D sample based on CST stress values and standard statistical method. The agreement between CPVI and HPVI was 90% (Figure. 24.12).

Trends, further challenges, and discussions

The trend is moving from fluid-only or structure-only models to FSI models including plaque components. For MRI-based modeling, 3D in vivo image resolution is still limited. Noninvasive methods to determine material properties, lumen surface conditions (inflammation) and flow pressure conditions remain to be challenging. 3D geometry reconstruction, mesh generation, model solution, and data analysis are labor-intensive and need to be integrated and automated.

Clinical validation of computational predictions is also a concern. Atherosclerosis takes a long time to grow and it is extremely hard to catch ruptured cases as the ultimate validation of computational (or any other) predictions. Histopathological analysis is currently regarded as the "gold standard" for validation of MRI tissue identification and is used in this chapter as the gold standard for computational plaque assessment. Long-term patient tracking data with the actual plaque progression and rupture rate can serve as a better in vivo 'gold standard' for predictive research. However, collection of 3D in vivo data with detailed plaque component information and development of an in vivo plaque assessment scheme require better resolutions and long-term effort (5–10 years or longer). A gold standard for in vivo plaque assessment has yet to be established.

Table 24.2. Histopathological plaque classifications and comparison with AHA classifications

HPVI	Plaque	Description	AHA classification
V = 0	Very stable	Normal or slight intimal thickening	Class I, some atherogenic lipoprotein and intimal thickening
V = 1	Stable	Moderate intimal thickening, no extracellular lipid, calcification or significant inflammation	Class II (fatty streak), III (preatheroma)
V = 2	Slightly unstable	Small lipid core (<30% of plaque size); calcification may be present; thick fibrous cap (>200 µm); little/no inflammation at plaque shoulders	Class IV, Vb, and Vc
V = 3	Moderately unstable	Moderate lipid core (30–40% of plaque size) and fibrous cap (65–200 µm); moderate intraplaque hemorrhage; moderate inflammation	Class Va
V = 4	Highly unstable	Large lipid core (>40%); thin fibrous cap (<65 µm); large intraplaque hemorrhage; extensive inflammation; evidence of previous plaque rupture	Class VI

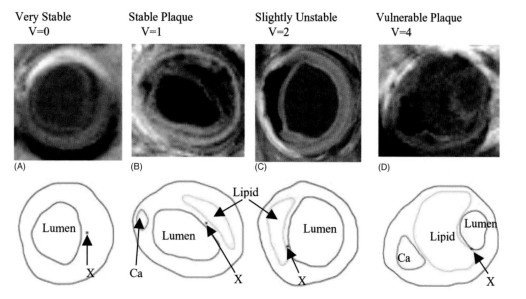

Figure 24.11 Magnetic resonance imaging and segmented contour plots (lower) of selected sample plaques with various degrees of vulnerability as classified by histopathological analysis. Critical sites are indicated by "X". (A) A remarkable stable plaque used as the baseline case; (b) a well-capped stable plaque, V = 1; (C) an unstable plaque with a large lipid core and thin cap; (D) a vulnerable plaque with a huge lipid-rich necrotic core, a separate calcium (Ca) deposit, and a very thin cap near lumen with many inflammatory cells. (Reproduced from Tang, D., Yang, C., Zheng, J., *et al.* (2005a). Local maximal stress hypothesis and computational plaque vulnerability index for atherosclerotic plaque assessment. *Annals of Biomedical Engineering*, **33**, 1789–801 with kind permission of Springer Science and Business Media.)

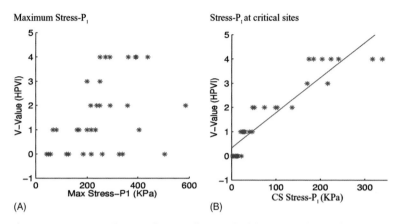

Figure 24.12 Stress-P$_1$ by critical site tracking method from critical sites shows much better correlation with histopathological plaque vulnerability index (HPVI) than global maximum Stress-P$_1$. Results are obtained from 34 2D MR images from human coronary plaques. $p < 0.0001$ for (B). (Reproduced from Tang, D., Yang, C., Zheng, J., *et al.* (2005a). Local maximal stress hypothesis and computational plaque vulnerability index for atherosclerotic plaque assessment. *Annals of Biomedical Engineering*, **33**, 1789–801 with kind permission of Springer Science and Business Media.)

Concluding remarks

Development in medical image technology has led to impressive progress in computational models and finite element methods for atherosclerotic plaque image analysis in the last 10–15 years. Image-based computational modeling is adding a new dimension (mechanical analysis) to athero-sclerostic plaque image analysis. With advanced imaging and computational modeling techniques, atherosclerotic plaques can be analyzed under fluid-structure interaction environment and critical flow and stress/strain conditions can be identified and used for more accurate plaque rupture risk assessment and predictions. Combination of imaging analysis, computational modeling, and clinical studies may lead to establishment of new industrial standard, gold standard for arterial disease assessment, and new noninvasive diagnostic and screening procedures.

Acknowledgements

Tang's research was supported in part by NSF grants DMS-0540684, DMS-0072873 and NIH grant NIH/NIBIB, 5 R01 EB004759 as part of the NSF/NIH Collaborative Research in Computational Neuroscience Program. Collaborations from Drs. Jie Zheng, Pamela K. Woodard, Jeffrey E. Saffitz, Gregorio A. Sicard, Fei Liu, Paul Chu and other coauthors in the papers cited are gratefully acknowledged.

REFERENCES

Bathe, K. J. (1996). *Finite Element Procedures*. New Jersey: Prentice Hall.

Bathe, K. J. (2002). *Theory and Modeling Guide*, Vols I & II: ADINA and ADINA-F. Watertown, MA: ADINA R & D, Inc.

Cheng, G. C., Loree, H. M., Kamm, R. D., Fishbein, M. C. and Lee, R. T. (1993). Distribution of circumferential stress in ruptured and stable atherosclerotic lesions, a structural analysis with histopathological correlation. *Circulation*, **87**, 1179–87.

Fuster, V. (Ed.). (1998). In J. F. Cornhill, R. E. Dinsmore, J. T. Fallon, W. Insull, P. Libby, S. Nissen, M. E. Rosenfeld, W. D. Wagner (co eds.), *The Vulnerable Atherosclerotic Plaque: Understanding, Identification, and Modification*. Armonk NY: Futura Publishing.

Fuster, V., Stein, B., Ambrose, J.A., *et al.*, (1990). Atherosclerotic plaque rupture and thrombosis, evolving concept. *Circulation,* **82** (Suppl. II), II-47–II-59.

Holzapfel, G.A., Stadler, M. and Schulze-Bause, C.A.J. (2002). A layer-specific three-dimensional model for the simulation of balloon angioplasty using Magnetic Resonance Imaging and mechanical testing. *Annals of Biomedical Engineering,* **30**, 753–67.

Huang, H., Virmani, R., Younis, H., *et al.* (2001). The impact of calcification on the biomechanical stability of atherosclerotic plaques. *Circulation,* **103**, 1051–6.

Kaazempur-Mofrad, M.R., Isasi, A.G., Younis, H.F., *et al.* (2004). Characterization of the atherosclerotic carotid bifurcation using MRI, finite element modeling, and histology. *Annals of Biomedical Engineering,* **32**, 932–46.

Kerwin, W., Hooker, A., Spilker, M., *et al.* (2003). Quantitative magnetic resonance imaging analysis of neovasculature volume in carotid atherosclerotic plaque. *Circulation,* **107**, 851–6.

Long, Q., Xu, X.Y., Ariff, B., *et al.* (2000). Reconstruction of blood flow patterns in a human carotid bifurcation: A combined CFD and MRI study. *Journal of Magnetic Resonance Imaging,* **11**, 299–311.

Long, Q., Ariff, B., Zhao, S.Z., *et al.* (2003). Reproducibility study of 3D geometrical reconstruction of the human carotid bifurcation from magnetic resonance images. *Magnetic Resonance in Medicine,* **49**, 665–74.

Long, Q., Xu, X.Y., Collins, M.W., Griffith, T.M. and Bourne, M. (1997). Fluid dynamics of the aortic bifurcation using magnetic resonance imaging and computational fluid dynamics. *Internal Medicine (Clinical and Laboratory),* **5**, 35–42.

Loree, H.M., Kamm, R.D., Stringfellow, R.G. and Lee, R.T. (1992). Effects of fibrous cap thickness on peak circumferential stress in model atherosclerotic vessels. *Circulation Research,* **71**, 850–8.

Suri, J.S. and Laxminarayan, S. (Eds.). (2003). *Angiography and Plaque Imaging: Advanced Segmentation Techniques.* New York: CRC Press.

Stary, H.C., Blankenhorn, D.H., Chandler, A.B., *et al.* (1992). A definition of the intima of human arteries and of its atherosclerosis-prone regions. A report from the Committee on Vascular Lesions of the Council on Arteriosclerosis, AHA. *Circulation,* **85**, 391–405.

Stary, H.C., Chandler, A.B., Glagov, S., *et al.* (1994). A definition of initial, fatty streak and intermediate lesions of atherosclerosis. A report from the Committee on Vascular Lesions of the Council on Arteriosclerosis, AHA. *Circulation,* **89**, 2462–78.

Stary, H.C., Chandler, A.B., Dinsmore, M.D., *et al.* (1995). Definitions of advanced types of atherosclerotic lesions and the histological classification of atherosclerosis. A report from the Committee on Vascular Lesions of the Council on Arteriosclerosis, AHA. *Circulation,* **92**, 1355–74.

Steinman, D.A. (2002). Image-based computational fluid dynamics modeling in realistic arterial geometries. *Annals of Biomedical Engineering,* **30**, 483–97.

Steinman, D.A., Thomas, J.B., Ladak, H.M., *et al.* (2002). Reconstruction of carotid bifurcation hemodynamics and wall thickness using computational fluid dynamics and MRI. *Magnetic Resonance in Medicine,* **47**,149–59.

Tang, D., Yang, C., Kobayashi, S. and Ku, D.N. (2001). Steady flow and wall compression in stenotic arteries: a 3-D thick-wall model with fluid-wall interactions. *Journal of Biomechanical Engineering,* **123**, 548–57.

Tang, D., Yang, C., Kobayashi, S. and Ku, D.N. (2004a). Effect of a lipid pool on stress/strain distributions in stenotic arteries: 3D FSI models. *Journal of Biomechanical Engineering,* **126**, 363–70.

Tang, D., Yang, C., Zheng, J., *et al.* (2004b). 3D Computational Mechanical Analysis for Human Atherosclerotic Plaques Using MRI-Based Models with Fluid-Structure Interactions. *Medical Image Computing and Computer Assisted Intervention,* **2**, 328–36.

Tang, D., Yang, C., Zheng, J., *et al.* (2004c). 3D MRI-based multi-component FSI models for atherosclerotic plaques, a 3D FSI model. *Annals of Biomedical Engineering,* **32**, 947–60.

Tang, D., Yang, C., Zheng, J., *et al.* (2005a). Local maximal stress hypothesis and computational plaque vulnerability index for atherosclerotic plaque assessment. *Annals of Biomedical Engineering,* **33**, 1789–801.

Tang, D., Yang, C., Zheng, J., *et al.* (2005b). Quantifying Effects of Plaque Structure and Material Properties on Stress Behaviors in Human Atherosclerotic Plaques Using 3D FSI Models. *Journal of Biomechanical Engineering,* **127**, 1185–94.

Tang, D., Yang, C., Zheng, J., *et al.* (2005c). Sensitivity analysis of 3D MRI-based models with fluid-structure interactions for human atherosclerotic coronary and carotid plaques. In: K.J. Bathe (Ed.), *Computational Solid and Fluid Mechanics.* Elsevier, New York, pp. 1009–13.

Williamson, S. D., Lam, Y., Younis, H. F., *et al.* (2003). On the sensitivity of wall stresses in diseased arteries to variable material properties. *Journal of Biomechanical Engineering*, **125**, 147–55.

Younis, H. F., Kaazempur-Mofrad, M. R., Chan, R. C., *et al.* (2004). Hemodynamics and wall mechanics in human carotid bifurcation and its consequences for atherogenesis: investigation of inter-individual variation. *Biomechanical Model Mechanobiology*, **3**, 17–32.

Yuan, C., Beath, B. W., Smith, L. H. and Hatsukami, T. S. (1998). Measurement of atherosclerotic carotid plaque size in vivo using high resolution Magnetic Resonance Imaging. *Circulation*, **98**, 2666–71.

Yuan, C., Hatsukami, T. S. and O'Brien, K. D. (2001a). High resolution magnetic resonance imaging of normal and atherosclerotic human coronary arteries ex vivo: discrimination of plaque tissue components. *Journal of Medical Investigation*, **49**, 491–9.

Yuan, C. and Kerwin, W. S. (2004). MRI of atherosclerosis. *Journal of Magnetic Resonance Imaging*, **19**, 710–19.

Yuan, C., Kerwin, W. S., Ferguson, M. S., *et al.* (2002). Contrast enhanced high resolution MRI for atherosclerotic carotid artery tissue characterization. *Journal of Magnetic Resonance Imaging*, **15**, 62–7.

Yuan, C., Mitsumori, L. M., Ferguson, M. S., *et al.* (2001b). In vivo accuracy of multispectral MR imaging for identifying lipid-rich necrotic cores and intraplaque hemorrhage in advanced human carotid plaques. *Circulation*, **104**, 2051–6.

Zhao, S. Z., Ariff, B., Long, Q., *et al.* (2002). Inter-individual variations in wall shear stress and mechanical stress distributions at the carotid artery bifurcation of healthy humans. *Journal of Biomechanics*, **35**, 1367–77.

25

Transcranial Doppler monitoring

Michael Gaunt

University of Cambridge, Cambridge CB2 2QQ, UK

Introduction

History and development of transcranial doppler (TCD)

The idea of investigating the intracranial circulation with ultrasound was first proposed in 1960 by Kaneko working in Osaka while developing the clinical uses of sonography (Kaneko, 1986; Satomursa and Kaneko, 1986). At that time the skull was considered a significant barrier to the penetration of ultrasound and the investigators chose to concentrate on investigating the extracranial circulation instead.

However the problem can be minimized by using a lower frequency of ultrasound and utilizing areas of the skull where the bone is thin enough to allow ultrasound waves to penetrate. Fortunately, one of the areas of thin bone is located in the temporal region and this area allows insonation of all the main cerebral arteries arising from the circle of Willis, namely the anterior cerebral, middle cerebral and posterior cerebral arteries. The middle cerebral artery (MCA) is particularly important as this is the main blood supply to the parietal area of the brain which contains the main motor and sensory cortices, the most important clinical areas affected by stroke.

The first transcranial Doppler recordings were performed by Rune Aaslid in the Department of Neurosurgery in Bern in the summer of 1981 utilizing a 2 MHz pulsed Doppler machine originally designed for cardiac use (Aaslid *et al.*, 1982).

Today, advances in microprocessor technology have enabled the development of specialized systems which have helped to establish TCD as a useful method for studying cerebral hemodynamics and detecting cerebral embolization in a wide variety of clinical and research situations.

Technical aspects of TCD

In order to interpret TCD data appropriately it is important to have an understanding of the principles that are used to obtain the Doppler signals and how they are processed and finally displayed for interpretation. As with all electronic imaging methods it is important to appreciate that the image one sees on the screen is the result of electronic filtering, amplification and processing to produce a clean crisp display. The reflected ultrasound signals contains a mass of information and how certain information is obtained, chosen and displayed in, is largely the result of technical choices made by the manufacturer. The same information obtained, processed and displayed differently may result in fundamentally different interpretations.

The Doppler principle as applied to TCD

TCD utilizes the Doppler principle to determine the direction and velocity of blood flow. The Doppler theory was first described by the Austrian physicist Christian Doppler in 1842 and describes the relationship between the velocity of

Carotid Disease: The Role of Imaging in Diagnosis and Management, ed. Jonathan Gillard, Martin Graves, Thomas Hatsukami and Chun Yuan. Published by Cambridge University Press. © Cambridge University Press 2007.

objects and the frequencies of transmitted and reflected sound waves (Doppler, 1842). In brief, if sound waves of a given frequency are transmitted toward a moving object, the frequency of the reflected waves depends, to certain extent, on the direction of movement of the object. If the object is moving toward the source the reflected waves will have a higher frequency, whereas if the object is moving away the reflected waves will have a lower frequency. The degree of frequency shift depends on the velocity of the object and therefore the velocity can be estimated if the frequency shift is known. If we concentrate on a single blood cell moving toward the probe, mathematically, the relationship is described by the following formulae:

$$f^1 = f^0 \left(\frac{V+c}{c} \right) = f^0 \left(\frac{1+V}{c} \right)$$

where f^1 is the frequency of ultrasound received by a red blood cell moving toward the source with a velocity, V, f^0 = frequency of transmitted wave and c = propagation velocity of ultrasound.

The movement of the blood cell affects the frequency of both the ultrasound wave received by the blood cell and that transmitted back to the probe receiver. f^1 is transmitted from the moving blood cell but during this time this cell moves a distance of $\frac{V}{f^1}$ while transmitting one entire wave. Therefore the actual wavelength (λ_2) will be shorter and therefore the frequency higher – f^2.

$$\lambda_2 = \left(\frac{c-V}{f^1} \right)$$

$$f^2 = \frac{c}{\lambda_2} = \left(\frac{f^1}{1 - \frac{V}{c}} \right) = f^0 \left(\frac{1 + \frac{V}{c}}{1 - \frac{V}{c}} \right)$$

The Doppler shift (f) is the difference in frequency between the transmitted frequency and the received frequency:

$$f = f^2 - f^0 = 2f^0 \frac{V}{c}$$

An object travelling with a velocity of 1 m/sec will give a shift of about 2.5 kHz at an f^0 of 2 MHz and 5 kHz if the Doppler frequency is 4 MHz. To simplify interpretation, on most TCD units, the velocity is expressed as cm/sec rather than kHz to enable comparison of readings which operate at different emission frequencies. However, this calculation of the velocity only applies if the object is travelling parallel to the line of insonation. Usually an angle exists between the direction of movement of the object and the line of insonation and this causes the measured velocity to be lower than the actual velocity. However if the angle of insonation ϕ is known, this effect can be corrected for using this formula:

$$V = \frac{c}{2\cos\phi} \frac{f}{f^0}$$

Unfortunately, it is not possible to measure the angle of insonation when using TCD, however, the most often insonated vessel, the MCA, runs perpendicular to the surface of the skull for a considerable distance from its origin (Aaslid et al., 1982). Insonating the artery from the posterior temporal window the angle of insonation is seldom greater than 30° which means that the measured velocity is at least 87% of the true velocity. Therefore absolute values for velocities measured by TCD have an inbuilt error which must be taken into account when analyzing MCA velocity data (Aaslid, 1992). Also, when performing serial velocity measurements at different times it is important to appreciate that variations in the angle of insonation may, in themselves, produce changes in velocity readings.

Specular reflection and backscatter of ultrasound

When ultrasound is directed at an object or interface which is larger than one wavelength in size the percentage reflection accurately predicts the amount of ultrasound reflected, this is known as specular reflection. However, if the object is smaller than one wavelength then the reflected ultrasound is back-scattered in all directions, nonspecular reflection, and the intensity of the ultrasound signal returning to the receiver will be reduced. For example, the TCD detection of emboli is based on the measurement of the backscatter (nonspecular reflection) from the emboli which is usually greater than the backscatter ultrasound reflected from normal flowing blood (Ringlstein *et al.*, 1998).

Sample volume, gating and dual gating

The sample volume is the spatial region from which the TCD detects the Doppler shifts. Most TCDs have a beam width of 3–4 mm that coincides with the diameters of the basal cerebral arteries. The axial component of the sample volume is determined by the technique of range gating. Pulses of ultrasonic waves are sent out from the transmitter at a preset pulse repetition frequency (PRF). A typical TCD transducer would send out bursts of ultrasound at approximately 10 μs duration and 70 μs intervals. The transmitter then stops and a set time elapses before the receiver switches on and receives returning Doppler shifts for a fixed duration. Only signals received during this time are used to determine the Doppler shift and these signals correspond to those signals reflected from anatomical structures at a certain depth. The depth can be altered by altering the time interval before the receiver receives signals. The length of the sample volume can be altered both by increasing the duration of transmission or receipt of signals. Most TCDs use long sample volumes (5–12 mm) in order to improve the signal-to-noise ratio and therefore ease the detection of the basal cerebral arteries (Aaslid, 1992). There is no ideal sample volume length but to optimize embolus detection most investigators recommend a sample volume length >3 mm and <10 mm (Ringlstein *et al.*, 1998).

The sensitivity of the sample volume is greatest at the center and weakest at the edges in all directions. Therefore objects which reflect a high proportion of incident ultrasound waves passing through the sample volume (e.g. air emboli) will be detected over a greater distance than other objects which reflect less ultrasound (particulate emboli) (Smith *et al.*, 1994) (Figure 25.1).

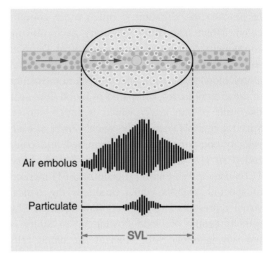

Figure 25.1 The sensitivity of the sample volume is greatest at its center and weakest at its edges. Air emboli are detected over a greater sample volume length (SVL) than particulate emboli (Smith *et al.* 1994)

Dual gating

Some TCD systems utilize the principles described above to sample Doppler shifts from two separate depths simultaneously, e.g. two points along the MCA. For example, the first sample volume would be focused deeply on the MCA at 55 mm, while the second sample volume would be focused more superficially on the MCA at 45 mm. This set-up is known as dual gating and helps differentiate embolic signals from artefact. A true embolus would first be detected passing through the deeper sample volume and then through the more superficial sample volume indicating propagation, while an artefact caused by probe movement would be seen simultaneously in both sample volumes at the same time (Smith *et al.*, 1996).

Velocity profiles and Doppler spectra

The Doppler equation derived above, was for a single blood cell reflecting one ultrasonic wave.

In practice the situation is much more complicated. When insonating an artery each moving component contributes to a mixture of Doppler shifts consisting of many frequencies. Within an artery, blood flows at a higher velocity in the center of the arterial lumen compared to blood flow near the walls of the artery which is much slower. Spectral analysis enables the signal power of each velocity component to be determined and color coded to give a visual computer display. Most TCDs use the fast Fourier transform (FFT) method of spectral analysis which produces the typical visual representation of blood flow velocity. The velocity profile of blood flowing in an artery is typically parabolic with most of the blood cells flowing with velocities in the upper half of the spectrum. The outline of this spectral display corresponds to the maximal Doppler shift and therefore, the maximal velocity component of the velocity profile $= V_{max}$. This in turn, corresponds with the velocity of blood flow in the center of the arterial lumen and is the more accurate measure for most monitoring purposes. The V_{max} is displayed in most commercially available instruments. Other indices include time-mean velocity which usually refers to the mean velocity of V_{max} and the time-averaged V_{max} which is determined by the area under the spectral curve (Matta, 2000).

The FFT method of spectral analysis is used in most TCD systems because it allows almost instantaneous detection and display of information in a form which is understandable to most observers. This is ideal for displaying velocity waveforms but the way the Fourier analysis is performed may have a significant impact on the detection of emboli. Data are analyzed according to frequency and time. Because most emboli are of very short duration (10–100 ms) if the time gaps between data sampling are long an embolus may occur during one of these gaps and not be displayed or recorded (Markus, 1995). The use of different time windows that overlap by at least 50% reduces the chance that emboli are missed. Also to obtain reasonable temporal resolution short time periods for data sampling should be used (5–10 ms). When these data lengths are used the spectral resolution of the FFT is 100–200 Hz. For embolus detection the lower the frequency resolution the stronger the embolic signal will appear in the display since it represents a greater percentage of the input data samples (Ringlstein *et al.*, 1998).

Volume flow

TCD measures the velocity of blood flow and not the volume of blood flow (Naylor *et al.*, 1991). This is because the diameter of the insonated artery cannot be determined accurately enough to enable calculation of absolute volume flow in milliliters. Although some authors have found a good correlation between measures of cerebral blood flow such as ^{133}Xe SPECT and regional mean cerebral transit time and TCD velocity values, an individual value can only be considered an indicator of the amount of blood flow and not an absolute measure (Sorteberg *et al.*, 1990; Naylor *et al.*, 1991). In the clinical situation this "indication" of blood flow can be used to detect large falls in cerebral blood flow known to be associated with neurological damage. During monitoring of carotid endarterectomy operations, a middle cerebral artery velocity (MCAV) of less than 10–15 cm/sec during carotid clamping has been associated with a flattening of the electroencephalogram (EEG) in some cases and therefore, has led to recommendations that the MCAV should be maintained above this level (Spencer, 1992; Steiger, 1992). However, due to the reasons explained above, the absolute values for MCAV can be inaccurate and Halsey suggested that the percentage fall in MCAV on carotid clamping is a more reliable indicator of ischemia. It was found that if the MCAV fell to less than 40% of its preclamp value this was associated with mild cerebral ischemia and less than 15% was severe ischemia (Halsey, 1993).

Pulsatility index and resistance index

These indices reflect characteristics of the Doppler shift velocity waveforms and indicate the degree of pulsatility of the waveform. If the proximal arteries are stenosed then the waveform will be dampened (flattened) and the pulsatility index (PI) value will be lower. However, if the proximal arteries are normal then pulsatility reflects distal cerebrovascular resistance and is complementary to the resistance index (RI). A simplified formula is used by most TCDs to calculate the PI which describes the maximal vertical excursion of the waveform divided by its mean amplitude:

$$PI = \frac{Vs - Ved}{Vm}$$

where Vs = peak systolic velocity, Vm = mean velocity and Ved = end-diastolic velocity.

The PI in the cerebral arteries of normal subjects varies from 0.5 to 1.1 (standard deviation 0.1–0.15) with no significant side to side or cerebral inter-arterial differences (Gosling and King, 1974).

The RI indicates the condition of arterial bed distal to the insonated artery and indicates the resistance to blood flow. It is described as the ratio of the maximum waveform excursion to the peak systolic velocity:

$$RI = \frac{Vs - Ved}{Vs}$$

The normal range for the cerebral arteries is between 0.55 and 0.75 (Pourcelot, 1974).

In general PI and RI correspond to each other during changes in resistance, however, caution is needed in interpretation with regard to the cause of any changes. For example, an increase in PI can be due to cerebral vasoconstriction or high intracranial pressure (Matta, 2000).

Doppler ultrasound detection of cerebral emboli

In addition to measuring the frequency of ultrasound waves returning to the Doppler receiver the amount of ultrasound is also measured and expressed as the amplitude or signal power. The amount of ultrasound reflected depends on both the size and the acoustic impedance of the substance being insonated.

Acoustic impedance (Z) is a measure of the resistance to sound passing through a medium and is a product of density (p) and velocity (c), i.e., $Z = pc$ and is expressed in units of $kg/m^2/sec$. High density materials have a high acoustic impedance while low density materials have a low acoustic impedance. The amount of sound that is reflected at an interface depends on the acoustic impedance change from one substance to another. A large difference in the acoustic impedance at the interface between two materials will result in a large amount of ultrasound being reflected. This is known as the reflection coefficient:

$$\alpha_R = \left(\frac{Z_2 - Z_1}{Z_2 + Z_1}\right)^2$$

α_R = reflection coefficient.
Z_1 = acoustic impedance of medium 1.
Z_2 = acoustic impedance of medium 2.

Multiplying this relation by 100 gives the percentage reflection of ultrasound waves at the interface. The same percentage is reflected whether going from a substance of high acoustic impedance to one of low impedance or vice versa. In the case of the blood/air interface the reflection is 99.9% and therefore air emboli in blood produce very high intensity signals which tend to overload the dynamic range of most commercial TCD systems producing aliasing. With particulate emboli consisting of platelet aggregates the acoustic impedance coefficients are similar, therefore the reflection is lower and particulate emboli produce lower intensity signals (Smith *et al.*, 1994).

Most TCD systems are set-up primarily to display cerebral blood velocities and because the back-scattered power of a Doppler signal from blood alone is fairly constant the dynamic range is not particularly high, e.g. 20–40 dB.

Air emboli can produce back-scattered power signals of 40–50 dB above the background blood signal and this overloads the dynamic range of most commercial TCD systems producing aliasing on the display. The air emboli signals can appear to extend outside the blood velocity envelope and can disappear off the top of the display and appear again at the bottom. In contrast most solid particulate emboli produce signals typically 10 dB above the background blood signal. These signals do not overload the system and high intensity signals are contained within the blood velocity envelope. However, very small air emboli do not overload the system while large particulate emboli may cause overload and therefore there is some overlap in the detection of air and particulate emboli which makes absolute differentiation difficult (Smith *et al.*, 1994).

Detection of different embolic materials using Doppler ultrasound

Clinically, the differentiation of air and particulate emboli can be very important as various studies have established that most air microemboli have few clinical consequences while particulate emboli can indicate imminent cerebral infarction and stroke (Gaunt *et al.*, 1994a; Horn *et al.*, 2005). However, these studies differentiated emboli by combining objective and subjective data to make reasonable assumptions as to their likely composition. This approach is perfectly valid from a practical point of view and allows clinical decisions to be made with regard to patient treatment but for future development it was realized that more accurate, automated methods of embolus detection and differentiation were required. A number of different investigators have explored different properties of the ultrasound signals produced by emboli to try and differentiate air and particulate emboli using Doppler criteria alone.

In 1995 leading investigators published certain criteria for the TCD detection of emboli (Consensus Committee of the Ninth International Cerebral Haemodynamic Symposium, 1995). These criteria were:

1. A Doppler microembolic signal is transient usually lasting less than 300 ms. Its duration depends on its time of passage through the Doppler sample volume.
2. The amplitude of a Doppler microembolic signal is usually at least 3 dB higher than that of the background blood flow signal and depends on the characteristics of the individual microembolus.
3. Within the appropriate dynamic range of bidirectional Doppler equipment, a signal is unidirectional within the Doppler velocity spectrum.
4. Depending on the equipment used and its own velocity, a microembolic signal is accompanied by a "snap", "chirp" or "moan" on the audible output.

Although these criteria accurately described what is commonly detected on most TCD systems when emboli occur, they still contained an element of subjectivity. A second consensus statement was published in 1998 which emphasized the effect of different TCD parameters on embolus detection and the need to standardize TCD equipment and recording methods in order to achieve meaningful results (Ringlstein *et al.*, 1998). The authors proposed that future research papers should state the following parameters:

1. Ultrasound device
2. Transducer type and size
3. Insonated artery
4. Insonation depth
5. Algorithms for signal intensity measurement
6. Scale settings
7. Detection threshold
8. Axial extension of sample volume
9. FFT size (number of points used)
10. FFT length (time)
11. FFT overlap
12. Transmitted ultrasound frequency
13. High-pass filter settings
14. Recording time.

These criteria emphasize the point that TCD machine settings have a profound effect on whether emboli are detected and whether the different composition of emboli can be differentiated.

Differentiating emboli and artefacts

An artefact which appears and sounds like an embolus can be produced by probe displacement or a variety of external electrical sources. In general bidirectional signals, i.e. signals above and below the baseline are frequently artefacts. However, embolic signals may also cause bidirectional signals particularly if they are gaseous in nature or with inadequate instrument settings. The dual-gating method described earlier is one method which can differentiate between emboli and artefacts (Smith *et al.*, 1996).

Differentiating solid and gaseous emboli

At present there is no method using Doppler criteria alone to absolutely differentiate between solid and gaseous emboli. As already described, gaseous emboli produce very high intensity signals which tend to overload the dynamic range of most TCD machines. This produces aliasing where particulate emboli produce more subtle high intensity signals that are usually contained within the blood velocity envelope.

FFT spectral analysis is not ideal for the differentiation of emboli because the temporal resolution is so poor. All emboli appear as very short high-intensity transients. Smith and colleagues increased the dynamic range of the TCD from 30 dB to 60 dB to prevent embolic signal overload and applied Wigner spectral analysis to try and differentiate air and particulate emboli on the basis of sample volume length (SVL) (Smith *et al.*, 1994). The sensitivity of the TCD sample volume to detect emboli is greater at its center and weaker at its edges. Air emboli reflect more ultrasound than particulate emboli and are detected both at the edges and the center of the sample volume. Particulate emboli reflect less ultrasound and are only detected in the center of the sample volume. Therefore, air emboli are detected for a longer length and time than particulate emboli, i.e. air emboli have a greater SVL. The use of Wigner analysis improved the differentiation of emboli but further studies showed there was still overlap between the SVL of air and particulate (Smith *et al.*, 1994). In addition, Wigner analysis was slow and laborious and had to be performed off-line and this limited its clinical application.

Dual frequency methods utilize the theory that the scattering properties of very small targets such as red blood cells change in a different way to the scattering properties of larger targets such as emboli as the frequency of the incident ultrasound is altered and this can also be used to differentiate emboli of different composition. Therefore two frequencies of ultrasound (e.g. 1.3 MHz and 2 MHz) are used to insonate the middle cerebral artery and the backscatter properties of emboli are compared at the two frequencies. Promising results have been obtained in vitro but clinical studies have indicated that current systems are still not accurate enough for use in clinical or research studies and further development work is needed (Markus and Punter, 2005).

Smith and colleagues noticed that as emboli pass through the TCD sample volume, air emboli change their velocity and position in the blood stream much more than particulate emboli whose position in the blood stream is fairly constant. One can imagine a bubble of air "fizzing" about the blood stream. This effect is known as frequency modulation and can be observed more easily if the time-domain of the TCD signal is expanded. So far there have been few attempts to apply this method in vivo but this property, combined with other methods may help differentiation in the future (Smith *et al.*, 1997).

TCD examination techniques

TCD sonography exploits three areas of the skull where the bone is relatively thin and therefore provides less of a barrier to the penetration of ultrasonic waves. These areas are known as acoustic windows and are located as follows: the transtemporal window (Aaslid *et al.*, 1982), the transorbital window (Spencer and Whisler, 1986) and the transoccipital window (Arnold and von Reutern, 1986). The transtemporal window is the most commonly used and is located over the temporal bone just superior to the zygomatic arch. The transtemporal window is used to insonate the middle cerebral artery and is the site used for most monitoring purposes.

Although radiological studies have shown that the transtemporal area is the most consistently radiolucent area of the skull (Tavares and Wood, 1976) (Figure 25.2) insonation is still impossible in approximately 10 subjects due to hyperostosis (Feinber *et al.*, 1990). This predominantly occurs in post-menopausal women and is due to a localized increase in the density of the inner table of the skull (Tavares and Wood, 1976).

The transorbital window utilizes the thin orbital plate of the frontal bone, the optic canal and/or the superior orbital fissure to insonate the intracranial portion of the internal carotid artery and the ophthalmic artery. Although attenuation is much less through this window and the carotid sinus may be insonated, the acoustic intensity needs to be carefully controlled to reduce exposure to the eye (Spencer and Whisler, 1986). Also the effects of prolonged insonation (2–4 hours) is unknown and therefore the application of this technique for intraoperative monitoring is restricted.

The transoccipital window provides access to the intracranial portions of the vertebral and basilar arteries by exploiting the gap between the cranium and the atlas. However, adequate access requires considerable neck flexion on the part of the patient which is uncomfortable for many patients and may be impossible in the older age group. This position of the neck is unsuitable for the performance of carotid endarterectomy and the insonation of these arteries would not be expected to detect any emboli which had their origin in the carotid artery.

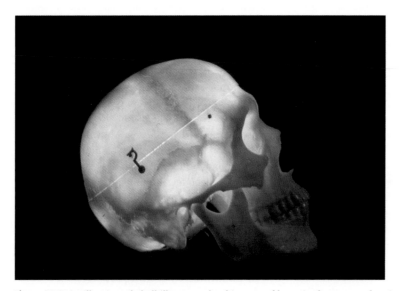

Figure 25.2 An illuminated skull illustrates the thin area of bone in the temporal region which is the main acoustic window for TCD monitoring.

Examination of the middle cerebral artery

The transtemporal window is divided into three regions: posterior, middle and anterior moving from the area just in front of the ear and above the zygomatic arch, forward (Fujioka and Douville, 1992). The posterior transtemporal window is the most commonly used but if no window is found the other regions should be investigated. The probe is placed on the posterior temporal area with some aqueous ultrasound coupling gel between the probe and the skin. The acoustic intensity is set to 100% of its maximum, the sample volume placed at a depth of 55 mm and the probe angled slightly forward and upward. From this position small alterations in depth and angle are made until a Doppler signal is obtained (Figure 25.3). The angle and position is further adjusted to obtain the maximum MCA velocity possible thereby

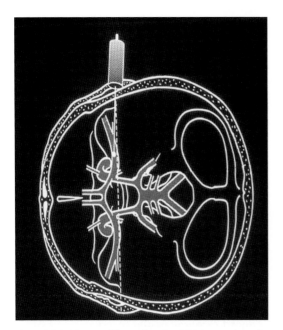

Figure 25.3 Diagram illustrating the TCD insonation of the middle cerebral artery of circle of Willis.

ensuring that the angle between the line of insonation and the direction of blood flow is as low as possible (see explanation above). For a positive identification of the MCA the following criteria should be satisfied (Fujioka and Douville, 1992):

1. With the probe positioned on the posterior temporal window the probe should be angled slightly anterior and superior.
2. The Doppler spectral signal obtained should have a positive deflection (indicating blood flow toward the probe), the systolic upstroke should be steep (except in cases of severe flow-limiting proximal stenoses) and the time-averaged mean velocity should be in the region of 55±12 cm/sec.
3. On increasing the depth (55–64 mm), the signal should bifurcate, with a negative deflecting signal becoming visible in addition to the positive deflection. This indicates the point of bifurcation of the internal carotid artery into the anterior cerebral artery (ACA) (negative deflection-flow away from the probe) and MCA (positive deflection-flow toward the probe). Increasing the depth further and angling the probe more anteriorly should yield a predominantly negative deflection indicating insonation of the anterior cerebral artery alone (65–70 mm).
4. On decreasing the depth, the MCA signal should be detectable to at least 45 mm although the angle of the probe may need to be adjusted to take account of bends in the artery. Only the MCA is detectable at these shallow depths because it runs outward toward the skull for 16–20 mm of its course before bifurcating.
5. Having identified the MCA and ACA, the probe should now be angled posteriorly and the depth increased to 60–70 mm and the posterior cerebral arteries identified. The P1 segment has a positive deflection but usually has a less steep systolic upstroke and velocity in the

region of 39±10 cm/sec. The P2 segment has a negative deflection and a velocity of 40 ± 10 cm/sec.

Exceptions to the criteria

It is probably safe to say that the only criterion which does not vary is the fact that blood flow in the MCA should always be towards the probe. However, anatomical variations and altered directions and velocities of flow due to disease can make positive vessel identification very difficult.

A very severe ipsilateral carotid stenosis or occlusion can reduce flow to such an extent that the direction of blood flow in the anterior cerebral artery is reversed providing a collateral blood supply. In such a case the bidirectional signal at the bifurcation is never obtained because the blood is still flowing toward the probe. This gives the impression that the MCA can be traced to a much greater depth than would be normally expected.

Alternatively, in cases of reduced ipsilateral carotid blood flow the amount of blood flowing through the posterior cerebral artery increases considerably. In such a patient the MCA signal is detectable but the systolic upstroke may be damped and the velocity reduced so that it does not resemble a typical MCA waveform. The P1 segment of the posterior cerebral is the strongest signal with a steep systolic upstroke and a higher blood flow velocity and therefore closely mimics the MCA, and can lead to monitoring of the wrong artery. However, the probe will be noted to be angled slightly posteriorly and if angled further posteriorly no other signals will be detected (Fujioka and Douville, 1992).

Clinical applications of TCD

There is now a wide range of clinical applications for the application of TCD monitoring (Table 25.1).

Table 25.1. Clinical applications of TCD (Hansen *et al.*, 1996; Vajda *et al.*, 1999; Sloan *et al.*, 2004)

Screening of children with sickle cell for stroke
Detecting vasospasm after subarachnoid hemorrhage
Detecting intracranial steno-occlusive disease
Vasomotor reactivity testing
Detection of cerebral circulatory arrest/brain death
Monitoring of carotid endarterectomy
Cerebral thrombolysis monitoring
Monitoring of cardiac surgery
Contrast enhanced assessment of right to left and extracardiac shunts
Hemorrhagic cerebrovascular disease
Hyperperfusion due to preeclampsia in pregnancy
Abnormal cerebral autoregulation in liver failure
Monitoring of treatment for hydrocephalus in children

Only the more major applications will be described in detail.

Extracranial vascular disease: carotid artery disease

A major cause of stroke is thromboembolism originating from stenotic arterial disease at the carotid bifurcation. Intervention to remove the stenosis by the operation of carotid endarterectomy or carotid angioplasty can prevent strokes but carotid artery disease is very common and not all patients will benefit from these invasive procedures particularly if they are asymptomatic. TCD can help in selection of appropriate patients for intervention by identifying patients with reduced cerebrovascular reserve and those patients with high-risk carotid plaques that are actively embolizing to the brain.

Reduced cerebrovascular reserve

A close relationship has been demonstrated between cerebral blood flow (CBF) and TCD

MCAV and this relationship can be used to identify patients where a stenosed carotid artery is significantly reducing blood supply to the brain. In a normal individual, CBF and MCAV changes by approximately 3% for every mmHg change in arterial carbon dioxide (PaCO$_2$) (Markwalder *et al.*, 1984). Hyperventilation can be used to reduce PaCO$_2$ and CO$_2$ rebreathing can be used to raise it and the effect on MCAV can be observed. The absence of a normal response indicates impaired cerebral blood supply and provides an indication for intervention on the carotid artery. Intravenous administration of acetazolamide can be used as an alternative method of raising CO$_2$ tension (Staszkiewicz *et al.*, 2000).

Silent cerebral embolization

Many patients have significant carotid artery stenosis but are either asymptomatic or describe symptoms which are atypical for embolic disease. The detection of silent cerebral emboli during monitoring of the ipsilateral MCA for 1–2 hours over several days has been demonstrated to identify a group of patients at higher risk of subsequent stroke than patients where no emboli are detected. These patients can be selected for carotid surgery or angioplasty (Markus and Mackinnon, 2005).

Monitoring of carotid angioplasty and stenting

Carotid angioplasty and stenting is an increasingly popular method of treating carotid stenosis and consists of inflating a balloon across the stenosis to obliterate it. Unfortunately manipulation of wires and catheters in the vicinity of unstable plaque as well as inflation and deflation of the angioplasty balloon can be associated with significant cerebral embolization causing strokes (Ackerstaff *et al.*, 2005). The use of different types of stents and embolus protection devices have been proposed to reduce this embolization and TCD monitoring has been used to assess the effectiveness of such devices (Vos *et al.*, 2005). So far different studies

have produced conflicting results with no overall benefit shown. Continuing TCD monitoring in the postprocedure period is also useful to detect thrombosis of the treated artery (Ackerstaff and Vos, 2004).

Monitoring of carotid endarterectomy

Monitoring of carotid endarterectomy has been one of the major applications of TCD monitoring and has been successful in detecting the major causes of perioperative strokes such as cerebral hypoperfusion, hyperperfusion and perioperative embolization.

TCD detection of hemodynamic complications – hypoperfusion, hyperperfusion

The operation of carotid endarterectomy involves clamping of the carotid arteries while the procedure is performed (Figure 25.4). CBF can be restored by the insertion of a temporary bypass shunt but this can cause complications and may be considered unnecessary in those patients where collateral blood flow around the circle of Willis maintains adequate CBF. TCD monitoring of the ipsilateral MCA can detect significant falls in MCAV and identify cerebral hypoperfusion and ischemia in those patients requiring shunt insertion (see previous explanation). Once the shunt is inserted continuous TCD monitoring can detect shunt malfunction which would not be otherwise detected and prevent ischemic stroke (Gaunt *et al.*, 1994a).

At the end of the operation when blood flow is restored through the carotid system TCD confirms improved perfusion of the cerebral hemisphere and continued patency of the operated artery. However, some patients with severe carotid stenosis, especially those with bilateral disease, may have impaired cerebrovascular autoregulation and carotid baroreceptor blood pressure control and have difficulty regulating the improved blood supply to the brain (Keunen *et al.*, 1994; Sigaudo-Roussel *et al.*, 2002). This can result in cerebral

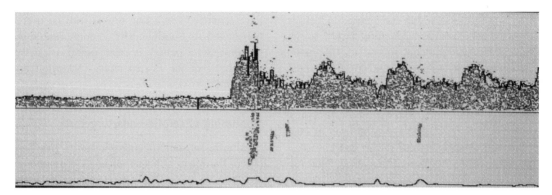

Figure 25.4 Intraoperative TCD trace showing the relative hypoperfusion during carotid clamping, the sudden increase in middle cerebral artery velocities on clamp release and the occurrence of typical overloading embolic signals suggestive of air.

edema and in severe cases intracranial hemorrhage. This scenario can be predicted by the TCD detection of sustained abnormally high MCAV in the postoperative period. Generally, a MCAV greater than 2.0–3.0 times the preoperative velocity indicates a high risk of hyperperfusion, and therapy to reduce the systemic blood pressure is indicated until the powers of cerebral autoregulation are regained (Keunen *et al.*, 2001).

TCD detection of perioperative embolization

Providing the correct MCA has been insonated and the TCD parameters are properly set-up, some degree of embolization is detectable during every carotid endarterectomy operation – indeed failure to detect any emboli is an indication that the wrong artery may have been monitored. The vast majority of these emboli represent air microbubbles and are associated with no significant neurological deficits. These emboli produce the typical high intensity signals and occur in showers after operative maneuvres such as shunt insertion or final restoration of flow and quickly clear and cease (Gaunt *et al.*, 1994a).

However, particulate emboli occurring during the initial dissection of the carotid artery represent unstable plaque causing cerebral embolization of plaque fragments or thrombus and these can be associated with the development of neurological deficits (Spencer *et al.*, 1990). These emboli tend to be of lower intensity than air emboli, and occur before the arterial system has been entered and, therefore, are unlikely to be air. Typically, these emboli occur when the carotid bifurcation itself is being dissected and therefore, dissection of this area should cease and carotid arteries proximal and distal to the area should be clamped and if necessary a shunt inserted. This maneuvre should stop the embolization and dissection can be completed in safety.

Particulate embolization occurring at the end of the operation after final restoration of flow is another ominous sign (Figure 25.5). After clamp release air emboli quickly clear within the first 30–60 seconds. Occasional air emboli may be detected after this time as tiny air bubbles are dislodged but their occurrence is random. If a persistent pattern of particulate emboli are detected after this time this represents the build-up of platelet thrombus on the endarterectomy site and subsequent cerebral embolization. Untreated, this pattern of persistent particulate embolization is associated with serious neurological deficits. This persistent embolization may be accompanied by a gradual fall in MCAV as carotid thrombus

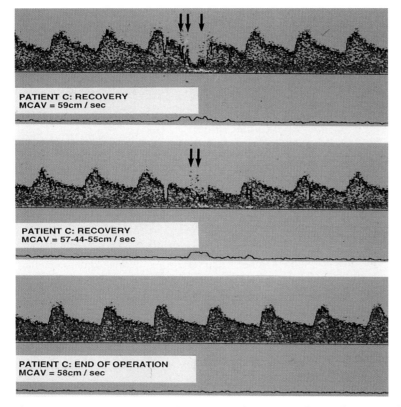

PATIENT C: RECOVERY
MCAV = 59cm / sec

PATIENT C: RECOVERY
MCAV = 57-44-55cm / sec

PATIENT C: END OF OPERATION
MCAV = 58cm / sec

Figure 25.5 A series of TCD traces after carotid endarterectomy showing large particulate emboli (arrows) which temporarily impair blood flow in the middle cerebral artery.

narrows the artery and reduces cerebral perfusion but this is not necessary for the development of neurological deficits which can result from particulate embolization alone (Gaunt *et al.*, 1994a,b).

One option for therapeutic intervention is to reopen the carotid artery and clear the thrombus, occasionally a technical error such as an intimal flap can be corrected but more commonly the thrombus has built up on the raw endarterectomy surface itself and is due to an abnormality in platelet aggregation. Therefore Leonard and colleagues proposed an alternative approach consisting of the intravenous administration of 10% Dextran 40 solution. Dextran reduces platelet aggregation and is started at a rate of 20 mls per hour and is

increased by 20 mls per hour every 10 minutes until the rate of TCD-detected embolization reduces and eventually stops. If embolization fails to respond to Dextran then reoperation is indicated (Lennard *et al.*, 1997).

Intracranial vascular disease

Subarachnoid hemorrhage

Cerebral vasospasm is the leading cause of morbidity and mortality in patients who survive a subarachnoid hemorrhage (SAH) and is sufficient to be clinically significant in approximately 20% of patients (Kassell *et al.*, 1990). TCD monitoring has become useful in diagnosing vasospasm before it becomes clinically apparent. Cerebral vasospasm is generally considered to be present if the MCAV is greater than 120 cm/sec or the ratio between the MCAV and maximal velocity in the internal carotid artery exceeds a ratio of 3. This ratio should decrease with effective treatment and daily TCD monitoring is a useful noninvasive way to detect this (Lindegaard et al., 1998).

Arteriovenous malformations

Characteristically these arteriovenous malformations have feeder vessels characterized by high blood flow velocity, low pulsatility, low perfusion pressure and decreased CO_2-reactivity which can be detected using TCD. Therapeutic embolization or resection of these lesions usually results in normalization of these parameters and this can be confirmed by TCD which also detects complications resulting from these treatments such as the hyperperfusion syndrome. Comparison of the feeding vessel and the corresponding normal vessel from the contralateral side is often useful (Fleischer et al., 1993).

Closed head injury

Episodes of hypoxemia, hypotension and reduced cerebral perfusion due to high intracranial pressure are associated with a poor outcome following closed head injury. TCD is useful as part of multimodal monitoring to detect these complications (Kirkpatrick et al., 1996). TCD can be used to detect changes in MCAV, pulsatility index and impaired cerebrovascular reserve. When cerebral autoregulation is functioning there is little change in MCAV during changes in CPP. However, in head-injured patients with impaired cerebral autoregulation, a positive linear correlation between MCAV and cerebral perfusion pressure is observed and this can be used to identify when autoregulation has failed (Czosnycka et al., 1996). In addition, as CPP falls, an increase in the PI as a result of a reduction in the diastolic blood flow velocity, gives an early warning of impending autoregulatory failure (Padayachee et al., 1987).

Cerebral vasospasm is another significant cause of morbidity and mortality following closed-head injury which can be diagnosed by TCD using the same criteria as for SAH.

Cardiac surgery

Monitoring during cardiac surgery was one of the earliest applications of TCD (Uekermann et al., 2005). Cognitive dysfunction following cardiac surgery has been reported in up to 60% of patients with perioperative strokes occurring in 5% (Murkin, 1993). TCD monitoring has been used to identify significant amounts of cerebral embolization occurring during cardiopulmonary bypass as well as episodes of cerebral hypo- and hyperperfusion (Katz et al., 1998).

Conclusion

The technique of transcranial Doppler has progressed from interesting research tool to an essential part of clinical practice. TCD is a convenient, noninvasive bedside test which can be used to monitor patients over many hours. TCD is able to detect two of the major causes of neurological deficits, i.e. abnormalities in blood flow and cerebral embolization. These two properties have made it a valuable practical tool to assist in the management and treatment of patients in a wide range of clinical disciplines. Research continues in even wider areas and more indications for TCD monitoring are still being discovered. However, those new to the field should take time to appreciate the technical limitations of the technique and not take what they see on the screen at face value.

REFERENCES

Aaslid, R. (1992). Developments and principles of transcranial Doppler. In *Transcranial Doppler*, ed.

D. W. Newell and R. Aaslid. New York: Raven Press, pp. 1–8.

Aaslid, R., Markwalder, T.-M. and Nornes, H. (1982). Non-invasive transcranial ultrasound recording of flow velocity in basal cerebral arteries. *Journal of Neurosurgery*, **57**, 769–74.

Ackerstaff, R. G. and Vos, J. A. (2004). TCD detected cerebral embolism in carotid endarterectomy versus angioplasty and stenting of the carotid bifurcation. *Acta Chirurgica Belgica*, **104**, 55–9.

Ackerstaff, R. G., Suttorp, M. J., van den Berg, J. C., *et al.* (2005). Prediction of early cerebral outcome by transcranial Doppler monitoring in carotid bifurcation angioplasty and stenting. *Journal of Vascular Surgery*, **41**, 618–24.

Arnold, B. J. and von Reutern, G. M. (1986). Transcranial Doppler sonography. Examination techniques and normal reference values. *Ultrasound in Medicine and Biology*, **12**, 115–23.

Consensus Committee of the Ninth International Cerebral Haemodynamic Symposium. (1995). Basic identification criteria of Doppler microembolic signals. *Stroke*, **26**, 1123.

Czosnycka, M., Smielewski, P., Kirkpatrick, P., *et al.* (1996). Monitoring of cerebral autoregulation in head injured patients. *Stroke*, **27**, 1829.

Doppler, C. A. (1842). Uber das farbige Licht der Doppelsterne und einiger anderer Gestirne des Himmels. *Abhandl Konigl Bohm Ges Wiss.*

Feinber, W. M., Devine, J. and Ledbetter, E. (1990). Clinical characteristics of patients with inadequate temporal windows. *The 4ᵗʰ International Intracranial hemodynamics symposium, Orlando, Fl.*

Fleischer, L. H., Young, W. L., Pile-Spellman, J., *et al.* (1993). Relationship of transcranial Doppler flow velocities and arteriovenous malformation feeding artery pressures. *Stroke*, **24**, 1897.

Fujioka, K. A. and Douville, C. M. (1992). Anatomy and freehand examination techniques. In *Transcranial Doppler*, ed. D. W. Newell and R. Aaslid. New York: Raven Press, pp. 9–31.

Gaunt, M. E., Martin, P. J., Smith, J. L., *et al.* (1994a). The clinical relevance of intraoperative embolisation detected by transcranial Doppler monitoring during carotid endarterectomy: a prospective study in 100 patients. *British Journal of Surgery*, **81**, 1435–9.

Gaunt, M. E., Ratliff, D. A., Martin, P. J., *et al.* (1994b). On-table diagnosis of incipient carotid thrombosis during carotid endarterectomy. *Journal of Vascular Surgery*, **20**, 104–7.

Gosling, R. G. and King, D. H. (1974). Arterial assessment by Doppler shift ultrasound. *Proceedings of the Royal Society of Medicine*, **60**, 447–9.

Hansen, W. F., Burnham, S. J., Svendsen, T. O., *et al.* (1996). Transcranial Doppler findings of cerebral vasospasm in pre-eclampsia. *Journal of Maternal Fetal Medicine*, **5**, 194.

Halsey, J. H., Jr. (1993). Monitoring blood flow velocity in the middle cerebral artery during carotid endarterectomy. In *Transcranial Doppler Ultrasonography*, ed. V. L. Babikan and L. R. Wechsler. St. Louis: Mosby-Year Book Inc, pp. 216–21.

Horn, J., Naylor, A. R., Laman, D. M., *et al.* (2005). Identification of patients at risk for ischaemic cerebral complications after carotid endarterectomy with TCD monitoring. *European Journal of Vascular and Endovascular Surgery*, **30**, 270–4.

Kaneko, Z. (1986). First steps in the development of the Doppler flowmeter. *Ultrasound in Medicine and Biology*, **12**, 187–95.

Kassell, N. F., Torner, J. C., Jane, J. A., *et al.* (1990). The international co-operative study on the timing of aneurysm surgery, part 1: overall management results. *Journal of Neurosurgery*, **7**, 18.

Katz, J. J., Mandell, M. S., House, R. M., *et al.* (1998). Cerebral blood flow velocity in patients with subclinical portal-systemic encephalopathy. *Anesthesia and Analgesia*, **86**, 1005.

Keunen, R. W., Eikelboom, B. C., Stegeman, D. F. and Ackerstaff, R. G. (1994). Chronic cerebral hypotension induces a downward shift of the cerebral autoregulation: a hypothesis based on TCD and OPG-GEE studies in ambulatory patients with occlusive cerebrovascular disease. *Neurological Research*, **16**, 413–16.

Keunen, R., Nijmeijer, H. W., Tavy, D., *et al.* (2001). An observational study of pre-operative transcranial Doppler examinations to predict cerebral hyperperfusion following carotid endarterectomies. *Neurological Research*, **23**, 593–8.

Kirkpatrick, P. J., Czosnycka, M. and Pickard, J. D. (1996). Multimodality monitoring in intensive care. *Journal of Neurology, Neurosurgery and Psychiatry*, **60**, 131.

Lennard, N., Smith, J., Dumville, J., *et al.* (1997). Prevention of post-operative thrombotic stroke after carotid endarterectomy: the role of transcranial

Doppler ultrasound. *Journal of Vascular Surgery*, **26**, 579–84.

Lindegaard, K. F., Nornes, H., Bakke, S. J., *et al.* (1998). Cerebral vasospasm after subarachnoid haemorrhage investigated by means of transcranial Doppler ultrasound. *Acta Neurochirurgica*, **24**, 81.

Markus, H. S. (1995). Importance of time-window overlap in the detection and analysis of embolic signals. *Stroke*, **26**, 2044–7.

Markus, H. S. and MacKinnon, A. (2005). Asymptomatic embolization detected by Doppler ultrasound predicts stroke risk in symptomatic carotid artery stenosis. *Stroke*, **36**, 971–5.

Markus, H. S. and Punter, M. (2005). Can transcranial Doppler discriminate between solid and gaseous microemboli? Assessment of a dual-frequency transducer system. *Stroke*, **36**, 1731–4.

Markwalder, T. M., Gromilund, P., Seiler, R. W., *et al.* (1984). Dependency of blood flow velocity in the middle cerebral artery on end-tidal carbon dioxide partial pressure – a transcranial ultrasound Doppler study. *Journal of Cerebral Blood Flow Metabolism*, **4**, 368.

Matta, B. (2000). Transcranial Doppler ultrasonography. *In Anaesthesia and Neurosurgery*, eds. J. E. Cottrell and D. S. Smith. St Louis: Mosby.

Murkin, J. M. (1993). Anaesthesia, the brain and cardiopulmonary bypass. *Annals of Thoracic Surgery*, **56**, 1461.

Naylor, A. R., Merrick, M. V., Slattery, J. M., *et al.* (1991). Parametric imaging of cerebrovascular reserve. 2. Reproducibility, response to CO_2 and correlation with middle cerebral artery velocities. *European Journal of Nuclear Medicine*, **18**, 259–64.

Padayachee, T. S., Parsons, S. and Theobald, R. (1987). The detection of microemboli in the middle cerebral artery during cardiac surgery using transcranial Doppler ultrasound: investigation using membrane and bubble oxygenation. *Annals of Thoracic Surgery*, **44**, 298–302.

Pourcelot, L. (1974). Applications cliniques de l'examen Doppler transcutane. Les colloques de l'Institut National de la Sante et de la Recherche Medicale. *Institut national de la Santé et de la recherche Médicale*, **34**, 213–40.

Ringlstein, E. B., Droste, D. W., Babikian, V. L., *et al.* (1998). Consensus on Microembolus Detection by TCD. *Stroke*, **29**, 725–9.

Satomura, S. and Kaneko, Z. (1986). Ultrasonic blood rheograph. *Proceedings of the 3rd International Conference on Medical Electronics; Tokyo, Japan, 1960*, pp. 254–8

Sigaudo-Roussel, D., Evans, D. H., Naylor, A. R., *et al.* (2002). Deterioration in carotid baroreflex during carotid endarterectomy. *Journal of Vascular Surgery*, **36**, 793–8.

Sloan, M. A., Alexandrov, A. V., Tegeler, C. H., *et al.* (2004). Assessment of transcranial Doppler ultrasonography: report of the Therapeutic and Technology Assessment Subcommittee of the American Academy of Neurology. *Neurology*, **62**, 1468–81.

Smith, J. L., Evans, D. H., Fan, L., Bell, P. R. F. and Naylor, A. R. (1996). Differentiation between emboli and artefacts using dual-gated transcranial Doppler ultrasound. *Ultrasound in Medicine and Biology*, **22**, 1031–6.

Smith, J. L., Evans, D. H., Fan, L., Thrush, A. J. and Naylor, A. R. (1994). Processing Doppler ultrasound signals from blood borne emboli. *Ultrasound in Medicine and Biology*, **20**, 455–62.

Smith, J. L., Evans, D. H. and Naylor, A. R. (1997). Analysis of the frequency modulation present in Doppler ultrasound signals may allow differentiation between particulate and gaseous cerebral emboli. *Ultrasound in Medicine and Biology*, **23**, 727–34.

Sorteberg, W., Langmoen, I. A., Lindegaard, K. F. and Nornes, H. (1990). Side-to-side differences and day-to-day variations of transcranial Doppler parameters in normal subjects. *Journal of Ultrasound in Medicine*, **9**, 403–9.

Spencer, M. P. (1992). Detection of cerebral arterial emboli. In *Transcranial Doppler*, eds. D. W. Newell and R. Aaslid. New York: Raven Press, pp. 215–30.

Spencer, M. P., Thomas, G. I. and Moehring, M. A. (1990). Detection of middle cerebral artery emboli during carotid endarterectomy using transcranial Doppler ultrasonography. *Stroke*, **21**, 415–23.

Spencer, M. P. and Whisler, D. (1986). Transorbital Doppler diagnosis of intracranial arterial stenosis. *Stroke*, **17**, 916–21.

Staszkiewicz, W., Antepowicz, W., Gatrusiewicz, A. and Gowlikowska, D. (2000). Assessment of cerebrovascular reserve in patients with carotid artery disease using transcranial Doppler and acetazolamide. *Neurologia i Neurochirurgia Polska*, **34**, 289–99.

Steiger, H. J. (1992). Monitoring for carotid surgery. In *Transcranial Doppler*, eds. D. W. Newell and R. Aaslid. New York: Raven Press, pp. 197–205.

Tavares, R. L. and Wood, E. H. (Eds.) (1976). *Diagnostic Neuroradiology* (Vol. 2). Baltimore: Williams and Wilkins, pp. 577–80.

Uekermann, J., Suchan, B., Doum, I., *et al.* (2005). Neuropsychological deficits after mechanical aortic valve replacements. *Journal of Heart Valve Disease*, **14**, 338–43.

Vajda, Z., Buki, A., Veto, F., *et al.* (1999). Transcranial Doppler-determined pulsatility index in the evaluation of endoscopic third ventriculostomy (preliminary data). *Acta Neurochirurgica* (Wien) **141**, 247–50

Vos, J. A., van den Berg, J. C., Ernst, S. M., *et al.* (2005). Carotid angioplasty and stent placement: comparison of transcranial Doppler US data and clinical outcome with and without filtering cerebral protection devices in 509 patients. *Radiology*, **237**, 374–5.

26

Imaging carotid disease: MR and CT perfusion

Jeroen van der Grond and Matthias J. P. van Osch

Leiden University Medical Center, Leiden, The Netherlands

Introduction

The presence of adequate cerebral circulation is important to maintain cerebral perfusion and brain function in patients with severe carotid artery disease (Powers, 1991; Klijn *et al.*, 1997; Caplan and Hennerici, 1998; Derdeyn *et al.*, 1999). The level of cerebral perfusion is influenced by many factors such as degree of ipsilateral stenosis, degree of contralateral stenosis, capacity of posterior circulation, the anatomical variants and completeness of the circle of Willis, the remaining vasomotor reactivity, which on itself is influenced by underlying pathology such as atherosclerosis or inflammatory processes, and capacity to reroute blood flow, for instance, via leptomeningeal anastomoses. Although Liebeskind correctly mentioned that the understanding of the cerebral circulation is improved by determining the extra- and intra-cranial collateral capacity (Liebeskind, 2003), the large number of confounding factors, mentioned above, makes it virtually impossible to predict which patients with carotid artery disease are at (high) risk for recurrent symptoms caused by hemodynamical factors. It has been shown that in patients with symptomatic severe internal carotid artery (ICA) stenosis carotid endarterectomy reduces the risk of recurrent stroke by removal of the atheromatous plaque (European Carotid Surgery Trialists' Collaborative Group, 1991; NASCET, 1991; Barnett *et al.*, 2000). Although in patients with occlusive disease of the ICA, the cause of stroke is primarily thromboembolic, the presence of hemodynamic impairment is also recognized as additional risk factor (Caplan and Hennerici, 1998; Grubb *et al.*, 1998). It was noted that improvement of cerebral blood flow (CBF) after carotid endarterectomy may further decrease stroke risk by a better wash out of cerebral embolism (Caplan and Hennerici, 1998). Several studies demonstrated impaired perfusion in patients with ICA stenosis (Silvestrini *et al.*, 1996; Detre *et al.*, 1998; Markus and Cullinane, 2001) and improvement of regional hemodynamics after carotid desobstruction, e.g. carotid endarterectomy (Schroeder *et al.*, 1987; Hartl *et al.*, 1994; Kluytmans *et al.*, 1998; Wiart *et al.*, 2000; Markus and Cullinane, 2001) carotid angioplasty (Markus *et al.*, 1996) or stent placement (Ogasawara *et al.*, 2003; Niesen *et al.*, 2004; Ko *et al.*, 2005). On the other hand, several other reports have been unable to detect any significant cerebral hemodynamic abnormality in a majority of patients with ICA stenosis (Powers *et al.*, 1987; Powers, 1991; Nighoghossian *et al.*, 1994). Although the importance of hemodynamic factors in the pathogenesis of cerebral ischemia in patients with carotid artery disease remains vague, it is accepted that the flow contribution of the stenosed artery to the total blood supply is decreased (Boysen *et al.*, 1970; Gordon *et al.*, 1995; Vanninen *et al.*, 1995; Blankensteijn *et al.*, 1997). In this respect, determination of the actual cerebral hemodynamical status at the tissue level in patients with carotid artery

Carotid Disease: The Role of Imaging in Diagnosis and Management, ed. Jonathan Gillard, Martin Graves, Thomas Hatsukami and Chun Yuan. Published by Cambridge University Press. © Cambridge University Press 2007.

disease remains one of the potential methods to determine the risk for recurrent, hemodynamically induced, symptoms in patients with carotid artery disease.

Available techniques

Different modalities, each with its own advantages and disadvantages, can be applied to measure cerebral perfusion. The modern day successor of the early radioisotope studies is single positron emission computed tomography (SPECT). An important improvement of SPECT over the early radioisotope studies is the possibility of 3D reconstruction. Moreover, the development of technetium (Tc)-labeled isotopes such as 99m Tc-labeled red blood cells to measure cerebral blood volume (CBV) or 99mTc-hexamethyl propylene amine oxime (HMPAO) to measure CBF refined the imaging of cerebral perfusion. Parallel to the development in SPECT imaging, positron emission tomography (PET) was developed, with the important advantage that it measures blood flow in a fully quantitative way. Since, in addition to the determination of CBF and CBV, oxygen extraction fraction (OEF), glucose and oxygen metabolism can be obtained, PET is one of the most complete modalities to determine the cerebral hemodynamic status. Due to its ability to quantitatively measure important metabolic and hemodynamic variables, PET is considered the gold standard imaging method. Still, a disadvantage of both methods is that they expose the patient to ionizing radiation. Moreover, SPECT has a poor spatial resolution, and PET is expensive and not widely available, which limits its use in routine clinical practice.

In the last decade several magnetic resonance imaging (MRI)-based perfusion techniques have been developed to evaluate tissue perfusion. More recently, with the introduction of the 32- and 64-slice computed tomography (CT), CT perfusion techniques have also become available.

Perfusion MRI

MRI offers two different approaches to measure the cerebral perfusion. The first technique, arterial spin labeling (ASL), exploits the water in blood as an endogenous tracer. Dynamic susceptibility contrast MRI (DSC-MRI or MR bolus tracking) is the alternative method. This method uses an intravenous injection of contrast agent, applied as an exogenous tracer. Both techniques have been used to study the CBF in patients with stenotic artery disease, showing their ability to provide important information on the hemodynamic status. However, both techniques suffer from quantification hazards when applied in patients with large vessel pathology. Careful experimental design is therefore essential. Implementation and quantification issues of both techniques will be discussed in the following paragraphs.

Arterial spin labeling (ASL)

ASL employs a spatial selective inversion proximal to the imaging slice and monitors the inflow of these labeled spins in the imaging slice (Figure 26.1) (Kwong et al., 1995; Alsop and Detre, 1998; Thomas et al., 2000; Barbier et al., 2001). The method is implemented as a subtraction technique: first an image is acquired without the spatial selective inversion: thereafter a second image is acquired with the inversion pulse switched on. When subtracting these two images, all static signals from the imaging slice are subtracted out, leaving only the contribution of the labeled spins that have entered the imaging slice. To achieve the elimination of all contributions of static signal, it is important to compensate for magnetization transfer effects. Because the quality of one subtraction image is too low, the procedure is repeated several times and all subtraction images are averaged (control and perfusion-weighted images are still interleaved). A delay between labeling and imaging is used to enable the labeled spins to reach the microvasculature and to exchange with the

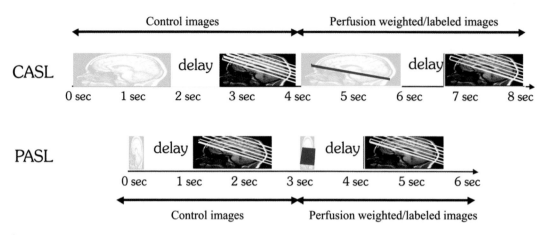

Figure 26.1 Time schedule of arterial spin labeling (ASL). Upper row shows the timing of a continuous ASL experiment: control and perfusion-weighted images are acquired interleaved both lasting about 4–5 s. Labeling is performed in an adiabatic labeling plane during the first 2 s for the perfusion-weighted images (indicated in red), whereas for the control image during the first 2 s no effective label is created, although equal magnetization transfer effects are caused. After a delay of 1 s acquisition is performed. Lower row shows the timing diagram of pulsed ASL. Label and control images both last only about 3 s and labeling is now achieved in 10 ms for a much larger region (again indicated in red).

tissue (Alsop and Detre, 1996). However, since the inverted spins will relax back to their equilibrium magnetization after labeling due to T_1 relaxation (time constant of approximately 1 s), too long a delay would lead to loss of the label and low-quality perfusion images. ASL techniques can be subdivided into two groups:

1. Continuous arterial spin labeling (CASL) employs a long adiabatic inversion pulse, approximately 2 s, which inverts the blood when flowing through a labeling plane. The efficiency of the labeling depends on the velocity in the arteries; on the angle of the vessel with respect to the labeling plane, and the compensation method for magnetization transfer effects (Werner *et al.*, 2005b).

2. Pulsed arterial spin labeling (PASL) is based on a short (typically 10 ms) spatial selective inversion pulse, which labels the blood in a large volume located proximal to the imaging slices. More than 10 different implementation versions of PASL have been described, like flow-sensitive alternating inversion recovery (FAIR),

quantitative imaging of perfusion using a single subtraction (QUIPSS), transfer insensitive labeling technique (TILT), echo-planar imaging and signal targeting with alternating RF (EPISTAR), double inversions with proximal labeling of both tag and control images (DIPLOMA), PULSAR, etc. Main differences between these implementations include differences in labeling regions and control for magnetization transfer effects. We refer to several reviews for further details (Calamante *et al.*, 1999; Barbier *et al.*, 2001; Golay *et al.*, 2004).

The main problems in quantifying CBF by means of ASL in patients with stenosis or occlusion of the main brain-feeding arteries are inter- and intrasubject differences in transport times of the label to the imaging slices and low signal-to-noise in hypoperfused regions. Longer transport times, often called transit delays, lead to delayed arrival of labeled spins and thereby an underestimation of CBF. Two different techniques have been proposed to correct for differences in transit delays. The first method involves the creation of a fixed duration of the bolus of labeled spins. For CASL this equals the labeling time, for PASL this is achieved by an additional saturation pulse applied to the labeling region after a certain delay (this technique is called QUIPSSII) (Alsop and Detre, 1996; Wong *et al.*, 1998). The delay between the labeling and saturation pulse should be applied before all labeled spins have left the labeling region for one brain-feeding artery. Finally, one should choose the delay between the end of labeling (for CASL) or the saturation pulse (QUIPSSII) and the imaging longer than the transit delay. This could be problematic in patients with large vessel obstructions, since this transit delay is a priori unknown. The other technique for circumventing quantification errors due to differences in transit time, is to perform imaging not at a single time point, but at several time points after labelling, e.g. ITS-FAIR and TURBO-TILT (Buxton *et al.*, 1998; Gunther *et al.*, 2001; Hendrikse *et al.*, 2003). This approach will monitor the inflow, relaxation and outflow of labeled spins and modeling resulting in quantitative CBF values. An example of such a multiinversion time technique in a patient with severe carotid artery disease of the right ICA is shown in Figure 26.2. This example shows that in patients with severe coronary artery disease, TURBO-TILT is well suited to visualize delayed flow that is being rerouted via primary or secondary collaterals. However, in patients with coronary artery disease, differences in transport times within a voxel or region-of-interest results in deviations from the model and may still lead to quantification errors (Figueiredo *et al.*, 2005). The low signal-to-noise in hypoperfused regions arises not only because of the low flow and thus low signal, but also due to the longer transport times that leads to significant loss of label due to relaxation. The limitations of measuring hypoperfusion by ASL can only be solved by imaging at higher magnetic field strengths. Higher field strengths do not only profit from the inherent higher signal-to-noise, but also lead to a longer T_1 relaxation time of blood that will limit the decay of the labeled spins before they enter the brain tissue. However, the quality of CBF measurement in white matter even at 3 Tesla is still limited.

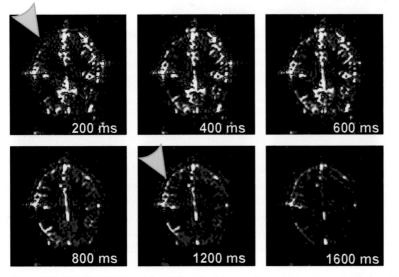

Figure 26.2 TURBO-TILT (multiinversion time) in a patient with severe carotid artery disease of the right internal carotid artery (ICA), showing delayed flow in the symptomatic hemisphere (arrowhead).

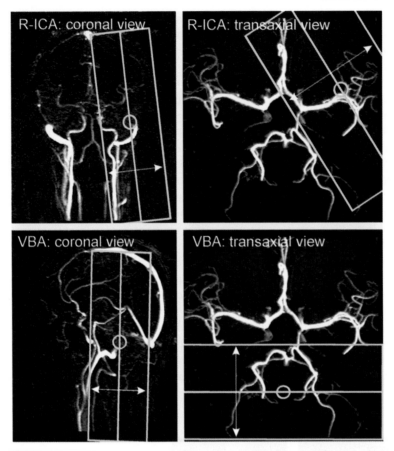

Figure 26.3 Orientation of labeling slab for selective labeling of the right internal carotid artery (ICA) and posterior circulation. The oblique sagittal labeling slab for selectively labeling of the ICA was planned using the maximum intensity projection (MIP) of the circle of Willis and the coronal phase contrast (PC) survey. The coronal labeling slab for selective labeling of the posterior circulation was planned using the MIP of the circle of Willis and the sagittal PC survey.

In patients with carotid artery disease, collateral flow is important to compensate for the decreased flow from the stenosed artery and to maintain adequate cerebral perfusion (Powers *et al.*, 1987; Powers, 1991). Although various studies have visualized the presence of collateral circulation in patients with ICA lesions (Mount and Taveras, 1957; Powers *et al.*, 1987; Norris *et al.*, 1990; Schomer *et al.*, 1994; Muller *et al.*, 1995; Baumgartner *et al.*, 1997; Henderson *et al.*, 2000; Hendrikse *et al.*, 2002), the actual contribution of these collateral arteries to the regional perfusion remains unknown. Thus far, no method has been able to quantify the actual contribution of individual collateral pathways on the brain tissue level. Recently, noninvasive selective ASL-MRI has been introduced, which is capable to combine flow territory information of the individual brain-feeding arteries with information of regional CBF (Hendrikse *et al.*, 2004). Selective ASL makes use of the fact that it is possible to limit the labeling pulses to single brain-feeding arteries.

This results in the visualization of an individual arterial flow territory, and therefore it enables the identification of cross flow from the asymptomatic hemisphere to the symptomatic hemisphere flow via the anterior communicating artery or from the posterior circulation to the anterior circulation via the posterior communicating artery (Davies and Jezzard, 2003; Hendrikse *et al.*, 2004; Taoka *et al.*, 2004; Werner *et al.*, 2005a). The first selective ASL methods were based on the use of a local surface coil with selective labeling of the ICA reached by the small penetration depth of this coil (Zaharchuk *et al.*, 1999; Trampel *et al.*, 2002). A more recent selective ASL approach is based on angulation of the labeling slab to reach selectivity for either a single ICA or the vertebrobasilar arteries (VBA) (Hendrikse *et al.*, 2004). An example of selective arterial label planning is shown in Figure 26.3. Planning of these labeling slabs is based on anatomical MRA studies of the brain vasculature. Recently, a CASL method for selective labeling of the anterior cerebral artery (ACA), middle cerebral artery (MCA) and posterior cerebral artery (PCA) has been introduced based on a rotating labeling frame

(Werner *et al.*, 2005a). Selective ASL perfusion territory measurements also offer the possibility to investigate the interindividual variability in flow territories in vivo, which were previously only visualized in postmortem studies (Van der Zwan *et al.*, 1992). Such information is essential in the diagnosis of presumed border-zone or watershed infarcts. Recently, Van Laar and coworkers have confirmed these postmortem findings in a large in vivo study using selective ASL, showing that the anatomy of the circle of Willis is an important confounder (Van Laar *et al.*, 2005). In patients with cerebrovascular disease selective ASL can demonstrate a decrease in perfusion territory with presence of steno-occlusive disease and increase in perfusion territory with presence of compensatory collateral flow. In addition to flow territory measurements the regional CBF contribution of each individual artery can be obtained. Figure 26.4 shows the changes in flow territories in a symptomatic patient with a right-sided severe stenosis, showing a significantly increased flow territory of the contralateral ICA caused by cross flow via the anterior communicating artery.

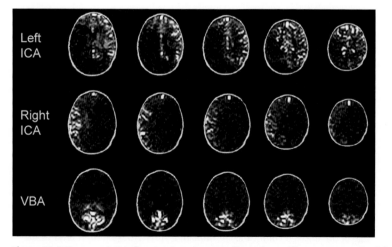

Figure 26.4 Representative flow territory images of a patient with a symptomatic right-sided internal carotid artery (ICA) stenosis of 90%, resulting from selective labeling of the stenosed ICA, contralateral ICA and vertebrobasilar arteries (VBA). Image courtesy of Dr. P.J. van Laar, University Medical Center Utrecht, the Netherlands.

Bolus tracking or dynamic susceptibility contrast MRI (DSC-MRI)

Bolus tracking or DSC-MRI is based on an intravenous injection of contrast agent and the monitoring of the first passage of this contrast agent through brain tissue and a brain-feeding artery (Figure 26.5) (Rempp *et al.*, 1995; Ostergaard *et al.*, 1996a,b). The contrast agent is rapidly injected into a vein of the patient's arm and is followed by a saline chaser to flush the contrast agent from the line. During and after injection of contrast agent, fast gradient or spin echo imaging measures the MR signal at a temporal resolution of approximately 1−2 s. Because the contrast agent consists of paramagnetic ions, the presence of contrast agent leads to local magnetic field inhomogeneities and thus to dephasing and loss of MR signal (Boxerman *et al.*, 1995). This loss in MR signal can be used to measure the concentration of the contrast agent. Selection of voxels located in or nearby a brain-feeding artery yields the arterial input function (AIF). This AIF represents the shape of the bolus of contrast agent when it enters the brain. Subsequently, for each voxel in the brain the measured passage of contrast agent through the brain tissue is deconvolved with the AIF, yielding the hemodynamic response function. From this response function, the CBF, CBV and the mean transit time (MTT) can be calculated (Zierler, 1962). The result of a DSC-MRI scan of a symptomatic patient with a severe stenosis is shown in Figure 26.6. Obtaining absolute quantitative values of the perfusion by means of DSC-MRI is cumbersome. Factors that influence accurate quantification include:

1. Dispersion of the input function. DSC-MRI assumes that the measured AIF equals the input function of the microvasculature. However, the AIF is measured in a large brain-feeding artery and the transport of the contrast agent from this location to the microvasculature

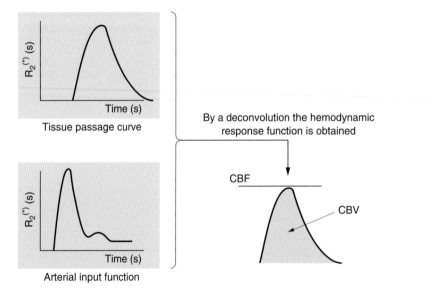

Figure 26.5 Schematic overview of the analysis of dynamic susceptibility contrast magnetic resonance imaging. Two curves are measured, the first passage of the injected contrast agent through a voxel or region-of-interest in the brain parenchyma and the first passage through a brain-feeding artery. Deconvolution of these two curves yields the hemodynamic response function. The maximum of this function equals the cerebral blood flow; the area under the curve is the cerebral blood volume.

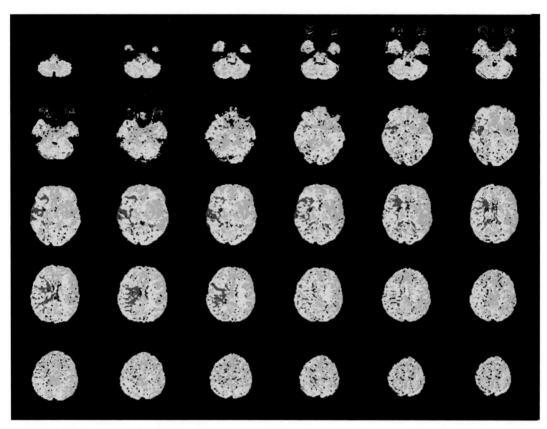

Figure 26.6 Whole brain cerebral blood flow (CBF) map of a patient with a severe stenosis of the right internal carotid artery (ICA), showing decreased CBF in the symptomatic hemisphere.

can easily lead to dispersion of the AIF. This is especially true in patients who suffer from large vessel pathology (Calamante *et al.*, 2003). Dispersion of the AIF between the AIF measurement and the microvasculature leads to an underestimation of the CBF (Calamante *et al.*, 2000).

2. Limited validation of contrast agent properties in brain tissue. Several theoretical studies have shown that the assumed linear relation between the transverse relaxation rate and the concentration of contrast agent is probably a simplification (Boxerman *et al.*, 1995; Kiselev *et al.*, 2001). However, good practical verification is still absent.

3. Partial volume effects on the input function. Since the spatial resolution of DSC-MRI is still limited, it is hard to identify voxels that are exclusively sensitive to arterial blood. For gradient echo imaging, such partial volume effects do not only affect the amplitude of the AIF, but also the shape (Osch *et al.*, 2001).

4. Poor temporal resolution. To achieve accurate CBF measurements a high temporal resolution (higher than 1.5 s) is essential (Van Osch *et al.*, 2003; Knutsson *et al.*, 2004).

5. Choice of deconvolution method. Deconvolution of noisy curves can easily result in errors and especially determining the maximum value of the response function

requires advanced algorithms. Although the first deconvolution algorithm showed good stability for noisy curves and was insensitive to the shape of the underlying response function, it resulted in erroneous results when the AIF and the tissue passage curve were delayed with respect to each other (Calamante et al., 2000; Wu et al., 2003). New deconvolution methods are less sensitive to delays (Vonken et al., 1999; Wu et al., 2003; Smith et al., 2004).

6. Postprocessing. When calculating perfusion values for regions-of-interest (ROI), two approaches can be used. First, one can calculate the perfusion values pixel-wise and average the perfusion values over the ROI. This involves deconvolution of very noisy curves that can affect the accuracy. Second, one can calculate the averaged passage over the ROI and deconvolve the averaged curve with the AIF. Although this last approach leads to less noisy curves and therefore a more accurate deconvolution, arrival time differences over the ROI can lead to erroneous broadening of the passage curve, leading to underestimation of the CBF.

The last five aspects are general to bolus-tracking MRI and several studies, that have shown good correlations between bolus-tracking MRI and perfusion imaging by PET or ASL (Li et al., 2000; Sakoh et al., 2000; Wirestam et al., 2000; Lin et al., 2001), indicate their influence can either be controlled for or considered to be small. However, the first factor is especially important in patients with stenosed or occluded arteries. In principle only a single AIF is used in bolus-tracking MRI, whereas in these patients it is questionable whether the input function for each flow territory only differs in timing but also in shape. One study that compared patients with an occlusion of the ICA with control subjects did not show altered CBF ipsilateral from the occlusion. This implies that no additional dispersion of the AIF occurred before the contrast agent entered the microvasculature. However, another study including patients with stenosed or occluded ICAs did show a lower CBF (Lythgoe et al., 2000). This different behavior can be explained by the fact that primary collaterals show little additional dispersion, whereas stenosed arteries could show significant dispersion (Calamante et al., 2003), or it could be explained by the use of a deconvolution technique that was sensitive to delays (in contrast to the first study). Finally, one study compared DSC-MRI with PET in patients with unilateral occlusion of the internal carotid artery (Lin et al., 2001). After correction of the AIF for partial volume effects, they showed reasonable agreement between both techniques.

Recently, it was proposed to measure the input function at the tissue level (Alsop et al., 2002; Calamante et al., 2004), i.e. an AIF is sought for each voxel in the brain tissue. This approach has the major advantage that the input function is measured much closer to the microvasculature, thereby eliminating dispersion errors. Furthermore, this approach ensures that each flow territory uses its own input function. However, due to partial volume effects it is doubtful whether such local AIF measurements yield the correct shape and amplitude of the input function (Van Osch et al., 2005). Therefore, more research should be performed on this subject before it is applied in clinical practice.

CT perfusion imaging

With the introduction of helical multislice CT scanners the development of CT perfusion (CTP) imaging has gained renewed attention. Perfusion CT is based on the same principle as bolus-tracking MRI: the technique involves the administration of a single-bolus dose of (iodinated) contrast material, followed by spiral CT imaging during the passage of the contrast bolus through the brain-feeding arteries and brain tissue (Axel, 1980). Quantitative maps of MTT, CBF and CBV are obtained. A limiting factor in the application of CTP is the speed of helical machines, which should at least be capable of imaging faster than one slice/s to sample the entire contrast passage with sufficient

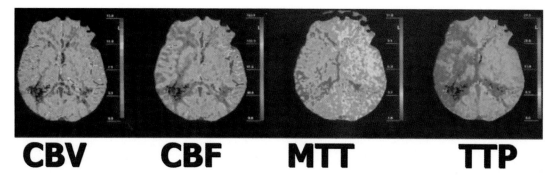

Figure 26.7 Example of computerized tomography perfusion in a patient with a right occluded internal carotid artery. The right middle cerebral artery (MCA) territory shows late arrival of contrast agent, prolonged mean transit time (MTT), and lowered cerebral blood flow (CBF). Also shown is the time-to-peak (TTP) image. Images courtesy of Dr. A. Waaijer, University Medical Center Utrecht, the Netherlands.

time resolution. A clear advantage of CTP over DSC-MRI is that the change in CTP signal intensity during the contrast bolus passage has a linear relationship with the signal intensity in Hounsfield units and is, therefore, quantitative and independent of, e.g. the radius of the vessel or the exact layout of the microvasculature. Corresponding to the quantitation techniques used in DSC-MRI, contrast time-concentration curves are obtained from an arterial region of interest, to provide the AIF. To correct for partial volume effects, the measured AIF is scaled with respect to the area under the curve of the venous output function as measured in a large vein, like the superior sagittal venous sinus. The corrected AIF is used to deconvolve the passage through a parenchymal pixel, resulting in the impulse function. From this impulse function the MTT can be calculated, whereas the CBV can be calculated from the area under the curve of the parenchymal passage and the corrected AIF (Nabavi *et al.*, 1999; Wintermark *et al.*, 2001). CBF can be subsequently calculated from the central volume principle ($CBF = CBV/MTT$) (Zierler, 1962). Similar to the problems in DSC-MRI, CTP has problems in differentiating between effects due to dispersion of the contrast bolus before entering the microvasculature and changes in the rate of blood flow. Furthermore, ambiguity is present in the choice of the

AIF: without knowledge of the flow territories, most studies employ a single AIF for all parenchymal tissue. In patients with severe carotid disease this might give rise to large errors, since the true input function can vary considerably between the different flow territories. However, perfusion CT is useful to evaluate the hemodynamic state of patients with chronic major cerebral artery occlusive disorders (Miyazawa *et al.*, 2005). Figure 26.7 shows CTP images in a symptomatic patient with a right occluded ICA. It is to be expected that due to the increasing availability of 32, 64 and more slice CT scanners, the application of CTP may even become greater than MRI perfusion. The use of contrast agents in CT is no major disadvantage since in most subjects CT contrast is delivered anyway. However, reduction of radiation dose will remain important for a more widespread use of CTP (Hirata *et al.*, 2005).

REFERENCES

Alsop, D. C. and Detre, J. A. (1996). Reduced transit-time sensitivity in noninvasive magnetic resonance imaging of human cerebral blood flow. *Journal of Cerebral Blood Flow Metabolism*, **16**, 1236–49.

Alsop, D. C. and Detre, J. A. (1998). Multisection cerebral blood flow MR imaging with continuous arterial spin labeling. *Radiology*, **208**, 410–16.

Alsop, D. C., Wedmid, A. and Schlaug, G. (2002). Defining a local input function for perfusion quantification with bolus contrast MRI. 659. *Proceedings of the ISMRM 10th annual meeting, Hawaii.*

Axel, L. (1980). Cerebral blood flow determination by rapid sequence computed tomography. *Radiology*, **137**, 679–86.

Barbier, E. L., Lamalle, L. and Decorps, M. (2001). Methodology of brain perfusion imaging. *Journal of Magnetic Resonance Imaging*, **13**, 496–520.

Barnett, H. J. M., Gunton, R. W., Eliasziw, M, *et al.* (2000). Causes and severity of ischemic stroke in patients with internal carotid artery stenosis. *Journal of the American Medical Association*, **283**, 1429–36.

Baumgartner, R. W., Baumgartner, I., Mattle, H. P. and Schroth, G. (1997). Transcranial color-coded duplex sonography in the evaluation of collateral flow through the circle of Willis. *AJNR. American Journal of Neuroradiology*, **18**, 127–33.

Blankensteijn, J. D., Van der Grond, J., Mali, W. P. T. M., and Eikelboom, B. C. (1997). Flow volume changes in the major cerebral arteries before and after carotid endarterectomy: an MR angiography study. *European Journal of Vascular and Endovascular Surgery*, **14**, 446–50.

Boxerman, J. L., Hamberg, L. M., Rosen, B. R. and Weisskoff, R. M. (1995). MR contrast due to intravascular magnetic susceptibility perturbations. *Magnetic Resonance in Medicine*, **34**, 555–66.

Boysen, G., Ladergaard-Pedersen, H. J., Valentin, N. and Engell, H. C. (1970). Cerebral blood flow and internal carotid artery flow during carotid surgery. *Stroke*, **1**, 253–60.

Buxton, R. B., Frank, L. R., Wong, E. C., *et al.* (1998). A general kinetic model for quantitative perfusion imaging with arterial spin labeling. *Magnetic Resonance in Medicine*, **40**, 383–96.

Calamante, F., Gadian, D. G. and Connelly, A. (2000). Delay and dispersion effects in dynamic susceptibility contrast MRI: simulations using singular value decomposition. *Magnetic Resonance in Medicine*, **44**, 466–73.

Calamante, F., Morup, M. and Hansen, L. K. (2004). Defining a local arterial input function for perfusion MRI using independent component analysis. *Magnetic Resonance in Medicine*, **52**, 789–97.

Calamante, F., Thomas, D. L., Pell, G. S., Wiersma, J. and Turner, R. (1999). Measuring cerebral blood flow using magnetic resonance imaging techniques. *Journal of Cerebral Blood Flow Metabolsim*, **19**, 701–35.

Calamante, F., Yim, P. J. and Cebral, J. R. (2003). Estimation of bolus dispersion effects in perfusion MRI using image-based computational fluid dynamics. *Neuroimage*, **19**, 341–53.

Caplan, L. R. and Hennerici, M. (1998). Impaired clearance of emboli (washout) is an important link between hypoperfusion, embolism, and ischemic stroke. *Archives of Neurology*, **55**, 1475–82.

Davies, N. P. and Jezzard, P. (2003). Selective arterial spin labeling (SASL): Perfusion territory mapping of selected feeding arteries tagged using two-dimensional radiofrequency pulses. *Magnetic Resonance in Medicine*, **49**, 1133–42.

Derdeyn, C. P., Grubb, R. L. J. and Powers, W. J. (1999). Cerebral hemodynamic impairment: methods of measurement and association with stroke risk. *Neurology*, **53**, 251–9.

Detre, J. A., Alsop, D. C., Vives, L. R., *et al.* (1998). Noninvasive MRI evaluation of cerebral blood flow in cerebrovascular disease. *Neurology*, **50**, 633–41.

European Carotid Surgery Trialists' Collaborative Group. (1991). MRC European Carotid Surgery Trial: interim results for symptomatic patients with severe (70–99%) or with mild (0–29%) carotid stenosis. *Lancet*, **337**, 1235–43.

Figueiredo, P. M., Clare, S. and Jezzard, P. (2005). Quantitative perfusion measurements using pulsed arterial spin labeling: effects of large region-of-interest analysis. *Journal of Magnetic Resonance Imaging*, **21**, 676–82.

Golay, X., Hendrikse, J. and Lim, T. C. (2004). Perfusion imaging using arterial spin labeling. *Topics in Magnetic Resonance Imaging*, **15**, 10–27.

Gordon, I. L, Stemmer, E. A. and Wilson, S. E. (1995). Redistribution of blood flow after carotid endarterectomy. *Journal of Vascular Surgery*, **22**, 349–58.

Grubb, R. L., Jr., Derdeyn, C. P., Fritsch, S. M., *et al.* (1998). Importance of hemodynamic factors in the prognosis of symptomatic carotid occlusion. *Journal of the American Medical Association*, **280**, 1055–60.

Gunther, M., Bock, M. and Schad, L. R. (2001). Arterial spin labeling in combination with a look-locker sampling strategy: inflow turbo-sampling EPI-FAIR (ITS-FAIR). *Magnetic Resonance in Medicine*, **46**, 974–84.

Hartl, W. H., Janssen, I. and Fürst, H. (1994). Effect of carotid endarterectomy on patterns of cerebrovascular reactivity in patients with unilateral carotid artery stenosis. *Stroke*, **25**, 1952–7.

Henderson, R. D., Eliasziw, M., Fox, A. J., Rothwell, P. M. and Barnett, H. J. M. (2000). Angiographically defined collateral circulation and risk of stroke in patients with severe carotid artery stenosis. *Stroke*, **31**, 128–32.

Hendrikse, J., Lu, H., van der Grond, J., Van Zijl, P. C. and Golay, X. (2003). Measurements of cerebral perfusion and arterial hemodynamics during visual stimulation using TURBO-TILT. *Magnetic Resonance in Medicine*, **50**, 429–33.

Hendrikse, J., Eikelboom, B. C. and Van der Grond, J. (2002). Magnetic resonance angiography of collateral compensation in asymptomatic and symptomatic internal carotid artery stenosis. *Journal of Vascular Surgery*, **36**, 799–805.

Hendrikse, J., van der Grond, J., Lu, H., van Zijl, P. C. and Golay, X. (2004). Flow territory mapping of the cerebral arteries with regional perfusion MRI. *Stroke*, **35**, 882–7.

Hirata, M., Murase, K., Sugawara, Y., Nanjo, T. and Mochizuki, T. (2005). A method for reducing radiation dose in cerebral CT perfusion study with variable scan schedule. *Radiation Medicine*, **23**, 162–9.

Kiselev, V. G. (2001). On the theoretical basis of perfusion measurements by dynamic susceptibility contrast MRI. *Magnetic Resonance in Medicine*, **46**, 1113–22.

Klijn, C. J. M., Kappelle, L. J., Tulleken, C. A. F. and van Gijn, J. (1997). Symptomatic carotid artery occlusion. A reappraisal of hemodynamic factors. *Stroke*, **28**, 2084–93.

Kluytmans, M., Van der Grond, J., Eikelboom, B. C. and Viergever, M. A. (1998). Long-term hemodynamic effects of carotid endarterectomy. *Stroke*, **29**, 1567–72.

Knutsson, L., Stahlberg, F. and Wirestam, R. (2004). Aspects on the accuracy of cerebral perfusion parameters obtained by dynamic susceptibility contrast MRI: a simulation study. *Magnetic Resonance Imaging*, **22**, 789–98.

Ko, N. U., Achrol, A. S., Chopra, M., *et al.* (2005). Cerebral blood flow changes after endovascular treatment of cerebrovascular stenoses. *AJNR. American Journal of Neuroradiology*, **26**, 538–42.

Kwong, K. K., Chesler, D. A., Weisskoff, R. M., *et al.* (1995). MR perfusion studies with T1-weighted echo planar imaging. *Magnetic Resonance in Medicine*, **34**, 878–87.

Li, T. Q., Guang, C. Z., Ostergaard, L., Hindmarsh, T. and Moseley, M. E. (2000). Quantification of cerebral blood flow by bolus tracking and artery spin tagging methods. *Magnetic Resonance Imaging*, **18**, 503–12.

Liebeskind, D S. (2003). Collateral circulation. *Stroke*, **34**, 2279–84.

Lin, W., Celik, A., Derdeyn, C., *et al.* (2001). Quantitative measurements of cerebral blood flow in patients with unilateral carotid artery occlusion: a PET and MR study. *Journal of Magnetic Resonance Imaging*, **14**, 659–67.

Lythgoe, D. J., Ostergaard, L., William, S. C., *et al.* (2000). Quantitative perfusion imaging in carotid artery stenosis using dynamic susceptibility contrast-enhanced magnetic resonance imaging. *Magnetic Resonance Imaging*, **18**, 1–11.

Markus, H. S, Clifton, A., Buckenham, T., Taylor, R. and Brown, M. M. (1996). Improvement in cerebral hemodynamics after carotid angioplasty. *Stroke*, **27**, 612–16.

Markus, H. and Cullinane, M. (2001). Severely impaired cerebrovascular reactivity predicts stroke and TIA risk in patients with carotid artery stenosis and occlusion. *Brain*, **124**(Pt. 3), 457–67.

Miyazawa, N., Arbab, A., Umeda, T. and Akiyama, I. (2005). Perfusion CT investigation of chronic internal carotid artery occlusion: comparison with SPECT. *Clinical Neurology and Neurosurgery*, **108**, 11–17.

Mount, L. A. and Taveras, J. M. (1957). Arteriographic demonstration of the collateral circulation of the cerebral hemispheres. *AMA. Archives of Neurology and Psychiatry*, **78**, 235–53.

Muller, M., Hermes, M., Bruckmann, H. and Schimrigk, K. (1995). Transcranial Doppler ultrasound in the evaluation of collateral blood flow in patients with internal carotid artery occlusion: correlation with cerebral angiography. *AJNR. American Journal of Neuroradiology*, **16**, 195–202.

Nabavi, D. G., Cenic, A., Craen, R. A., *et al.* (1999). CT assessment of cerebral perfusion: experimental validation and initial clinical experience. *Radiology*, **213**, 141–9.

NASCET North American Symptomatic Carotid Endarterectomy Trial Steering Committee. (1991). North American Symptomatic Carotid Endarterectomy Trial. Methods, patient characteristics, and progress. *Stroke*, **22**, 711–20.

Niesen, W. D., Rosenkranz, M., Eckert, B., *et al.* (2004). Hemodynamic changes of the cerebral circulation after stent-protected carotid angioplasty. *AJNR. American Journal of Neuroradiology*, **25**, 1162–7.

Nighoghossian, N., Trouillas, P., Philippon, B., Itti, R. and Adeleine, P. (1994). Cerebral blood flow reserve assessment in symptomatic versus asymptomatic high-grade internal carotid artery stenosis. *Stroke*, **25**, 1010–13.

Norris, J. W., Krajewski, A. and Bornstein, N. M. (1990). The clinical role of the cerebral collateral circulation in carotid occlusion. *Journal of Vascular Surgery*, **12**, 113–18.

Ogasawara, K., Yukawa, H., Kobayashi, M., *et al.* (2003). Prediction and monitoring of cerebral hyperperfusion after carotid endarterectomy by using single-photon emission computerized tomography scanning. *Journal of Neurosurgery*, **99**, 504–10.

Osch, M. J. P., Vonken, E. J., Bakker, C. J. G. and Viergever, M. A. (2001). Correcting partial volume artifacts of the arterial input function in quantitative cerebral perfusion MRI. *Magnetic Resonance in Medicine*, **45**, 477–85.

Ostergaard, L., Sorensen, A. G., Kwong, K. K., *et al.* (1996a). High resolution measurement of cerebral blood flow using intravascular tracer bolus passages. Part II: Experimental comparison and preliminary results. *Magnetic Resonace in Medicine*, **36**, 726–36.

Ostergaard, L., Weisskoff, R. M., Chesler, D. A., Gyldensted, C. and Rosen, B. R. (1996b). High resolution measurement of cerebral blood flow using intravascular tracer bolus passages. Part I: Mathematical approach and statistical analysis. *Magnetic Resonance in Medicine*, **36**, 715–25.

Powers, W. J. (1991). Cerebral hemodynamics in ischemic cerebrovascular disease. *Annals of Neurology*, **29**, 231–40.

Powers, W. J., Press, G. A. and Grubb, R. L., Jr. (1987). The effect of hemodynamically significant carotid artery disease on the hemodynamic status of the cerebral circulation. *Annals of Internal Medicine*, **106**, 27–35.

Rempp, K. A., Brix, G., Wenz, F., *et al.* (1994). Quantification of regional cerebral bloodflow and volume with dynamic susceptibility contrast-enhanced MR imaging. *Radiology*, **193**, 637–41.

Sakoh, M., Rohl, L., Gyldensted, C., Gjedde, A. and Ostergaard, L. (2000). Cerebral blood flow and blood volume measured by magnetic resonance imaging bolus tracking after acute stroke in pigs. Comparison with 15O H2O positron emission tomography. *Stroke*, **31**, 1958–64.

Schomer, D. F., Marks, M. P., Steinberg, G. K., *et al.* (1994). The anatomy of the posterior communicating artery as a risk factor for ischemic cerebral infarction. *New England Journal of Medicine*, **330**, 1565–70.

Schroeder, T., Sillesen, H., Sorensen, O. and Engell, H. C. (1987). Cerebral hyperperfusion following carotid endarterectomy. *Journal of Neurosurgery*, **66**, 824–9.

Silvestrini, M., Troisi, E., Matteis, M., Cupini, L. M. and Caltagirone, C. (1996). Transcranial Doppler assessment of cerebrovascular reactivity in symptomatic and asymptomatic severe carotid stenosis. *Stroke*, **27**, 1970–3.

Smith, M. R., Lu, H., Trochet, S. and Frayne, R. (2004). Removing the effect of SVD algorithmic artifacts present in quantitative MR perfusion studies. *Magnetic Resonance in Medicine*, **51**, 631–4.

Taoka, T., Iwasaki, S., Nakagawa, H., *et al.* (2004). Distinguishing between anterior cerebral artery and middle cerebral artery perfusion by color-coded perfusion direction mapping with arterial spin labeling. *AJNR. American Journal of Neuroradiology*, **25**, 248–51.

Thomas, D. L., Lythgoe, M. F., Pell, G. S., Calamante, F. and Ordidge, R. J. (2000). The measurement of diffusion and perfusion in biological systems using magnetic resonance imaging. *Physics in Medicine and Biology*, **45**, R97–138.

Trampel, R., Mildner, T., Goerke, U., *et al.* (2002). Continuous arterial spin labeling using a local magnetic field gradient coil. *Magnetic Resonance in Medicine*, **48**, 543–6.

Van der Zwan, A., Hillen, B., Tulleken, C. A. F., *et al.* (1992). Variability of the territories of the major cerebral arteries. *Journal of Neurosurgery*, **77**, 927–40.

Van Laar, P. J., Hendrikse, J. and Golay, X., *et al.* (2005). In vivo flow territory mapping of major brain feeding arteries. *Neuroimage*, **29**, 136–44.

van Osch, M. J., van der Grond, J. and Bakker, C. J. (2005). Partial volume effects on arterial input functions: Shape and amplitude distortions and their correction. *Journal of Magnetic Resonance Imaging*, **22**, 704–9.

van Osch, M. J., Vonken, E. J., Wu, O., *et al.* (2003). Model of the human vasculature for studying the influence of contrast injection speed on cerebral perfusion MRI. *Magnetic Resonance in Medicine*, **50**, 614–22.

Vanninen, R., Koivisto, K., Tulla, H., Manninen, H. and Partanen, K. (1995). Hemodynamic effects of carotid endarterectomy by magnetic resonance flow quantification. *Stroke*, **26**, 84–9.

Vonken, E. P. A., Beekman, F. J., Bakker, C. J. G. and Viergever, M. A. (1999). Maximum likelihood estimation of cerebral blood flow in dynamic susceptibility contrast MRI. *Magnetic Resonance in Medicine*, **41**, 343–50.

Werner, R., Norris, D. G., Alfke, K., Mehdorn, H. M. and Jansen, O. (2005a). Continuous artery-selective spin labeling (CASSL). *Magnetic Resonance in Medicine*, **53**, 1006–12.

Werner, R., Norris, D. G., Alfke, K., Mehdorn, H. M. and Jansen, O. (2005b). Improving the amplitude-modulated control experiment for multislice continuous arterial spin labeling. *Magnetic Resonance in Medicine*, **53**, 1096–102.

Wiart, M., Berthezène, Y., Adeleine, P., *et al.* (2000). Vasodilatory response of border zones to acetazolamide before and after endarterectomy. An echo planar imaging-dynamic susceptibility contrast-enhanced MRI study in patients with high-grade unilateral internal carotid artery stenosis. *Stroke*, **31**, 1561–5.

Wintermark, M., Maeder, P., Thiran, J. P., Schnyder, P. and Meuli, R. (2001). Quantitative assessment of regional cerebral blood flows by perfusion CT studies at low injection rates: a critical review of the underlying theoretical models. *European Radiology*, **11**, 1220–30.

Wirestam, R., Ryding, E., Lindgren, A., *et al.* (2000). Absolute cerebral blood flow measured by dynamic susceptibility contrast MRI: a direct comparison with Xe-133 SPECT. *Magma*, **11**, 96–103.

Wu, O., Ostergaard, L., Koroshetz, W. J., *et al.* (2003). Effects of tracer arrival time on flow estimates in MR perfusion-weighted imaging. *Magnetic Resonance in Medicine*, **50**, 856–64.

Wu, O., Ostergaard, L., Weisskoff, R. M., *et al.* (2003). Tracer arrival timing-insensitive technique for estimating flow in MR perfusion-weighted imaging using singular value decomposition with a block-circulant deconvolution matrix. *Magnetic Resonance in Medicine*, **50**, 164–74.

Wong, E. C., Buxton, R. B. and Frank, L. R. (1998). Quantitative imaging of perfusion using a single subtraction (QUIPSS and QUIPSS II). *Magnetic Resonance in Medicine*, **39**, 702–8.

Zaharchuk, G., Ledden, P. J., Kwong, K. K., *et al.* (1999). Multislice perfusion and perfusion territory imaging in humans with separate label and image coils. *Magnetic Resonance in Medicine*, **41**, 1093–8.

Zierler, K. L. (1962). Theoretical basis of indicator-dilution methods for measuring flow and volume. *Circulation Research*, **10**, 393–407.

27

Near infrared spectroscopy in carotid endarterectomy

Pippa G. Al-Rawi and Peter J. Kirkpatrick

Addenbrooke's Hospital, Cambridge, UK

Introduction

The use of in vivo tissue near infrared spectroscopy (NIRS) in humans was first described more than 25 years ago by F.F. Jöbsis (Jöbsis, 1977). The technique is based on the concept that light of wavelengths 680–1000 nm is able to penetrate human tissue and is absorbed by the chromophores oxyhemoglobin (HbO$_2$), deoxyhemoglobin (Hb) and cytochrome oxidase. Changes in the detected light levels can therefore represent changes in concentrations of these chromophores. The noninvasive nature of the technique led to its first clinical application for monitoring the cerebral oxygenation status of premature infants (Brazy et al., 1985). Since then it has become an established research tool with numerous applications (Ferrari et al., 1986; Brown et al., 1993; Aldrich et al., 1994; Villringer et al., 1994; Lam et al., 1996; Elwell et al., 1997; Tamura et al., 1997; Nollert et al., 2000; Watanabe et al., 2002; Vernieri et al., 2004).

Whilst its clinical use for monitoring the brain has been well established in neonates, where transillumination is possible due to the thin skull and small dimensions, clinical application of NIRS for monitoring the adult brain has been hampered by the fact that it must be applied in reflectance mode (Young et al., 2000). This has resulted in concerns about quantification, the volume and type of tissue being illuminated, and most

significantly the issue of signal contamination by the extracranial tissue layers (Harris et al., 1994; Germon et al., 1995; Schwarz et al., 1996; Litscher and Schwarz, 1997; Kirkpatrick et al., 1998a; Germon et al., 1999; Kytta et al., 1999). A number of algorithms have been applied to try to overcome these issues, and techniques such as time resolved, phase resolved and spatially resolved spectroscopy have been developed (Miwa et al., 1995; Oda et al., 1996; Delpy and Cope, 1997; Al-Rawi et al., 2001).

To be clinically useful, NIRS devices should not only reliably detect changes in cerebral oxygenation but must also be insensitive to concentration changes occurring in the extracerebral tissues. Recent technical advances have led to the development of instruments that detect changes in optical attenuation of several wavelengths of light, with the potential to derive a tissue oxygen saturation from spontaneous Hb and HbO$_2$ signal changes (Hazeki and Tamura, 1988; Fantini et al., 1995; Al-Rawi et al., 2001).

The use of NIRS to evaluate cerebral oxygenation changes has been reported in a variety of medical and neurosurgical conditions, including those associated with disturbed cerebral circulation (du Plessis et al., 1995; Kurth et al., 1995; Liem et al., 1995; Kirkpatrick et al., 1995a; Al-Rawi et al., 1999). Despite initial enthusiasm for the technique, there remain many practical as well as theoretical limitations to overcome. It is important

Carotid Disease: The Role of Imaging in Diagnosis and Management, ed. Jonathan Gillard, Martin Graves, Thomas Hatsukami and Chun Yuan. Published by Cambridge University Press. © Cambridge University Press 2007.

to understand both the assumptions on which NIRS is based and the limitations of this technology in order to interpret the results correctly.

In this chapter we will look at the application of NIRS during carotid endarterectomy. We will demonstrate our own use of this technique in combination with other monitoring modalities.

Principles

The theory behind NIRS is described in detail elsewhere (Cope and Delpy, 1988; Piantadosi, 1989; Wyatt et al., 1990). The basic principle is that near infrared light (delivered via optodes placed on the skin) penetrates the scalp and brain tissue and is subjected to scatter and absorption within the various tissues. Whilst some of these media can be considered to have a fixed concentration (e.g. bone, melanin, bilirubin, lipids, water), and hence fixed scattering and absorption, the concentration of Hb and HbO_2 may vary with time or with oxygenation status. Cytochrome oxidase, the terminal enzyme of the respiratory chain, also contributes to the near infrared spectrum of cortical tissue (Wray et al., 1988).

Assuming constant scattering properties and applying knowledge of the absorption spectra for oxy- and deoxyhemoglobin, measurements of light attenuation are converted into concentrations of these chromophores using a modified Beer-Lambert law, which includes a differential path-length factor to account for scattering within the tissue, and can be defined as:

$$\Delta A = L \bullet \Delta \mu a$$

where,
A = light attenuation
L = differential pathlength, and
μa = absorption scattering coefficient

This concept works very well in the infant head where the skull is thin enough to allow trans-illumination of light from one side to the other. In the adult, the relative thickness of scalp, skull and brain prevents transmission spectroscopy

and NIRS must be used in reflectance mode, with the optodes situated on the same side of the head. Reflectance mode oximetry is dependent upon a proportion of the light reflected having passed through cerebral tissue. The human head is comprised of multiple tissue layers, all of which have varying scattering properties and contain concentrations of light-absorbing compounds, which may change independently (Dehghani and Delpy, 2000). This results in the introduction of unknown, nonlinear variables for light absorption and scattering coefficients (Okada et al., 1997). Various algorithms have been applied in attempts at quantification, but claims as to their accuracy remain controversial (Harris and Bailey, 1993; Schwarz et al., 1996; Litscher and Schwarz, 1997; Kytta et al., 1999; Komiyama et al., 2001).

Extracranial contamination

Although it has been demonstrated that transcranial NIRS is sensitive to oxygenation changes in cerebral tissues (Germon et al., 1994), most spectrometers are sensitive to changes in extracerebral oxygenation which can profoundly influence estimates of cerebral oxygenation (Germon et al., 1995). Studies have demonstrated that despite using large optode distances there is still a major contribution from the extracranial tissues to the NIRS signal (Germon et al., 1999). Conditions in which changes in extracerebral oxygenation may seem unlikely should not therefore be taken for granted. Significant changes in extracerebral oxygenation in the scalp have been detected during the performance of functional activation tasks. Even in the absence of extracerebral oxygenation changes the extracerebral tissues may confound attempts at calibration and quantification of changes in cerebral oxygenation. Mathematical in vitro modelling has attempted to predict the distribution of light through the extracerebral layers (Hiraoka et al., 1993). Multilayer studies have highlighted the influence that superficial tissue layers can have on light distribution in tissues and provide further evidence for the underestimation of transcranial measurements of changes in concentration. Additionally, mathematical simulations using Monte Carlo techniques have indicated that the clear cerebrospinal fluid layer surrounding the brain can act as an optical short-cut for light as it passes through the tissues resulting in the near infrared light completely bypassing the cerebral compartment (Firbank *et al.*, 1995; Okada *et al.*, 1995). In any NIRS study, it is essential to consider whether the changes detected could be due, even in part, to extracerebral contamination. Either extracerebral changes must be shown to be insignificant or their effect eliminated. Developed algorithms need correction factors applying not only for the confounding effect of extracranial signals but also concerning the effects of hemodilution, temperature, underlying CSF layers, and blood pressure.

Instrumentation

NIRS instrumentation has continued to evolve. Early machines were large and cumbersome, showed considerable drift and were prone to both movement and light artefacts. In reality they were really only useful as trend monitors. Evaluation of the technology culminated in the mid-nineties with numerous publications assessing several devices in different clinical scenarios. Current commercial machines detect changes in optical attenuation of a number of wavelengths of light, are compact, portable and enable noninvasive measurements of cerebral oxygenation at the bedside (McKeating *et al.*, 1997; Al-Rawi *et al.*, 2001; Yoshitani *et al.*, 2002; Dullenkopf *et al.*, 2003). However, it should be recognized that values obtained from different instruments are likely to give different cerebral tissue oxygen saturations because the data are being derived from different volumes of tissue (Delpy and Cope, 1997). Of the current techniques on offer, spatially resolved spectroscopy appears to be the most promising.

Spatially resolved spectroscopy

Spatially resolved spectroscopy has been described in a number of publications (Matcher *et al.*, 1993; Al-Rawi *et al.*, 2001). Spatial resolution relies upon the measurement of the attenuation gradient as a function of source-detector separation. Using a modified diffusion equation, a product of the absorption and scattering coefficients is calculated (Suzuki *et al.*, 1999). Treating the tissue as homogeneous, the scattering coefficient can be assumed to be a constant (k) in the near infrared wavelength. In order to increase the accuracy of the calculation however, a wavelength dependency for the scattering coefficient is derived in the form of:

$$k(1 - h\lambda)$$

where, λ = wavelength and h is the normalized slope of the scattering coefficient along λ (Matcher *et al.*, 1993). From here, the relative absorption coefficients and thus the relative concentrations of HbO_2 and Hb can be obtained.

NIRO 300

The NIRO 300 (Hamamatsu Photonics K.K., Hamamatsu City, Japan) is a noninvasive bedside monitor which gives simultaneous measurement of tissue oxygen index (TOI) and hemoglobin concentration changes (Suzuki *et al.*, 1999; Al-Rawi *et al.*, 2001).

The instrument is based on technology employed in the earlier NIRO 500 and a prototype spatially resolved spectrometer (Al-Rawi *et al.*, 1999). Four wavelengths of light (775, 810, 850, and 910 nm, respectively) are delivered by four pulsed laser diodes and scattered light is detected by three closely placed photodiodes (Figure 27.1). The concentration changes of the chromophores oxyhemoglobin (HbO_2), deoxyhemoglobin (Hb), total hemoglobin and cytochrome oxidase are measured by conventional differential

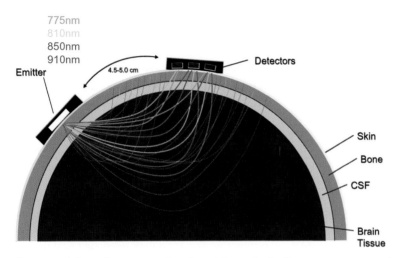

Figure 27.1 Schematic representation of spatially resolved reflectance spectroscopy in the NIRO 300.

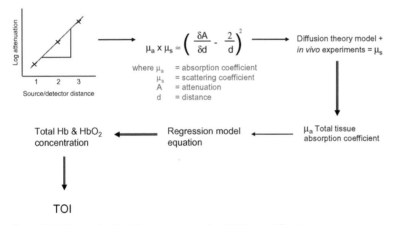

Figure 27.2 Theory behind tissue oxygen index (TOI) quantification.

spectroscopy using a modified Beer-Lambert law (Delpy *et al.*, 1988; Patterson *et al.*, 1989), whilst the basic principle behind calculation of the tissue oxygenation index is spatially resolved reflectance spectroscopy (Delpy *et al.*, 1988; Matcher *et al.*, 1993; Al-Rawi *et al.*, 1999). The basic measurement made is the rate of increase of light attenuation with respect to source/detector spacing and TOI is calculated from this using photon diffusion theory (Suzuki *et al.*, 1999). The hemoglobin and cytochrome concentration changes are measured by the middle photodiode, whilst TOI is measured by using all three (Figure 27.2).

TOI is the ratio of oxygenated to total tissue hemoglobin and can be expressed as:

$$TOI = \frac{HbO_2}{HbO_2 + Hb} \times 100$$

Clinical neuromonitoring in carotid surgery

It is known that patients undergoing carotid endarterectomy often suffer brief periods of cerebral ischemia during cross-clamping of the internal carotid artery (ICA) (Chan *et al.*, 1992; Kirkpatrick *et al.*, 1995b). The reliable detection of compromised regional cerebral perfusion therefore plays an important role in the management of patients undergoing carotid surgery. The decision for selective use of an intraluminal shunt in patients operated on under general anaesthesia needs to be based on accurate and reliable neuromonitoring. Monitoring devices with a high sensitivity must identify those patients who are unable to tolerate carotid cross-clamping due to insufficient collateral circulation and require insertion of an intraluminal shunt to prevent ischemia. However the monitoring must also demonstrate a high specificity in order to identify those patients with sufficient collateral circulation. This will help prevent potential complications, such as a higher rate of embolism, caused by routine shunt insertion (Kuroda *et al.*, 1996). Furthermore, the monitoring technique must satisfy such basic requirements as ease of use and interpretation as well as being noninvasive, in order to qualify for routine use. Many established forms of neuromonitoring require technical expertise and experience in interpreting the results (Cheng *et al.*, 1997). NIRS is an attractive alternative as a continuous, noninvasive measurement that is both safe and simple to apply.

A number of papers concerning the use of NIRS in carotid endarterectomy have been published. A variable decrease in cerebral saturation has been shown to occur following cross-clamping. Williams *et al.* (1994a) reported that a decrease in cerebral oxygen saturation is accompanied by a significant decrease in middle cerebral artery flow velocity and that even minor changes in oxygen saturation are suspected to represent relatively serious ischemia. They also showed in 33 patients, that a fall of 5% or more in cerebral oxygen saturation following application of cross clamps

was accompanied by a decrease in mean middle cerebral artery blood velocity of at least 60% (Williams *et al.*, 1994b). Hirofumi *et al.* (2003) in 19 patients undergoing carotid endarterectomy without a vascular shunt showed that ipsilateral cerebral oxygen saturation, measured by the INVOS 4100 (Somanetics Corporation, Troy MI), during cross-clamping caused a significant decrease of 19.1% from an average baseline of 49.5% which was accompanied with a significant decrease in ipsilateral electroencephalogram (EEG) main frequency. However, no neurological deterioration occurred in this group of patients. Several other reports have shown that the ipsilateral cerebral oxygen saturation decreased significantly during carotid cross-clamping. Duffy *et al.* compared regional oxygen saturation (rSO$_2$) using the INVOS 3100 with somatosensory evoked potentials (SEP) and concluded that rSO$_2$ fell by 5.6% on clamping, with a sensitivity of 50% and a specificity of 96%. They considered a decrease in rSO$_2$ of 10% clinically significant (Duffy *et al.*, 1997). Likewise Carlin *et al.* showed a drop of 7.2% (INVOS 3100) (Carlin *et al.*, 1998) with carotid clamping and Samra *et al.* a fall of 7.4% (range +2.6 to −28.6%, INVOS 3100) (Samra *et al.*, 1996). Using a different NIRS machine (Critikon) and comparing it to transcranial Doppler (TCD) and cerebral venous oxygen saturation (SjO$_2$) Williams *et al.* showed that derived cerebral oxygenation fell by 8.4% (Williams *et al.*, 1995).

During awake carotid endarterectomy, the changes in mental state have been used to indicate the accurate meaning of the cerebral oxygen saturation data. Samra *et al.* showed that a decrease in cerebral oxygen saturation during cross-clamping was greatest in patients with neurological symptoms (19.3%) than those without (7.3% decrease) (Samra *et al.*, 2000). They concluded that a baseline cerebral oxygen saturation of more than 61% and its decrease by less than 6.9–7.3% of the preclamp baseline is the safe range, whilst a cerebral saturation of less than 54–56.1% and a decrease by more than 15.6–18.2% predicted neurological compromise. A sensitivity of 80% and a specificity of 82.2% for clinical deterioration were calculated using a fall in cerebral oxygenation of 20%.

In one of the few studies that have attempted to define a threshold for ischemia with NIRS, Mille *et al.* (2004) calculated the %Δ rSO$_2$ from baseline to 2 minutes after clamping the common carotid artery (CCA) and/or ICA and identified a cut-off of 11.7% for neurological complication. The sensitivity and specificity for this threshold was calculated at 75% and 77%, respectively. However they went on to define a cut-off of >20% as clinically relevant, since a drop >20% was associated with neurological complications in 37% of patients, while a drop ≤20% was associated with neurological complications in only 2%. The sensitivity and specificity for a 20% threshold was 30% and 98%, respectively.

Beese *et al.* using the INVOS, compared SEP with rSO$_2$ to detect severe cerebral ischemia requiring shunt placement (Beese *et al.*, 1998). A significant decrease in rSO$_2$ was seen in patients without loss of cortical SEP (from 64.9 to 60.9%) as well as in patients with loss of cortical SEP (from 65.8 to 56.1%). The difference between the decrease seen in the two groups was significant, although they were unable to determine a threshold for rSO$_2$ due to marked individual variability of rSO$_2$ and the derived changes.

By using bilateral cerebral oximetry, Samra *et al.* demonstrated a significant but variable drop in the ipsilateral cerebral oxygen saturation without neurologic dysfunction in patients undergoing carotid endarterectomy under regional anaesthesia (Samra *et al.*, 1996). However they were unable to determine the critical cerebral oxygen saturation or change in saturation that requires the insertion of a shunt.

However, in most of these studies no attempt has been made to address the issue of extracerebral contamination of the NIRS signal, and only absolute decreases in cerebral oxygen saturation have been quoted.

During carotid endarterectomy, segregation of the NIRS signal between intra- and extracranial vascular territories is possible, by staged application

of vascular clamps to the external and internal carotid arteries (Graham *et al.*, 1986; Jorgensen and Schroeder, 1992; Kirkpatrick *et al.*, 1996; Lam *et al.*, 1997). In this way, the NIRO 500 has been used successfully to monitor patients undergoing carotid endarterectomy under general anaesthesia (Kirkpatrick *et al.*, 1995b). It was demonstrated that once the extracranial component was subtracted, a threshold for severe critical ischemia could be defined (Lam *et al.*, 1997; Kirkpatrick *et al.*, 1998b). An intraoperative drop in mean flow velocity to <40% of baseline, accompanied by a sustained fall in cerebral function monitoring was adopted as the criteria for severe cerebral ischemia. Ipsilateral frontal NIRS recorded the total difference in concentrations of oxyhemoglobin and deoxyhemoglobin (Total ΔHb_{diff}). Using interrupted time series analysis following clamping of the external and internal carotid arteries, the different vascular components of total ΔHb_{diff} (i.e. ECA ΔHb_{diff} and ICA ΔHb_{diff}) could be identified (Figure 27.3). All patients who demonstrated an ICA ΔHb_{diff} of >6.8 μmol/l showed severe cerebral ischemia. This threshold was used to guide the selective use of an interoperative carotid artery shunt.

Evaluation of the NIRO 300 as a monitor of cerebral ischemia

Our routine multimodal monitoring during carotid endarterectomy includes frontal cutaneous laser Doppler flowmetry (LDF), transcranial Doppler mean flow velocity (FV), measurements of the ipsilateral middle cerebral artery and mean arterial blood pressure (ABP) (Kirkpatrick *et al.*, 1995b). The LDF (Moor Instruments Ltd, Axminster, UK) is modified to use light in the visible spectrum (wavelength 650 nm) in order to avoid any interference to the NIRS signal (Lam *et al.*, 1997). We have incorporated the NIRO 300 into this multimodal monitoring system, enabling documentation of cerebral hemodynamic changes under highly controlled conditions (Al-Rawi *et al.*, 2001) (Figure 27.4).

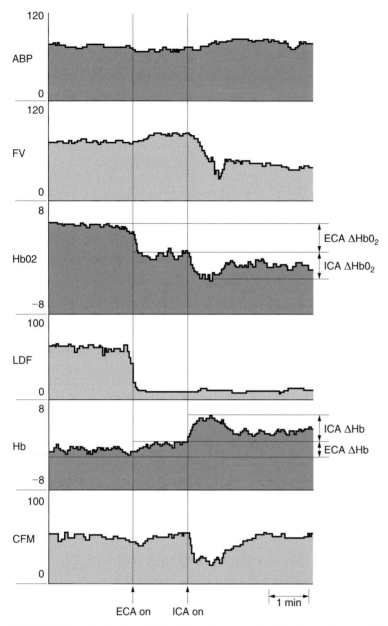

Figure 27.3 Graphic display of data obtained from a patient during elective carotid endarterectomy. The vertical lines demonstrate time of application of vascular clamps. On sequential clamping of the external carotid artery (ECA) and internal carotid artery (ICA), biphasic and reciprocal changes in oxyhemoglobin (HbO$_2$) and oxyhemoglobin (Hb) were seen. The ΔHbO$_2$ specific to ICA clamping can be resolved (ICA ΔHbO$_2$). The corresponding ICA ΔHb$_{diff}$ was calculated at 7.26 μmol/L. ECA ΔHb$_{diff}$ = [ECA ΔHbO$_2$] − [ECA ΔHb]. ICA ΔHb$_{diff}$ = [ICA ΔHbO$_2$] − [ICA ΔHb].

Abbreviations: 27.3 ABP# = mean arterial blood pressure (mmHg); FV = mean ipsilateral middle cerebral artery flow velocity (cm/sec); HbO$_2$ = oxyhemoglobin concentration (μmol/L); LDF = frontal cutaneous laser Doppler flow (arbitrary units); Hb = deoxyhemoglobin concentration (μmol/L); CFM = cerebral function monitoring.

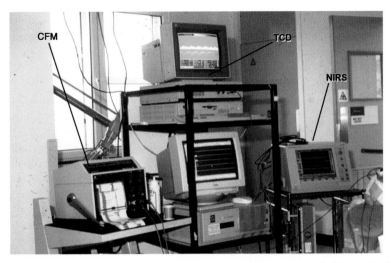

Figure 27.4 Routine intraoperative multimodal monitoring set-up, including cerebral function monitoring (CFM), transcranial Doppler (TCD), laser Doppler flow (LDF) and near infrared spectroscopy (NIRS).

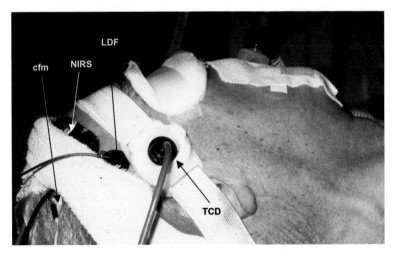

Figure 27.5 Position of the monitoring probes on the ipsilateral side showing cerebral function monitoring (cfm), transcranial Doppler (TCD), laser Doppler flow (LDF) and near infrared spectroscopy (NIRS).

Method

In 167 patients undergoing elective carotid endarterectomy, monitoring was applied after induction of anaesthesia, when the patient entered theatre. NIRS optodes were placed high on the ipsilateral forehead to avoid the prominent temporalis muscle, and sufficiently lateral from the midline to avoid the superior saggital sinus. Optode spacing was kept at 5 cm. Care was taken to ensure no hair was present between optodes and skin (Figure 27.5). Sequential clamping of the external and internal carotid arteries (ECA followed by ICA) was performed intraoperatively, allowing a sufficient time interval (≈2 minutes) for accurate assessment of the extracranial contribution to the NIRS signal (Kirkpatrick *et al.*, 1998b). Simultaneous measurement of hemoglobin concentration and TOI changes (ΔTOI) were assessed by observing changes in LDF (ΔLDF) and FV (ΔFV), in order to identify the extracerebral and intracerebral contribution to the NIRS signal (Kirkpatrick *et al.*, 1998a,b). Timing of intraoperative events and in particular the timing of vascular clamp applications was accurately documented. Data signals from all the monitored parameters were digitized and collected on computer using specialized multimodality software (Czosnyka *et al.*, 1994; Smielewski *et al.*, 1997). Maximum physiological stability is generally observed at the time of application of clamps rather than removal, therefore data from this period were used for analysis. In order to account for baseline variation in TOI, interrupted time series analysis was applied (Lam *et al.*, 1997; Kirkpatrick *et al.*, 1998b). From this data a baseline threshold of 2% was derived and therefore a ΔTOI greater than 2% was considered significant.

Results

Typical data obtained during carotid endarterectomy for an individual patient are demonstrated in Figure 27.6. Sequential clamping was performed with the ECA clamp being applied before the ICA clamp. As expected, the typical biphasic changes seen with the chromophores HbO_2 and Hb upon sequential clamping correspond to the patterns we have previously identified with the NIRO 500, and ΔTOI was only associated with ICA-related chromophore changes (Kirkpatrick *et al.*, 1996; Lam *et al.*, 1997). These observations lend support to the contention that ΔTOI is largely derived from the intracranial (ICA) vascular bed. The HbO_2 and Hb values derived by the NIRO 300 cannot reliably be taken to represent the intracranial compartment in the same way.

The values obtained before and after clamping of the internal carotid artery are shown in Table 27.1. Mean percentage change in TOI from baseline to post-ICA clamping (%ΔTOI) was −8.2 (± 9.0).

We found that changes in tissue oxygen index correlated with changes in intracranial blood flow, but not with cutaneous skin flow. Notably, ΔTOI was not seen without an associated ΔFV. The sensitivity and specificity of change in tissue oxygen index to intracranial changes (as detected by TCD) was 87.5 and 100%, respectively (Al-Rawi *et al.*, 2001).

Most importantly we were able to define a %ΔTOI threshold of −13%, above which no patients showed any evidence of ischemia (Figure 27.7). The threshold for %ΔTOI of −13 provided 100% sensitivity and 93.2% specificity for patients satisfying the preset criteria cerebral ischemia (Table 27.2) (Al-Rawi *et al.*, 2006).

Conclusion

As a monitor of cerebral oxygenation, NIRS has an obvious advantage. It allows for continuous, noninvasive monitoring, it is easy to use and can register complex mechanisms of oxygen balance in the brain. The probes can be applied and readings monitored without the need for expertise. Having a continuous, real-time measure of cerebral perfusion can potentially identify critical ischemic events before they manifest clinically and, in some cases, before other monitors have documented changes. However a number of issues need to be addressed before routine use for monitoring the adult brain during carotid endarterectomy can be recommended. The representation of regional cerebral oxygen saturation as an absolute value could be misleading since no reliable data regarding normal values exist. Additionally, the clinician is unable to check the accuracy of the given numeric values. The enduring issue surrounding the use of NIRS in the adult brain is extracranial contamination (Kirkpatrick *et al.*,

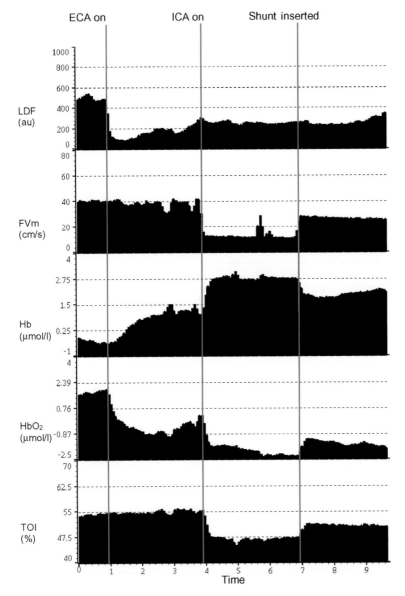

Figure 27.6 Graphic display of data obtained from a patient during elective carotid endarterectomy. The vertical lines demonstrate time of application of vascular clamps. Both Hb and HbO$_2$ show significant concentration changes on both external carotid artery (ECA) and internal carotid artery (ICA) clamping. LDF can be seen to fall only when the ECA clamp is applied. The drop in FV is seen to be specific to ICA clamping, as is the drop in TOI. On insertion of an ICA vascular shunt, FV and TOI were restored to values approaching baseline levels.

Abbreviations: LDF = frontal cutaneous laser Doppler flow; FV = mean ipsilateral middle cerebral artery flow velocity; HbO$_2$ = oxyhemoglobin concentration; Hb = deoxyhemoglobin concentration; TOI = tissue oxygen index.

Table 27.1. Summary of baseline and % change (%Δ) in mean flow velocity (mFV; cm/s), mean arterial blood pressure (ABP; mmHg) and tissue oxygen index (TOI; %) during sequential clamping of the internal carotid artery (ICA)

	Baseline (mean ± SD)	Post-ICA clamping (mean ± SD)
TOI (%)	68 ± 8.96 (range 46–93.6)	64.1 ± 10.3 (range 40.6–93)
FVm (cm/s)	37.8 ± 13.18 (range 17.2–76)	28.8 ± 13.7 (range 4.54–92.4)
ABPm (mmHg)	89.1 ± 14.3 (range 60.9–121)	89.3 ± 17.2 (range 53.4–114)

Table 27.2. Contingency table of sustained fall in cerebral function monitoring (CFM) by change in tissue oxygen index (ΔTOI) greater than −13% upon internal carotid artery (ICA) clamping. Sensitivity of ΔTOI to detect cerebral ischemia (at threshold of %ΔTOI ≤ −13%) = 100%, and specificity = 93.2%

	Fall in CFM	No fall in CFM	Total
ΔTOI ≤ −13%	31	10	**41**
ΔTOI > −13%	0	126	**126**
Total	**31**	**136**	**167**

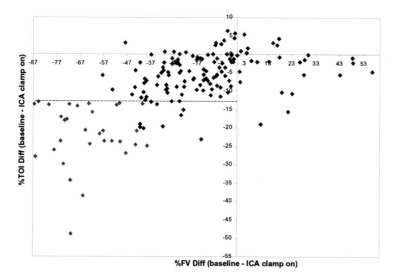

Figure 27.7 Scatterplot comparing percentage change in middle cerebral artery flow velocity (%ΔFV) with percentage change in tissue oxygen index (%ΔTOI) from baseline to postapplication of ICA clamp for 167 patients. Patients exhibiting a sustained fall in ipsilateral cerebral function monitoring are marked in red. Dotted line indicates ΔTOI −13% level.

1998a). Previous work has demonstrated that despite using large optode distances there is still a major contribution from the extracranial tissue to the NIRO signal (Lam *et al.*, 1997; Germon *et al.*, 1999). Our approach has been to sequentially clamp the ECA and ICA during carotid endarterectomy, allowing the opportunity to separate the intracranial and extracranial signal contributions and to identify changes in the cutaneous circulation affecting the NIRS measurements (Kirkpatrick *et al.*, 1995b; Kirkpatrick *et al.*, 1998b). Of the available NIRS instruments, the NIRO 300 appears to most reliably reflect changes in cerebral tissue oxygenation to a high degree of sensitivity and specificity by extracting extracerebral contamination from the calculated tissue oxygen index and a threshold for cerebral ischemia during carotid endarterectomy has been defined. NIRS is an evolving technology that holds significant potential for technical advancement. Improvements in the methodology, quantitative accuracy and regional specificity will increase its clinical applicability.

REFERENCES

Al-Rawi, P. G., Smielewski, P. and Kirkpatrick, P. J. (2001). Evaluation of a near infrared spectrometer (NIRO 300) for the detection of intracranial oxygenation changes in the adult head. *Stroke*, **32**, 2492–500.

Al-Rawi, P. G., and Kirkpatrick, P. J. Tissue Oxygen Index (TOI): Thresholds for cerebral ischaemia using infrared spectroscopy. *Stroke*, in press.

Al-Rawi, P. G., Smielewski, P., Hobbiger, H., Ghosh, S. and Kirkpatrick, P. J. (1999). Assessment of spatially resolved spectroscopy during cardiopulmonary bypass. *Journal of Biomedical Optics*, **4**, 208–16.

Aldrich, C. J., D'Antona, D., Wyatt, J. S., *et al.* (1994). Fetal cerebral oxygenation measured by near infrared spectroscopy shortly before birth and acid-base status at birth. *Obstetrics and Gynaecology*, **84**, 861–6.

Beese, U., Langer, H., Lang, W. and Dinkel, M. (1998). Comparison of near-infrared spectroscopy and somatosensory evoked potentials for the detection of cerebral ischaemia during carotid endarterectomy. *Stroke*, **29**, 2032–7.

Brazy, J. E., Lewis, D. V., Mitnik, M. H. and Jöbsis, F. F. (1985). Non invasive monitoring of cerebral oxygenation in preterm infants: preliminary observations. *Paediatrics*, **75**, 217–25.

Brown, R., Wright, G. and Royston, D. (1993). A comparison of two systems for assessing cerebral venous oxyhaemoglobin saturation during cardiopulmonary bypass in humans. *Anaesthesia*, **48**, 697–700.

Carlin, R. E., McGraw, D. J., Calimlim, J. R. and Mascia, M. F. (1998). The use of near-infrared cerebral oximetry in awake carotid endarterectomy. *Journal of Clinical Anesthesia*, **10**, 109–13.

Chan, K.-H., Miller, J. D., Dearden, N. M., Andrews, P. J. D. and Midgley, S. (1992). The effect of changes in cerebral perfusion pressure upon middle cerebral artery blood flow velocity and jugular bulb venous oxygen saturation after severe brain injury. *Journal of Neurosurgery*, **77**, 55–61.

Cheng, M. A., Theard, M. A. and Tempelhoff, R. (1997). Anesthesia for carotid endarterectomy: a survey. *Journal of Neurosurgical Anaesthesiology*, **9**, 211–16.

Cope, M. and Delpy, D. T. (1988). System for long-term measurement of cerebral blood and tissue oxygenation on newborn infants by near infra-red transillumination. *Medical and Biological Engineering and Computing*, **26**, 289–94.

Czosnyka, M., Whitehouse, H., Smielewski, P., *et al.* (1994). Computer supported multimodal bed-side monitoring for neuro intensive care. *Journal of Clinical Monitoring and Computing*, **11**, 223–32.

Dehghani, H. and Delpy, D. T. (2000). Near infrared spectroscopy of the adult head: effect of scattering and absorbing obstructions in the CSF layer on light distribution in the tissue. *Applied Optics*, **39**, 4721–9.

Delpy, D. T. and Cope, M. (1997). Quantification in tissue near-infrared spectroscopy. *Philosophical Transactions of the Royal Society of London. Series B*, **352**, 649–59.

Delpy, D. T., Cope, M., van der Zee, P., *et al.* (1988). Estimation of optical pathlength through tissue from direct time of flight measurement. *Physics in Medicine and Biology*, **33**, 1433–42.

du Plessis, A. J., Newburger, J., Jonas, R. A., *et al.* (1995). Cerebral oxygenation supply and utilisation during infarct cardiac surgery. *Annals of Neurology*, **37**, 488–97.

Duffy, C. M., Manninen, P. H., Chan, A. and Kearns, C. F. (1997). Comparison of cerebral oximeter and evoked potential monitoring in carotid endarterectomy. *Canadian Journal of Anaesthesia*, **44**, 1077–81.

Dullenkopf, A., Frey, B., Baenziger, O., Gerber, A. and Weiss, M. (2003). Measurement of cerebral oxygenation state in anaesthetized children using the INVOS 5100 cerebral oximeter. *Paediatric Anaesthesia*, **13**, 384–91.

Elwell, C. E., Matcher, S. J., Tyszczuk, L., Meek, J. H. and Delpy, D. T. (1997). Measurement of cerebral venous saturation in adults using near infrared spectroscopy. *Advances in Experimental Medicine and Biology*, **411**, 453–60.

Fantini, S., Franceschini, M. A., Maier, J. S., *et al.* (1995). Frequency-domain multichannel optical detector for non-invasive tissue spectroscopy and oximetry. *Optical Engineering*, **34**, 32–42.

Ferrari, M., De Marchis, C. and Giannini, I. (1986). Cerebral blood volume and haemoglobin oxygen saturation monitoring in the neonatal brain by near infrared spectroscopy. *Advances in Experimental Medicine and Biology*, **200**, 203–11.

Firbank, M., Schweiger, M. and Delpy, D. T. (1995). Investigation of light piping through clear regions of scattering objects. *Proceedings of SPIE*, **2389**, 167–73.

Germon, T. J., Evans, D. H., Barnett, N., *et al.* (1999). Cerebral near infrared spectroscopy: emitter-detector separation must be increased. *British Journal of Anaesthesia*, **82**, 831–7.

Germon, T. J., Kane, N. M., Manara, A. R. and Nelson, R. J. (1994). Near-infrared spectroscopy in adults: effects of extracranial ischaemia and intracranial hypoxia on estimation of cerebral oxygenation. *British Journal of Anaesthesia*, **73**, 503–6.

Germon, T. J., Young, A. E. R., Manara, A. R., *et al.* (1995). Extracerebral absorption of near infrared light influences the detection of increased cerebral oxygen monitored by near infrared spectroscopy. *Journal of Neurology, Neurosurgery and Psychiatry*, **58**, 477–9.

Graham, A. M., Gewetz, B. L. and Zarins, C. K. (1986). Predicting cerebral ischaemia during carotid endarterectomy. *Archives of Surgery*, **121**, 595–8.

Harris, D. N. and Bailey, S. M. (1993). Near infrared spectroscopy in adults. Does the INVOS 3100 really measure intracerebral oxygenation? *Anaesthesia*, **48**, 694–6.

Harris, D. N., Cowans, F. M. and Wertheim, D. A. (1994). Near infrared spectroscopy in the temporal region: strong influence of external carotid artery. *Advances in Experimental Medicine and Biology*, **345**, 825–8.

Hazeki, O. and Tamura, M. (1988). Quantitative analysis of haemoglobin oxygenation state of brain *in situ* by near-infrared spectrophotometry. *Journal of Applied Physiology*, **64**, 796–802.

Hiraoka, M., Firbank, M. and Essenpries, M. (1993). A Monte Carlo investigation of optical pathlength in inhomogeneous tissue and its application to near infrared spectroscopy. *Physics in Medicine and Biology*, **38**, 1859–76.

Hirofumi, O., Otone, E., Hiroshi, I., *et al.* (2003). The effectiveness of regional cerebral oxygen saturation monitoring using near-infrared spectroscopy in carotid endarterectomy. *Journal of Clinical Neuroscience*, **10**, 79–83.

Jorgensen, L. G. and Schroeder, T. V. (1992). Transcranial Doppler for detection of cerebral ischemia during carotid endarterectomy. *European Journal of Vascular Surgery*, **6**, 142–7.

Jöbsis, F. F. (1977). Non-invasive infrared monitoring of cerebral and myocardial oxygen sufficiency and circulatory parameters. *Science*, **198**, 1264–7.

Kirkpatrick, P. J., Smielewski, P., Al-Rawi, P. and Czosnyka, M. (1998a). Resolving extra- and intracranial signal changes during adult near infrared spectroscopy. *Neurological Research*, **20**, S19–S22.

Kirkpatrick, P. J., Lam, J. M. K., Al-Rawi, P. G., Smielewski, P. and Czosnyka, M. (1998b). Defining thresholds for critical ischaemia by using near-infrared spectroscopy in the adult brain. *Journal of Neurosurgery*, **89**, 389–94.

Kirkpatrick, P. J., Smielewski, P., Czosnyka, M., Menon, D. K. and Pickard, J. D. (1995a). Near infrared spectroscopy use in patients with head injury. *Journal of Neurosurgery*, **83**, 963–70.

Kirkpatrick, P. J., Smielewski, P., Whitfield, P., *et al.* (1995b). An observational study of near infrared spectroscopy during carotid endarterectomy. *Journal of Neurosurgery*, **82**, 756–63.

Kirkpatrick, P. J., Smielewski, P., Lam, J. M. K. and Al-Rawi, P. G. (1996). Use of near infrared spectroscopy for the clinical monitoring of adult brain. *Journal of Biomedical Optics*, **1**, 363–72.

Komiyama, T., Quaresima, V., Shigematsu, H. and Ferrari, M. (2001). Comparison of two spatially resolved near-infrared photometers in the detection of tissue oxygen saturation: poor reliability at very low oxygen saturation. *Clinical Science*, **101**, 715–18.

Kuroda, S., Houkin, K., Abe, H., Hoshi, Y. and Tamura, M. (1996). Near-infrared monitoring of cerebral oxygenation state during carotid endarterectomy. *Surgical Neurology*, **45**, 450–8.

Kurth, C. D., Steven, J. M. and Nicholson, S. C. (1995). Cerebral oxygenation during pediatric surgery using deep hypothermic circulatory arrest. *Anaesthesiology*, **82**, 74–82.

Kytta, J., Ohman, J., Tanskanen, P. and Randell, T. (1999). Extracranial contribution to cerebral oximetry in brain dead patients: a report of six cases. *Journal of Neurosurgical Anaesthesiology*, **11**, 252–4.

Lam, J. M. K., Kirkpatrick, P. J., Al-Rawi, P., Smielewski, P. and Pickard, J. D. (1996). Internal and external carotid contribution to near infrared spectroscopy (NIRS) during carotid endarterectomy (CE). *Journal of Neurology, Neurosurgery and Psychiatry*, **61**, 553.

Lam, J. M. K., Smielewski, P., Al-Rawi, P., *et al.* (1997). Internal and external carotid contributions to near-infrared spectroscopy during carotid endarterectomy. *Stroke*, **28**, 906–11.

Liem, K. D., Hopman, J. C. W., Oeseburg, B., *et al.* (1995). Cerebral oxygenation and haemodynamics during induction of extracorporeal membrane oxygenation as investigated by near infrared spectroscopy. *Paediatrics*, **95**, 555–61.

Litscher, G. and Schwarz, G. (1997). Transcranial cerebral oximetry – is it clinically useless at this moment to interpret absolute values obtained by the INVOS 3100 cerebral oximeter? *Biomedizinische Technik*, **42**, 74–7.

Matcher, S. J., Kirkpatrick, P. J., Nahid, K., Cope, M. and Delpy, D. T. (1993). Absolute quantification methods in tissue near infrared spectroscopy. *Proceedings of SPIE*, **2389**, 486–95.

McKeating, E. G., Monjardino, J. R., Signorini, D. F., Souter, M. J. and Andrews, P. J. D. (1997). A comparison of the INVOS 3100 and the Critikon 2020 near-infrared spectrophotometer as monitors of cerebral oxygenation. *Anaesthesia*, **52**, 136–40.

Mille, T., Tachimiri, M. E., Klersy, C., *et al.* (2004). Near infrared spectroscopy monitoring during carotid endarterectomy: which threshold value is critical? *European Journal of Vascular and Endovascular Surgery*, **27**, 646–50.

Miwa, M., Ueda, Y. and Chance, B. (1995). Development of time resolved spectroscopy system for quantitative non-invasive tissue measurement. *Proceedings of SPIE*, **2389**, 142–9.

Nollert, G., Jonas, R. A. and Reichart, B. (2000). Optimising cerebral oxygenation during cardiac surgery: a review of experimental and clinical investigations with near infrared spectrophotometry. *Thoracic and Cardiovascular Surgeon*, **48**, 247–53.

Oda, M., Yamashita, Y., Nishimura, G. and Tamura, M. (1996). A simple and novel algorithm for time resolved multiwavelength oximetry. *Physics in Medicine and Biology*, **40**, 2093–108.

Okada, E., Firbank, M., Schweiger, M., *et al.* (1995). A theoretical and experimental investigation of the effect of sulci on light propagation in brain tissue. *Proceedings of SPIE*, **2626**, 2–8.

Okada, E., Firbank, M., Schweiger, M., *et al.* (1997). Theoretical and experimental investigation of near-infrared light propagation in a model of the adult head. *Applied Optics*, **36**, 21–31.

Patterson, M. S., Chance, B. and Wilson, B. C. (1989). Time resolved reflectance and transmittance for the noninvasive measurement of tissue optical properties. *Applied Optics*, **28**, 2331–6.

Piantadosi, C. A. (1989). Near infrared spectroscopy: principles and application to non-invasive assessment of tissue oxygenation. *Journal of Critical Care*, **4**, 308–18.

Samra, S. K., Dorje, P., Zelenock, G. B. and Stanley, J. C. (1996). Cerebral oximetry in patients undergoing carotid endarterectomy under regional anaesthesia. *Stroke*, **27**, 49–55.

Samra, S. K., Dy, E. A., Welch, K., *et al.* (2000). Evaluation of a cerebral oximeter as a monitor of cerebral ischaemia during carotid endarterectomy. *Anaesthesiology*, **93**, 970.

Schwarz, G., Litscher, G., Kleinert, R. and Jobstmann, R. (1996). Cerebral oximetry in dead subjects. *Journal of Neurosurgical Anesthesiology*, **8**, 189–93.

Smielewski, P., Czosnyka, M., Zabolotny, W., *et al.* (1997). A computing system for the clinical and experimental investigation of cerebrovascular reactivity. *International Journal of Clinical Monitoring and Computing*, **14**, 185–98.

Suzuki, S., Takasaki, S., Ozaki, T. and Kobayashi, Y. (1999). A tissue oxygenation monitor using NIR spatially resolved spectroscopy. *Proceedings of SPIE*, **3597**, 582–92.

Tamura, M., Hoshi, Y. and Okada, F. (1997). Localised near-infrared spectroscopy and functional optical imaging of brain activity. *Philosophical Transactions of the Royal Society of London. Series B*, **352**, 737–42.

Vernieri, F., Tibuzzi, F., Pasqualetti, P., *et al.* (2004). Transcranial Doppler and near-infrared spectroscopy can evaluate the haemodynamic effect of carotid artery occlusion. *Stroke*, **35**, 64–70.

Villringer, A., Planck, J., Stodieck, S., *et al.* (1994). Non invasive assessment of cerebral haemodynamics and tissue oxygenation during activation of brain function in human adults using near infrared spectroscopy. *Advances in Experimental Medicine and Biology*, **345**, 559–65.

Watanabe, E., Nagahori, Y. and Mayanagi, Y. (2002). Focus diagnosis of epilepsy using near-infrared spectroscopy. *Epilepsia*, **43** (Suppl. 9), 50–5.

Williams, I. M., Mead, G., Picton, A. J., *et al.* (1995). The influence of contralateral carotid stenosis and occlusion on cerebral oxygen saturation during carotid artery surgery. *European Journal of Vascular and Endovascular Surgery*, **10**, 198–206.

Williams, I. M., Picton, A., Farrell, A., *et al.* (1994a). Light reflective cerebral oximetry and jugular bulb venous oxygen saturation during carotid endarterectomy. *British Journal of Surgery*, **81**, 1291–5.

Williams, I. M., Vohra, R., Farrell, A., *et al.* (1994b). Cerebral oxygen saturation, transcranial Doppler ultrasonography and stump pressure in carotid surgery. *British Journal of Surgery*, **81**, 960–4.

Wray, S., Cope, M., Delpy, D. T., Wyatt, J. S. and Reynolds, E. O. R. (1988). Characterisation of the near infrared absorption spectra of cytochrome aa3 and haemoglobin for the non-invasive monitoring of cerebral oxygenation. *Biochimica et Biophysica Acta*, **933**, 184–92.

Wyatt, J. S., Cope, M., Delpy, D. T., *et al.* (1990). Quantification of cerebral blood volume in newborn infants by near infrared spectroscopy. *Journal of Applied Physiology*, **68**, 1086–91.

Yoshitani, K., Kawaguchi, M., Tatsumi, K., Kitaguchi, K. and Furuya, H. (2002). A comparison of the INVOS 4100 and the NIRO 300 near-infrared spectrometers. *Anesthesia and Analgesia*, **94**, 586–90.

Young, A. E. R., Germon, T. J., Barnett, N. J., Manara, A. R. and Nelson, R. J. (2000). Behaviour of near-infrared light in the adult human head: implications for clinical near-infrared spectroscopy. *British Journal of Anaesthesia*, **84**, 38–42.

28

Single photon emission computed tomography (SPECT)

Kuniaki Ogasawara

Iwate Medical University, Morioka, Japan

Introduction

Brain single-photon emission computed tomography (SPECT) has been widely used to assess regional brain perfusion and can also quantify regional cerebral blood flow (CBF) and regional cerebral hemodynamic reserve by measuring cerebrovascular reactivity to acetazolamide. The relationship between the brain perfusion using SPECT and the risk of stroke recurrence in patients with symptomatic carotid disease or the risk for cerebral hyperperfusion or hyperperfusion syndrome after carotid endarterectomy has been investigated.

In this chapter, the utility of SPECT in the evaluation of carotid disease and interventions are discussed.

Cerebrovascular reactivity to acetazolamide and outcome in patients with symptomatic carotid artery occlusion

The hemodynamic effects of an occlusive lesion on the distal circulation have been categorized into three stages (Powers *et al.*, 1987; Derdeyn *et al.*, 1999). Occlusive lesions often have no effect on the distal circulation (stage 0, normal cerebral hemodynamics). When the perfusion pressure distal to the lesion begins to fall, however, reflex vasodilatation maintains normal blood flow (stage 1). This response is known as autoregulation.

Autoregulatory vasodilatation can be detected using two basic strategies (Norrving *et al.*, 1982). The first involves quantitative measurements of resting CBF and cerebral blood volume (CBV). CBV increases with autoregulatory vasodilatation and the CBV/CBF ratio, which means the vascular transit time of red blood cells, increases. The second method relies on measurements of CBF at rest and following a vasodilatory stimulus. An absent or diminished response indicates autoregulatory vasodilatation. When autoregulatory vasodilatation is not adequate to maintain normal CBF, CBF begins to fall. In this situation, the brain can increase the amount of oxygen it extracts from the blood (oxygen extraction fraction [OEF]) to maintain normal cerebral oxygen metabolism. This stage (stage 2) of hemodynamic compromise has been termed "misery perfusion" (Baron *et al.*, 1981). While evidence indicates that patients with "misery perfusion" are at high risk of recurrent ischemic stroke (Yamauchi *et al.*, 1996; Grubb *et al.*, 1998), OEF can be directly measured only by positron emission tomography (PET) at present. On the other hand, diminished response to a vasodilatory stimulus accompanied by reduction in the resting CBF, which can be quantified by SPECT, theoretically indicates reduction of cerebral perfusion pressure below the lower limit of autoregulation, that is "misery perfusion" (Kuroda *et al.*, 1993).

A prospective study demonstrated that reduced regional cerebrovascular reactivity (rCVR) to

Carotid Disease: The Role of Imaging in Diagnosis and Management, ed. Jonathan Gillard, Martin Graves, Thomas Hatsukami and Chun Yuan. Published by Cambridge University Press. © Cambridge University Press 2007.

acetazolamide determined quantitatively using ^{133}Xe SPECT is significantly associated with an increased risk of stroke recurrence in patients with symptomatic occlusion of the middle cerebral artery (MCA) or internal carotid artery (ICA) (Ogasawara *et al.*, 2002b). In addition, resting rCBF was found to predict recurrent stroke in patients with symptomatic occlusion of the MCA or ICA, although the parameter is not as strong a predictor as rCVR. A further prospective study using a similar method also demonstrated that decreased rCVR to acetazolamide is associated with a higher risk of subsequent ischemic stroke (Kuroda *et al.*, 2001). Conversely, studies by Yokota *et al.* that defined hemodynamic compromise based on qualitative (relative) CBF measured using N-isopropyl-p-[^{123}I]-iodoamphetamine (^{123}I-IMP) failed to demonstrate an association of hemodynamic failure and stroke risk (Yokota *et al.*, 1998). Thus, it was possible that the two SPECT methodologies, cerebrovascular reactivities to acetazolamide measured quantitatively and qualitatively, did not identify the same patients as having hemodynamic compromise and a high risk of recurrent stroke. rCVR to acetazolamide was divided in the MCA territory ipsilateral to the occluded artery on the basis of two different methodologies: CBF% change obtained quantitatively from ^{133}Xe SPECT and asymmetry index (AI)% change obtained qualitatively from ^{123}I-IMP SPECT, and I divided patients with unilateral ICA or MCA occlusion into two groups within each SPECT methodology (normal or decreased CBF% change and AI% change) (Ogasawara *et al.*, 2002a). As a result, cumulative recurrence-free survival rates for patients with decreased CBF% change were significantly lower than for those with normal CBF% change. There was no significant difference in cumulative recurrence-free survival rates between patients with decreased AI% change and those with normal AI% change. Only decreased CBF% change was a significant independent predictor of stroke recurrence. Thus, these findings demonstrated that while decreased cerebrovascular reactivity to acetazolamide determined

quantitatively by ^{133}Xe SPECT is an independent predictor of the risk of subsequent stroke in patients with symptomatic carotid artery occlusion, the qualitative method using ^{123}I-IMP SPECT is a poor predictor of the risk of subsequent stroke in this type of patient. Forty one percent of patients with decreased AI% change had normal ipsilateral CBF% change, and 16% of patients with normal AI% change had decreased ipsilateral CBF% change. These findings indicated that the two SPECT methodologies (quantitative assessment using ^{133}Xe SPECT and qualitative assessment using ^{123}I-IMP SPECT) do not always identify the same patients as possessing hemodynamic compromise. Because relative ^{123}I-IMP uptake normalized by contralateral uptake compared with relative CBF normalized by contralateral CBF shows a linear relationship (Nakano *et al.*, 1989; Ogasawara *et al.*, 2003a,b), the following factors, rather than difference in the tracer, may explain this disparity. First, normal ipsilateral CBF% change with decreased AI% change may occur when CBF increases asymmetrically after administration of acetazolamide (Yonas *et al.*, 1998; Ogasawara *et al.*, 2003b), and the qualitative assessment may incorrectly identify the ipsilateral cerebral hemodynamics as a "significant" compromise when CBF% change in the contralateral side is relatively higher than the ipsilateral side. Second, patients with unilateral ICA occlusion, especially with collateral circulation through the anterior communicating artery, may demonstrate hemodynamic disturbance in both hemispheres (Yamauchi *et al.*, 1990, 1996). Further, mild and diffuse arteriosclerosis may impair cerebral hemodynamics on the contralateral side despite absence of lesion on angiography (Yamauchi *et al.*, 1996; Yonas *et al.*, 1998). Thus, the hemisphere ipsilateral to the occluded artery may be deemed normal when the value of the contralateral hemisphere is used as an internal control (Ogasawara *et al.*, 2003b).

Evidence indicates that cerebrovascular reactivity spontaneously improves in approximately half of patients with unilateral ICA occlusion, predominantly during the first few months after the onset of ischemic symptoms, provided no interval stroke occurs (Widder *et al.*, 1994). In one study, rCVR returned to normal levels at 2-year follow-up in 44% of the stroke recurrence-free survivors with ICA occlusion and reduced rCVR at entry (Ogasawara *et al.*, 2002b). On the other hand, rCVR did not normalize during follow-up in any of the stroke recurrence-free survivors with MCA occlusion and reduced rCVR at entry. These findings suggest that cerebral hemodynamics impaired by MCA occlusion may remain in the long-term, unlike those impaired by ICA occlusion. Spontaneous improvement of hemodynamic failure following major cerebral artery occlusion probably depends on the development of collateral circulation. While collaterals across the circle of Willis and/or from the external carotid artery often perfuse an area distal to an occluded ICA, only pial or meningeal to pial collaterals are available to patients with MCA occlusion. Thus, the essentially inadequate development of collaterals to the distal circulation in MCA occlusion may result in longstanding hemodynamic failure. Also, in patients with carotid occlusion, Klijn *et al.* have reported that the presence of leptomeningeal collateral pathways is associated with impaired cerebral hemodynamics and a high risk of recurrent cerebral ischemic events (Klijn *et al.*, 2000).

Preoperative prediction and early detection of cerebral hyperperfusion after carotid endarterectomy

Most complications following carotid endarterectomy are ischemic in nature, either secondary to embolization or to inadequate cerebral protection in patients with poor collateral supply (Hosoda *et al.*, 2001). Postoperative neurological dysfunction may also be related to cerebral hyperperfusion, which is defined as a major increase in ipsilateral CBF well above the metabolic demands of the brain tissue following removal of carotid stenosis (Sundt *et al.*, 1981; Piepgras *et al.*, 1988). Cerebral hyperperfusion syndrome is

characterized by unilateral headache, face and eye pain, seizures, and focal symptoms related to cerebral edema or intracerebral hemorrhage (Sundt *et al.*, 1981; Bernstein *et al.*, 1984; Solomon *et al.*, 1986; Piepgras *et al.*, 1988). The incidence of this condition is relatively low (0.4–1.8%), but the prognosis for patients with intracerebral hemorrhage is poor (Solomon *et al.*, 1986; Schroeder *et al.*, 1987; Piepgras *et al.*, 1988; Pomposelli *et al.*, 1988; Jansen *et al.*, 1994; Riles *et al.*, 1994; Ouriel *et al.*, 1999).

Investigators have proposed mechanisms for development of post-carotid endarterectomy hyperperfusion (Bernstein *et al.*, 1984). In cases with severe ICA stenosis and deficient collateral circulation, hemispheric perfusion pressure is severely reduced distal to the ICA stenosis. This may result in reduction of perfusion pressure below the compensatory capacity of autoregulatory mechanisms, thus leading to maximal dilation of resistance vessels and chronic hypoperfusion or "misery perfusion". After restoration of normal perfusion pressure following carotid endarterectomy, chronically impaired autoregulatory mechanisms may require several days to adjust to the new steady state, resulting in hyperperfusion in the interim. This hypothesis is similar to the "normal perfusion pressure breakthrough" theory described by Spetzler *et al.* (1978).

Risk factors for this syndrome include long-standing hypertension, high-grade stenosis, poor collateral blood flow and contralateral carotid occlusion, which often impairs cerebral hemodynamic reserve (Reigel *et al.*, 1987). Actually, postoperative hyperperfusion is observed only in patients with reduced preoperative cerebrovascular reactivity to acetazolamide (Yoshimoto *et al.*, 1997; Hosoda *et al.*, 2001; Ogasawara *et al.*, 2003). Further, decreased cerebrovascular reactivity to acetazolamide is a significant independent predictor of postcarotid endarterectomy hyperperfusion (Ogasawara *et al.*, 2003). Thus, preoperative assessment of CBF with acetazolamide challenge using SPECT can identify patients at risk for postcarotid endarterectomy hyperperfusion. However, while postcarotid endarterectomy hyperperfusion is not observed in patients with normal preoperative cerebrovascular reactivity to acetazolamide, patients with impaired cerebral hemodynamic reserve do not always develop postcarotid endarterectomy hyperperfusion (Yoshimoto *et al.*, 1997; Hosoda *et al.*, 2001; Ogasawara *et al.*, 2003). In fact, the incidence of postcarotid endarterectomy hyperperfusion in patients with reduced preoperative CVR ranges from 20 to 70% (Yoshimoto *et al.*, 1997; Hosoda *et al.*, 2001; Ogasawara *et al.*, 2003). A recent study using SPECT and intraoperative transcranial cerebral oxygen saturation monitoring using near-infrared spectroscopy demonstrated that decreased preoperative cerebrovascular reactivity to acetazolamide and decreased regional cerebral oxygen saturation during ICA clamping were significant independent predictors of postcarotid endarterectomy hyperperfusion (Komoribayashi *et al.*, 2006). All patients with reduced preoperative cerebrovascular reactivity to acetazolamide and reduced regional cerebral oxygen saturation developed postcarotid endarterectomy hyperperfusion. In addition, all these patients recovered from surgery without new major neurological deficits, and postoperative computerized tomography (CT) scan or magnetic resonance imaging (MRI) did not detect additional ischemic lesions. These findings suggest that in addition to impairment of cerebrovascular autoregulation due to chronic ischemia, acute ischemia during clamping of the ICA, even when it is not so severe as the brain is damaged, contributes to the pathogenesis of postcarotid endarterectomy hyperperfusion (Komoribayashi *et al.*, 2006).

Several investigators have suggested that acute ischemia and reperfusion by clamping and declamping of the ICA may produce oxygen-derived free radicals (Soong *et al.*, 1996; Weigand *et al.*, 1999; Holm *et al.*, 2001). The free radicals may impair cerebrovascular autoregulation, resulting in postischemic hyperperfusion or brain edema (Phillis and Sen, 1993; Karibe *et al.*, 1994). In addition, pretreatment with a novel free radical scavenger, edaravone (Mitsubishi-Tokyo

Pharmaceuticals Inc, Tokyo, Japan), which is widely used in Japan to improve functional outcomes in patients suffering from acute ischemic stroke (The Edaravone Acute Brain Infarction Study Group, 2003), can prevent development of cerebral hyperperfusion after carotid endarterectomy (Ogasawara *et al.*, 2004). Thus, free radicals produced by clamping and declamping of the ICA may deteriorate further cerebrovascular autoregulation that is already impaired by preoperative chronic ischemia. This process likely culminates in postcarotid endarterectomy hyperperfusion.

Several studies with postoperative SPECT or intraoperative transcranial Doppler monitoring demonstrated that patients without cerebral hyperperfusion immediately after carotid endarterectomy does not exhibit hyperperfusion or hyperperfusion syndrome after that (Dalman *et al.*, 1999; Ogasawara *et al.*, 2003). In contrast, 11–25% of patients with cerebral hyperperfusion immediately after carotid endarterectomy show progressive increases in CBF and development of hyperperfusion syndrome (Figure 28.1). In the remaining patients with cerebral hyperperfusion immediately after carotid endarterectomy, CBF decreases and hyperperfusion resolves by the third postoperative day (Figure 28.2). Thus, persistence of hyperperfusion greater than several days is associated with development of hyperperfusion syndrome. Most authors have reported that signs or symptoms of hyperperfusion occur between 3 and 8 days after carotid endarterectomy (Harrison *et al.*, 1991; Penn *et al.*, 1995; Breen *et al.*, 1996; Yoshimoto *et al.*, 1997; Shinno *et al.*, 1998; Dalman *et al.*, 1999). In addition, Henderson *et al.* demonstrated that hemorrhage due to hyperperfusion occurred between 3 and 8 days after carotid endarterectomy (Henderson *et al.*, 2001). Therefore, a SPECT study performed between the first and third postoperative day could be advocated for the timely and reliable identification of patients at risk for hyperperfusion syndrome.

On SPECT images obtained between the first and third postoperative day, the presence or absence of crossed cerebellar hypoperfusion as well as

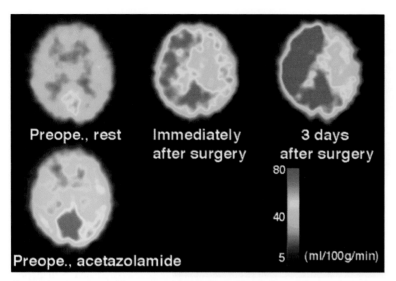

Figure 28.1 A 70-year-old woman with symptomatic right internal carotid artery stenosis (95%) exhibiting hyperperfusion syndrome after carotid endarterectomy. Preoperative SPECT showing poor acetazolamide-induced increases in right middle cerebral artery perfusion (left). Hyperperfusion was observed on SPECT immediately after carotid endarterectomy (middle). SPECT performed on the third postoperative day demonstrated worsening hyperperfusion (right). This patient developed confusion and left motor weakness 5 days after surgery.

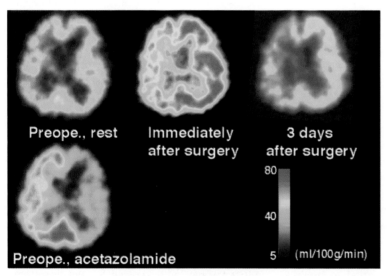

Figure 28.2 A 71-year-old man with symptomatic left internal carotid artery stenosis (95%) and asymptomatic right internal carotid artery stenosis (99%). Preoperative SPECT showing poor acetazolamide-induced increases in left middle cerebral artery perfusion (left). Hyperperfusion was observed on SPECT immediately after left carotid endarterectomy (middle). This patient developed a transient ischemic attack with left motor weakness on the third postoperative day. SPECT performed immediately after the transient ischemic attack showed resolution of hyperperfusion in the left hemisphere and hypoperfusion in the right hemisphere (right).

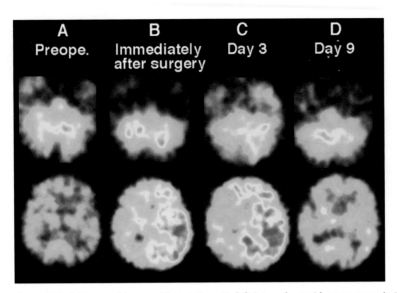

Figure 28.3 A 72-year-old man with symptomatic left internal carotid artery stenosis (95%) and symptomatic right internal carotid artery stenosis (95%). (A) Preoperative perfusion in the bilateral cerebral hemispheres was reduced compared with that in the cerebellum. (B) While perfusion in the left cerebral hemisphere was markedly increased immediately after carotid endarterectomy, perfusion in the bilateral cerebellar hemispheres remained equal. (C) Hyperperfusion in the left cerebral hemisphere persisted, and right cerebellar hemispheric perfusion was reduced on the third postoperative day. (D) Hyperperfusion in the left cerebral hemisphere and hypoperfusion in the right cerebellar hemisphere resolved on the ninth postoperative day.

that of cerebral hyperperfusion is important. In one case, SPECT performed immediately after carotid endarterectomy revealed no crossed cerebellar hypoperfusion despite the presence of cerebral hyperperfusion, and symptoms due to cerebral hyperperfusion (e.g. hyperperfusion syndrome) developed on the day after appearance of crossed cerebellar hypoperfusion (Ogasawara et al., 2005) (Figure 28.3). Therefore, the preceding crossed cerebellar hypoperfusion may suggest development of occult hyperperfusion syndrome as a result of reduction of cerebral metabolism due to cerebral hyperperfusion.

Most authors recommend strict control of blood pressure in the postoperative period to prevent hyperperfusion syndrome (Sundt et al., 1981; Solomon et al., 1986; Reigel et al., 1987; Piepgras et al., 1988; Mansoor et al., 1996; Yoshimoto et al., 1997; Dalman et al., 1999). Dalman et al. (1999) and Ogasawara et al. (2003) reported that although

11–25% of patients with postcarotid endarterectomy hyperperfusion were symptomatic with aggressive control of blood pressure, none experienced intracerebral hemorrhage. This stands in contrast to the 2% incidence of intracerebral hemorrhage in patients undergoing carotid endarterectomy without aggressive postoperative blood pressure control (Dalman et al., 1999).

Carotid artery disease and other vascular atherosclerotic disease such as coronary artery disease or lower extremity atherosclerotic occlusive disease have similar risk factors and often coexist. In addition, 30% of patients with carotid artery disease had bilateral lesions (Ogasawara et al., 2003). Patients with postcarotid endarterectomy hyperperfusion may experience ischemic events involving other atherosclerotic steno-occlusive lesions, likely secondary to relative hypotensive while undergoing aggressive blood pressure control (Ogasawara et al., 2003) (Figure 28.2).

Thus, in patients with concomitant vascular atherosclerotic disease, postcarotid endarterectomy CBF measurement should dictate who should receive aggressive blood pressure control to minimize the risk of relative hypotension in these patients. CBF measurements can also determine appropriate withdrawal of blood pressure control in patients with ischemic events related to other atherosclerotic steno-occlusive lesions.

REFERENCES

Baron, J. C., Bousser, M. G., Rey, A., Guillard, A., Comar, D. and Castaigne, P. (1981). Reversal of focal "misery-perfusion syndrome" by extra-intracranial arterial bypass in hemodynamic cerebral ischemia. A case study with 15O positron emission tomography. *Stroke*, **12**, 454–9.

Bernstein, M., Fleming, J. F. and Deck, J. H. (1984). Cerebral hyperperfusion after carotid endarterectomy: a cause of cerebral hemorrhage. *Neurosurgery*, **15**, 50–6.

Breen, J. C., Caplan, L. R., DeWitt, L. D., *et al.* (1996). Brain edema after carotid surgery. *Neurology*, **46**, 175–81.

Dalman, J. E., Beenakkers, I. C., Moll, F. L., Leusink, J. A. and Ackerstaff, R. G. (1999). Transcranial Doppler monitoring during carotid endarterectomy helps to identify patients at risk of postoperative hyperperfusion. *European Journal of Vascular and Endovascular Surgery*, **18**, 222–7.

Derdeyn, C. P., Grubb, R. L. Jr. and Powers, W. J. (1999). Cerebral hemodynamic impairment: methods of measurement and association with stroke risk. *Neurology*, **53**, 251–9.

Grubb, R. L. Jr., Derdeyn, C. P., Fritsch, S. M., *et al.* (1998). Importance of hemodynamic factors in the prognosis of symptomatic carotid occlusion. *Journal of the American Medical Association*, **280**, 1055–60.

Harrison, P. B., Wong, M. J., Belzberg, A. and Holden, J. (1991). Hyperperfusion syndrome after carotid endarterectomy. CT changes. *Neuroradiology*, **33**, 106–10.

Henderson, R. D., Phan, T. G., Piepgras, D. G. and Wijdicks, E. F. (2001). Mechanisms of intracerebral hemorrhage after carotid endarterectomy. *Journal of Neurosurgery*, **95**, 964–9.

Holm, J., Nilsson, U., Waters, N., Waters, S. and Jonsson, O. (2001). Production of free radicals measured by spin trapping during operations for stenosis of the carotid artery. *European Journal of Surgery*, **167**, 4–9.

Hosoda, K., Kawaguchi, T., Shibata, Y., *et al.* (2001). Cerebral vasoreactivity and internal carotid artery flow help to identify patients at risk for hyperperfusion after carotid endarterectomy. *Stroke*, **32**, 1567–73.

Jansen, C., Sprengers, A. M., Moll, F. L., *et al.* (1994). Prediction of intracerebral haemorrhage after carotid endarterectomy by clinical criteria and intraoperative transcranial Doppler monitoring: results of 233 operations. *European Journal of Vascular Surgery*, **8**, 220–5.

Karibe, H., Chen, S. F., Zarow, G. J., *et al.* (1994). Mild intraischemic hypothermia suppresses consumption of endogenous antioxidants after temporary focal ischemia in rats. *Brain Research*, **27**, 12–18.

Klijn, C. J., Kappelle, L. J., van Huffelen, A. C., *et al.* (2000). Recurrent ischemia in symptomatic carotid occlusion: prognostic value of hemodynamic factors. *Neurology*, **55**, 1806–12.

Komoribayashi, N., Ogasawara, K., Kobayashi, M., *et al.* (2006). Cerebral hyperperfusion after carotid endarterectomy is associated with preoperative hemodynamic impairment and intraoperative cerebral ischemia. *Journal of Cerebral Blood Flow and Metabolism.*

Kuroda, S., Houkin, K., Kamiyama, H., *et al.* (2001). Long-term prognosis of medically treated patients with internal carotid or middle cerebral artery occlusion: Can acetazolamide test predict it? *Stroke*, **32**, 2110–16.

Kuroda, S., Kamiyama, H., Abe, H., *et al.* (1993). Acetazolamide test in detecting reduced cerebral perfusion reserve and predicting long-term prognosis in patients with internal carotid artery occlusion. *Neurosurgery*, **32**, 912–18.

Mansoor, G. A., White, W. B., Grunnet, M. and Ruby, S. T. (1996). Intracerebral hemorrhage after carotid endarterectomy associated with ipsilateral fibrinoid necrosis: a consequence of the hyperperfusion syndrome? *Journal of Vascular Surgery*, **23**, 147–51.

Nakano, S., Kinoshita, K., Jinnouchi, S., Hoshi, H. and Watanabe, K. (1989). Comparative study of regional cerebral blood flow images by SPECT using xenon-133, iodine-123 IMP, and technetium-99m HM-PAO. *Journal of Nuclear Medicine*, **30**, 157–64.

Norrving, B., Nilsson, B. and Risberg, J. (1982). rCBF in patients with carotid occlusion. Resting and hypercapnic flow related to collateral pattern. *Stroke*, **13**, 155–62.

Ogasawara, K., Inoue, T., Kobayashi, M., *et al.* (2004). Pretreatment with the free radical scavenger edaravone prevents cerebral hyperperfusion after carotid endarterectomy. *Neurosurgery*, **55**, 1060–7.

Ogasawara, K., Ito, H., Sasoh, M., *et al.* (2003a). Quantitative measurement of regional cerebrovascular reactivity to acetazolamide using 123I-N-isopropyl-p-iodoamphetamine autoradiography with SPECT: validation study using H2 15O with PET. *Journal of Nuclear Medicine*, **44**, 520–5.

Ogasawara, K., Kobayashi, M., Komoribayashi, N., *et al.* (2005). Transient crossed cerebellar diaschisis secondary to cerebral hyperperfusion following carotid endarterectomy. *Annals of Nuclear Medicine*, **19**, 321–4.

Ogasawara, K., Ogawa, A., Terasaki, K., *et al.* (2002a). Use of cerebrovascular reactivity in patients with symptomatic major cerebral artery occlusion to predict 5-year outcome: comparison of xenon-133 and iodine-123-IMP single-photon emission computed tomography. *Journal of Cerebral Blood Flow and Metabolism*, **22**, 1142–8.

Ogasawara, K., Ogawa, A. and Yoshimoto, T. (2002b). Cerebrovascular reactivity to acetazolamide and outcome in patients with symptomatic internal carotid or middle cerebral artery occlusion: a xenon-133 single-photon emission computed tomography study. *Stroke*, **33**, 1857–62.

Ogasawara, K., Okuguchi, T., Sasoh, M., *et al.* (2003b). Qualitative versus quantitative assessment of cerebrovascular reactivity to acetazolamide using iodine-123-N-isopropyl-p-iodoamphetamine SPECT in patients with unilateral major cerebral artery occlusive disease. *AJNR. American Journal of Neuroradiology*, **24**, 1090–5.

Ogasawara, K., Yukawa, H., Kobayashi, M., *et al.* (2003). Prediction and monitoring of cerebral hyperperfusion after carotid endarterectomy by using single-photon emission computerized tomography scanning. *Journal of Neurosurgery*, **99**, 504–10.

Ouriel, K., Shortell, C. K., Illig, K. A., Greenberg, R. K. and Green, R. M. (1999). Intracerebral hemorrhage after carotid endarterectomy: incidence, contribution to neurologic morbidity, and predictive factors. *Journal of Vascular Surgery*, **29**, 82–9.

Penn, A. A., Schomer, D. F. and Steinberg, G. K. (1995). Imaging studies of cerebral hyperperfusion after carotid endarterectomy: Case report. *Journal of Neurosurgery*, **83**, 133–7.

Phillis, J. W. and Sen, S. (1993). Oxypurinol attenuates hydroxyl radical production during ischemia/reperfusion injury of the rat cerebral cortex: an ESR study. *Brain Research*, **628**, 309–12.

Piepgras, D. G., Morgan, M. K., Sundt, T. M. Jr., Yanagihara, T. and Mussman, L. M. (1988). Intracerebral hemorrhage after carotid endarterectomy. *Journal of Neurosurgery*, **68**, 532–6.

Pomposelli, F. B., Lamparello, P. J., Riles, T. S., *et al.* (1988). Intracranial hemorrhage after carotid endarterectomy. *Journal of Vascular Surgery*, **7**, 248–55.

Powers, W. J., Press, G. A., Grubb, R. L. Jr., Gado, M. and Raichle, M. E. (1987). The effect of hemodynamically significant carotid artery disease on the hemodynamic status of the cerebral circulation. *Annals of Internal Medicine*, **106**, 27–34.

Reigel, M. M., Hollier, L. H., Sundt, T. M. Jr., *et al.* (1987). Cerebral hyperperfusion syndrome: a cause of neurologic dysfunction after carotid endarterectomy. *Journal of Vascular Surgery*, **5**, 628–34.

Riles, T. S., Imparato, A. M., Jacobowitz, G. R., *et al.* (1994). The cause of perioperative stroke after carotid endarterectomy. *Journal of Vascular Surgery*, **19**, 206–16.

Schroeder, T., Sillesen, H., Boesen, J., Laursen, H. and Sorensen, P. (1987). Intracerebral hemorrhage after carotid endarterectomy. *European Journal of Vascular Surgery*, **1**, 51–60.

Shinno, K., Ueda, S., Uno, M., *et al.* (1998). Hyperperfusion syndrome following carotid endarterectomy: evaluation using diffusion-weighted magnetic resonance imaging – case report. *Neurologia Medico-Chirurgica, (Tokyo)*, **38**, 557–61.

Solomon, R. A., Loftus, C. M., Quest, D. O. and Correll, J. W. (1986). Incidence and etiology of intracerebral hemorrhage following carotid endarterectomy. *Journal of Neurosurgery*, **64**, 29–34.

Soong, C. V., Young, I. S., Hood, J. M., *et al.* (1996). The generation of byproducts of lipid peroxidation following carotid endarterectomy. *European Journal of Vascular and Endovascular Surgery*, **12**, 455–8.

Spetzler, R. F., Wilson, C. B., Weinstein, P., *et al.* (1978). Normal perfusion pressure breakthrough theory. *Clinical Neurosurgery*, **25**, 651–72.

Sundt, T. M. Jr., Sharbrough, F. W., Piepgras, D. G., *et al.* (1981). Correlation of cerebral blood flow and electroencephalographic changes during carotid endarterectomy: with results of surgery and hemodynamics of cerebral ischemia. *Mayo Clinic Proceedings*, **56**, 533–43.

The Edaravone Acute Brain Infarction Study Group. (2003). Effect of a novel free radical scavenger, edaravone (MCI-186), on acute brain infarction: randomized, placebo-controlled, double-blind study at multicenters. *Cerebrovascular Disease*, **15**, 222–9.

Weigand, M. A., Laipple, A., Plaschke, K., *et al.* (1999). Concentration changes of malondialdehyde across the cerebral vascular bed and shedding of L-selectin during carotid endarterectomy. *Stroke*, **30**, 306–11.

Widder, B., Kleiser, B. and Krapf, H. (1994). Course of cerebrovascular reactivity in patients with carotid artery occlusions. *Stroke*, **25**, 1963–7.

Yamauchi, H., Fukuyama, H., Kimura, J., Konishi, J. and Kameyama, M. (1990). Hemodynamics in internal carotid artery occlusion examined by positron emission tomography. *Stroke*, **21**, 1400–6.

Yamauchi, H., Fukuyama, H., Nagahama, Y., *et al.* (1996). Evidence of misery perfusion and risk for recurrent stroke in major cerebral arterial occlusive diseases from PET. *Journal of Neurology, Neurosurgery and Psychiatry*, **61**, 18–25.

Yokota, C., Hasegawa, Y., Minematsu, K. and Yamaguchi, T. (1998). Effect of acetazolamide reactivity on corrected long-term outcome in patients with major cerebral artery occlusive diseases. *Stroke*, **29**, 640–4.

Yonas, H., Pindzola, R. R., Meltzer, C. C. and Sasser, H. (1998). Qualitative versus quantitative assessment of cerebrovascular reserves. *Neurosurgery*, **42**, 1005–10.

Yoshimoto, T., Houkin, K., Kuroda, S., Abe, H. and Kashiwaba, T. (1997). Low cerebral blood flow and perfusion reserve induce hyperperfusion after surgical revascularization: case reports and analysis of cerebral hemodynamics. *Surgical Neurology*, **48**, 132–9.

29

Monitoring carotid interventions with xenon CT

Andrew Carlson and Howard Yonas

University of New Mexico, Albuquerque NM, USA

Introduction

Our knowledge of cerebral hemodynamics during carotid occlusion is derived from several pathophysiologically different clinical situations understood via myriad imaging and assessment modalities. This leads to what, at the outset, seems to be a vast and conflicting body of literature regarding the field. Our goal here is first, to carefully explore the physiologic information gained in these various clinical situations and second, to apply these principles, in so far as the available evidence allows, to patient care. It is important to understand that each of these disparate situations and technologies seek to offer some insight into the large picture of how cerebral blood flow (CBF) responds to various challenges. By focusing too closely on the minutia of any particular situation or technology without incorporating the alternate perspectives offered by other situations or technologies, one runs the risk of losing understanding of this larger picture.

There are two clinical scenarios in which we have gained our most extensive understanding of cerebral hemodynamics in relation to carotid occlusion. One is when the carotid artery is intentionally occluded as a test of tolerance to permanent occlusion (balloon test occlusion or BTO). The other involves the study of patients that present with chronic carotid occlusion who are objects of study in order to assess their risk for future stroke. Patients undergoing BTO are initially asymptomatic and temporary occlusion of the carotid provides the most "pure" study of cerebral hemodynamics – i.e. the physiological response to an abrupt carotid occlusion. The patient found with a symptomatic carotid occlusion and without a massive infarction has undergone hemodynamic adaptation and our measurements are directed at understanding the degree of hemodynamic compromise that may persist. Between these extremes are many examples including occlusion in acute carotid dissection, cross-clamping during carotid endarterectomy and the response to a progressive reduction of perfusion pressure.

Many methods have been and are currently used to assess cerebral hemodynamics. They vary from neurological examination during BTO to specialized technology available at only a few centers. During BTO, it is necessary to determine if the CBF to a given region is adequate to maintain brain function not only at the moment but also during subsequent subtle challenges such as may occur during sleep with blood pressure reduction and CO_2 retention. Simple technologies include measuring the clinical response to the tilt table, blood pressure reduction, or BTO. Electroencephalogram (EEG) may be a correlated technology, measuring gross brain activity. Direct measurements of CBF by [133]xenon or stable xenon computerized tomography (CT) or other methods appear to be the most reliable measure of the adequacy of flow. Other techniques including transcranial Doppler (TCD), cerebral

Carotid Disease: The Role of Imaging in Diagnosis and Management, ed. Jonathan Gillard, Martin Graves, Thomas Hatsukami and Chun Yuan. Published by Cambridge University Press. © Cambridge University Press 2007.

angiography, and various types of magnetic reso-nance imaging (MRI) are proxy measures for this value. For a thorough review of the various brain perfusion technologies available with comparison and specific descriptions, the reader is referred to an excellent recent review article (Wintermark et al., 2005).

The gold standard for understanding the extent of hemodynamic compromise involves the measurement of multiple metabolic parameters with positron emission tomography (PET). PET measures CBF and several variables that are interrelated in a consistent and predictable manner to decreasing perfusion pressure. During progressive chronic occlusion, CBF is initially maintained as the perfusion pressure falls due to vasodilation that results in an increase of cerebral blood volume (CBV). Only when perfusion pressure continues to fall after a maximum CBV is reached does the CBF begin to fall (loss of autoregulation) and metabolism is maintained by a progressive rise of the tissue oxygen extraction fraction (OEF). Metabolism becomes compromised only when CBF falls below the ischemic threshold of about 18 cc/100 gm/min at which point OEF is maximal and unable to maintain metabolism (cerebral rate of metabolism of oxygen or glucose $CMRO_2$/CMRGlu) (Powers et al., 1987).

Because PET using radiolabeled oxygen (required for the aforementioned measurements) is an expensive technology that is not widely available, alternate methodologies and strategies are employed to attempt to arrive at similar observations. One common strategy utilizes the response of a flow measurement to a vasodilatory challenge. Assuming that CBV has become maxi-mal, a test that increases tissue acidosis would demonstrate no significant increase of flow in a compromised area but a normal vasodilatory response elsewhere. This response can be measured in many different ways, either using quantitative values or various ratios of reduction compared to baseline or to normal tissue, therefore leading to seemingly conflicting and inconsistent results.

We must, however, remember that the wide view of our subject matter does assemble into a cohesive whole, and though results may seem confusing or conflicting, we must carefully try to understand the specifics of the clinical scenario and the specific modality being used in order to better fit these results into our growing corpus of knowledge.

Balloon Test Occlusion

Introduction

The study of the clinical tolerance to trial carotid occlusion combined with an examination of the associated changes of cerebral hemodynamics has been driven by the need to more accurately risk-stratify patients in whom sacrifice of the carotid artery is being considered. Several neck and skull-base pathologies require consideration of carotid sacrifice including: vascular problems such as intercavernous internal carotid artery (ICA) aneurysms, giant intracranial aneurysms, carotid-cavernous fistula, or some carotid dissections; neoplasia involving the neck, ICA, or skull base; or trauma resulting in uncontrollable hemorrhage (American Society of Interventional and Therapeutic Neuroradiology, 2001). Based on extensive review of case series, neurologic morbid-ity and mortality is high for sacrifice of the ICA if no selection criteria are employed, with estimates around 25% (Linskey et al., 1994; Reilly, 1995) for infarction and 12% for death (Linskey et al., 1994). In addition, these rates may vary between various surgical or endovascular methods of carotid occlu-sion (Standard et al., 1995). Many methods and modalities have been used to assess cerebral hemodynamics in order to improve the safety of occlusion. Patients who fail test occlusion and are believed to be at high risk for subsequent stroke have benefited from extracranial-intracranial (EC-IC) bypass (Barnett et al., 1994, Field et al., 2003).

The earliest tests of a patient's ability to tolerate carotid occlusion were based on manual compression of the common carotid artery and clinical indicators (Matas, 1911). Currently, endovascular occlusion of the internal carotid with an intraarterial balloon is the standard method (Field *et al.*, 2003). Recent evidence suggests that a clinical BTO exam may not be sensitive enough to reliably predict ischemic event following occlusion (Marshall *et al.*, 2002), though the preferred secondary modality is controversial. An understanding of cerebral hemodynamics during BTO is key to understanding the validity of these various modalities.

Cerebral physiology in occlusion

Normal CBF is around 54 cc/100 gm/min, with a standard deviation of 12 cc/100 gm/min (Yonas *et al.*, 1991). Patients with regional CBF values that fall with BTO from normal to between 20 and 30 cc/100 gm/min are below normal limits, but above the ischemic threshold. The vascular region that experiences a fall of flow into this range is presumed to be experiencing a failure of autoregulation with CBV being maximal and OEF being near maximum. These patients are believed to be at higher risk of postocclusion infarct, presumably due to inadequate circle of Willis collateral flow (Witt *et al.*, 1994; Marshall *et al.*, 2002). Though these values were initially thought to be somewhat relative, current evidence suggests that absolute values in this range are independent predictors for stroke (Marshall *et al.*, 2002). In addition, autoregulation predicts that decreasing cerebral perfusion pressure (CPP) causes reflex vasodilation in order to maintain CBF. This response has been well characterized after BTO by observing significant decrease in CBF by [133]xenon flow (Gupta *et al.*, 2002) and decreased pulsatility index by TCD (Bhattacharjee *et al.*, 1999). Around 40 mmHg, the vasculature no longer responds to the vasodilatory challenge of acetazolamide and probably represents the state of maximal autoregulatory dilation (Okudaira *et al.*, 1996).

Patients can be generally divided into three groups based on CBF response to BTO. Around 5–10% of patients will be unable to tolerate even brief occlusion without developing a focal neurological deficit and will predictably suffer stroke with permanent carotid occlusion. These patients presumably have regional CBF to levels less than 20 cc/100 gm/min. Another 10–15% will tolerate clinical occlusion, but retain CBF values between 20 and 30 cc/100 gm/min. These patients have a marginal hemodynamic status and though they may be able to tolerate occlusion for some period of time, any metabolic or hemodynamic challenge will likely lead to transient ischemic attack (TIA) or stroke. The final 80% are likely to be at low risk for infarction after occlusion (Linskey *et al.*, 1994).

Despite these generalizations, there remains a great deal of variability in the individual patient's CBF response to BTO. Witt *et al.* (1994) analyzed quantitative CBF data obtained with Xenon CT CBF technology prior to and during BTO, and classified 11 separate response patterns based on symmetry and degree of CBF change after BTO. This type of evaluation is relevant because qualitative assessments of CBF are far more widely available and utilized than quantitative studies. Only 27% of patients had no baseline asymmetry and postocclusion asymmetry with lower values on the side ipsilateral to the occlusion (the most expected response, and that which both qualitative and quantitative measurements can detect). Many patients, however exhibited quite different responses, ranging from baseline asymmetry and lower CBF on the ipsilateral side (18%), to no asymmetry at any stage (19%), to various responses with contralateral decreased CBF (6% after occlusion, 18% baseline, and 10% during occlusion and at baseline). The errors associated with qualitative data are most evident in the cases in which asymmetry developed due to a rise of flow on the nonoccluded side or due to the symmetric but significant drop of flow. The former would be labeled as abnormal and the latter as normal. In conclusion, regions that develop a reduction of flow to the 20–30 cc/100 gm/min range, as only detected with quantitative CBF, were only marginally related to asymmetry values derived by a qualitative assessment of symmetry. The causes postulated for these varying responses to BTO are myriad and include occlusive vascular disease, congenital variants of the circle of Willis collateral channels, autonomic changes in the vasculature, small vessel disease, vasospasm, or other intracranial pathology such as tumor influences. In addition, normal CBF values are likely to be reduced in the aging population (Linskey *et al.*, 1994). TCD velocity data supports this observed wide variability in responses (Eckert *et al.*, 1998).

Response to occlusion also likely varies temporally as various adaptive processes develop. Some patients with impaired collateral will initially have a dramatic ipsilateral CBF reduction, but flow will improve despite persistent occlusion at different rates (Barker *et al.*, 1993; Eckert *et al.*, 1998). After BTO, there may be a transient hyperemic period as autoregulation responds to the increased flow (Gupta *et al.*, 2002). This phenomenon has also been observed during carotid clamping in carotid endarterectomy as discussed later (Pascazio *et al.*, 1999). Late onset of neurologic symptoms after BTO has been described. It is unclear whether these are related to delayed hemodynamic aberrations or vascular injury that resulted in the immediate or delayed development of emboli (Eckert *et al.*, 1998).

Despite the fact that most patients who fail BTO will either not have carotid sacrifice or will have extracranial-intracranial (EC-IC) bypass, there are still strokes found in outcome studies. The patterns and timing of infarction are illustrative of the disordered hemodynamics present. Marshall *et al.* (2002) report that all strokes in patients failing BTO ($n = 7$) occurred ipsilateral to the occlusion, but that only one appeared to represent a "borderzone" infarction. Two occurred at greater than 1 month from occlusion. Another series reported 20% immediate infarct, 60% in 48 hours, and 20% later than 48 hours (Reilly, 1995). It is thought that this late infarct population represents patients with CBF in the 20–30 cc/100 gm/min group who have minimal cerebrovascular reserve and severely diminished flow pulsatility. In this situation, even

minor changes such as transient hypoxia, hypotension, or hypercarbia, all of which can occur in patients with sleep apnea, can be a cause for infarction. With a diminution of pulsatility even a microembolus can cause a cessation of flow and infarction. The various methods which exist to attempt to identify this high-risk subgroup will be discussed in the next section.

Methods of prediction of stroke after carotid sacrifice

Though performing BTO with clinical examination has been shown to significantly reduce morbidity and mortality from carotid occlusion compared to untested controls (Linskey *et al.*, 1994), it is nonetheless imperfect. Clinical examination alone has been shown to have a negative predictive value (NPV) 70% and positive predictive value (PPV) 33% (Marshall *et al.*, 2002). The same study showed that a more sustained attention test increases these values to NPV of 90% and decreases to PPV 25%. These values excluded patients who were felt to be at high risk "primarily by clinical criteria" who received EC-IC bypass. The addition of a secondary cerebrometabolic challenge such as induced hypotension may increase the sensitivity of the clinical exam (Standard *et al.*, 1995; Field *et al.*, 2003), though it is also not ideal. False negative tests have been reported in which strokes subsequently developed despite hypotensive BTO with clinical examination (rate 15%) (Dare *et al.*, 1998). Table 29.1 summarizes the clinical outcome-based studies assessing stroke risk by various modalities.

Clearly patients who cannot clinically tolerate BTO should not undergo carotid sacrifice without EC-IC bypass. To identify who among the remaining group is at moderate risk, quantitative CBF measurements have shown the best utility. Marshall reported the largest series of patients who did not fail clinical testing but demonstrated CBF < 30 cc/100 gm/min who still had permanent occlusion. Five out of 12 patients with CBF < 30 cc/100 gm/min had stroke while 0/11 with higher

Table 29.1. Results of studies assessing ischemic outcome after balloon test occlusion

Study	N	Population	Mean follow-up	Protocol for failure	Technique (n)	Stroke/high-risk patients with patent EC-IC bypass (PPV)	Stroke/high-risk patients without EC-IC bypass	Stroke/low-risk patients (NPV)	Comments
Field, 2003	26	Cavernous sinus aneurysm. All passed clinical BTO	15.3 m	EC-IC bypass for clinical failure or CBF <30 mL/100 g/m	Quantitative Xe CT CBF	1/8	0/0	0/16 (100%)	
Marshall, 2002	33	Aneurysm (30), Tumor (1), Trauma (2)	34 m	EC-IC if failure "Primarily by clinical criteria" (excluded from further analysis)	Standard clinical testing (33); Sustained attention testing (18); Quantitative 133Xe CBF (23)	1/8 (graft failure); 0/0; 0/0	1/7 (33%); 2/8 (25%); 5/12 (42%)	7/23 (70%); 1/10 (90%); 0/11 (100%)	Only trial to intentionally occlude patients with BTO failure
Van Rooij, 2000	29	Large or giant carotid aneurysm	21 m	EC-IC offered if clinical failure or venous phase asymmetry	Clinical, EEG (4); Clinical, angiography for venous phase asymmetry (25)	0/0; 0/4	0/0; 1/1 (100%)	2/4 (50%); 0/17 (100%)	
Standard, 1995	47	Aneurysm (36), tumor (5), head/neck carcinoma (6)	? (longest reported 5m)	One patient with EC-IC bypass, remainder no occlusion	Hypotensive challenge	0/1	1/1 (occluded in error) (100%)	1/19 (95%)	No long-term follow-up
Larson, 1995	58	ICA aneurysm	76 m	EC-IC offered for clinical failure or perfusion asymmetry	Clinical, some with hypotension; HMPAO SPECT (10)	0/1; 1/1	0/0; 0/0	11/55 (80%)	Numbers not separately reported for SPECT or hypotension. Strokes and mortality reported separately.

Table 29.1. (cont.)

Study	N	Population	Mean follow-up	Protocol for failure	Technique (n)	Stroke/high-risk patients with patent EC-IC bypass (PPV)	Stroke/high-risk patients without EC-IC bypass (PPV)	Stroke/low-risk patients (NPV)	Comments
Linskey, 1994	30	Vascular (14), cavernous sinus neoplasm (9), cervical neoplasm (7), temporal bone neoplasm (1)	1.3 y	No occlusion unless emergency	Clinical, quantitative Xe CT CBF	0/0	1/1 (100%)	3/30 (90%)	Only one of the strokes in the negative group was clinically significant, two additional strokes thought to be unrelated
Brunberg, 1994	20	Aneurysm or skull base tumor	? (short-term)	Only one failure, occluded due to emergency	Quantitative PET CBF	0/0	1/1 (100%)	0/8 (100%)	
Vazquez Anon, 1992	40	Giant intracavernous aneurysm	4.7 y	EC-IC if failure unless emergency	Clinical, angiogram (all), 133 Xe (13), TCD (10)	0/5	3/3 (100%)	1/35 (97%)	Only false negative was screened by angiogram and thought to be embolic. It resolved with anticoagulation.

values did. By multivariate analysis, CBF < 30 cc/ 100 gm/min was the only factor independently associated with stroke. Recommendations from this study for BTO protocol consist of 30-minute BTO with 15 minutes of normotension and 15 minutes of induced hypotension to 60–70% of baseline mean arterial pressure (MAP). If neurologic signs or CBF < 30 cc/100 gm/min is observed at any time, EC-IC bypass with repeat BTO after is indicated (Marshall *et al.*, 2002). This method was then prospectively cross-validated in a homogeneous population of patients with cavernous sinus aneurysms. Field *et al.*, 2003 used EC-IC to bypass all patients who failed clinical BTO or showed CBF < 30 cc/100 gm/min by xenon CT CBF. Again, no patients with CBF > 30 cc/100 gm/min had stroke, while 1/8 patients in the moderate-risk group who all had EC-IC bypass developed late onset ischemia. PET using oxygen15-labeled H_2O has also been used to identify CBF 25–35 cc/ 100 gm/min and negative results seem to safely identify low-risk patients (Brunberg *et al.*, 1994). Though small study populations, these studies show the potentially significant impact of using quantitative flow methodologies.

Other imaging modalities which are more widely available have been used with varying success. Single positron emission computed tomography (SPECT) imaging using labeled radionucleotides such as Tc-99m L,L-ethyl cysteinate dimer (Tc-99m EDC) or Tc-99m hexamethyl propyleneamine oxime (Tc-99m HMPAO) report positive results. Advantages are the wide availability and speed of results, though these methods have been criticized due to the inherent qualitative nature of the values they yield – either relative to preocclusion values or contralateral hemispheric values (Marshall *et al.*, 2002). Witt (1994) demonstrated that an asymmetry index of 10% as commonly employed in SPECT studies showed 16% specificity for areas of CBF < 30 cc/100 gm/min while an index of 45% was needed to attain a 61% sensitivity. Additionally, none of these methods have yet to be prospectively validated with any outcome studies. Most examine only correlation with clinical symptomatology.

The largest study used primarily clinical criteria, but added HMPAO SPECT late in the study period. No breakdown was given of this small group (Larson *et al.*, 1995). Other very small studies report positive results with these relative changes (Peterman *et al.*, 1991; Eckard *et al.*, 1992; Larson *et al.*, 1995; Yamamoto *et al.*, 2002) though there was no control for comparison. In addition, other clinical studies show poor predictive value of these methods (Monsein *et al.*, 1991; Origitano *et al.*, 1994).

TCD monitoring has also been used to assess cerebral hemodynamics during BTO. Advantages include accessibility and the ability to monitor values continuously, which may detect delayed changes or adaptation not otherwise observable (Eckert *et al.*, 1998). Disadvantages include wide patient-to-patient variability of normal values and reliance on relative values. Estimates for critical reduction in mean blood flow velocity (MBFV) range from 30 to 65% (Giller *et al.*, 1994; Eckert *et al.*, 1998). Eckert reported no complications with MBFV and pulsatility index reductions of < 30% and symptoms in all patients with reductions > 50%. Though TCD values have been correlated with CBF values (Kofke *et al.*, 1995), other data only show moderate correlation of TCD values with angiographic findings (Hetzel *et al.*, 2000) or even with clinical exam (Giller *et al.*, 1994). Despite the questionable ability of TCD to detect hemodynamic changes, currently the primary drawback is lack of outcome assessment.

Direct vascular assessments such as patency of collateral vessels or carotid stump pressure provide insight into hemodynamics, but their ability to adequately predict high-risk subgroups has not been confirmed. One study incorporated angiogram for collateral patency in addition to [133]xenon CT but there was no independent assessment of its utility (Vazquez Anon *et al.*, 1992). The largest study using angiography measured venous phase asymmetry as a proxy measure of collateral flow and found good initial results (no strokes in 17 patients deemed low risk) (van Rooij *et al.*, 2000). Assessing the carotid stump pressure as a measure of collateral circulation and ability to tolerate permanent carotid occlusion is attractive due to the ease of testing and the intuitive nature of the test. Experimentally, however, this has proven to be an unreliable measure. Conflicting results are observed with stump pressure as it relates to asymmetry. By Tc-99m HMPAO SPECT (Morishima *et al.*, 1998; Kaminogo *et al.*, 1999) stump pressure < 40 mmHg may correlate with decreased regional oxygen saturation, though there is no prospective clinical validation of this utility. Using xenon CT CBF, though there was a significant association between a reduced stump pressure and compromised flow, the range of values was too wide to be of clinical utility (Steed *et al.*, 1990; Barker *et al.*, 1993).

Finally, many additional technologies have been employed; some with potential promise, but these tests have no prospective outcome validation, and often seek validation via other measurements which may themselves have serious limitations. For example, local oxygenation as measured by near infrared spectroscopy has been correlated with lower stump pressures (Takeda *et al.*, 2000) and with asymmetry on Tc-99m HMPAO SPECT (Kaminogo *et al.*, 1999). Also, crossed cerebellar diaschisis may be associated with HMPAO SPECT abnormalities (Nathan *et al.*, 1994). Finally, EEG has been used, but shows only changes in brain function, which have poor and late correlation with CBF patterns (Morioka *et al.*, 1989; Origitano *et al.*, 1994). In one series it was only able to detect patients with clinical symptoms (Herkes *et al.*, 1993), while another reported both a false positive and a false negative compared to clinical exam (Cloughesy *et al.*, 1993). These studies clearly do not currently offer enough evidence to incorporate their use into routine clinical practice.

Technical notes

Field's protocol used 7000-U intravenous heparin during balloon catheter insertion, and daily aspirin (325 mg) started 24 hours after occlusion and continued for life. A variety of catheters exist, and

the shape of the balloon is key for preserving vessel integrity. Excessive inflation may damage the intima while under inflation risks not completely occluding flow. Distal injection of heparinized saline is also now common practice during the BTO to avoid emboli. In addition, the test location should be the same as the permanent occlusion location to avoid unexpected collateral flow or differing hemodynamic response (Field *et al.*, 2003). Placing the occlusion distal to collateral circulation is necessary to achieve complete stagnation of flow – essential in order to promote clot maturation without embolism.

Complications of temporary BTO are not negligible, but are acceptable given the benefit of identification of patients unable to tolerate permanent sacrifice. Relatively early experience from the University of Pittsburgh showed an overall procedural complication rate of 3.2% in 500 patients. Only 1.6% were symptomatic and 0.4% had permanent neurologic deficit. Advances in endovascular technology and technique undoubtedly continuously increase the safety of this procedure.

Symptomatic carotid occlusion

Introduction

Though a landmark randomized surgical trial showed that when all patients with symptomatic ICA or middle cerebral artery (MCA) stenosis or occlusion were randomized to EC-IC bypass (1985), that there was no demonstrable benefit of the bypass procedure, symptomatic carotid occlusion, however, is associated with a severely elevated subsequent stroke risk and patients with ICA and MCA stenosis remained at high risk for both embolic and hemodynamic stroke. Clearly, even patients with only carotid occlusion may have a heterogeneous hemodynamic response to occlusion, primarily dependent upon the quality of the collateral supply available via the circle of Willis at the time of occlusion and perhaps dependent upon the duration of time available for additional collateral development. Fortunately, a number of measurements of cerebral hemodynamics have evolved in the past two decades making it now possible to identify a high-risk subgroup for whom bypass surgery may still have a therapeutic role. This group can only be defined based on a better understanding of cerebral hemodynamics rather than by angiographic definition of vascular anatomy.

Cerebral physiology in symptomatic carotid occlusion

Parametric studies of cerebral hemodynamics in patients with symptomatic carotid occlusion have defined a predictable and progressive series of compensatory mechanisms designed to prevent ischemic injury despite a fall of blood pressure. First, an autoregulatory dilation occurs in response to decreasing CPP thereby maintaining CBF (stage I). Second, OEF is increased in response to failure of autoregulation and decreasing CBF thereby maintaining $CMRO_2$ and tissue function (stage II). Stage III occurs with the failure of the remaining circulation to maintain metabolism so that metabolic parameters ($CMRO_2$ and CMRglu) begin to fall associated with the onset of neurological deficit (Powers et al., 1989; Derdeyn et al., 1999) (Figure 29.1). What has been learned over the past two decades is that patients can persist in stage II for extended periods of time leaving them susceptible to small potentially cumulative injuries that can occur with even mild transient hemodynamic challenges.

Currently the OEF only derived by specially equipped PET facilities has become the measurement upon which many authorities have based the study of both the selection of high-risk patients as well as the study of the possible efficacy of bypass surgery (Derdeyn et al., 2002; Grubb et al., 2003; Yamauchi et al., 2004). The COSS (carotid occlusion surgery study) is in fact a multicenter, randomized, controlled trial currently underway to test this hypothesis (Grubb et al., 2003). While the

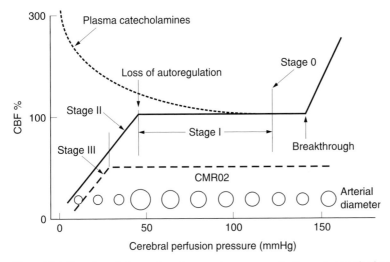

Figure 29.1 Overview of stages of cerebrovascular response to decreasing cerebral perfusion pressure. Stage I: autoregulatory vasodilation. Cerebral blood volume increases while metabolism is preserved. Stage II: failure of autoregulation. Oxygen extraction fraction increases to maintain metabolism. Stage III: threshold for tissue adaptation is exceeded and metabolism begins to fall. Catecholamines increase dramatically. (Reproduced from Nemoto et al. (2004) *Journal of Cerebral Blood Flow Metabolism*, **24**, 1081–9.) (CBF = cerebral blood flow; $CMRO_2$ = cerebral rate of metabolism of oxygen.)

St. Louis Stroke Study established that an elevated OEF indicates a patient at increased ischemic risk (Grubb *et al.*, 1998), the fact that even a small stroke in the deep white will be associated with a fall of OEF despite no improvement in the degree of hemodynamic compromise makes it necessary for the sensitivity and specificity of OEF to be better defined (Kuroda *et al.*, 2006 in press). This means that OEF is a biphasic measurement with both a rise and a fall, potentially despite a progression of the hemodynamic compromise (Figure 29.2). The importance of these observations is apparent from an examination of the data from the St. Louis Carotid Trial that reported that while an elevated CBV was predictive of an increased stroke rate that an elevated OEF with a normal CBV was not (Derdeyn *et al.*, 2002). This state at the end of stage II insufficiency has been termed marginal ischemia (Nemoto *et al.*, 2004) or matched hypometabolism (Kuroda *et al.*, 2006 in press). Additionally, these changes are probably variable depending on the course of occlusion (acute vs. chronic). As the tissue descends into ischemic territory, increasing levels of circulating plasma catecholamines have been observed to accompany the rise in $CMRO_2$ (Nemoto *et al.*, 2004).

A powerful, potentially widely available alternative method for assessing hemodynamic stress has proven to be the indirect assessment of chemoregulatory state by measuring the cerebral vasodilatory response (CVR) to acetazolamide or CO_2. Many modalities exist to measure these changes and the reproducibility and applicability for stroke prediction will be discussed in the next section. Three responses representing various stages of hemodynamic failure are observed with vasodilatory challenge (Derdeyn *et al.*, 1999): first, the CVR may be decreased compared to normal controls. This situation represents the cerebral vasculature nearing the end of the autoregulatory curve. Second, there may be no response to vasodilatory challenge indicating that maximal vasodilation has been achieved. Third, there may be a paradoxical reduction in flow compared to baseline. This "steal" phenomenon is likely due to vasculature

which is maximally dilated and dependent upon blood supply via pial collaterals from adjacent vascular territories (Yonas *et al.*, 1997). The changes of CVR are monophasic throughout the full range of hemodynamic compromise ranging from positive to negative values in contrast to the biphasic rise and fall of OEF near the end of adaptation (Figure 29.2) (Nemoto *et al.*, 2004).

This biphasic response is controversial, but both intuitive and supported by developing evidence. As tissue begins to fail and metabolism falls off in stage III, it stands to reason that the adaptive capacity of oxygen extraction would likewise fall off. Several recent studies support this hypothesis with observed "normal" OEF values in patients expected to be in advanced hemodynamic failure by measurement of CVR (Nemoto *et al.*, 2004; Kuroda *et al.*, 2006 in press). In addition, preliminary work has started to explore the dynamic nature of OEF. Correlation is observed between the CBF response to vasodilatory challenge (acetazolamide), and OEF reactivity to a similar challenge ($p = 0.0001$) (Nemoto *et al.*, 2004). The implications of this observation are powerful. As OEF falls, when measured as a "snapshot" by PET, theoretically normal values could in fact be demonstrating severe stage II disease progressing into stage III (Kuroda *et al.*, 2006 in press). At baseline, OEF may or may not be related to CVR as one study found no relationship (Nemoto *et al.*, 2004) and another found a weak, nonlinear relationship ($p = 0.02$) (Yamauchi *et al.*, 2004). Despite these correlations, it is important to point out that OEF varies significantly within the normal range from somewhere around 30–50%, impeding the ability to make strong linear associations.

Metabolic response of the brain in symptomatic carotid occlusion has also been characterized by MR spectroscopy. Ipsilateral to the occlusion, decreased N-acetyl aspartate (NAA) levels have been observed in comparison to the unaffected side and to defined normal controls (Rutgers *et al.*, 2003). These changes have also been correlated with changes in $CMRO_2$ (Tsuchida *et al.*, 2000). This may indicate neuronal loss and may also be

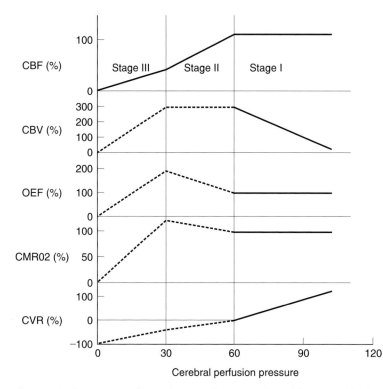

Figure 29.2 The response of several commonly measured variables to steadily decreasing cerebral perfusion pressure. Note the biphasic response of oxygen extraction fraction (OEF) during the transition from stage II to stage III compared to the monophasic (though negative) decrease in CVR indicating steal. (Reproduced from Nemoto *et al.* (2004) *Journal of Cerebral Blood Flow and Metabolism*, **24**, 1081–9.) (CBF = cerebral blood flow; CBV = cerebral blood volume; CMRO$_2$ = cerebral rate of metabolism of oxygen; CVR = cerebral vasodilatory response.)

related to neurologic symptoms, as asymptomatic patients do not show this decrease (Lythgoe *et al.*, 2001). Interestingly, this decrease in NAA is independent of cerebral perfusion or vasoreactivity. In addition, concentrations of choline and creatinine are not affected in these long-term symptomatic patients (which is an important observation as several studies have used various ratios to describe these metabolic changes). It is hypothesized that in the setting of subacute occlusion or infarct that these metabolites would correlate with cerebral perfusion (Rutgers *et al.*, 2003).

Over a period of time, there is clearly adaptation to the state of carotid occlusion. Empiric evidence

for this is both observational and experimental. First, strokes tend to occur during the first 6 months after symptoms begin (Widder *et al.*, 1994; Ogasawara *et al.*, 2002). It has also been shown that CVR may return to normal levels over a period of months to years in patients with symptomatic occlusion and no stroke (Ogasawara *et al.*, 2002). This is probably related to the formation of collateral flow either via the circle of Willis, ophthalmic artery, or leptomeningeal vessels. In general, flow via the circle of Willis is considered the primary channel, and with failure of this route, collaterals may form via the ophthalmic artery or leptomeningeal vessels (Powers *et al.*, 1987). Flow reversal across the anterior communicating artery is seen frequently in carotid occlusion (82%), as is collateral flow via the ophthalmic artery (74%) (Tan *et al.*, 2002). Apruzzese *et al.*, 2001 observed that CBF as observed by contrast-enhanced MRI is higher in grey matter than white matter ipsilateral to the occlusion, hypothesizing that grey matter has more ready access to adjacent pial collaterals. CO_2 reactivity has been shown to change over time, and is one reason hypothesized as to why investigators have found disparate results regarding its ability to predict stroke (Klijn *et al.*, 2000).

Observation of the regional patterns of stroke in carotid occlusion also lends further understanding to the hemodynamic response and patterns in carotid occlusion. Carotid occlusion has been associated with infarcts in the external border zone (or territorial watershed areas), internal border zone (the white matter of the centrum semiovale and corona radiata), and also major vascular territories (Bisschops *et al.*, 2003). Territorial infarcts are usually from thrombotic sources, and though associated with stenosis and occlusion, are more variable (Klijn *et al.*, 2000). Advanced hemodynamic compromise, on the other hand, significantly increases the prevalence of infarcts in the so called "internal border zones" presumably between the cortical and periventricular penetrating vessels. Decreased CO_2 or acetazolamide reactivity has been associated with infarcts in the internal border zone (Isaka *et al.*, 1997; Bisschops *et al.*, 2003) and Firlik *et al.* (1997) demonstrated a maximal steal phenomenon in the deep white matter. These have been described as small (<1.5 cm) "rosarylike" lesions in the centrum semiovale (Krapf *et al.*, 1998). An additional area lateral to the ventricles, possibly representing the same internal border zone, has been associated with increased OEF (Derdeyn *et al.*, 2001a). A proposed alternative mechanism for these internal border zone infarcts is impaired washout of microemboli which form in an ulcerated lesion, an occluded stump, or from various flow and vessel aberrations. These would normally be able to be cleared by adequate CPP, but in advanced hemodynamic compromise, become lodged in the above mentioned areas and cannot be cleared.

Predicting stroke in symptomatic carotid occlusion

Studies assessing stroke risk stratification have used varying modalities and have been heterogeneous in terms of methodology and participants, though two primary modalities have demonstrated promising data. The most widely accepted method is measurement of increased OEF by PET (stage II hemodynamic insufficiency). Several major prospective studies have positively correlated increased OEF values with stroke risk (Yamauchi *et al.*, 1996, 1999; Grubb *et al.*, 1998; Derdeyn *et al.*, 2002). Yamauchi's (Yamauchi *et al.*, 1996) study measured quantitative values for OEF but was limited by a heterogeneous patient population and high exclusion rate (Derdeyn *et al.*, 1999), though showed stroke in 4/7 patients with increased OEF compared to 2/33 without. Five-year follow-up of this group revealed stroke in 5/7 patients with increased OEF and 6/33 without. Relative risk for all stroke was 7.2 (95% CI 2.0–25.5) and ipsilateral stroke was 6.4 (95% CI 1.6–26.1) (Yamauchi *et al.*, 1999). This yields a PPV of 71% and NPV of 82%. The St. Louis Carotid Occlusion Study (STLCOS) (Grubb *et al.*, 1998) was more methodologically sound (Derdeyn *et al.*, 1999); being a prospective, blinded, longitudinal cohort study. The authors demonstrated that by multivariate analysis, only age and increased OEF were correlated with stroke risk but it utilized a qualitative assessment of OEF. The age-adjusted relative risk for increased OEF was 6.0 (95% CI 1.7–21.6) for all stroke and 7.3 (95% CI 1.6–33.4) for ipsilateral stroke (Grubb *et al.*, 1998). Reanalysis of this data has shown that several methods for calculating OEF are probably comparable, but by multivariate analysis, a count-based quantitative method was the most predictive (Derdeyn *et al.*, 2001b). A more recent small study showed that the highest rate of strokes (10 strokes in 19 patients) occur in patients with high CBV and high OEF when compared to normal control or contralateral hemispheric values (Derdeyn et al., 2002). These study results are important, but clearly not definitive. Even in the STLCOS, stroke occurred in 12/39 patients with increased OEF and 3/42 without (Grubb et al., 1998). This indicates a sensitivity of 80%, specificity of 59%, PPV of 31%, and NPV of 93% – clearly inadequate given the devastating nature of missed tests and the potentially unnecessary further intervention with false positives.

Though "normal" OEF is around 30% (Powers et al., 1987), this value varies significantly, and as OEF begins to fall off in the state of matched hypometabolism, false normal values may occur in patients with severe disease (Nemoto et al., 2004; Kuroda et al., 2006 in press). Preliminary data supporting this have identified a population which has a very high increase in OEF in response to acetazolamide (OEF reactivity) despite "normal" baseline OEF. Though prospective validation is lacking, this population exhibited the most severe subcortical white matter infarction in the study (Nemoto et al., 2004). These limitations emphasize the need for complimentary techniques for accurate stroke prediction.

The second primary method which has been associated with increased stroke risk is quantitative measurement of the cerebrovascular response to a vasodilatory challenge. It must be pointed out that there are two distinct endpoints that these modalities are measuring, which accounts for some of the seeming confusion and conflicting results in the literature. The primary tactic, for which more convincing data is accumulating, measures CBF quantitatively and by identifying a state of "steal." As described in the previous section, it identifies stage II hemodynamic insufficiency (vasodilation has been exhausted and CVR is negative). The other methods employ qualitative technologies that also "measure" vasodilatory response but do so by examining changes of ratios between sides. This group is more heterogeneous in terms of hemodynamic compromise, and will, predictably, exhibit conflicting results (Yonas et al., 1997, 1998).

Xenon CT CBF has been used to detect patients exhibiting misery perfusion (stage II) using acetazolamide challenge. Two studies retrospectively combined two thresholds in symptomatic mixed carotid occlusion and stenosis patients. The first (Yonas et al., 1993) showed that CBF reduction of $>5\%$ (steal) and baseline CBF of 45 cc/100 gm/min was correlated with 12.6 times higher risk of stroke ($p = 0.0007$). An extension study from the same group (Webster et al., 1995) reported that the steal phenomenon alone was associated with stroke (in patients with carotid occlusion only 10/38 in the steal group compared to 0/26 in the normal reactivity group had a stroke [$p = 0.003$]) (PPV 26%, NPV 100%).

This association has been validated prospectively, with patients exhibiting decreased CBF and CVR (defined as the "steal" described above, but using a different classification system) showing significantly higher number of subsequent strokes (RR 3.6, 95% CI 1.9–34.4 for all stroke and RR 8.0, 95% CI 1.9–34.4 for ipsilateral stroke) (Kuroda et al., 2001). The authors of the former two studies admit that the cut-off for defining steal was arbitrary and stress the need for large studies to further prospectively define or validate this value. Another group has proposed a value of 6.65% for reduced CBF response as having utility at detecting increased OEF (100% sensitivity, 89% specificity, 50% PPV, and 100% NPV) (Yamauchi et al., 2004). It should be noted that regional quantitative CBF obtained with ^{133}xenon CBF has relatively poor resolution compared with xenon CT CBF thereby making it more difficult to discern the focal low flow values that can occur after acetazolamide. Though more low-risk patients are detected using the acetazolamide reactivity test, better false negative rates are reported, indicating that fewer high-risk patients are being missed.

Various SPECT methods have been employed using acetazolamide or CO_2 with varying results (Bushnell et al., 1991; Matsuda et al., 1991; Burt et al., 1992; Hirano et al., 1994; Ogasawara et al., 2002), though few have attempted to predict stroke risk (Hasegawa et al., 1992; Yokota et al., 1998;

Ogasawara *et al.*, 2002). Using quantitative ^{133}xenon SPECT CBF, low regional cerebrovascular reactivity to acetazolamide has been prospectively shown to correlate with increased risk of stroke (17.4% annual risk in low regional cerebrovascular reactivity compared to 3.3% in normal regional cerebrovascular reactivity, $n = 70$) (Ogasawara *et al.*, 2002). On the other hand, in two studies using qualitative data obtained with 123I-IMP SPECT, neither found a correlation with stroke, though each had major limitations. In Hasegawa's study there were no cerebrovascular events in the 51 patients, though reductions in vasodilatory capacity were seen in 20 (Hasegawa *et al.*, 1992). In the second study from this group (Yokota *et al.*, 1998), methodology was superior (prospective and blinded) though lesions and patients were still heterogeneous. Again, no significance by multivariate analysis was found between acetazolamide reactivity and stroke. In addition, all these imaging modalities are limited by the use of relative values such as the asymmetry index. As previously discussed, it has been clearly shown that hemodynamic response can be quite variable in both hemispheres leading to misleading values for asymmetry index (Witt *et al.*, 1994). Furthermore, in direct comparison between methods, quantitative analysis has been shown to be necessary to accurately characterize the hemodynamic state (asymmetry index showed 61% sensitivity, 75% specificity, and 50% PPV for stroke prediction) (Yonas *et al.*, 1998). Though attempts have been made to address this problem by using semiquantitative techniques (Imaizumi *et al.*, 2002), so far it has only been correlated with PET OEF values rather than outcomes.

Since CBV is an additional variable reflecting the degree of autoregulatory dilation (Yamauchi *et al.*, 2004), intuitively it would be an additional candidate to easily predict stroke risk. Unfortunately empirically this value has proven to demonstrate extreme variability in terms of measurement modalities and person-to-person changes. There are also complex contributions from many vascular sources and it has been

suggested that this value is of limited or no clinical utility for these reasons (Derdeyn *et al.*, 2002). Some authors use the CBV to CBF ratio (or vascular mean transit time), but this has been found to have no correlation with stroke (Powers *et al.*, 1989).

TCD has yielded mixed results regarding the ability to predict stroke using CO_2 reactivity. Klijn *et al.* (2000) found no prognostic significance of CO_2 reactivity as measured by inhaled CO_2 while Vernieri *et al.* (2001) found that low breath holding index (BHI) (< 0.69) was predictive for stroke (hazard ratio [HR] of 10.1, 95% CI 2.1–49.9). In addition, Kleiser and Widder (1992) reported positive correlation of reduced or absent increase in flow after inhaled CO_2 with stroke or TIA. The most recent study prospectively showed a highly significant correlation of reactivity $< 20\%$ (exhausted response) with any ipsilateral ischemic event (K-M log rank 7.81 $p = 0.0052$) in carotid occlusion patients (Markus and Cullinane, 2001). Though methodologies and techniques for inducing hypercapnea differ, there are many possible explanations for differing results. One may be the changing nature of CO_2 reactivity over time. Several authors have shown increasing CO_2 reactivity over time, presumably in response to the development of collateral flow (Hasegawa *et al.*, 1992; Widder *et al.*, 1994; Klijn *et al.*, 2000). There are also practical limitations of the CO_2 techniques in that they may cause systemic side effects such as hypertension and yield variable results. Also patient selection may play a role as some studies included asymptomatic patients or patients with stenosis or occlusion while others did not.

Extent of collateral circulation has been assessed in a number of ways, but is probably of limited clinical utility, as it is not correlated with the hemodynamic state (Powers *et al.*, 1987). Counting the number of patent channels by TCD correlated with increased stroke risk in one study with annual stroke risk varying from 32.7% with no collateral channels to 0% annual risk with 3 or more (Vernieri *et al.*, 2001). In contrast, the presence of leptomeningeal collaterals probably indicates poor large vessel collateral circulation, and has been associated with increased risk of stroke (HR 4.1, 95% CI 1.3–13.3) (Klijn *et al.*, 2000). An indirect method of measuring adequate collateral flow may be offered by DSC-MRI's ability to measure time-to-peak (TTP) flow (Nasel *et al.*, 2001). Clinical studies are lacking at this point.

Blood oxygen level-dependent (BOLD) MRI has shown promise initially in detecting response to acetazolamide (Kleinschmidt *et al.*, 1995), and more recently in quantifying both CBV and OER. In theory, this seems appropriate as the BOLD images are dependent on contributions from CBF, CBV, and $CMRO_2$ (Kavec *et al.*, 2004). Normal values have been defined for grey matter CBV ($n=4$) 3.49 ± 0.42 mL/100 g. The slope of the value for grey matter volume versus CBV gives a normal OER of 40% (similar to Powers' OEF value of 30%). In patients with occlusion ($n=5$), increased grey matter CBV was weakly associated with elevated OER (Kavec *et al.*, 2004). Clinical applications have not yet been defined.

Finally, clinical symptomatology (stroke or TIA) is clearly related to stroke risk. Estimates range from 1.3 to 3.3% annual stroke risk if asymptomatic to 16.7–18.5% with stroke or TIA (Powers *et al.*, 2000; Vernieri *et al.*, 2001). Specific symptoms may have some limited clinical utility in stroke prediction also. If symptoms are stereotypically cerebral in origin and posturally related as opposed to retinal, the risk of stroke or TIA is significantly increased (hazard ratio 5.0, 95% CI 1.4–17.2) (Klijn *et al.*, 2000). A small ($n=13$) recent study has shown some promise for using a head-up tilt test to detect patients with OEF $>53.3\%$. Sensitivity was reported as 60% and specificity was reported as 100% to detect this OEF value (Sakaguchi *et al.*, 2005). Despite these observations, there are limitations to only clinical symptoms, and even these patients probably have some degree of early hemodynamic compromise which may be significant in terms of stroke risk (Gur *et al.*, 1996; Apruzzese *et al.*, 2001).

Cerebral hemodynamics in other carotid occlusive conditions

Carotid dissection

Carotid dissection is in some respects the clinical correlate of BTO in that it may produce a sudden occlusion. It differs in that there are often varying degrees of stenosis rather than complete sudden occlusion and there are nearly always intimal abnormalities which serve as sources for emboli. Though initial small studies regarding stroke pattern in carotid dissection showed a mix of embolic and hemodynamic patterns (Weiller *et al.*, 1991), large prospective studies have since shown that the vast majority of strokes represent embolic sources (Steinke *et al.*, 1996; Lucas *et al.*, 1998; Benninger *et al.*, 2004). Nonetheless, there is probably a hemodynamic element to the development of these embolic strokes due to low flow states and the inability to clear small emboli that would be inconsequential with normal flow dynamics. Understanding of cerebral hemodynamics is also complicated by the fact that up to 20% of dissections are bilateral or may include vertebral dissections (Guillon *et al.*, 1998). Though the distribution of embolic and hemodynamic patterns is similar between patients with complete occlusion and stenosis, multiple infarcts are more common with occlusion (Lucas *et al.*, 1998). Most carotid dissections are associated with some type of ischemic symptomatology (50–95%), and this risk is increased in high-grade stenosis and occlusion (Baumgartner *et al.*, 2001; Schievink, 2001). These figures are likely overestimated as there are likely many patients with asymptomatic dissection or other pain symptoms which are not diagnosed as caused by dissection. Dissections of the intracranial portion of the ICA are more rare, and may have worse outcomes probably due to the formation of more severe hemodynamic ischemic patterns than occur with extracranial dissections (Chaves *et al.*, 2002).

As with BTO, clinical response to occlusion due to dissection is dependent on the ability of immediate recruitment of collateral flow. Mortality rates are around 5%, probably representing the proportion of the population with absent collateral via the circle of Willis. For survivors of the initial stroke event the prognosis is reasonably good with three quarters of patients making good functional recovery. Better outcomes can also be expected in the long-run because up to two thirds of dissections exhibit some spontaneous restoration of flow (Schievink, 2001). These outcomes are worse than in patients with stroke from chronic carotid occlusion, probably due to the acute onset of the vessel narrowing and the ability to injure due to recurrent emboli as well as compromised hemodynamics (Milhaud *et al.*, 2002).

Carotid occlusion during carotid endarterectomy

Though a comprehensive discussion regarding hemodynamics in patients with stenosis and the treatment with carotid endarterectomy is outside the scope of this chapter, several points can be made regarding carotid cross-clamping during carotid endarterectomy. As with carotid BTO, the cerebral vasculature is subjected to a sudden occlusion of flow, however this flow may have already been significantly decreased by the stenosis. In this respect the physiology may be more closely related to the changes in chronic carotid occlusion. Patients currently undergoing carotid endarterectomy typically already have stenosis of >70% as this group has been shown to benefit most from the procedure (Barnett *et al.*, 1998; ECST, 1998). Immediately after cross-clamping of the carotid, there is a fall in CPP to the ipsilateral ICA. This has been shown to be associated with a stump pressure reduction of around 31 mmHg in the distal ICA. Over the following 10 s, a further decrease of around 11 mmHg concurrent with a rise in MCA velocity, measured by TCD, indicates autoregulatory dilation (McCulloch *et al.*, 2003). Normally, after unclamping, there is a return to normal velocities,

which are typically somewhat elevated compared to before-clamping (Pascazio *et al.*, 1999). This is a transient hyperemic response indicating the slight lag of the autoregulatory response in restoring normal flow values.

Some patients show an exaggerated lag in this response or even steal phenomena (Pascazio *et al.*, 1999), indicating poor collateral circulation and chronic impaired hemodynamics (exhaustion of vasodilatory reserve). This delay in autoregulatory adaption is associated with postoperative ischemic complications (Halsey, 1992; Pascazio *et al.*, 1999). These patients may require shunting during the procedure if the flow does not return to normal within 5 minutes (Halsey, 1992). Furthermore, a small select population is unable to tolerate even brief occlusion similar to as with BTO. In the case of chronic stenosis, however, these patients likely exhibit some evidence of ischemic disease from their chronic state of uncompensated decreased CPP (Pascazio *et al.*, 1999). These again, are the patients with absent circle of Willis collateral flow. These patients clearly require shunting for the procedure (Halsey, 1992). Extensive literature also exists regarding the utility of EEG correlating with CBF intraoperatively in predicting patients who may need shunt (Sundt *et al.*, 1974, 1981). EEG changes clearly correlate with CBF values from 10 to 20 cc/100 gm/min (Messick *et al.*, 1987), and it has been proposed that shunting is unnecessary if intraoperative EEG remains normal during cross-clamping (Messick *et al.*, 1984). As the occlusion time during carotid endarterectomy is relatively short and stroke risk is associated with decreased hemodynamic parameters, it is presumed that most strokes are hemodynamic in origin (Halsey, 1992). In addition, the use of heparinized saline and the restoration of robust flow serve to decrease the embolic risk. There is, alternatively, a small risk of primarily embolic stroke associated with the use of shunt, and therefore it should be restricted to patients with documented hemodynamic insufficiency (Halsey, 1992).

Conclusion: the role of EC-IC bypass

Though the operation quickly passed from favor after a large ($n = 1377$) randomized controlled trial of EC-IC bypass compared to best medical treatment for symptomatic carotid occlusion found no improvement in outcomes, our increasingly sophisticated understanding of cerebral hemodynamics suggests that the bypass study examined the benefit of bypass surgery in the wrong patient group. The primary reason for the failure of EC-IC in the 1985 study is thought to be that the overall risk of stroke is relatively low and only a minority of patients in the bypass study had any compromise of hemodynamics. The risk of surgery to restore flow, though low (2.5% mortality), was of no benefit in the majority of the study population who do not have impaired hemodynamics (EC/IC Bypass Study Group, 1985). EC-IC bypass should theoretically be indicated in patients with poor cerebral hemodynamic reserve. In acute carotid occlusion, these are patients who fail BTO either clinically or by demonstrating CBF < 30 mL/100 g/m. In chronic carotid occlusion, these are patients probably somewhere in stage II hemodynamic impairment, demonstrating increased OEF or very poor CVR. The ambiguity of defining this subgroup has sparked extensive physiologic research into cerebral hemodynamics and has ultimately resulted in the undertaking of a new EC-IC bypass trial which is currently underway. This trial will examine whether EC-IC bypass will be effective in the subgroup at highest risk of stroke with increased OEF (Adams et al., 2001). This large collaborative trial may open the way for wider applicability of this operation.

Theoretically, the physiologic mechanism of EC-IC bypass is sound. This trial will now begin to apply this theory to clinical practice. In both the situation of poor flow during BTO and impaired hemodynamics in symptomatic carotid occlusion there is a mechanical loss of CBF to brain tissue due to poor collateral circulation. By transposing a more robust source of blood flow to the distal MCA, CBF should be gradually restored to tissue in this territory. Empiric evidence using multiple modalities shows that EC-IC bypass indeed restores CBF to impaired tissue to normal or near normal levels (Yamashita et al., 1996; Ueno et al., 2001; Neff et al., 2004). These tissues are maximally compensated in terms of vasodilation and even metabolic response (stage II or III). By restoring an adequate vascular conduit, CPP is increased, and these patients should theoretically improve in terms of hemodynamic insufficiency (to stage I or 0). Besides CBF, other advanced changes of hemodynamic insufficiency such as increased OEF (Muraishi et al., 1993) and vasodilatory capacity (Karnik et al., 1992) have been shown to reverse with bypass. These and other cerebrometabolic changes are likely to continue to improve over months to years of restored flow (Murata et al., 2003).

There may even be an additional bonus to the already promising future for patients with symptomatic carotid occlusion and poor hemodynamics. These patients have been reported to display some degree of dementia even in the absence of cortical infarction. Decreased neuropsychologic test scores have shown significant independent correlation with elevated OEF and decreased $CMRO_2$. Most importantly, these changes have been shown to reverse after EC-IC bypass indicating improvement of cognitive impairment with restoration of normal CBF (Sasoh et al., 2003).

The hemodynamic physiology of carotid occlusion has been extensively studied in many disparate clinical situations, yet yields many correlating points. In addition, the clinical response to these situations has been meticulously documented by dedicated physicians and researchers. We must remember, however that these observations are simply many different perspectives on the ultimate goal of understanding CBF. Each added perspective offers new insights into this picture, though it is often challenging to conceptualize exactly how it fits. Through understanding basic physiology, we continue to progress in our understanding to a point where there are new and effective therapeutic prospects to better treat our patients.

REFERENCES

Adams, H. P., Jr., Powers, W. J., Grubb, R. L., Jr., Clarke, W. R. and Woolson, R. F. (2001). Preview of a new trial of extracranial-to-intracranial arterial anastomosis: the carotid occlusion surgery study. *Neurosurgery Clinics of North America*, **12**, 613–24, ix–x.

American Society of International and Therapeutic Neuroradiology (2001). Carotid artery balloon test occlusion *AJNR. American Journal of Neuroradiology*, **22**, S8–9.

Apruzzese, A., Silvestrini, M., Floris, R., *et al.* (2001). Cerebral hemodynamics in asymptomatic patients with internal carotid artery occlusion: a dynamic susceptibility contrast MR and transcranial Doppler study. *AJNR. American Journal of Neuroradiology*, **22**, 1062–7.

Barker, D. W., Jungreis, C. A., Horton, J. A., Pentheny, S. and Lemley, T. (1993). Balloon test occlusion of the internal carotid artery: change in stump pressure over 15 minutes and its correlation with xenon CT cerebral blood flow. *AJNR. American Journal of Neuroradiology*, **14**, 587–90.

Barnett, D. W., Barrow, D. L. and Joseph, G. J. (1994). Combined extracranial-intracranial bypass and intraoperative balloon occlusion for the treatment of intracavernous and proximal carotid artery aneurysms. *Neurosurgery*, **35**, 92–7; discussion 97–8.

Barnett, H. J., Taylor, D. W., Eliasziw, M., *et al.* (1998). Benefit of carotid endarterectomy in patients with symptomatic moderate or severe stenosis. North American Symptomatic Carotid Endarterectomy Trial Collaborators. *New England Journal of Medicine*, **339**, 1415–25.

Baumgartner, R. W., Arnold, M., Baumgartner, I., *et al.* (2001). Carotid dissection with and without ischemic events: local symptoms and cerebral artery findings. *Neurology*, **57**, 827–32.

Benninger, D. H., Georgiadis, D., Kremer, C., *et al.* (2004). Mechanism of ischemic infarct in spontaneous carotid dissection. *Stroke*, **35**, 482–5.

Bhattacharjee, A. K., Tamaki, N., Wada, T., Hara, Y. and Ehara, K. (1999). Transcranial Doppler findings during balloon test occlusion of the internal carotid artery. *Journal of Neuroimaging*, **9**, 155–9.

Bisschops, R. H., Klijn, C. J., Kappelle, L. J., Van Huffelen, A. C. and Van Der Grond, J. (2003). Association between impaired carbon dioxide reactivity and ischemic lesions in arterial border zone territories in patients with unilateral internal carotid artery occlusion. *Archives of Neurology*, **60**, 229–33.

Brunberg, J. A., Frey, K. A., Horton, J. A., *et al.* (1994). 15O H2O positron emission tomography determination of cerebral blood flow during balloon test occlusion of the internal carotid artery. *AJNR. American Journal of Neuroradiology*, **15**, 725–32.

Burt, R. W., Witt, R. M., Cikrit, D. F. and Reddy, R. V. (1992). Carotid artery disease: evaluation with acetazolamide-enhanced Tc-99m HMPAO SPECT. *Radiology*, **182**, 461–6.

Bushnell, D. L., Gupta, S., Barnes, W. E., *et al.* (1991). Evaluation of cerebral perfusion reserve using 5% CO2 and SPECT neuroperfusion imaging. *Clinical Nuclear Medicine*, **16**, 263–7.

Chaves, C., Estol, C., Esnaola, M. M., *et al.* (2002). Spontaneous intracranial internal carotid artery dissection: report of 10 patients. *Archives of Neurology*, **59**, 977–81.

Cloughesy, T. F., Nuwer, M. R., Hoch, D., *et al.* (1993). Monitoring carotid test occlusions with continuous EEG and clinical examination. *Journal of Clinical Neurophysiology*, **10**, 363–9.

Dare, A. O., Chaloupka, J. C., Putman, C. M., Fayad, P. B. and Awad, I. A. (1998). Failure of the hypotensive provocative test during temporary balloon test occlusion of the internal carotid artery to predict delayed hemodynamic ischemia after therapeutic carotid occlusion. *Surgical Neurology*, **50**, 147–55; discussion 155–6.

Derdeyn, C. P., Grubb, R. L., Jr. and Powers, W. J. (1999). Cerebral hemodynamic impairment: methods of measurement and association with stroke risk. *Neurology*, **53**, 251–9.

Derdeyn, C. P., Khosla, A., Videen, T. O., *et al.* (2001a). Severe hemodynamic impairment and border zone-region infarction. *Radiology*, **220**, 195–201.

Derdeyn, C. P., Videen, T. O., Grubb, R. L., Jr. and Powers, W. J. (2001b). Comparison of PET oxygen extraction fraction methods for the prediction of stroke risk. *Journal of Nuclear Medicine*, **42**, 1195–7.

Derdeyn, C. P., Videen, T. O., Yundt, K. D., *et al.* (2002). Variability of cerebral blood volume and oxygen extraction: stages of cerebral haemodynamic impairment revisited. *Brain*, **125**, 595–607.

Eckard, D. A., Purdy, P. D. and Bonte, F. J. (1992). Temporary balloon occlusion of the carotid artery combined with brain blood flow imaging as a test to predict tolerance prior to permanent carotid sacrifice. *AJNR. American Journal of Neuroradiology*, **13**, 1565–9.

Eckert, B., Thie, A., Carvajal, M., Groden, C. and Zeumer, H. (1998). Predicting hemodynamic ischemia by transcranial Doppler monitoring during therapeutic balloon occlusion of the internal carotid artery. *AJNR. American Journal of Neuroradiology*, **19**, 577–82.

ECST (1998). Randomised trial of endarterectomy for recently symptomatic carotid stenosis: final results of the MRC European Carotid Surgery Trial (ECST). *Lancet*, **351**, 1379–87.

Field, M., Jungreis, C. A., Chengelis, N., *et al.* (2003). Symptomatic cavernous sinus aneurysms: management and outcome after carotid occlusion and selective cerebral revascularization. *AJNR. American Journal of Neuroradiology*, **24**, 1200–7.

Firlik, A. D., Kaufmann, A. M., Wechsler, L. R., *et al.* (1997). Quantitative cerebral blood flow determinations in acute ischemic stroke. Relationship to computed tomography and angiography. *Stroke*, **28**, 2208–13.

Giller, C. A., Mathews, D., Walker, B., Purdy, P. and Roseland, A. M. (1994). Prediction of tolerance to carotid artery occlusion using transcranial Doppler ultrasound. *Journal of Neurosurgery*, **81**, 15–19.

Grubb, R. L., Jr., Derdeyn, C. P., Fritsch, S. M., *et al.* (1998). Importance of hemodynamic factors in the prognosis of symptomatic carotid occlusion. *Journal of the American Medical Association*, **280**, 1055–60.

Grubb, R. L., Jr., Powers, W. J., Derdeyn, C. P., Adams, H. P., Jr. and Clarke, W. R. (2003). The carotid occlusion surgery study. *Neurosurgical Focus*, **14**, e9.

Guillon, B., Levy, C. and Bousser, M. G. (1998). Internal carotid artery dissection: an update. *Journal of the Neurological Sciences*, **153**, 146–58.

Gupta, D. K., Young, W. L., Hashimoto, T., *et al.* (2002). Characterization of the cerebral blood flow response to balloon deflation after temporary internal carotid artery test occlusion. *Journal of Neurosurgical Anesthesiology*, **14**, 123–9.

Gur, A. Y., Bova, I. and Bornstein, N. M. (1996). Is impaired cerebral vasomotor reactivity a predictive factor of stroke in asymptomatic patients? *Stroke*, **27**, 2188–90.

Halsey, J. H., Jr. (1992). Risks and benefits of shunting in carotid endarterectomy. The International Transcranial Doppler Collaborators. *Stroke*, **23**, 1583–7.

Hasegawa, Y., Yamaguchi, T., Tsuchiya, T., Minematsu, K. and Nishimura, T. (1992). Sequential change of hemodynamic reserve in patients with major cerebral artery occlusion or severe stenosis. *Neuroradiology*, **34**, 15–21.

Herkes, G. K., Morgan, M., Grinnell, V., *et al.* (1993). EEG monitoring during angiographic balloon test carotid occlusion: experience in sixteen cases. *Clinical and Experimental Neurology*, **30**, 98–103.

Hetzel, A., Von Reutern, G., Wernz, M. G., Droste, D. W. and Schumacher, M. (2000). The carotid compression test for therapeutic occlusion of the internal carotid artery. Comparison of angiography with transcranial Doppler sonography. *Cerebrovascular Disease*, **10**, 194–9.

Hirano, T., Minematsu, K., Hasegawa, Y., *et al.* (1994). Acetazolamide reactivity on 123I-IMP single photon emission computed tomography in patients with major cerebral artery occlusive disease: correlation with positron emission tomography parameters. *Journal of Cerebral Blood Flow and Metabolism*, **14**, 763–70.

Imaizumi, M., Kitagawa, K., Hashikawa, K., *et al.* (2002). Detection of misery perfusion with split-dose 123I-iodoamphetamine single-photon emission computed tomography in patients with carotid occlusive diseases. *Stroke*, **33**, 2217–23.

Isaka, Y., Nagano, K., Narita, M., Ashida, K. and Imaizumi, M. (1997). High signal intensity on T2-weighted magnetic resonance imaging and cerebral hemodynamic reserve in carotid occlusive disease. *Stroke*, **28**, 354–7.

Kaminogo, M., Ochi, M., Onizuka, M., Takahata, H. and Shibata, S. (1999). An additional monitoring of regional cerebral oxygen saturation to HMPAO SPECT study during balloon test occlusion. *Stroke*, **30**, 407–13.

Karnik, R., Valentin, A., Ammerer, H. P., Donath, P. and Slany, J. (1992). Evaluation of vasomotor reactivity by transcranial Doppler and acetazolamide test before and after extracranial-intracranial bypass in patients with internal carotid artery occlusion. *Stroke*, **23**, 812–17.

Kavec, M., Usenius, J. P., Tuunanen, P. I., Rissanen, A. and Kauppinen, R. A. (2004). Assessment of cerebral hemodynamics and oxygen extraction using dynamic susceptibility contrast and spin echo blood oxygenation level-dependent magnetic resonance imaging: applications to carotid stenosis patients. *Neuroimage*, **22**, 258–67.

Kleinschmidt, A., Steinmetz, H., Sitzer, M., Merboldt, K. D. and Frahm, J. (1995). Magnetic resonance imaging of regional cerebral blood oxygenation changes under acetazolamide in carotid occlusive disease. *Stroke*, **26**, 106–10.

Kleiser, B. and Widder, B. (1992). Course of carotid artery occlusions with impaired cerebrovascular reactivity. *Stroke*, **23**, 171–4.

Klijn, C. J., Kappelle, L. J., Van Huffelen, A. C., *et al.* (2000). Recurrent ischemia in symptomatic carotid occlusion: prognostic value of hemodynamic factors. *Neurology*, **55**, 1806–12.

Kofke, W. A., Brauer, P., Policare, R., *et al.* (1995). Middle cerebral artery blood flow velocity and stable xenon-enhanced computed tomographic blood flow during balloon test occlusion of the internal carotid artery. *Stroke*, **26**, 1603–6.

Krapf, H., Widder, B. and Skalej, M. (1998). Small rosary-like infarctions in the centrum ovale suggest hemodynamic failure. *AJNR. American Journal of Neuroradiology*, **19**, 1479–84.

Kuroda, K., Shiga, T., Houkin, K., *et al.* (2006 in press). Cerebral oxygen metabolism and neuronal integrity in patients with impaired vasoreactivity due to occlusive carotid artery disease. *Stroke*.

Kuroda, S., Houkin, K., Kamiyama, H., *et al.* (2001). Long-term prognosis of medically treated patients with internal carotid or middle cerebral artery occlusion: can acetazolamide test predict it? *Stroke*, **32**, 2110–16.

Larson, J. J., Tew, J. M., Jr., Tomsick, T. A. and Van Loveren, H. R. (1995). Treatment of aneurysms of the internal carotid artery by intravascular balloon occlusion: long-term follow-up of 58 patients. *Neurosurgery*, **36**, 26–30; discussion 30.

Linskey, M. E., Jungreis, C. A., Yonas, H., *et al.* (1994). Stroke risk after abrupt internal carotid artery sacrifice: accuracy of preoperative assessment with balloon test occlusion and stable xenon-enhanced CT. *AJNR. American Journal of Neuroradiology*, **15**, 829–43.

Lucas, C., Moulin, T., Deplanque, D., Tatu, L. and Chavot, D. (1998). Stroke patterns of internal carotid artery dissection in 40 patients. *Stroke*, **29**, 2646–8.

Lythgoe, D., Simmons, A., Pereira, A., *et al.* (2001). Magnetic resonance markers of ischaemia: their correlation with vasodilatory reserve in patients with carotid artery stenosis and occlusion. *Journal of Neurology, Neurosurgery, and Psychiatry*, **71**, 58–62.

Markus, H. and Cullinane, M. (2001). Severely impaired cerebrovascular reactivity predicts stroke and TIA risk in patients with carotid artery stenosis and occlusion. *Brain*, **124**, 457–67.

Marshall, R. S., Lazar, R. M., Young, W. L., *et al.* (2002). Clinical utility of quantitative cerebral blood flow measurements during internal carotid artery test occlusions. *Neurosurgery*, **50**, 996–1004; discussion 1004–5.

Matas, R. (1911). Testing the efficiency of the collateral circulation as preliminary to the occlusion of the internal carotid artery: experience in 500 cases. *Annals of Surgery*, **53**, 1–43.

Matsuda, H., Higashi, S., Kinuya, K., *et al.* (1991). SPECT evaluation of brain perfusion reserve by the acetazol-amide test using Tc-99m HMPAO. *Clinical Nuclear Medicine*, **16**, 572–9.

McCulloch, T. J., Thompson, C. L. and Dunne, V. (2003). Cerebral hemodynamics immediately following carotid occlusion. *Journal of Neurosurgical Anesthesiology*, **15**, 126–30.

Messick, J. M., Jr., Casement, B., Sharbrough, F. W., *et al.* (1987). Correlation of regional cerebral blood flow (rCBF) with EEG changes during isoflurane anesthesia for carotid endarterectomy: critical rCBF. *Anesthesiology*, **66**, 344–9.

Messick, J. M., Jr., Sharbrough, F. and Sundt, T., Jr. (1984). Selective shunting on the basis of EEG and regional CBF monitoring during carotid endarterectomy. *International Anesthesiology Clinics*, **22**, 137–45.

Milhaud, D., De Freitas, G. R., Van Melle, G. and Bogousslavsky, J. (2002). Occlusion due to carotid artery dissection: a more severe disease than previously suggested. *Archives of Neurology*, **59**, 557–61.

Monsein, L. H., Jeffery, P. J., Van Heerden, B. B., *et al.* (1991). Assessing adequacy of collateral circulation during balloon test occlusion of the internal carotid artery with 99mTc-HMPAO SPECT. *AJNR. American Journal of Neuroradiology*, **12**, 1045–51.

Morioka, T., Matsushima, T., Fujii, K., *et al.* (1989). Balloon test occlusion of the internal carotid artery with monitoring of compressed spectral arrays (CSAs) of electroencephalogram. *Acta Neurochirurgica (Wien)*, **101**, 29–34.

Morishima, H., Kurata, A., Miyasaka, Y., Fujii, K. and Kan, S. (1998). Efficacy of the stump pressure ratio as a guide to the safety of permanent occlusion of the internal carotid artery. *Neurological Research*, **20**, 732–6.

Muraishi, K., Kameyama, M., Sato, K., *et al.* (1993). Cerebral circulatory and metabolic changes following EC/IC bypass surgery in cerebral occlusive diseases. *Neurological Research*, **15**, 97–103.

Murata, Y., Katayama, Y., Sakatani, K., Fukaya, C. and Kano, T. (2003). Evaluation of extracranial-intracranial arterial bypass function by using near-infrared spectroscopy. *Journal of Neurosurgery*, **99**, 304–10.

Nasel, C., Azizi, A., Wilfort, A., Mallek, R. and Schindler, E. (2001). Measurement of time-to-peak parameter by use of a new standardization method in patients with stenotic or occlusive disease of the carotid artery. *AJNR. American Journal of Neuroradiology*, **22**, 1056–61.

Nathan, M. A., Bushnell, D. L., Kahn, D., Simonson, T. M. and Kirchner, P. T. (1994). Crossed cerebellar diaschisis associated with balloon test occlusion of the carotid artery. *Nuclear Medicine Communications*, **15**, 448–54.

Neff, K. W., Horn, P., Dinter, D., *et al.* (2004). Extracranial-intracranial arterial bypass surgery improves total brain blood supply in selected symptomatic patients with unilateral internal carotid artery occlusion and insufficient collateralization. *Neuroradiology*, **46**, 730–7.

Nemoto, E. M., Yonas, H., Kuwabara, H., *et al.* (2004). Identification of hemodynamic compromise by cerebrovascular reserve and oxygen extraction fraction in occlusive vascular disease. *Journal of Cerebral Blood Flow and Metabolism*, **24**, 1081–9.

Ogasawara, K., Ogawa, A. and Yoshimoto, T. (2002). Cerebrovascular reactivity to acetazolamide and outcome in patients with symptomatic internal carotid or middle cerebral artery occlusion: a xenon-133 single-photon emission computed tomography study. *Stroke*, **33**, 1857–62.

Okudaira, Y., Arai, H. and Sato, K. (1996). Cerebral blood flow alteration by acetazolamide during carotid balloon occlusion: parameters reflecting cerebral perfusion pressure in the acetazolamide test. *Stroke*, **27**, 617–21.

Origitano, T. C., Al-Mefty, O., Leonetti, J. P., Demonte, F. and Reichman, O. H. (1994). Vascular considerations and complications in cranial base surgery. *Neurosurgery*, **35**, 351–62; discussion 362–3.

Pascazio, L., Regina, G., Perilli, F., *et al.* (1999). Investigation on cerebral hemodynamics in patients with carotid disease receiving carotid endarterectomy. *Clinical Hemorheology Microcirculation*, **21**, 395–403.

Peterman, S. B., Taylor, A., Jr. and Hoffman, J. C., Jr. (1991). Improved detection of cerebral hypoperfusion with internal carotid balloon test occlusion and 99mTc-HMPAO cerebral perfusion SPECT imaging. *AJNR. American Journal of Neuroradiology*, **12**, 1035–41.

Powers, W. J., Derdeyn, C. P., Fritsch, S. M., *et al.* (2000). Benign prognosis of never-symptomatic carotid occlusion. *Neurology*, **54**, 878–82.

Powers, W. J., Press, G. A., Grubb, R. L., Jr., Gado, M. and Raichle, M. E. (1987). The effect of hemodynamically significant carotid artery disease on the hemodynamic status of the cerebral circulation. *Annals of International Medicine*, **106**, 27–34.

Powers, W. J., Tempel, L. W. and Grubb, R. L., Jr. (1989). Influence of cerebral hemodynamics on stroke risk: one-year follow-up of 30 medically treated patients. *Annals of Neurology*, **25**, 325–30.

Reilly, P. L. (1995). Tests of tolerance to carotid artery occlusion. In *Quantitative Cerebral Blood Flow Measurements Using Stable Xenon/CT: Clinical Applications*, ed. M. Tomonaga, A. Tanaka and H. Yonas. Armonk, NY: Futura publishing company, Inc.

Rutgers, D. R., Van Osch, M. J., Kappelle, L. J., Mali, W. P. and Van Der Grond, J. (2003). Cerebral hemodynamics and metabolism in patients with symptomatic occlusion of the internal carotid artery. *Stroke*, **34**, 648–52.

Sakaguchi, M., Kitagawa, K., Oku, N., *et al.* (2005). Critical analysis of hemodynamic insufficiency by head-up tilt in patients with carotid occlusive disease. *Circulation Journal*, **69**, 971–5.

Sasoh, M., Ogasawara, K., Kuroda, K., *et al.* (2003). Effects of EC-IC bypass surgery on cognitive impairment in patients with hemodynamic cerebral ischemia. *Surgical Neurology*, **59**, 455–60; discussion 460–3.

Schievink, W. I. (2001). Spontaneous dissection of the carotid and vertebral arteries. *New England Journal of Medicine*, **344**, 898–906.

Standard, S. C., Ahuja, A., Guterman, L. R., *et al.* (1995). Balloon test occlusion of the internal carotid artery with hypotensive challenge. *AJNR. American Journal of Neuroradiology*, **16**, 1453–8.

Steed, D. L., Webster, M. W., Devries, E. J., *et al.* (1990). Clinical observations on the effect of carotid artery occlusion on cerebral blood flow mapped by xenon computed tomography and its correlation with carotid artery back pressure. *Journal of Vascular Surgery*, **11**, 38–43; discussion 43–4.

Steinke, W., Schwartz, A. and Hennerici, M. (1996). Topography of cerebral infarction associated with carotid artery dissection. *Journal of Neurology*, **243**, 323–8.

Sundt, T. M., Jr., Sharbrough, F. W., Anderson, R. E. and Michenfelder, J. D. (1974). Cerebral blood flow measurements and electroencephalograms during carotid endarterectomy. *Journal of Neurosurgery*, **41**, 310–20.

Sundt, T. M., Jr., Sharbrough, F. W., Piepgras, D. G., *et al.* (1981). Correlation of cerebral blood flow and electroencephalographic changes during carotid endarterectomy: with results of surgery and hemodynamics of cerebral ischemia. *Mayo Clinic Proceedings*, **56**, 533–43.

Takeda, N., Fujita, K., Katayama, S. and Tamaki, N. (2000). Cerebral oximetry for the detection of cerebral ischemia during temporary carotid artery occlusion. *Neurologia Medico-Chirurgica (Tokyo)*, **40**, 557–62; discussion 562–3.

Tan, T.Y., Schminke, U., Lien, L.M., Eicke, B.M. and Tegeler, C.H. (2002). Extracranial internal carotid artery occlusion: the role of common carotid artery volume flow. *Journal of Neuroimaging*, **12**, 144–7.

The EC/IC Bypass Study Group (1985). Failure of extracranial-intracranial arterial bypass to reduce the risk of ischemic stroke. Results of an international randomized trial. *New England Journal of Medicine*, **313**, 1191–200.

Tsuchida, C., Kimura, H., Sadato, N., *et al.* (2000). Evaluation of brain metabolism in steno-occlusive carotid artery disease by proton MR spectroscopy: a correlative study with oxygen metabolism by PET. *Journal of Nuclear Medicine*, **41**, 1357–62.

Ueno, M., Nishizawa, S., Toyoda, H., *et al.* (2001). Assessment of cerebral hemodynamics before and after revascularization in patients with occlusive cerebrovascular disease by means of quantitative IMP-SPECT with double-injection protocol. *Annals of Nuclear Medicine*, **15**, 209–15.

Van Rooij, W.J., Sluzewski, M., Metz, N.H., *et al.* (2000). Carotid balloon occlusion for large and giant aneurysms: evaluation of a new test occlusion protocol. *Neurosurgery*, **47**, 116–21; discussion 122.

Vazquez Anon, V., Aymard, A., Gobin, Y.P., *et al.* (1992). Balloon occlusion of the internal carotid artery in 40 cases of giant intracavernous aneurysm: technical aspects, cerebral monitoring, and results. *Neuroradiology*, **34**, 245–51.

Vernieri, F., Pasqualetti, P., Matteis, M., *et al.* (2001). Effect of collateral blood flow and cerebral vasomotor reactivity on the outcome of carotid artery occlusion. *Stroke*, **32**, 1552–8.

Webster, M.W., Makaroun, M.S., Steed, D.L., *et al.* (1995). Compromised cerebral blood flow reactivity is a predictor of stroke in patients with symptomatic carotid artery occlusive disease. *Journal of Vascular Surgery*, **21**, 338–44; discussion 344–5.

Weiller, C., Mullges, W., Ringelstein, E.B., Buell, U. and Reiche, W. (1991). Patterns of brain infarctions in internal carotid artery dissections. *Neurosurgical Reviews*, **14**, 111–13.

Widder, B., Kleiser, B. and Krapf, H. (1994). Course of cerebrovascular reactivity in patients with carotid artery occlusions. *Stroke*, **25**, 1963–7.

Wintermark, M., Sesay, M., Barbier, E., *et al.* (2005). Comparative overview of brain perfusion imaging techniques. *Stroke*, **36**, e83–99.

Witt, J.P., Yonas, H. and Jungreis, C. (1994). Cerebral blood flow response pattern during balloon test occlusion of the internal carotid artery. *AJNR. American Journal of Neuroradiology*, **15**, 847–56.

Yamamoto, Y., Nishiyama, Y., Toyama, Y., *et al.* (2002). Preliminary results of Tc-99m ECD SPECT to evaluate cerebral collateral circulation during balloon test occlusion. *Clinical Nuclear Medicine*, **27**, 633–7.

Yamashita, T., Nakano, S., Ishihara, H., *et al.* (1996). Surgical modulation of the natural course of collateral circulation in chronic ischemic patients. *Acta Neurologica Scandinavica Supplementum*, **166**, 74–8.

Yamauchi, H., Fukuyama, H., Nagahama, Y., *et al.* (1996). Evidence of misery perfusion and risk for recurrent stroke in major cerebral arterial occlusive diseases from PET. *Journal of Neurology, Neurosurgery, and Psychiatry*, **61**, 18–25.

Yamauchi, H., Fukuyama, H., Nagahama, Y., *et al.* (1999). Significance of increased oxygen extraction fraction in five-year prognosis of major cerebral arterial occlusive diseases. *Journal of Nuclear Medicine*, **40**, 1992–8.

Yamauchi, H., Okazawa, H., Kishibe, Y., *et al.* (2004). Oxygen extraction fraction and acetazolamide reactivity in symptomatic carotid artery disease. *Journal of Neurology, Neurosurgery, and Psychiatry*, **75**, 33–7.

Yokota, C., Hasegawa, Y., Minematsu, K. and Yamaguchi, T. (1998). Effect of acetazolamide reactivity on corrected long-term outcome in patients with major cerebral artery occlusive diseases. *Stroke*, **29**, 640–4.

Yonas, H., Darby, J.M., Marks, E.C., Durham, S.R. and Maxwell, C. (1991). CBF measured by Xe-CT: approach to analysis and normal values. *Journal of Cerebral Blood Flow and Metabolism*, **11**, 716–25.

Yonas, H., Kromer, H. and Jungreis, C. (1997). Compromised vascular reserves does predict subgroups with carotid occlusion and an increased stroke risk. *Journal of Stroke and Cerebrovascular Disease*, **6**, 458.

Yonas, H., Pindzola, R.R., Meltzer, C.C. and Sasser, H. (1998). Qualitative versus quantitative assessment of cerebrovascular reserves. *Neurosurgery*, **42**, 1005–10; discussion 1011–12.

Yonas, H., Smith, H.A., Durham, S.R., Pentheny, S.L. and Johnson, D.W. (1993). Increased stroke risk predicted by compromised cerebral blood flow reactivity. *Journal of Neurosurgery*, **79**, 483–9.

30

Vascular imaging and the clinical development of new pharmaceuticals

James H. Revkin[1] and David S. Lester[2]

[1]Pfizer Inc, New London CT, USA
[2]Pfizer Inc, New York NY, USA

Introduction

Cardiovascular disease now represents the leading cause of death and disability globally (Mackay and Mensah, 2004). Clinical trials designed to image vessel wall structure can be useful in the late clinical development of therapies targeting vascular disease and atherosclerosis. This review discusses the use of vascular imaging data to advance the development of new therapies from the perspective of the pharmaceutical industry. It will discuss the technologies currently used in large phase 3 studies, as well as the technical, clinical, and regulatory considerations that must be addressed for the purpose of drug development and regulatory approval.

In North America a number of marketed drug therapies have approved indications for use in slowing the progression of atherosclerosis (see Table 30.1). The regulatory registration for those indications was based upon imaging data from placebo-controlled clinical trials, some of which were large enough to demonstrate differences in the frequency of cardiovascular events. The efficacy of these antiatherosclerotic therapies, particularly statins, has led to the development of clinical guidelines and standards of care that preclude the possibility of conducting long-term placebo controlled trials to demonstrate antiatherosclerotic efficacy. If vascular imaging techniques are to be used in clinical drug development, they must be powerful enough to be capable of detecting meaningful differences in atheroma burden between new therapies and powerful active control therapies.

The challenge for the pharmaceutical industry, medical science, and regulatory agencies will be to work together to find better ways to expedite the development of safe and effective new antiatherosclerotic treatments that reduce residual risk of cardiovascular morbidity and mortality. The current paradigm of conducting large cardiovascular morbidity and mortality studies to assess clinical efficacy, the gold standard for clinical trials, requires many years of follow-up and very large investments of resources. To demonstrate an incremental clinical benefit of new therapies above and beyond the current standard of care (by measuring hard cardiovascular events, nonfatal myocardial infarction, stroke, and cardiovascular death, in a secondary prevention population) requires between 10 000 and 15 000 subjects, followed for 5 years or more. Vascular imaging methods that are capable of detecting early, clinically important, changes in vessel structure could be used in clinical programs to develop novel therapies in a much more efficient manner with less overall morbidity and mortality

Carotid Disease: The Role of Imaging in Diagnosis and Management, ed. Jonathan Gillard, Martin Graves, Thomas Hatsukami and Chun Yuan. Published by Cambridge University Press. © Cambridge University Press 2007.

Table 30.1. Lipid-lowering therapies with USA product information that includes data from vascular imaging studies

Compound name	Imaging modality: imaging endpoints	Modality: trial acronym for studies described in Clinical Pharmacology section of Product information	Study acronym: studies demonstrating reduction in clinical events or relative risk (p-value)	Indication granted
Lovastatin (Mevacor)	QCA: MLD, percent stenosis, percent of progressors, Percent with new lesions. Carotid ultrasound: IMT	QCA: CCAIT MARS FATS IMT: ACAPS	ACAPS (0.04)	CAD: slow progression of CAD
Pravastatin (Pravachol)	QCA: MLD. Carotid ultrasound: IMT.	QCA: PLAC I REGRESS CIMT: PLAC II REGRESS KAPS	PLAC I PLAC II REGRESS KAPS Pooled (0.001)	CHD: slow progression of CAD
Simvastatin (Zocor)	QCA: MLD Percent stenosis Percent with progression and regress Percent of new lesions.	QCA: MAAS	None	None
Fluvastatin (Lescol)	QCA: MLD.	QCA: LCAS	LCAS (trend but not significant)	CHD: slow progression of CAD
Niacin (Niaspan) in combination with bile acid resin (colestipol)	QCA: Percent of progressors. Percent of regressors	QCA: CLAS FATS	FATS (RR 0.27)	CAD: slow progression or promote regression of CAD

Abbreviations: QCA = quantitative coronary angiography; MLD = minimum lumen diameter; IMT = carotid intima-media thickness.
Studies: ACAPS = Asymptomatic Carotid Artery Progression Study (Furberg, 1994); CCAIT = Canadian Coronary Atherosclerosis Intervention Trial (Waters, 1994); FATS (Brown, 1990) = Familial Atherosclerosis Treatment Study; KAPS (Salonen, 1995) = Kupio Atherosclerosis Study; LCAS (Herd, 1997) = Lipoprotein and Coronary Atherosclerosis Study; MAAS = Multicentre Anti-Atheroma Study (MAAS, 1994); MARS = Monitored Atherosclerosis Regression Study (Hodis, 1996); PLAC I and II (Furberg, 1995) = Pravastatin Limitation of Atherosclerosis in the Coronary and Carotid Arteries; REGRESS (de Groot, 1995) = Regression Growth Evaluation Statin Study.

(Sankatsing *et al.*, 2005). Sufficient data exists to support the design of clinical development programs that include vascular imaging studies, to supplement other efficacy and safety data including lipids and biomarkers. A successful regulatory submission will depend upon the weight of the evidence of the imaging data combined with data from other clinically relevant endpoints.

Choice of vascular imaging technologies and endpoints

Issues to be addressed in choosing a particular vascular imaging modality for clinical drug development include: (1) whether imaging changes of vessel wall structure reflect the pathophysiology of atherosclerosis; (2) whether there is a relationship between atheroma burden measured by that technology and clinical events; and (3) whether treatment that can cause a change in vessel wall structure detected by imaging can also alter clinical outcomes. Espeland *et al.* recently reviewed the utility of carotid ultrasound as a clinical research tool to monitor atherosclerosis progression (Espeland *et al.*, 2005). He discussed the concept of surrogacy with respect to imaging data, and using the clinical (Boissel *et al.*, 1992) and statistical (Prentice *et al.*, 1989) criteria that are required for research data to be considered clinically meaningful. Those criteria were defined as follows:

Clinical criteria

- Efficiency: the surrogate marker should be easier to measure and progress at a faster rate than the gold standard.
- Linkage: the quantitative and qualitative relationship between the surrogate marker and the gold standard should be established based on epidemiological and clinical studies.

- Congruency: the surrogate should be able to measure both risk and benefit such that, with an intervention, an anticipated benefit should be deducible from the measured changes in the surrogate Statistical Criteria.
For a given intervention:
- The intervention should affect the distribution of the true endpoint (the gold standard).
- The intervention should affect the distribution of the surrogate marker.
- The distribution of the true endpoint should be dependent on the surrogate marker's distribution.
- The surrogate marker should fully account for the impact of the treatment on the true endpoint.

If one looks at established vascular imaging technologies, there is considerable evidence that both conventional X-ray angiography and ultrasound, meet these criteria. The following is a discussion of data that now exists with respect to angiography and intra- and extravascular ultrasound, to support their use in clinical trials for the development of antiatherosclerotic therapies.

Angiography

Historically, vascular imaging was first used as a tool, for the purpose of clinical diagnosis. The first vascular imaging studies utilized contrast angiography to detect luminal disease, its severity, and potential targets for clinical intervention and revascularization. Contrast angiography was considered the gold standard to confirm the presence of clinically significant coronary luminal stenoses that were causing the signs and symptoms of atherosclerosis. Clinically, the degree of angiographic severity of a lesion was typically a subjective determination. With the development of quantitative methods to analyze angiographic images, it became possible to measure the progression or regression of atherosclerosis measured as lumen diameter or percent stenosis, leading to its utilization in clinical trials (Reiber *et al.*, 1985; Brown *et al.*, 1977, 1993a). Using quantitative coronary angiography (QCA) it was established in placebo-controlled clinical trials that there was a correlation between the change in the severity of angiographic coronary artery disease and clinical outcomes. A number of comprehensive reviews of the use of QCA to assess the clinical efficacy of pharmacologic and nonpharmacologic therapies have shown consistent trends whereby reductions in low-density lipoprotein cholesterol (LDL-C), increases in high-density lipoprotein cholesterol (HDL-C), and a reduction in the frequency of cardiovascular events are accompanied by a reduced rate of atherosclerosis progression or actual atherosclerosis regression (Brown *et al.*, 1993b; Rossouw *et al.*, 1995). Across these studies, different primary endpoints were chosen including changes in minimal lumen diameter, percent stenosis, percentages of progressors/regressors in treatment groups, and numbers of new lesions. It is apparent that in suitably powered and well-designed trials, quantitative angiographic measures of changes in coronary artery lumen diameter, were capable of detecting clinically meaningful treatment differences.

As coronary angiography and acute coronary intervention became more widespread, and with the execution of clinical trials evaluating the treatment of acute coronary artery occlusion, with either surgical revascularization or thrombolytic therapy, it became apparent that more than half of coronary occlusions were occurring in nonstenotic lesions. It appeared that atheroma burden, in the form of "vulnerable plaque" could be clinically important even though it might be undetectable, as a stenotic lesion, using coronary angiography (Falk *et al.*, 1995). With the work of Glagov *et al.*, atherosclerosis became understood as a disease of vessel wall remodeling and that only in the more advanced disease, did it encroach upon the vessel lumen (Glagov *et al.*, 1987). It is now understood that QCA has important limitations: (1) it can only detect advanced lesions that encroach upon the coronary lumen, and; (2) with the replacement of film by digital imaging, digital QCA has less spatial resolution, increasing the variability of the measures, making its use in clinical research, less

likely to detect treatment differences through time, particularly in studies with an active control treatment (Brown, 2002).

Ultrasound

With the development of ultrasound imaging technology, it became possible to assess the presence and severity of clinical vascular disease within the vessel wall, which was undetectable by X-ray angiography. Clinically, ultrasound was initially used noninvasively, in vascular beds accessible to extravascular ultrasound energy. Ultrasound could assess vascular lumen diameter or identify the presence of plaque, in the carotid arteries of patients felt to be at risk of, or who had sustained, cerebrovascular events, transient ischemic attacks, or stroke. It was also used to identify vascular abnormalities such as vessel wall dissection, hematoma, and aneurysms. As was the case with contrast angiography, the development of quantitative measures of ultrasound images permitted the conduct of clinical trials, both observational and interventional, to assess the clinical risk of cardiovascular morbidity and mortality and antiatherosclerotic treatment efficacy.

A host of long-term epidemiologic studies of various populations in both North America and Europe consistently demonstrated a relationship between baseline measures of carotid intima media thickening (IMT) and recognized cardiac risk factors including age, hypertension, smoking, diabetes, and lipid disorders. In most studies, subjects with larger measures of carotid IMT had an increased risk of developing stroke, nonfatal myocardial infarction, or cardiac death (Salonen *et al.*, 1991; Chambless *et al.*, 1997, 2000; Bots *et al.*, 1997; O'Leary *et al.*, 1999). A long-term follow-up (average of 8.8 years) of subjects who participated in the Cholesterol Lowering Atherosclerosis Study (CLAS), a 2-year study with both QCA and carotid ultrasound, comparing lipid-lowering therapy and diet-to-diet alone, demonstrated a relationship between the rate of progression of IMT thickening and clinical events (Hodis *et al.*, 1998). In that study, for every 0.03 mm/year increase in carotid IMT, there was an increase in the relative risk for nonfatal myocardial infarction or coronary death of 2.2 (95% CI, 1.4–3.6). Absolute IMT was also a predictor of outcomes. Carotid measures of IMT, in that study, were better predictors than coronary angiography or lipid levels. Ultrasound measures of carotid IMT have been suggested as a clinical tool to refine risk stratification in both the National Cholesterol Education-Adult Treatment Panel III clinical guidelines (NCEP, 2002) and more formally by the International Task Force for Prevention of Coronary Heart Disease, as an "emerging risk factor" that can be used to provide additional predictive information (Assmann *et al.*, 2005).

Carotid ultrasound has been used in a large number of studies comparing treatments in the areas of hypertension, atherosclerosis, diabetes, and estrogen replacement therapy. For the most part, these studies looked at changes in carotid IMT as the primary endpoint. Different analytical methodologies were used. Some studies simply looked at the mean or maximal far wall IMT of the common carotid artery, comparing baseline to end-of-study measures. Other investigators took the mean of the maximal IMT of multiple segments and multiple walls, with different angles of sonographic interrogation of the target segments. There is no general agreement on the optimal methodology of measuring coronary IMT though there is agreement on the importance of sonographic and reader training, the standardization of equipment and software, and the importance of a comprehensive quality assurance program. Despite differences in analytic methodologies, as was the case with QCA, there has been a consistent trend in which salutary changes in lipid levels and a reduction in cardiovascular events are paralleled by a reduction in the rate of IMT thickening. In a meta-analysis of seven HMG-CoA reductase inhibitor (statin) lipid-treatment studies cardiovascular event frequency was calculated where a change in the mean IMT thickening rate of

−0.012 mm/year (−0.016, −0.007, 95% confidence interval [CI]) was associated with an odds ratio of 0.48 (0.30, 0.78, 95% CI) (Espeland *et al.*, 2005). Espeland concluded that for clinical trials of statin therapy, carotid ultrasound measures of IMT met the criteria for surrogacy for cardiovascular events.

A promising imaging modality, that also gives information about vessel wall thickness, is coronary intravascular ultrasound (IVUS). The intravascular location and higher frequency of the ultrasound transducer, gives high resolution of coronary artery vessel wall cross-sectional area. The automated pullback system used to obtain serial tomographic data, permitting the measurement of vessel wall volume, essentially eliminates the operator variability that can be problematic during image acquisition with a hand-held extravascular ultrasound transducer. While IVUS has not yet generated the large clinical datasets of QCA or carotid ultrasound, there is accumulating evidence to suggest that IVUS-measured changes in atheroma burden are clinically meaningful. In IVUS studies performed on normal hearts that served as transplant donor organs, it was noted that, as was the case with carotid ultrasound, there was a relationship between age, and IVUS measures of atheroma burden (Tuzcu *et al.*, 1995, 2001). There has also been a demonstration of a relationship between IVUS measures of vessel wall cross-sectional area and cardiovascular risk. In a small retrospective study of just under 60 subjects with angiographic evidence of coronary artery disease, von Birgelen *et al.*, demonstrated a relationship between changes in IVUS measures of left main coronary artery cross-sectional area and risk factors for coronary heart disease (CHD), risk scores of the subjects, using either of three widely accepted risk scoring models, and a relationship between cardiovascular events and IVUS measures of disease progression (von Birgelen *et al.*, 2004). A number of IVUS lipid studies have now been completed, that show reductions in LDL-C with associated reductions in IVUS measures of atheroma burden (Schartl *et al.*, 2001; Nissen *et al.*,

2004; Tardif *et al.*, 2004). The relatively short duration of these studies, has precluded the demonstration of a direct, within-trial, statistically significant relationship between changes in IVUS measures of atheroma burden and clinical events. Of interest is the observation that three trials of secondary prevention in different populations, a carotid ultrasound study (Taylor *et al.*, 2002), a coronary IVUS study (Nissen *et al.*, 2004), and a morbidity and mortality study (Cannon *et al.*, 2004), with identical treatment arms comparing moderate and high-dose statin regimens, showed nearly identical responses in LDL-C lowering. In the high-dose statin therapy arms, the carotid ultrasound study showed a regression of atherosclerosis measured as IMT, the coronary IVUS study showed a halt in atherosclerosis progression, and the morbidity and mortality study showed a clinically significant reduction in cardiovascular events. While this evidence is indirect, it supports the argument that ultrasound measures of vessel wall thickness in both coronary and carotid arteries are clinically meaningful and can be used in drug development.

Future directions in vascular imaging

A number of new imaging modalities are being developed. One approach is to focus on monitoring changes in plaque composition. Related efforts will focus on understanding the factors that lead to plaque converting from a stable to unstable or vulnerable state. The methodology that is most advanced in assessing plaque composition is vascular magnetic resonance imaging (MRI) targeting the carotid artery and/or aorta. A small number of groups are developing this technology and to date there have been two intervention studies using MRI to measure changes in atheroma volume (Zhao *et al.*, 2001; Corti *et al.*, 2002) and one small study demonstrating changes in plaque composition, specifically the lipid core, due to therapeutic intervention (Hatsukami *et al.*, 2005).

There have been a number of studies focusing on the validation of the technique. Histological analysis of excised plaque has been compared and mapped to MRI of the same excised samples showing that the MRI image does compare favorably to the histology gold standard (Yuan *et al.*, 2005). In addition, there are ongoing studies to determine the ability to use this technology for clinical trials, including variability of the quantitative capabilities, semiautomated analysis to reduce reader variability and establishment of fixed imaging sequences (Rutt *et al.*, 2004; Saam *et al.*, 2005). The transition from 1.5T to 3.0T MRI provides opportunities in the early clinical development phases of drug development and in differentiating competitive therapies (Hinton *et al.*, 2003). It may ultimately be used in pivotal phase 3 trials.

Other methodologies that may play a role in development of therapies include:

1. [18]Fluoro-deoxyglucose Positron Emission Tomography (FDG-PET) which could be useful upon earlier development as an indicator of therapeutic action on plaque inflammation (Rudd *et al.*, 2002; Dunphy *et al.*, 2005).
2. Ultrasmall paramagnetic iron oxide particles (USPIO), which can also be used as indicators of plaque inflammation (Corot *et al.*, 2004).
3. Novel ultrasound contrast reagents (Villanueva *et al.*, 2004).
4. Molecular imaging of apoptosis in plaques (Choudhury *et al.*, 2004).
5. Infrared invasive and noninvasive (thermography) imaging (Bhatia *et al.*, 2003).
6. Multislice CT has potential for coronary analyses and with the advancement of this technology may prove to be a noninvasive alternative to IVUS (Moselewski *et al.*, 2004).

The success of these modalities in enhancing drug development in early or late stages, will depend upon the characteristics of the imaging technology, the endpoints that they can detect, and the clinical relevance of the data. If one looks at the development and acceptance of QCA and carotid IMT technologies as paradigms and then considers the need to detect efficacy on top of current standards of pharmacologic care rather than placebo controls, one can appreciate the amount of new imaging research that will need to be accomplished.

Regulatory challenges in reference to vascular imaging

There is substantial scientific evidence that imaging endpoints can be used in clinical drug development. It is important to recognize that regulatory agencies of different countries have different attitudes toward the submission of clinical trial data imaging to assess clinical efficacy. The primary issue is whether or not images of vascular structure are clinically relevant and can be used as valid surrogate markers of clinical benefit. Two different regulatory perspectives are now described.

U.S. Food and Drug Administration (FDA) Metabolic Division

At a symposium regarding regulatory issues in the approval of new drugs for the treatment of disorders of metabolism and dyslipidemia, a representative of the U.S. Food and Drug Administration (FDA) stated, with regard to surrogate (vascular imaging) endpoint studies,

For changes in vascular anatomy as assessed by a particular method of imaging to be acceptable as a surrogate for reduction in risk for atherosclerotic events, mechanistic plausibility must be demonstrated as well as adequate evidence that the imaging method accurately reflects the disease process…and must clearly be supported by epidemiologic, pathologic, and clinical evidence linking changes in the "picture" of the vessel, by whatever method used, to changes in the clinical course of atherosclerotic vascular disease (Isaacsohn *et al.*, 2004).

The FDA representative indicated that the "burden to validate the method(s) chosen is on

the sponsor" and suggested strategies that might fulfill that requirement including the following (Isaacsohn *et al.*, 2004):

1. Characterizing the minimum clinically meaningful change measurable by the technique used.
2. Characterizing the sensitivity and specificity of the measured changes as a predictor of change in risk.
3. Considering defining the degree of clinically meaningful change by relating it to the alteration of a validated biomarker (e.g. LDL cholesterol) or a proved clinically effective dose of another antiatherosclerosis agent.
4. Vascular effects must be documented using at least two different imaging modalities.
5. The imaging results should be supported by other biomarker effects.

European Medicines Agency (EMEA), Committee for Medicinal Products for Human Use (CHMP)

At this time, the EMEA does not recognize data provided by imaging techniques to have clinical significance:

Although target organ damage of heart, brain, kidneys and, in particular blood vessels is presumably and plausibly associated with morbidity and mortality, the prognostic value of these drug effects with regard to morbidity and mortality remains to be established; this holds particularly true for changes in IMT and plaque stability. For the time being, the effect of a particular drug (or combination of drugs) on the arteriosclerotic burden at a particular site cannot be considered as a valid surrogate for cardiovascular morbidity and mortality…these parameters are not considered as surrogates for hard clinical endpoints, but they may constitute appropriate secondary endpoints to support information on progression or regression of atherosclerosis. (CHMP, 2004)

A number of pharmaceutical companies have submitted QCA and IMT data to the USA and Canadian drug regulatory authorities to supplement clinical study information and/or for supplemental indications that their therapies could slow the progression of atherosclerosis.

At this time five lipid-lowering drugs have USA product information that includes imaging data from clinical studies and/or indications to alter the progression of atherosclerosis (see Table 30.1).

From the perspective of the pharmaceutical industry, because of the regulatory challenges noted above, the use of vascular imaging data to support a regulatory submission for approval should include scientific support for the technical and clinical elements that serve as the basis for the conduct of vascular imaging studies in human subjects.

Elements of technical validation

The technical validation elements to be addressed in a regulatory submission should have background information on the hardware, analytical software, training, data processing, data transfer, and quality control.

Hardware: in the conduct of a multicenter imaging study, a detailed description of the hardware used should be provided, including data provided by the manufacturer or from the published literature, outlining the characteristics of the hardware, background studies showing how the image measurements correlate with physical measures (e.g. phantoms).

Image acquisition: the technical aspects of image acquisition particular to the trial should be outlined including an outline of the image acquisition protocol (instrument calibration, number of vascular segments imaged, imaging sequence, etc.), how technicians (e.g. sonographers) were trained and certified, who trained them, and quality-control measures that were employed during the conduct of the study. Information should be provided describing how new technicians were trained and certified during the conduct of the study, particularly in studies of longer than 1 year in duration, since technician turnover can be expected. There should be a description of the media used on which the image data is recorded and the file format used. The technical document should describe how the image data is sent or transmitted to the image-reading center.

Image analysis: measures of vessel structure (e.g. wall thickness, lumen diameter) can be made manually or using semiautomated methods. In either instance data should be provided regarding the hardware (computer workstations) and software (operating systems and image analysis software) used in the image reading center. The validation of the software needs to be reviewed. The training used for the readers should be described, as well as the credentials of the trainers, and the procedures that will be used in instances of reader turnover. Quality control measures (e.g. procedures for review and over-reads throughout the conduct of the trial) need to be outlined. Intra- and interreader variability should be described. If serial imaging will be done during the conduct of a study, there should be a description of the reading process including whether the images will all be read at one time by the same reader at the end of the study, or at intervals, periodically, or as images are acquired during the conduct of the study.

It is important that the image reading center or core-lab and the sponsor can demonstrate the integrity of the acquired imaging data and measurements. The software and data management applications used for any imaging program should be evaluated to ensure that they are consistent with the U.S. Department of Health and Human Services FDA guidelines outlined in Title 21 Code of Federal Regulations Part 11 (21 CFR Part 11) pertaining to electronic records, signatures, and submissions (CDER, 2003). In addition to the raw image data, the reading center must be able to demonstrate that they have records of time stamped, annotated images showing the actual measurements that were made and an identification of the reader. The data management system must have the ability to show any measurement changes that were edited.

Such changes need to be documented, time stamped, and it must be possible to identify who made the changes so that there is an audit trail. Computer network security procedures need to be outlined as well as file backup and data storage procedures.

Elements of clinical validation

The sponsor of clinical imaging studies should be able to demonstrate the extent to which the imaging data provided is clinically meaningful. Assuming that a treatment effect can be demonstrated by imaging, the regulators will want to know what is the minimal clinically meaningful change in the primary endpoint. For any imaging measure of atheroma burden, the sponsor should provide evidence that shows the quantitative distribution of the primary and/or secondary imaging endpoints in various populations at risk of cardiovascular disease and the relationship of those measures to other parameters including cardiac risk factors such as smoking, diabetes, lipid parameters and other biomarkers. It will be important to provide supporting evidence that changes in the primary endpoints are related to cardiovascular morbidity and mortality. As noted

previously, at the time of this publication, the EMEA only recognizes imaging data as potential secondary endpoints. The basis for US FDA and Canadian approval of supplemental indications to slow the progression of atherosclerosis were based on QCA and/or carotid IMT studies rested largely upon the demonstration of reductions in clinical events that paralleled the differences in treatment effects as measured by percent stenosis, minimal lumen diameter, percent of progressors or regressors, or changes in carotid IMT. Those studies were all placebo-controlled trials, a paradigm that is generally not ethically acceptable at this time, because of current treatment guidelines and a better appreciation of cardiovascular risk and the benefits of treatment.

If antiatherosclerosis drug development is to advance, industry, academia, and regulators will need to partner to adopt new paradigms that will permit one to assess drug safety and efficacy on shorter timelines (see Figure 30.1).

Assuming that vascular imaging technologies can permit the identification and quantification of clinically meaningful endpoints and if that data is accepted by regulatory authorities for registration and approval, it may be possible to provide new therapies to patients sooner, and at less cost.

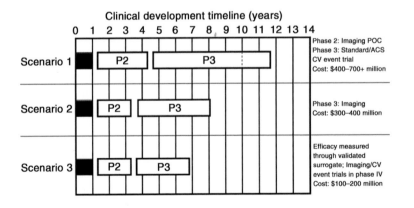

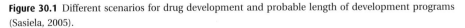

Figure 30.1 Different scenarios for drug development and probable length of development programs (Sasiela, 2005).

REFERENCES

Assmann, G., Cullen, P., Fruchart, J-C., *et al.* for the International Task Force for Prevention of Coronary Heart Disease. (2005). Implications of emerging risk factors for therapeutic intervention. *Nutrition, Metabolism, and Cardiovascular Disease*, **15**, 373–81.

Bhatia, V., Bhatia, R., Dhindsa, S. and Dhindsa, M. (2003). Imaging of the vulnerable plaque: New modalities. *Southern Medical Journal*, **95**, 1142–7.

Boissel, J. P., Collet, J. P., Moleur, P. and Haugh, M. (1992). Surrogate endpoints: a basis for a rational approach. *European Journal of Clinical Pharmacology*, **43**, 235–44.

Bots, M. L., Hoes, A. W., Koudstaal, P. J., Hofman, A. and Grobbee, D. E. (1997). Common carotid intima-media thickness and risk of stroke and myocardial infarction: the Rotterdam Study. *Circulation*, **96**, 1432–7.

Brown, B. G., Albers, J. J., Fisher, L. D., *et al.* (1990). Regression of coronary artery disease as a result of intensive lipid-lowering therapy in men with high levels of apolipoprotein B. *New England Journal of Medicine*, **323**, 1289–98.

Brown, B. G., Bolson, E., Frimer, M. and Dodge, H. T. (1977). Quantitative coronary arteriography: estimation of dimensions, hemodynamic resistance, and atheroma mass of coronary artery lesions using the arteriogram and digital computation. *Circulation*, **55**, 329–37.

Brown, B. G., Hillger, L. A. and Lewis, C. (1993a). A maximum confidence approach for measuring progression and regression of coronary artery disease in clinical trials. *Circulation*, **87** (Suppl. II.), II-66-II-73.

Brown, B. G., Zhao, X-Q., Sacco, D. E. and Albers, J. J. (1993b). Lipid lowering and plaque regression. New insights into prevention of plaque disruption and clinical events in coronary disease. *Circulation*, **87**, 1781–91.

Cannon, C. P., Braunwald, E., McCabe, C. H., *et al.* (2004). Intensive versus moderate lipid lowering with statins after acute coronary syndromes. *New England Journal of Medicine*, **350**, 1495–504.

Center for Drug Evaluation and Research (CDER), Division of Drug Information. (2003). *Guidance for Industry Part 11, Electronic Records; Electronic Signatures-Scope and Application*. U.S. Dept. of Health and Human Services, FDA, http://www.fda.gov/cder/guidance/5667fnl.htm, HFD-240, Rockville, MD.

Chambless, L. E., Folsom, A. R., Clegg, L. X., *et al.* (2000). Carotid wall thickness is predictive of incident clinical stroke: The Atherosclerosis Risk in Communities (ARIC) Study. *American Journal of Epidemiology*, **151**, 478–87.

Chambless, L. E., Heiss, G. and Folsom, A. R. (1997). Association of coronary heart disease incidence with carotid arterial wall thickness and major risk factors: the Athersclerosis Risk in Communities (ARIC) Study, 1987–1993. *American Journal of Epidemiology*, **146**, 483–94.

Choudhury, R. P., Fuster, V. and Fayad, Z. A. (2004). Molecular, cellular and functional imaging of athero-thrombosis. *Nature Reviews Drug Discovery*, **3**, 913–25.

Committee for Medicinal Products for Human Use (CHMP) (2004). *Note for guidance on clinical investigation of medicinal products in the treatment of lipid disorders*. European Medicines Agency (EMEA), Publication CPMP/EWP/3020/03. London, UK.

Corot, C., Petry, K. G., Trivedi, R., *et al.* (2004). Macrophage imaging in central nervous system and carotid atherosclerotic plaque using ultrasmall superparamagnetic iron oxide in magnetic resonance imaging. *Investigative Radiology*, **39**, 619–23.

Corti, R., Fuster, V., Fayad, Z. A., *et al.* (2002). Lipid lowering by simvastatin induces regression of human atherosclerotic lesions: two years' follow-up by high-resolution noninvasive magnetic resonance imaging. *Circulation*, **106**, 2884–7.

de Groot, E., Jukema, J. W., van Boven, A. J., *et al.* (1995). Effect of pravastatin on progression and regression of coronary atherosclerosis and vessel wall changes in carotid and femoral arteries: a report from the Regression Growth Evaluation Statin Study. *American Journal of Cardiology*, **76**, 40C–6C.

Dunphy, M. P., Freima, A., Larson, S. M. and Strauss, H. W. (2005). Association of vascular 18FDG-PET uptake with vascular calcification. *Journal of Nuclear Medicine*, **46**, 1278–84.

Espeland, M. A., O'Leary, D. H., Terry, J. G., *et al.* (2005). Carotid intimal-media thickness as a surrogate for cardiovascular disease events in trials of HMG-CoA reductase inhibitors. *Current Controlled Trials in Cardiovascular Medicine*, **6**, 3.

Furberg, C. D., Adams, H. P., Applegate, W. B., *et al.* (1994). Effect of lovastatin on early carotid atherosclerosis and cardiovascular events. *Circulation*, **90**, 1679–87.

Hatsukami, T., Zhao, X-Q., Kraiss, L. W., *et al.* (2005). Assessment of rosuvastatin treatment on carotid atherosclerosis in moderately hypercholesterolemic subjects using high-resolution magnetic resonance imaging. *European Heart Journal*, **26** (Abstract Suppl.), 626.

Falk, E., Shah, P. K. and Fuster, V. (1995). Coronary plaque disruption. *Circulation*, **92**, 657–71.

Furberg, C. D., Pitt, B., Byington, R. P., Park, J. S. and McGovern, M. E. (1995). Reduction in coronary events during treatment with pravastatin. PLAC I and PLAC II Investigators. Pravastatin Limitation of Atherosclerosis in the Coronary Arteries. *American Journal of Cardiology*, **76**, 60C–3C.

Glagov, S., Weisenberg, E., Zarins, C. K., *et al.* (1987). Compensatory enlargement of human atherosclerotic coronary arteries. *New England Journal of Medicine*, **316**, 1371–5.

Herd, J. A., Ballantyne, C. M., Farmer, J. A., *et al.* (1997). Effects of fluvastatin on coronary atherosclerosis in patients with mild to moderate cholesterol elevations (Lipoprotein and Coronary Atherosclerosis Study LCAS). *American Journal of Cardiology*, **80**, 278–86.

Hinton, D. P., Wald, L. L., Pitts, J. and Schmitt, F. (2003). Comparison of cardiac MRI on 1.5 and 3.0 Tesla clinical whole body systems. *Investigative Radiology*, **38**, 436–42.

Hodis, H. N., Mack, W. J., LaBree, L., *et al.* (1996). Reduction in carotid arterial wall thickness using lovastatin and dietary therapy. *Annals of Internal Medicine*, **124**, 548–56.

Hodis, H. N., Mack, W. J., LaBree, L., *et al.* (1998). The role of carotid arterial intima-media thickness in predicting clinical coronary events. *Annals of Internal Medicine*, **128**, 262–9.

Isaacsohn, J. L., Troendle, A. J. and Orloff, D. G. (2004). Regulatory issues in the approval of new drugs for diabetes mellitus, dyslipidemia, and the metabolic syndrome. *American Journal of Cardiology*, **93** (11A), 49C–52C.

MAAS Investigators. (1994). Effect of simvastatin on coronary atheroma: the Multicentre Anti-Atheroma Study (MAAS). *Lancet*, **344**, 633–8.

Mackay, J. and Mensah, G. A. (2004). *The Atlas of Heart Disease and Stroke*. Geneva, Switzerland: World Health Organization.

Moselewski, F., Ropers, D., Pohle, K., *et al.* (2004). Comparison of measurement of cross-sectional coronary atherosclerotic plaque and vessel areas by 16-slice multidetector computed tomography versus intravascular ultrasound. *American Journal of Cardiology*, **94**, 1294–7.

National Cholesterol Education Program Expert Panel (NCEP). (2002). *Detection, evaluation, and treatment of high blood cholesterol in adults (Adult Treatment Panel III): Final Report*. National Heart, Lung, and Blood Institute. National Institutes of Health. NIH Publication No. 02–5215. P II-25.

Nissen, S. E., Tuzcu, E. M., Schoenhagen, P., *et al.* (2004). Effect of intensive compared with moderate lipid-lowering therapy on progression of coronary atherosclerosis: a randomized controlled trial. *Journal of the American Medical Association*, **291**, 1071–80

O'Leary, D. H., Polak, J. F., Kronmal, R. A., *et al.* (1999). Carotid-artery intima and media thickness as a risk factor for myocardial infarction and stroke in older adults. Cardiovascular Health Study Collaborative Research Group. *New England Journal of Medicine*, **340**, 14–22.

Prentice, R. L. (1989). Surrogate endpoints in clinical trials: definition and operational criteria. *Statistics in Medicine*, **8**, 431–40.

Reiber, J. H. C., Serruys, P. W., Kooijman, C. J., *et al.* (1985). Assessment of short-, medium-, and long-term variations in arterial dimensions from computer-assisted quantitation of coronary cine-angiograms. *Circulation*, **71**, 280–8.

Rossouw, J. E. (1995). Lipid-lowering interventions in angiographic trials. *American Journal of Cardiology*, **76**, 86C–92C.

Rudd, J. H., Warburton, E. A., Fryer, T. D., *et al.* (2002). Imaging atherosclerotic plaque inflammation with 18F-flourodeoxyglucose positron emission tomography. *Circulation*, **105**, 2708–11.

Rutt, B. K., Clarke, S. E. and Fayad, Z. A. (2004). Atherosclerotic plaque characterization by MR imaging. *Current Drug Targets. Cardiovascular and Haemotological Disorders*, **4**, 147–59.

Saam, T., Ferguson, M. S., Yarnykh, V. L., *et al.* (2005). Quantitative evaluation of carotid plaque composition by in vivo MRI. *Arteriosclerosis, Thrombosis and Vascular Biology*, **25**, 234–9.

Salonen, R., Nyyssonen, K., Porkkala, E., *et al.* (1995). Kuopio Atherosclerosis Prevention Study (KAPS). A population-based primary preventive trial of the effect of LDL lowering on atherosclerotic progression in carotid and femoral arteries. *Circulation*, **92**, 1758–64.

Salonen, J. T. and Salonen, R. (1991). Ultrasonographically assessed carotid morphology and the risk of coronary heart disease. *Arteriosclerosis and Thrombosis*, **11**, 1245–9.

Sankatsing, R. R., de Groot, E. and Jukema, J. W. (2005). Surrogate markers for atherosclerotic disease. *Current Opinion in Lipidology*, **16**, 434–41.

Sasiela, W. J. *The need for biomarkers in drug development. Cardiovascular biomarkers and surrogate endpoints symposium.* Sponsored by University of Montréal, 23 September, 2005. Bethesda, MD, USA

Schartl, M., Bocksch, W., Koschyk, D. H., *et al.* (2001). Use of intravascular ultrasound to compare effects of different strategies of lipid-lowering therapy on plaque volume and composition in patients with coronary artery disease. *Circulation*, **104**, 387–92.

Tardif, J. C., Gregoire, J., L'Allier, P. L., for the Avasimibe and Progression of Lesions on Ultrasound (A-PLUS) Investigators. (2004). Effects of the acyl coenzyme A:cholesterol acyltransferase inhibitor avasimibe on human atherosclerotic lesions. *Circulation*, **110**, 3372–7.

Taylor, A. J., Kent, S. M. and Flaherty, P. J. (2002). ARBITER: Arterial Biology for the Investigation of the Treatment Effects of Reducing Cholesterol: a randomized trial comparing the effects of atorvastatin and pravastatin on carotid intima medial thickness. *Circulation*, **106**, 2055–60.

Tuzcu, E. M., Hobbs, R. E., Rincon, G., *et al.* (1995). Occult and frequent transmission of atherosclerotic coronary disease with cardiac transplantation. Insights from intravascular ultrasound. *Circulation*, **91**, 1706–13.

Tuzcu, E. M., Kapadia, S. R., Tutar, E., *et al.* (2001). High prevalence of coronary atherosclerosis in asymptomatic teenagers and young adults: evidence from intravascular ultrasound. *Circulation*, **103**, 2705–10.

Villanueva, F. S., Wagner, W. R., Vannan, M. A. and Narula, J. (2004). Targeted ultrasound imaging using microbubbles. *Cardiology Clinics*, **22**, 283–91.

von Birgelen, C., Hartmann, M., Mintz, G. S., *et al.* (2004). Relationship between cardiovascular risk as predicted by established risk scores versus plaque progression as measured by serial intravascular ultrasound in left main coronary arteries. *Circulation*, **110**, 1579–85.

Waters D., Higginson, L. and Gladstone, P. (1994). Effects of monotherapy with an HMG-CoA reductase inhibitor on the progression of coronary atherosclerosis as assessed by serial quantitative arteriography. *Circulation*, **89**, 959–68.

Yuan, C., Hatsukami, T. S. and Cai, J. (2005). MRI plaque tissue characterization and assessment of plaque stability. *Studies in Health Technology and Informatics*, **113**, 55–74.

Zhao, X-Q., Yuan, C., Hatsukami, T. S., *et al.* (2001). Effects of prolonged intensive lipid lowering therapy on the characteristics of carotid atherosclerotic plaques in vivo by MRI. *Arteriosclerosis, Thrombosis and Vascular Biology*, **21**, 1623–9.

31

Monitoring pharmaceutical interventions with conventional ultrasound (IMT)

John R. Crouse

Wake Forest University School of Medicine, Winston-Salem NC, USA

Background

Doppler ultrasound was validated in the mid 1970s as a means of quantifying tight stenosis of the extracranial carotid arteries (Barnes *et al.*, 1976) and thus of identifying individuals at risk for cerebrovascular events. In the early 1980s, as reviewed previously (Crouse and Thompson, 1993), several investigators demonstrated associations of cardiovascular risk factors with Doppler-quantified extracranial carotid stenosis (e.g. Hennerici *et al.*, 1981; Postiglione *et al.*, 1985; Lo *et al.*, 1986; Josse *et al.*, 1987) and of stenosis with a 5.5-fold increased risk of incident stroke and a 3-fold increased risk of coronary disease compared to individuals without stenosis (Chambers and Norris, 1986). However, although Doppler ultrasound accurately identifies stenosis of the extracranial carotid arteries, in 1982 Blankenhorn and Curry reviewed the evidence that imaging lumens of arteries and stenosis (angiography, Doppler) underestimated the underlying pathology and that therefore only autopsy provided an accurate evaluation of the pathogenesis, prevalence, and prognosis of atherosclerosis (Blankenhorn and Curry, 1982). This observation provided rationale for early studies that used B-mode ultrasound to quantify wall thickness of the extracranial carotid arteries, and investigation utilizing noninvasive imaging of walls of arteries

led to a paradigm shift in the population-based investigation of arterial disease. Development of methods that were not invasive and provided information on arterial walls rather than lumens enabled quantification of the impact of risk factors on subclinical disease (before the occurrence of clinical events), and of subclinical disease on clinical outcome for the first time. Identification of subclinical disease also enabled investigators to distinguish between risk factors for underlying atherosclerosis and those for development of symptoms.

As a means of imaging chronic stable atherosclerotic vascular disease, B-mode ultrasound of the extracranial carotid arteries (extracranial carotid intima-media thickness [IMT]) has many advantages, and IMT has been related to a number of risk factors, some of which are well recognized risk factors for cardiovascular disease and some of which are novel (Bonithon-Kopp *et al.*, 1991; Heiss *et al.*, 1991; O'Leary *et al.*, 1992; Howard *et al.*, 1996; Bots *et al.*, 1997; Wilson *et al.*, 1997; Gariepy *et al.*, 1998; Schott *et al.*, 2004). As might be expected, IMT relates better to the integrated experience of past risk factor burden than to current risk factor exposure. B-mode can also be used to define rates of progression of IMT (e.g. Zureik *et al.*, 1991; Salonen and Salonen, 1993; Willeit *et al.*, 2000; Chambless *et al.*, 2002; Crouse *et al.*, 2002; Van der Meer *et al.*, 2003;

Carotid Disease: The Role of Imaging in Diagnosis and Management, ed. Jonathan Gillard, Martin Graves, Thomas Hatsukami and Chun Yuan. Published by Cambridge University Press. © Cambridge University Press 2007.

Mackinnon *et al.*, 2004) and the influence of risk factors and interventions (e.g. on lipids, diabetes, blood pressure) on progression rates (Bots *et al.*, 2003b). IMT is associated with prevalent coronary artery (Craven *et al.*, 1990; O'Leary *et al.*, 1992; Burke *et al.*, 1995) and cerebrovascular (O'Leary *et al.*, 1992; Chambless *et al.*, 1996) disease as well as incident coronary artery disease (Salonen and Salonen, 1993; Bots *et al.*, 1997; Hodis *et al.*, 1998; O'Leary *et al.*, 1999; Chambless *et al.*, 2003), stroke (Manolio *et al.*, 1996; Bots *et al.*, 1997; O'Leary *et al.*, 1999; Chambless *et al.*, 2004), and all cause mortality (Fried *et al.*, 1998). More recently, investigators have quantified the heritability of and genetic polymorphisms associated with IMT (Zannad and Benetos, 2003; Humphries and Morgan, 2004; Manolio *et al.*, 2004). Although carotid IMT relates both to risk factors and to outcome, the magnitude of the relation of risk factors to IMT and to outcome is not always the same, leading to development of hypotheses related to the generation of clinical events vis-à-vis the atherosclerosis substrate (Sharrett *et al.*, 1999).

This chapter deals with both established correlates of IMT as well as new findings and formulations of data derived from this technology. The reliability and validity of the method are now well described as are relationships with risk factors, although new risk factors (including genetic markers and hereditary influences) continue to be tested for associations with IMT. Although associations with progression of IMT are more difficult to demonstrate, these, too, are well established. Differences in progression are now routinely used to define surrogate outcomes for clinical trials of behavioral and pharmacologic intervention; the Food and Drug Administration (FDA) accepts this as a valid marker of atherosclerosis change. Also of considerable interest are insights that B-mode ultrasound provides into the process of vascular remodeling. This review also discusses the associations of IMT with prevalent as well as incident coronary artery and cerebrovascular disease. Finally, strengths and weaknesses of this method are discussed.

Methodology

B-mode ultrasound imaging equipment has reached a mature stage of development. The echo principle relies on time delay to return from a pulsed ultrasound reflected from echodense targets. Using an assumed value for the speed of propagation of the ultrasound energy between the source and the target, the reflectance time is translated into an index of distance from these targets to the tip of the ultrasound probe placed against the skin. Generally the transducer produces 2–3 cycle pulses of about 10 MHz ultrasound which results in an axial resolution of approximately 100–200 μm. Thus distances between structures that exceed this distance (e.g. arterial adventitia and lumen: distance is 550–1000 μm in healthy arteries and up to 3000 μm in diseased arteries) can be reliably measured, and changes in this distance over time can be ascertained.

The extent of deviation of wall thicknesses from normal can be quantified based on wall thicknesses at individual sites or on composite measures based on sums or averages of measurements across multiple sites (e.g. the near and far walls of the internal carotid, bifurcation, and common carotid from the right and left sides, 2). Since the far wall of the common carotid artery is easiest to visualize and most reproducibly measured with the least missing data (Crouse *et al.*, 1992), many investigators have chosen this as their index of analysis. However, plaques tend to develop at areas of turbulence associated with bifurcations, and the area of the bulb and internal carotid may therefore provide additional information and more broadly reflect disease burden. Such composite measures also provide greater statistical power and efficiency, and are recommended as primary outcome measures for most clinical research studies (Espeland *et al.*, 1996, 2003; Bots *et al.*, 2003b), although by formal testing information from the common carotid alone is also valuable (Espeland *et al.*, 1999a). When multiple sites are the focus of analysis, multivariate (maximum likelihood) methods are necessary to minimize biases associated with occasionally nonvisualized sites (Espeland *et al.*, 1999b).

Reproducibility

Early analyses used B-mode ultrasound in case-control and cross-sectional studies to quantify associations of IMT with risk factors and with coronary artery disease. Cross-sectional associations are relatively easy to demonstrate because of the wide cross-sectional dispersion of levels of independent variables (age, blood pressure, cholesterol, etc.) and the magnitude and consistency of the biologic response. However, the role of risk factors in progression and of interventions on progression cannot be determined from cross-sectional studies. Studies of progression require a higher level of reproducibility, more demanding techniques and highly standardized protocols that include the definition of anatomic landmarks, control of probe interrogation angle, and careful circumferential scanning of segments to identify the maximum wall thickness. Figure 31.1 defines the extracranial carotid arterial segments that can be interrogated with B-mode ultrasound (Kanters *et al.*, 1997). This diagram identifies the anatomic landmark (tip of flow divider) relative to the segments of interest that are defined above.

There are four important sources of variability in quantification of IMT (particularly for multi-center studies): choice of number of segments to measure, choice of equipment, sonographer error, and reader error. The number of sites chosen for analysis varies from study to study. Averages of several measurements taken from any single individual should provide greater reproducibility than any individual measurement (Crouse and Thompson, 1993). This formulation (together with the greater representativeness that multiple measurements provide, see above) provides rationale for obtaining multiple measurements from the left and right sides at three locations (common carotid, bifurcation, internal carotid) and from both near and far walls. Others have argued

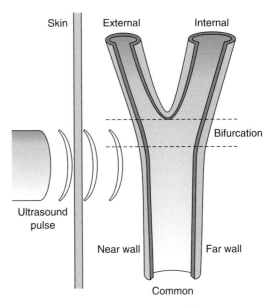

Figure 31.1 Schematic representation of the common carotid artery, the bifurcation, the internal carotid artery, and the external carotid artery. (Reproduced from Kanters S. D. *et al.* (1997). *Stroke*, **28**, 665–71.)

in favor of taking measurements from only the common carotid artery or only the far wall of the common carotid artery. IMT at this site can be quantified with a greater degree of reliability and at less cost in time and money than other sites. However, more recent studies have shown greater ability than previous studies to obtain information from the internal carotid and bifurcation (IMT data were available in >95% of the screening and randomization visits on all segments except the left internal near wall [92.9%], and right internal near wall [88.6%] in a recent clinical trial) (Bots *et al.*, 2003a). As discussed above, statistical methods are available to minimize the impact of missing data (missing at random) by using maximum likelihood techniques (Espeland *et al.*, 1999b). Moreover, since progression rates of various walls and sites of the carotid artery are correlated with one another (Espeland *et al.*, 2003), inclusion of several sites improves power as well as representativeness.

Investigators have also discussed the relative strengths and weaknesses of using information from the far wall alone as opposed to that from both the near and far walls. Although validity of near wall measurements may be questioned, the association that near wall IMT has with prevalent and incident cardiovascular disease is similar to that for the far wall (Bots *et al.*, 2000b; Espeland *et al.*, 2003). As noted above, if appropriate statistical methods are used, the greater information provided by measurement across more sites should provide greater statistical power and efficiency (Crouse and Thompson, 1993).

A second source of variability rests in the ultrasound equipment. Many large multicenter epidemiologic studies and clinical trials have purchased uniform equipment and provided centralized standardization across clinical sites to avoid this problem. Central ultrasound sites that draw on multiple clinical sites for multicenter studies also provide greater equipment uniformity at reduced cost (Crouse *et al.*, 2004).

Sonographer characteristics have potential to introduce significant variability into ultrasound readings, and, to reduce this, investigators have used standard angles for ultrasound interrogation. Sonographer variability can also be reduced in multicenter studies by centralized training, and certification based on acquiring a prespecified number of adequate exams. Centralized sonography suites that accommodate patients from several surrounding clinical sites also provide a means of reducing sonographer variability (Crouse *et al.*, 2004), however, the operator dependence of the B-mode technique is one of its enduring drawbacks.

Variability between readers can also be substantial, and for longitudinal studies this can be reduced by reading all studies from a protocol by a single reader toward the end of the protocol to avoid "reader drift", automated image quantification; training and retraining of readers as well as sonographers; an ongoing quality control program for both instrumentation and personnel;

and central reading sites for multicenter trials. The importance of "batch reading" of baseline and follow-up examinations for longitudinal investigation cannot be stressed enough. In one recently reported clinical trial, reader drift over the course of the trial resulted in the appearance of an outcome that was the opposite of that obtained if the data were controlled for reader drift either by contemporaneous reading of a standard set of scans or by batch reading at the end of the trial (Zanchetti *et al.*, 2004). Recently a number of studies have recruited patients in the USA and Europe, and the protocols outlined above represent approaches implemented in order to overcome the substantial challenges encountered in these international studies (Bots *et al.*, 2003a; Crouse *et al.*, 2004).

Reliability can be expressed in several ways. For cross-sectional or case-control studies often only a single estimate of IMT is available and reliability of a single reader or multiple readers reading a single frame of an ultrasound exam can be compared, or the entire tape of the exam can be reviewed twice to estimate the reliability of quantification of the maximum. In some protocols the sonographer identifies the maximum wall thickness and freezes the frame for the reader to read, and in other protocols the sonographer carries out a more extensive circumferential scan of the arteries and the reader chooses the maximum thickness. For longitudinal studies the greatest source of variability is neither in the reader nor the sonographer, but in the repositioning and overall reevaluation of the participant. Since this is the most relevant comparison for determination of change over time, estimations of reliability of the overall positioning/scanning/ reading process are necessary for planning of longitudinal studies. The estimate of reliability together with the anticipated progression rate are used to estimate sample sizes for epidemiologic studies or clinical trials.

Reliability can be discussed in terms of correlation coefficients or mean absolute differences of repeat measurements. Table 31.1 presents

Table 31.1. Mean intima-media thickness (IMT), arithmetic difference, correlation coefficient, and correlation coefficient of reliability at baseline by endpoint

Endpoint	Average of measurements (mm) Mean ± SD	Arithmetic difference (mm) n	Mean ± SD	Absolute difference (mm) Mean ± SD	Median	95th percentile	Reliability R	Lower bound
CBM$_{max}$	1.198 ± 0.256	2227	0.004 ± 0.141	0.101 ± 0.099	0.076	0.288	0.859	0.850
M$_{max}$	1.135 ± 0.206	2227	0.005 ± 0.108	0.077 ± 0.075	0.057	0.211	0.872	0.864
T$_{max}$	1.799 ± 0.576	2227	0.015 ± 0.390	0.254 ± 0.296	0.158	0.818	0.794	0.781
Near wall	1.119 ± 0.216	2227	0.006 ± 0.140	0.102 ± 0.096	0.077	0.279	0.809	0.796
Far wall	1.149 ± 0.247	2227	0.004 ± 0.141	0.097 ± 0.101	0.071	0.297	0.851	0.841
Common	1.042 ± 0.171	2227	0.003 ± 0.099	0.069 ± 0.070	0.053	0.192	0.847	0.837
Bifurcation	1.325 ± 0.309	2227	0.008 ± 0.191	0.137 ± 0.133	0.098	0.404	0.826	0.815
Internal	1.020 ± 0.282	2227	0.002 ± 0.258	0.165 ± 0.196	0.108	0.554	0.659	0.639
Right	1.145 ± 0.235	2227	0.002 ± 0.138	0.098 ± 0.098	0.089	0.280	0.841	0.831
Left	1.125 ± 0.225	2227	0.009 ± 0.143	0.100 ± 0.103	0.071	0.290	0.815	0.803

From: Tang R., Hennig M., Thomasson B., *et al.* (2000). Baseline reproducibility of B-mode ultrasonic measurement of carotid artery IMT: the European Lacidipine Study on Atherosclerosis (ELSA). *Journal of Hypertension*, **18**, 197–201.

reliability data from a recent publication (Tang *et al.*, 2000). In general within-reader or within-sonographer variability is considerably less than interreader or intersonographer variability, and both can be controlled with suitable protocols and training.

Validity

Pignoli *et al.* were the first to evaluate the validity of the B-mode quantification of wall thickness in vitro and in vivo. Their experiments focused on the aorta and common carotid arteries and indicated that IMT obtained from B-mode imaging did not differ significantly from the histologic IMT (Pignoli *et al.*, 1986). Wong *et al.* (Wong *et al.*, 1993) performed similar measurements on carotid and femoral arteries and concluded that B-mode imaging of IMT on the far (deeper) wall compared well with histology. Gamble *et al.* (1993) carried out in vitro and *in situ* experiments in the common carotid arteries of cadavers. These indicated that B-mode

imaging of the artery wall correlated best with the combined intimal-medial-adventitial thickness as measured from histologic sections but that increased wall thickness due to intimal atherosclerotic thickening still correlated well with the thickness obtained from B-mode images. Thickness measurements from the far (deeper) wall of a vessel were more clearly defined and valid than those from the near (shallower) wall, due to the basic physical principles used in constructing B-mode images (Wong *et al.*, 1993).

Some investigators have advocated use of "plaque" rather than IMT as a primary index of disease since some increase in IMT may result from hyperplasia rather than atherosclerosis per se (Crouse, 1993). In theory, this approach has merit; however, in practice different investigators have proposed different definitions of "plaque" (most characterize "plaque" as a lesion whose IMT is 50% greater than a normal appearing nearby segment [Salonen *et al.*, 1988], whereas others identify "plaque" as present if there is a localized thickening ≥1.2 mm [Markussis *et al.*, 1992]). Investigators

Table 31.2. Mean wall thicknesses for black and white men and women (adapted from Howard *et al.*, 1993)

	Black women			Black men			White women			White men		
	45y	55y	65y	45y	55y	65y	45y	55y	65y	45y	55y	65y
Common	0.57	0.67	0.73	0.62	0.71	0.83	0.54	0.62	0.70	0.58	0.67	0.76
Bifurcation	0.65	0.77	0.87	0.70	0.84	0.98	0.62	0.74	0.90	0.69	0.83	1.00
Internal	0.55	0.60	0.68	0.56	0.63	0.77	0.52	0.60	0.67	0.56	0.69	0.77

who prefer use of IMT argue that information about "plaque" is captured through IMT since the "maximum" IMT is generally measured at the site of a "plaque". Furthermore, "plaque" does not appear to add information about associations with risk factors or with prevalent or incident disease that is not available from measurement of IMT alone (Bots *et al.*, 2003b). Spence and colleagues have also advocated use of "3D ultrasound" for quantification of plaque volume using B-mode. This method is reliable and has face validity; however, measures of wall area or volume depend heavily on lumen area and use of these measures in epidemiologic studies may be fraught with problems. In addition, at the present time published validation of the method relies on artificial phantoms rather than endarterectomy specimens (Ainsworth *et al.*, 2005).

Characterization of plaque composition from B-mode images has also been advocated by some investigators (El-Barghouty *et al.*, 1996), because of the well-described association of unstable plaque with acute events (Davies, 1996); however, such characterization is complex and difficult. The methods described above for assessing IMT evolved from validation studies on normal or near-normal arteries in which the lumen-intima and media-adventitia boundaries were clearly defined. When complex plaques are present, these boundaries may become less well defined and other boundaries may develop within the wall that can change the fundamental principles underlying the IMT measurement process and decrease the reproducibility. Current investigations are under

way to explore further the potential of ultrasonic B-mode imaging in the characterization of athero-sclerotic plaque composition (Sztajzel *et al.*, 2005).

Normative values for intima-media thicknesses

Critical to interpretation of B-mode ultrasound data was development of normative data from several National Institutes of Health funded multicenter epidemiologic studies that evaluated healthy individuals ranging in age from 45 to 64 (Arteriosclerosis Risk In Communities study [ARIC]) and from 65 to 94 (Cardiovascular Health Study [CHS]) (Howard *et al.*, 1993). Table 31.2 demonstrates that the median IMT increases with age, is higher in men than in women, and is higher in the bifurcation than in the common and internal carotid arteries. The "normal" thickness at the bifurcation for 55-year-old men and women is approximately 830 μm and 740 μm, respectively.

Associations of cardiovascular disease risk factors with IMT

It is both a strength and a weakness of the B-mode method that IMT represents an index of chronic stable disease: on the one hand the method is powerful for quantifying associations of IMT with lifetime risk factor exposure (Wilson *et al.*, 1997), however, in contrast to measures of vascular function, it is not possible to use this technique to evaluate rapid change with, for instance, short-term exposure to a dietary intervention (as is possible with measures of vascular function). Well-recognized risk factors for clinical manifestations of coronary artery disease include age, male gender, menopausal status, cigarette smoking, diabetes, hypertension, elevated low density lipoprotein cholesterol, and depressed high density lipoprotein cholesterol, and all of these have been shown to be related to increased extracranial carotid IMT (Salonen *et al.*, 1988; Bonithon-Kopp *et al.*, 1991; Heiss *et al.*, 1991; O'Leary *et al.*, 1992; Howard *et al.*, 1996; Bots *et al.*, 1997; Wilson *et al.*, 1997; Gariepy *et al.*, 1998; Ebrahim *et al.*, 1999; Espeland *et al.*, 1999a; Anand *et al.*, 2000; Schott *et al.*, 2004). In addition, a number of "non-traditional" risk factors have been associated with increased IMT. These include passive smoking (Diez-Roux *et al.*, 1995), ethnic factors (D'Agostino *et al.*, 1996), elevated homocysteine levels (Selhub *et al.*, 1995), dietary saturated fat intake (Tell *et al.*, 1994), postprandial lipids (Boquist *et al.*, 1999) factors related to thrombosis (Tracy *et al.*, 1995) and thrombolysis (Salomaa *et al.*, 1995), past *Chlamydia pneumoniae* infection (Melnick *et al.*, 1993), elevated levels of E selectin and intercellular adhesion molecule 1 (ICAM-1) (Hwang *et al.*, 1997), C-reactive protein (Hak *et al.*, 1999; Van der Meer *et al.*, 2002; Wang *et al.*, 2002; Cao *et al.*, 2003), psychosocial factors (Lynch *et al.*, 1997), asymmetric dimethylarginine (Miyazaki *et al.*, 1999), the metabolic syndrome (Anand *et al.*, 2003; McNeill *et al.*, 2004), insulin sensitivity (Howard *et al.*, 1996), and inflammatory disease states (Nagata-Sakurai *et al.*, 2003; Raitakari *et al.*, 2003). Childhood risk factors have also been related to IMT in adults (Li *et al.*, 2003; Raitakari *et al.*, 2003). Sharrett *et al.* noted only a weak association of high density lipoprotein cholesterol (HDL-C) and triglycerides with IMT but a strong association with incident cardiovascular events, leading them to speculate that these risk factors might be involved in the transition from atheroma to atherothrombosis (Sharrett *et al.*, 1999). It has been speculated that different risk factors might

impact to a greater or lesser extent on different segments (common carotid vs. bifurcation vs. internal carotid), but the data for this have been inconsistent (reviewed in Espeland *et al.*, 1999a).

A number of genetic variants have been studied for their relation to carotid IMT, including those associated with angiotensin 1 converting enzyme, apolipoprotein E, angiotensinogen and angiotensin II type 1 receptor, methylene tetra-hydrofolate reductase, paraoxonase, nitric oxide synthase, various genes related to lipid and lipoprotein levels (e.g. hepatic lipase), and genetic variants related to hemostatic and inflammatory factors, interleukins and immune response, platelet receptors, and oxidative pathways (Zannad and Benetos, 2003; Humphries and Morgan, 2004; Manolio *et al.*, 2004). Of these, the 6A allele of the matrix metalloproteinase 3 (MMP3) 5A/6A promoter polymorphism has been associated with higher IMT and stenosis in all studies examining it (e.g. Gnasso *et al.*, 2000). Other markers are under active investigation in this exciting new approach to quantification of the genetics of atherosclerosis.

To the extent that all of these risk factors are heritable, it is not surprising that IMT is heritable as well; the availability of noninvasive means of imaging arterial walls provides an excellent opportunity to quantify the magnitude of this effect. Duggirala *et al.* were among the first to estimate heritability of 86–92% for internal carotid IMT in 46 sibships in Mexico City (Duggirala *et al.*, 1996). Xiang *et al.* also found high heritability estimates of 72% for the common carotid artery. Subsequently, heritability estimates of 21–67% have been derived by various groups (Xiang *et al.*, 2002). Table 31.3, from Manolio *et al.* (Manolio *et al.*, 2004), summarizes heritability of various carotid artery phenotypes in nine studies reported through 2003 (Duggirala *et al.*, 1996; Zannad *et al.*, 1998; Hunt *et al.*, 2002; Jartti *et al.*, 2002; Lange *et al.*, 2002; North *et al.*, 2002; Xiang *et al.*, 2002; Fox *et al.*, 2003; Swan *et al.*, 2003).

Table 31.3. Heritability of various carotid artery phenotypes

Reference	CC IMT		IC IMT		Plaque	
	Unadjusted or minimally adjusted (%)	Adjusted for CVD risk factors	Unadjusted or minimally adjusted (%)	Adjusted for CVD risk factors	Unadjusted or minimally adjusted (%)	Adjusted for CVD risk factors
Duggirala *et al.*, 1996	86	92	87	86		
Zannad *et al.*, 1998		30–33				
Hunt *et al.*, 2002					29	23
North *et al.*, 2002		21				
Jartti *et al.*, 2002	36					
Lange *et al.*, 2002	32	41				
Xiang *et al.*, 2002	72	64				
Fox *et al.*, 2003	67	38	43	35		
Swan *et al.*, 2003	31					

CVD indicates cardiovascular disease.

Progression of intima-media thickness

Salonen *et al.* were the first to define progression rates of IMT in a population of individuals in Finland in 1990. They observed that several cardiovascular disease risk factors were related to IMT progression including age, low-density lipoprotein (LDL) cholesterol, pack-years of smoking, white blood cell count, and platelet aggregability (Salonen and Salonen, 1990). More recently Chambless *et al.* analyzed data from the ARIC study to identify diabetes, smoking, HDL-C, pulse pressure, white blood cell count, and fibrinogen as risk factors for progression (Chambless *et al.*, 2002). The average annual change in mean common carotid IMT in this study for black women, black men, white women, and white men, respectively was 8.4, 7.4, 9.1, and 8.6 μm, respectively. Other population-based studies (Zureik *et al.*, 1999; Willeit *et al.*, 2000; Van der Meer *et al.*, 2003; Mackinnon *et al.*, 2004) generally agree that traditional risk factors for cardiovascular events are related to IMT progression and that progression in healthy individuals is approximately 10 μm per year.

Nontraditional risk factors have also been associated with more rapid progression of atherosclerosis, including passive smoking (Howard *et al.*, 1996), factors related to thrombosis and thrombolysis (Salonen and Salonen, 1990; Willeit *et al.*, 2000; Chambless *et al.*, 2002; Johnson *et al.*, 2005; Sabeti *et al.*, 2005), monocyte count (Johnson *et al.*, 2005), hs-C reactive protein and serum amyloid A (Van der Meer *et al.*, 2002; Schillinger *et al.*, 2005), human immunodeficiency virus infection (Hsue *et al.*, 2004), psychosocial stress (Lynch *et al.*, 1997), and abdominal obesity (Lakka *et al.*, 2001a) and the metabolic syndrome (Wallenfeldt *et al.*, 2004, 2005). Cardiorespiratory fitness (Lakka *et al.*, 2001b), dietary fiber (Wu *et al.*, 2003), and exercise (Nordstrom *et al.*, 2003) as well as higher plasma levels of antioxidant vitamins (Dwyer *et al.*, 2004) have been associated with slower IMT progression.

Patients with coronary artery disease have also been shown to progress their IMT more rapidly than patients free of coronary artery disease (CAD) (Crouse *et al.*, 2002). In this study of patients with coronary status defined at coronary angiography, patients with no CAD had progression rates of about 10 μm/yr for the common, bifurcation, and internal carotid arteries, and patients with CAD had progression rates of about 30 μm/yr in these segments. Of interest, the impact of risk factors on progression was greater in patients with CAD than in those free of CAD. For example, patients with a high concentration of HDL-cholesterol (54–127 mg/dl) increased their IMT at about 10 μm/yr whether they had CAD or no CAD. However, patients with low concentrations of HDL cholesterol (15–34 mg/dl) progressed at <10 μm/yr if they did not have CAD but at 77 μm/yr if they had CAD.

Clinical trials

The FDA has recently accepted change in progression of IMT measured by B-mode ultrasound as an index of improvement in vascular risk (Black, 2002). A recent publication has summarized the associations between IMT change and clinical events (Espeland et al., 2005). Typically, it takes 1–3 years to show differences in rates of progression of IMT between intervention and placebo groups or between different interventions. Clinical trials of lipid-lowering regimens, antihypertensive interventions, diabetes intervention, and lifestyle management have shown variable effects. The first clinical trial to evaluate the effect of a pharmacologic intervention on progression of IMT was the Cholesterol Lowering Atherosclerosis study published by Blankenhorn et al. in 1993 (Blankenhorn et al., 1993). This study compared colestipol-niacin therapy with placebo in 78 patients with CAD who had carotid ultrasound studies at baseline, 2, and 4 years. Computerized analysis of the far wall of the common carotid was used to define the outcome. Placebo-treated patients progressed at a rate of about 25 μm/yr whereas colestipol-niacin treated patients showed no progression and in fact had smaller IMT at the end of the study. Subsequently an additional 12 studies have been reported. Eleven of these have evaluated statin treatment either compared to placebo (Furberg et al., 1994; Crouse et al., 1995; Salonen et al., 1995; Hodis et al., 1996; Mercuri

et al., 1996; De Groot et al., 1998; MacMahon et al., 1998; Hedblad et al., 2001), probucol (Sawayama et al., 2002) or in a comparator fashion (atorvastatin vs. pravastatin [Taylor et al., 2002], atorvastatin vs. simvastatin [Smilde et al., 2001]) and one has evaluated the incremental impact of niacin added to statin treatment (Taylor et al., 2004). These trials have consistently shown that cholesterol lowering retards the rate of progression or is associated with net regression of IMT. In two of these trials (Smilde et al., 2001; Taylor et al., 2002) more intensive lipid lowering was associated with more dramatic reduction of IMT progression. Addition of niacin to underlying statin therapy resulted in absence of progression in the group administered niacin whereas the group not taking niacin showed progression (Taylor et al., 2004). LDL apheresis has also been associated with retardation of progression of carotid atherosclerosis (Koga et al., 1999).

In addition, ten clinical trials have evaluated effects of antihypertensive therapy on IMT progression compared to diuretic or placebo (Borhani et al., 1996; Zanchetti et al., 1998, 2002, 2004; MacMahon et al., 2000; Pitt et al., 2000; Lonn et al., 2001; Simon et al., 2001; Hoogerbrugge et al., 2002; Sawayama et al., 2002; Wiklund et al., 2002). In general, these trials have shown that antihypertensive treatment slows progression compared to placebo or diuretic; however, these trials are more difficult to interpret than lipid-lowering trials because antihypertensive therapy often acutely changes intravascular volume. Since IMT varies inversely with acute changes in intravascular volume, it becomes difficult to distinguish between acute changes in IMT due to physiologic alterations in blood volume as opposed to long-term changes in atherosclerosis burden.

Intensive diabetes management has been shown to retard progression of IMT in patients with type 1 diabetes (Nathan et al., 2003) whereas rosiglitazone, metformin, and acarbose have shown benefit in patients with type 2 diabetes (Hanefeld et al., 2004; Matsumoto et al., 2004; Sidhu et al., 2004).

Hormone replacement has been associated with variable effects on IMT progression

(De Kleijn *et al.*, 1999; Hodis *et al.*, 2001; Angerer *et al.*, 2002b; Byington *et al.*, 2002).

Lifestyle interventions with weight loss, exercise, and stress reduction (Karason *et al.*, 1999; Haney *et al.*, 2000; Fontana *et al.*, 2004; Wildman *et al.*, 2004) have been shown to retard progression of IMT but treatment with omega-3 fatty acids does not (Angerer *et al.*, 2002a). Two of three studies evaluating the effects of antioxidant vitamins or B complex intervention have shown a beneficial effect on IMT (Vermeulen *et al.*, 2000; Marcucci *et al.*, 2003; Salonen *et al.*, 2003). Treatments with aspirin (Ranke *et al.*, 1993) and other antiplatelet agents (Kodama *et al.*, 2000) have also been shown to have a beneficial effect.

Associations of intima-media thickness with symptomatic vascular disease

Since atherosclerosis is a generalized phenomenon and there are strong associations between symptomatic manifestations of cerebrovascular and coronary artery disease (stroke and heart attack), it is no surprise that carotid IMT and IMT progression have been independently associated with prevalent symptomatic coronary artery (Craven *et al.*, 1990; O'Leary *et al.*, 1992; Salonen *et al.*, 1994; Burke *et al.*, 1995; Chambless *et al.*, 1996; Bots *et al.*, 1997; Kallikazaros *et al.*, 1999; Crouse *et al.*, 2002) and cerebrovascular (O'Leary *et al.*, 1992; Burke *et al.*, 1995; Chambless *et al.*, 1996; Bots *et al.*, 1997) disease. For prevalent carotid IMT the odds ratios are 2.84 and 2.56 for prevalent coronary artery and cerebrovascular disease, respectively, when comparing the highest with the lowest internal carotid IMT quartile (O'Leary *et al.*, 1992). Of interest, increased IMT has also been associated with cerebral white matter lesions (Bots *et al.*, 1993; Manolio *et al.*, 1994) which have themselves been associated with neurological abnormalities (Price *et al.*, 1997).

Increased IMT as identified by B-mode ultrasound of the extracranial carotid arteries is also a predictor of incident coronary events (Salonen and Salonen, 1993; Bots *et al.*, 1997; Chambless *et al.*, 1997; Hodis *et al.*, 1998; O'Leary *et al.*, 1999; Psaty *et al.*, 1999; Del Sol *et al.*, 2001; Chambless *et al.*, 2003) and stroke (Manolio *et al.*, 1996; Bots *et al.*, 1997; O'Leary *et al.*, 1999; Del Sol *et al.*, 2001; Chambless *et al.*, 2004) or the combined endpoint (O'Leary *et al.*, 1999; Del Sol *et al.*, 2001) (Figure 31.2), as well as incident white matter lesions (Vermeer *et al.*, 2003). In the most recent analyses from the ARIC study, addition of IMT together with several other "nontraditional" risk markers to a roster of traditional risk factors improved the area under the receiver operating curve (ROC) for incident coronary heart disease in men but not women (and IMT was also important when not combined with other nontraditional risk factors [Chambless *et al.*, 2003]). In the CHS, IMT was also independently related to incident coronary events (Psaty *et al.*, 1999).

IMT is also logically related to incident stroke. In ARIC, addition of IMT to a basic model including traditional risk factors increased the area under the ROC curve for stroke, but this was only statistically significant when combined with a marker of peripheral vascular disease (Chambless *et al.*, 2004). In the CHS (Manolio *et al.*, 1996), 14% of incident strokes in an older population occurred in the 6% of the population with the greatest carotid stenosis (>50%), and "hypoechoic" plaque (of an ultrasound density comparable to or less than that of the vessel lumen, and perhaps indicative of "vulnerable" plaque) conferred additional risk (Polak *et al.*, 1998). In the Rotterdam Study, age, sex, prior cardiovascular disease, and traditional risk factors correctly predicted 17% of all subjects with incident disease whereas when only the IMT was used 14% of all subjects with incident disease were correctly predicted (Del Sol *et al.*, 2001). Finally, a report has presented evidence for an independent association of IMT with all-cause mortality (Fried *et al.*, 1998).

Since IMT reflects a chronic stable index of disease, lifestyle or pharmacologic modifications that alter risk of incident disease rapidly (e.g. lipid lowering) are not rapidly reflected in changes

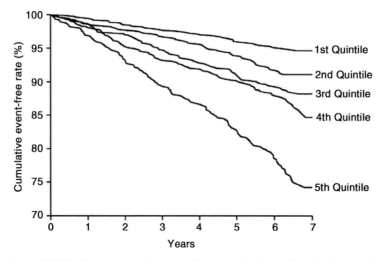

Figure 31.2 Unadjusted cumulative event-free rates for the combined end-point of myocardial infarction or stroke according to quintile of combined intima-media thickness. (Reproduced from O'Leary D. H, *et al.* (1999). *New England Journal of Medicine*, **340**, 14–22. Copyright © 1999 Massachusetts Medical Society.)

in IMT. Thus current IMT might not reflect the acute impact of risk factor treatment on events, and progression of IMT might better predict incident disease. Hodis has reported that progression of IMT is a stronger risk factor for incident coronary events than baseline coronary stenosis or progression of coronary stenosis (Hodis *et al.*, 1998). This observation has not been replicated, perhaps because of the challenges inherent in quantification of IMT progression.

Use of B-mode ultrasound to define arterial dimensions

In addition to IMT, B-mode ultrasound is capable of defining arterial lumen diameter and interadventitial diameter. As previously shown by Glagov *et al.* in the coronary arteries (Glagov *et al.*, 1987), increased IMT of the common carotid is associated with increased rather than decreased lumen diameter (Crouse *et al.*, 1994), and most risk factors that are associated with increased IMT (aging, male gender, cigarette smoking, hypertension, diabetes) are also associated with increased common carotid

lumen diameter (LDL cholesterol is the exception and is associated with smaller arterial lumens in the common carotid artery) (Bonithon-Kopp *et al.*, 1996; Crouse *et al.*, 1996; Polak *et al.*, 1996). Of interest, these relations do not seem to apply at the bifurcation or the internal carotid artery where increased IMT is associated with no change or even a constriction of the artery and more dramatic lumen narrowing than in the common carotid. These observations have recently been extended to compare patients with and without defined coronary artery disease: although associations of lumens and IMT are similar between coronary cases and controls in the common carotid, there is a suggestion of a greater tendency to lumen compromise with increasing IMT in the internal carotid for patients with CAD compared to CAD-free controls (Terry *et al.*, 2003).

Summary

The transformation of ultrasound from a clinical tool for identifying the few individuals at risk for incident stroke by virtue of extracranial carotid stenosis to its use as an epidemiologic tool for quantifying subclincial atherosclerosis in large populations of individuals and as an index of outcome for clinical trials represents a paradigm shift in clinical investigation. Of equal importance is the underlying utility of the ability to observe walls of arteries in healthy individuals and the development of disease in walls of arteries. The simple harmless nature of this investigation has led to an explosion in its use in epidemiologic studies of associations with risk factors (including genetic factors) and with clinical (coronary and cerebro-vascular) outcome. Endorsement of IMT as a "surrogate outcome" has vastly expanded the options for performing clinical trials. New insights into vascular biology have emerged from studies of vascular remodeling. Thus B-mode ultrasound has clearly become a mature technology for quantification and monitoring of the extent and progression of IMT of the extracranial carotid arteries. It is useful to consider the strengths and weaknesses of the use of this method:

Advantages	Disadvantages
Noninvasive, valid, reliable, inexpensive; high level of resolution	Images carotid arteries rather than coronary; operator dependent
Index of chronic stable disease	Not a measure of arterial function; acute physiologic change alters IMT
Visualizes wall thickness	Not a good tool for identifying arterial lumens, "plaque" or plaque volume or composition
Biologic validity: relates to risk factors and events in epidemiologic studies; FDA-recognized clinical outcome for clinical trials	Not a good tool for identifying individual risk

As discussed above, the chief advantage of the method is its noninvasive character; it has also been proven to be valid and reliable and is relatively inexpensive. The reliability and level of resolution are such that differences in progression rates of 20 μm/year between groups comprised of 100–200 individuals can be detected. Perhaps the most important disadvantage of the technique is its limitation to imaging the carotid rather than the coronary arteries, although the potential implications for stroke are obvious. The fact that a sonographer is needed to acquire images is also a relative disadvantage compared, for example, to magnetic resonance imaging or computerized tomography.

That IMT represents a chronic stable measure of disease is both a strength and a weakness. The stability of the measurement enhances its validity for quantifying the impact of chronic risk factor exposure; however, changes in risk factors due, for example, to acute modification of behavior and/or pharmacologic interventions, might result in acute improvements in risk factor profiles but not IMT, and associations of IMT with current risk factor levels might therefore be misleading. Furthermore, to the extent that these changes in risk factors acutely reduced the risk of incident cardiovascular disease but not IMT, the contemporaneously measured IMT might overestimate risk. For acute change clearly a measure of vascular function (e.g. vascular reactivity) would be better, and vascular function can identify changes related to very acute exposure over short periods of time. In fact, short-term changes in arterial lumen diameter associated, for instance, with antihypertensive therapy, can acutely change the IMT (if the wall area remains the same and the lumen diameter decreases then the IMT will increase) leading to challenges in interpretation of acute effects of certain agents in clinical trials. For these reasons change in IMT over 1 or 2 years might provide a better index of incident vascular events, but this has been tested only infrequently.

The measurement of wall thickness (rather than wall area or volume) is also both a strength and a weakness. Differences in wall thicknesses between individuals are, for the most part (with the caveat above), not influenced by arterial diameter. Wall area, by contrast, is heavily influenced by lumen diameter, and two individuals with the same wall thickness but different arterial lumen diameters would have different wall areas, not indicative of disease but of body size. On the other hand, the limitation of the B-mode method for imaging cross-sectional areas prevents accurate estimation of "plaque" or plaque volume. The B-mode method is similarly poor at accurately quantifying plaque composition, which is a key component in disease development. Furthermore, there is not universal agreement as to how best to quantify IMT, whether to measure wall thicknesses in multiple segments and walls, or whether to focus on the far wall of the common carotid only.

Finally, the method has biologic validity as IMT relates to risk factors and clinical events in a manner anticipated from current understanding of these relationships with atherosclerosis defined in other ways. This has supported characterization of IMT by the FDA as a valid marker for impact of pharmacologic agents. However, the correlation of IMT with clinical outcome is not strong enough to advocate its use for identifying individuals at risk of clinical events. Longitudinal measurements with sequential B-mode exams might be better, but these are hampered by the operator dependence of the method.

In summary, use of B-mode ultrasound to quantify IMT represents a mature technology for quantification of arterial disease that has enlarged research opportunities. Whereas previously estimates of arterial disease were only available from highly biased populations, now healthy individuals can be investigated to determine associations of risk factors with disease, of disease with outcome, and of the impact of risk factor modification on disease progression. The strengths of the method outweigh its weaknesses. New technologies will likely provide significant advances over the B-mode technology; however, each of the new technologies will also have weaknesses, and at present B-mode ultrasound continues to provide a tool for important new scientific discovery.

REFERENCES

Ainsworth, C. D., Blake, C. C., Tamayo, A., *et al.* (2005). 3D ultrasound measurement of change in carotid plaque volume: a tool for rapid evaluation of new therapies. *Stroke*, **36**, 1904–9.

Anand, S. S., Yusuf, S., Vuksan, V., *et al.* (2000). Differences in risk factors, atherosclerosis, and cardiovascular disease between ethnic groups in Canada: the Study of Health Assessment and Risk in Ethnic groups (SHARE). *Lancet*, **356**, 279–84.

Anand, S. S., Yi, Q., Gerstein, H., *et al.* (2003). Study of Health Assessment and Risk in Ethnic Groups; Study of Health Assessment and Risk Evaluation in Aboriginal Peoples Investigators. Relationship of metabolic syndrome and fibrinolytic dysfunction to cardiovascular disease. *Circulation*, **108**, 420–5.

Angerer, P., Kothny, W., Stork, S. and von Schacky, C. (2002a). Effect of dietary supplementation with omega-3 fatty acids on progression of atherosclerosis in carotid arteries. *Cardiovascular Research*, **54**, 183–90.

Angerer, P., Stork, S., Kothny, W. and von Schacky, C. (2002b). Effect of postmenopausal hormone replacement on atherosclerosis in femoral arteries. *Maturitas*, **41**, 51–60.

Barnes, R. W., Bone, G. E., Reinertson, J., *et al.* (1976). Noninvasive ultrasonic carotid angiography: prospective validation by contrast arteriography. *Surgery*, **80**, 328–35.

Black, D. M. (2002). Introduction to conference on vascular imaging. *American Journal of Cardiology*, **89** (Suppl. B), 1B–3B.

Blankenhorn, D. H. and Curry, P. J. (1982). The accuracy of arteriography and ultrasound imaging for atherosclerosis measurement. *Archives of Pathology and Laboratory Medicine*, **106**, 483–9.

Blankenhorn, D. H., Selzer, R. H., Crawford, D. W., *et al.* (1993). Beneficial effects of colestipol-niacin therapy on the common carotid artery. *Circulation*, **88**, 20–8.

Bonithon-Kopp, C., Touboul, P. J., Berr, C., Magne, C. and Ducimetiere, P. (1996). Factors of carotid arterial enlargement in a population aged 59 to 71 years. The EVA Study. *Stroke*, **27**, 654–60.

Bonithon-Kopp, C., Scarabin, P. Y. and Taquet, A. (1991). Risk factors for early carotid atherosclerosis in middle-aged French women. *Arteriosclerosis and Thrombosis*, **11**, 966–72.

Boquist, S., Ruotolo, G., Tang, R., *et al.* (1999). Alimentary lipemia, postprandial triglyceride-rich lipoproteins, and common carotid intima-media thickness in healthy, middle-aged men. *Circulation*, **100**, 723–8.

Borhani, N. O., Mercuri, M., Borhani, P. A., *et al.* (1996). Final outcome results of the Multicenter Isradipine Diuretic Atherosclerosis Study (MIDAS). A randomized controlled trial. *Journal of the American Medical Association*, **276**, 785–91.

Bots, M. L., van Swieten, J. C., Breteler, M. M. B., *et al.* (1993). Cerebral white matter lesions and atherosclerosis in the Rotterdam Study. *Lancet*, **341**, 1232–7.

Bots, M. L., de Jong, P. T. V. M., Hofman, A. and Grobbee, D. E. (1997). Left, right, near or far wall common carotid intima-media thickness measurements: associations with cardiovascular disease and lower extremity arterial atherosclerosis. *Journal of Clinical Epidemiology*, **50**, 801–7.

Bots, M. L., Hoes, A. W., Koudstaal, P. J., Hofman, A. and Grobbee, D. E. (1997). Common carotid intima-medial thickness and risk of stroke and myocardial infarction. The Rotterdam Study. *Circulation*, **96**, 1432–7.

Bots, M. L., Evans, G. W., Riley, W., *et al.* (2003a). The Osteoporosis Prevention and Arterial effects of Tibolone (OPAL) study: design and baseline characteristics. *Controlled Clinical Trials*, **24**, 752–75.

Bots, M. L., Evans, G. W., Riley, W. A. and Grobbee, D. E. (2003b). Carotid intima-media thickness measurements in intervention studies: design options, progression rates, and sample size considerations: a point of view. *Stroke*, **34**, 2985–94.

Burke, G. L., Evans, G. W., Riley, W. A., *et al.* (1995). Arterial wall thickness is associated with prevalent cardiovascular disease in middle-aged adults. The Atherosclerosis Risk in Communities (ARIC) study. *Stroke*, **26**, 386–91.

Byington, R. P., Furberg, C. D., Herrington, D. M., *et al.* (2002). Heart and Estrogen/Progestin Replacement Study Research Group. Effect of estrogen plus progestin on progression of carotid atherosclerosis in postmenopausal women with heart disease: HERS B-mode substudy. *Arteriosclerosis, Thrombosis and Vascular Biology*, **22**, 1692–7.

Cao, J. J., Thach, C., Manolio, T. A., *et al.* (2003). C-reactive protein, carotid intima-media thickness, and incidence of ischemic stroke in the elderly. The Cardiovascular Health Study. *Circulation*, **108**, 166–70.

Chambers, B. R. and Norris, J. W. (1986). Outcome in patients with asymptomatic neck bruits. *New England Journal of Medicine*, **315**, 860–5.

Chambless, L. E., Shahar, E., Sharrett, A. R., *et al.* (1996). Association of transient ischemic attack/stroke symptoms assessed by standardized questionnaire and algorithm with cerebrovascular risk factors and carotid artery wall thickness. *American Journal of Epidemiology*, **144**, 857–66.

Chambless, L. E., Heiss, G., Folsom, A. R., *et al.* (1997). Association of coronary heart disease incidence with carotid arterial wall thickness and major risk factors: the Atherosclerosis Risk in Communities (ARIC) study, 1987–1993. *American Journal of Epidemiology*, **146**, 483–94.

Chambless, L. E., Folsom, A. R., Davis, V., *et al.* (2002). Risk factors for progression of common carotid atherosclerosis: the Atherosclerosis Risk in Communities Study, 1987–1988. *American Journal of Epidemiology*, **155**, 38–47.

Chambless, L. E., Folsom, A. R., Sharrett, A. R., *et al.* (2003). Coronary heart disease risk prediction in the Atherosclerosis Risk in Communities (ARIC) study. *Journal of Clinical Epidemiology*, **56**, 880–90.

Chambless, L. E., Heiss, G., Shahar, E., Earp, M. J. and Toole, J. (2004). Prediction of ischemic stroke risk in the Atherosclerosis Risk in Communities Study. *American Journal of Epidemiology*, **160**, 259–69.

Craven, T. E., Ryu, J. E., Espeland, M. A., *et al.* (1990). Evaluation of the associations between carotid artery atherosclerosis and coronary artery stenosis: A case control study. *Circulation*, **82**, 1230–42.

Crouse, J. R. (1993). B-mode in clinical trials: Answers and questions. *Circulation*, **88**, 319–21.

Crouse, J. R. and Thompson, C. J. (1993). An evaluation of methods for imaging and quantifying coronary and carotid lumen stenosis and atherosclerosis. *Circulation*, **87** (Suppl. II), II-17–II-33.

Crouse, J. R., Byington, R. P., Bond, M. G., *et al.* (1992). Pravastatin, Lipids, and Atherosclerosis in the Carotid Arteries: Design features of a clinical trial with atherosclerosis outcome. *Controlled Clinical Trials*, **13**, 495–506.

Crouse, J. R. III, Goldbourt, U., Evans, G., *et al.* (1994). Arterial enlargement in the Atherosclerosis Risk in Communities (ARIC) Cohort. *Stroke*, **25**, 1354–9.

Crouse, J. R., Byington, R. P., Bond, M. G., *et al.* (1995). Pravastatin, Lipids, and Atherosclerosis in the Carotid

Arteries (PLAC-II). *American Journal of Cardiology*, **75**, 455–9.

Crouse, J. R. III, Goldbourt, U., Evans, G., *et al.* (1996). Risk Factors and Segment Specific Carotid Arterial Enlargement in the Atherosclerosis Risk in Communities (ARIC) Cohort. *Stroke*, **27**, 69–75.

Crouse, J. R., Tang, R., Espeland, M. A., *et al.* (2002). Associations of extracranial carotid atherosclerosis progression with coronary status and risk factors in patients with and without coronary artery disease. *Circulation*, **106**, 2061–6.

Crouse, J. R., Grobbee, D. E., O'Leary, D. H., *et al.* (2004). Measuring effects on intima media thickness: an evaluation of rosuvastatin in subclinical atherosclerosis – the rationale and methodology of the METEOR study. *Cardiovascular Drugs and Therapy*, **18**, 231–8.

D'Agostino, R. B., Burke, G., O'Leary, D., *et al.* (1996). Ethnic differences in carotid wall thickness. *Stroke*, **27**, 1744–9.

Davies, M. J. (1996). Stability and instability: two faces of coronary atherosclerosis. The Paul Dudley White Lecture 1995. *Circulation*, **94**, 2013–20.

De Groot, E., Jukema, J. W., Montauban van Swijndregt, A. D., *et al.* (1998). B-mode ultrasound assessment of pravastatin treatment effect on carotid and femoral artery walls and its correlations with coronary arteriographic findings: a report of the Regression Growth Evaluation Statin Study (REGRESS). *Journal of the American College of Cardiology*, **31**, 1561–7.

De Kleijn, M. J., Bots, M. L., Bak, A. A., *et al.* (1999). Hormone replacement therapy in perimenopausal women and 2-year change of carotid intima-media thickness. *Maturitas*, **32**, 195–204.

Del Sol, A. I., Moons, K. G., Hollander, M., *et al.* (2001). Is carotid intima-media thickness useful in cardiovascular disease risk assessment? *Stroke*, **32**, 1532–8.

Diez-Roux, A. V., Nieto, F. J., Comstock, G. W., Howard, G. and Szklo, M. (1995). The relationship of active and passive smoking to carotid atherosclerosis 12–14 years later. *Preventive Medicine*, **24**, 48–55.

Duggirala, R., Gonzalez Villalpando, C., O'Leary, D. H., Stern, M. P. and Blangero, J. (1996). Genetic basis of variation in carotid artery wall thickness. *Stroke*, **27**, 833–7.

Dwyer, J. H., Paul-Labrador, M. J., Fan, J., *et al.* (2004). Progression of carotid intima-media thickness and plasma antioxidants: the Los Angeles Atherosclerosis Study. *Arteriosclerosis, Thrombosis and Vascular Biology*, **24**, 313–19.

Ebrahim, S., Papacosta, O., Whincup, P., *et al.* (1999). Carotid plaque, intima media thickness, cardiovascular risk factors, and prevalent cardiovascular disease in men and women: the British Regional Heart Study. *Stroke*, **30**, 841–50.

El-Barghouty, N., Nicolaides, A., Behal, V., Geroulakos, G. and Androulakis, A. (1996). The identification of the high risk carotid plaque. *European Journal of Vascular and Endovascular Surgery*, **11**, 470–8.

Espeland, M. A., Craven, T. E., Riley, W. A., *et al.* (1996). Reliability of longitudinal ultrasonographic measurements of carotid intimal-medial thicknesses. *Stroke*, **27**, 480–5.

Espeland, M. A., Tang, R., Terry, J. G., *et al.* (1999a). Associations of risk factors with segment specific intimal-medial thickness of the extracranial carotid artery. *Stroke*, **30**, 1047–55.

Espeland, M. A., Craven, T. E., Miller, M. E. and D'Agostino, R. (1999b). Modeling multivariate longitudinal data that are incomplete. *Annals of Epidemiology*, **9**, 196–205.

Espeland, M. A., Evans, G. W., Wagenknecht, L. E., *et al.* (2003). Site-specific progression of carotid artery intimal-medial thickness. *Atherosclerosis*, **171**, 137–43.

Espeland, M. A., O'Leary, D. H., Terry, J. G., *et al.* (2005). Carotid intimal-media thickness as a surrogate for cardiovascular disease events in trials of HMG-CoA reductase inhibitors. *Current Controlled Trials in Cardiovascular Medicine*, **6**, 1–6.

Fontana, L., Meyer, T. E., Klein, S. and Holloszy, J. O. (2004). Long-term calorie restriction is highly effective in reducing the risk for atherosclerosis in humans. *Proceedings of the National Academy of Sciences USA*, **101**, 6659–63.

Fox, C. S., Polak, J. F., Chazaro, I., *et al.* (2003). Genetic and environmental contributions to atherosclerosis phenotypes in men and women: heritability of carotid intima-media thickness in the Framingham Heart Study. *Stroke*, **34**, 397–401.

Fried, L. P., Kronmal, R. A., Newman, A. B., *et al.* (1998). Risk factors for 5-year mortality in older adults. The Cardiovascular Health Study. *Journal of the American Medical Association*, **279**, 585–92.

Furberg, C. D., Adams, H. P., Applegate, W. B., *et al.* (1994). Effect of lovastatin on early carotid atherosclerosis and cardiovascular events. *Circulation*, **90**, 1679–87.

Gamble, G., Beaumont, B., Smith, H., *et al.* (1993). B-mode ultrasound images of the carotid artery wall: correlation of ultrasound with histological measurements. *Atherosclerosis*, **102**, 163–73.

Gariepy, J., Salomon, J., Denarie, N., *et al.* (1998). Sex and topographic differences in associations between large-artery wall thickness and coronary risk profile in a French working cohort: the AXA Study. *Arteriosclerosis, Thrombosis and Vascular Biology*, **18**, 584–90.

Glagov, S., Weisenberg, E., Zarins, C. K., Stankunavicius, R. and Kolettis, G. J. (1987). Compensatory enlargement of human atherosclerotic coronary arteries. *New England Journal of Medicine* **316**, 1371–5.

Gnasso, A., Motti, C., Irace, C., *et al.* (2000). Genetic variation in human stromelysin gene promoter and common carotid geometry in healthy male subjects. *Arteriosclerosis, Thrombosis and Vascular Biology*, **20**, 1600–5.

Hak, A. E., Stehouwer, C. D., Bots, M. L., *et al.* (1999). Associations of C-reactive protein with measures of obesity, insulin resistance, and subclinical atherosclerosis in healthy, middle-aged women. *Arteriosclerosis, Thrombosis and Vascular Biology*, **19**, 1986–91.

Hanefeld, M., Chiasson, J. L., Koehler, C., *et al.* (2004). Acarbose slows progression of intima-media thickness of the carotid arteries in subjects with impaired glucose tolerance. *Stroke*, **35**, 1073–8.

Haney, C., Rainforth, M. and Salerno, J. (2000). Effects of stress reduction on carotid atherosclerosis in hypertensive African Americans. *Stroke*, **31**, 568–73.

Hedblad, B., Wikstrand, J., Janzon, L., Wedel, H. and Berglund, G. (2001). Low-dose metoprolol CR/XL and fluvastatin slow progression of carotid intima-media thickness: Main results from the Beta-Blocker Cholesterol-Lowering Asymptomatic Plaque Study (BCAPS). *Circulation*, **103**, 1721–6.

Heiss, G., Sharrett, A. R., Barnes, R., *et al.* (1991). Carotid atherosclerosis measured by B-mode ultrasound in populations: Associations with cardiovascular risk factors in the ARIC study. *American Journal of Epidemiology*, **134**, 250–6.

Hennerici, M., Aulich, A., Sandmann, W. and Freund, H. J. (1981). Incidence of asymptomatic extracranial arterial disease. *Stroke*, **12**, 750–8.

Hodis, H. N., Mack, W. J., LaBree, L., *et al.* (1996). Reduction in carotid arterial wall thickness using lovastatin and dietary therapy. *Annals of Internal Medicine*, **124**, 549–56.

Hodis, H. N., Mack, W. J., LaBree, L., *et al.* (1998). The role of carotid arterial intima-media thickness in predicting clinical coronary events. *Annals of International Medicine*, **128**, 262–9.

Hodis, H. N., Mack, W. J., Lobo, R. A., *et al.* (2001). Estrogen in the Prevention of Atherosclerosis Trial Research Group. Estrogen in the prevention of atherosclerosis. A randomized, double-blind, placebo-controlled trial. *Annals of Internal Medicine*, **135**, 939–53.

Hoogerbrugge, N., de Groot, E., de Heide, L. H., *et al.* (2002). Doxazosin and hydrochlorothiazide equally affect arterial wall thickness in hypertensive males with hypercholesterolaemia (the DAPHNE study). Doxazosin Atherosclerosis Progression Study in Hypertensives in the Netherlands. *The Netherlands Journal of Medicine*, **60**, 354–61.

Howard, G., Sharrett, A. R., Heiss, G., *et al.* (1993). Carotid artery intimal-medial thickness distribution in general populations as evaluated by B-mode ultrasound. *Stroke*, **24**, 1297–304.

Howard, G., O'Leary, D. H., Zaccaro, D., *et al.* (1996). Insulin sensitivity and atherosclerosis. *Circulation*, **93**, 1809–17.

Howard, G., O'Leary, D. H., Zaccaro, D., *et al.* (1996). Insulin sensitivity and atherosclerosis. *Circulation*, **93**, 1809–17.

Hsue, P. Y., Lo, J. C., Franklin, A., *et al.* (2004). Progression of atherosclerosis as assessed by carotid intima-media thickness in patients with HIV infection. *Circulation*, **109**, 1603–8.

Humphries, S. E. and Morgan, L. (2004). Genetic risk factors for stroke and carotid atherosclerosis: insights into pathophysiology from candidate gene approaches. *The Lancet Neurology*, **3**, 227–36.

Hunt, K. J., Duggirala, R., Goring, H. H., *et al.* (2002). Genetic basis of variation in carotid artery plaque in the San Antonio Family Heart Study. *Stroke*, **33**, 2775–80.

Hwang, S., Ballantyne, C. M., Sharrett, A. R., *et al.* (1997). Circulating adhesions molecules VCAM-1, ICAM-1 and E-selectin in carotid atherosclerosis and incident coronary heart disease cases. The Atherosclerosis Risk in Communities (ARIC) Study. *Circulation*, **96**, 4219–25.

Jartti, L., Ronnemaa, T., Kaprio, J., *et al.* (2002). Population-based twin study of the effects of migration from Finland to Sweden on endothelial function and intima-media thickness. *Arteriosclerosis, Thrombosis and Vascular Biology*, **22**, 832–7.

Johnsen, S. H., Fosse, E., Joakimsen, O., *et al.* (2005). Monocyte count is a predictor of novel plaque formation: a 7-year follow-up study of 2610 persons without carotid plaque at baseline: the Tromso Study. *Stroke*, **36**, 715–19.

Josse, M. O., Touboul, P. J., Mas, J. L., Laplane, D. and Bousser, M. G. (1987). Prevalence of asymptomatic internal carotid artery stenosis. *Neuroepidemiology*, **6**, 150–2.

Kallikazaros, I., Tsioufis, C., Sideris, S., Stefanadis, C. and Toutouzas, P. (1999). Carotid artery disease as a marker for the presence of severe coronary artery disease in patients evaluated for chest pain. *Stroke*, **30**, 1002–7.

Kanters, S. D., Algra, A., van Leeuwen, M. S. and Banga, J. D. (1997). Reproducibility of in vivo carotid intima-media thickness measurements: a review. *Stroke*, **28**, 665–71.

Karason, K., Wikstrand, J., Sjostrom, L. and Wendelhag, I. (1999). Weight loss and progression of early athero-sclerosis in the carotid artery: a four-year controlled study of obese subjects. *International Journal of Obesity and Related Metabolic Disorders*, **23**, 948–56.

Kodama, M., Yamasaki, Y., Sakamoto, K., *et al.* (2000). Antiplatelet drugs attenuate progression of carotid intima-media thickness in subjects with type 2 diabetes. *Thrombosis Research*, **97**, 239–45.

Koga, N., Watanabe, K., Kurashige, Y., Sato, T. and Hiroki, T. (1999). Long-term effects of LDL apheresis on carotid arterial atherosclerosis in familial hypercholesterolae-mic patients. *Journal of Internal Medicine*, **246**, 35–43.

Lakka, T. A., Lakka, H. M., Salonen, R., Kaplan, G. A. and Salonen, J. T. (2001a). Abdominal obesity is associated with accelerated progression of carotid atherosclerosis in men. *Atherosclerosis*, **154**, 497–504.

Lakka, T. A., Laukkanen, J. A., Rauramaa, R., *et al.* (2001b). Cardiorespiratory fitness and the progression of carotid atherosclerosis in middle-aged men. *Annals of Internal Medicine*, **134**, 12–20.

Lange, L. A., Bowden, D. W., Langefeld, C. D., *et al.* (2002). Heritability of carotid artery intima-medial thickness in type 2 diabetes. *Stroke*, **33**, 1876–81.

Li, S., Chen, W., Srinivasan, S. R., *et al.* (2003). Childhood cardiovascular risk factors and carotid vascular changes in adulthood: the Bogalusa Heart Study. *Journal of the American Medical Association*, **290**, 2271–6.

Lo, L. Y., Ford, C. S., McKinney, W. M. and Toole, J. F. (1986). Asymptomatic bruit, carotid and vertebrobasilar transient ischemic attacks – a clinical and ultrasonic correlation. *Stroke*, **17**, 65–8.

Lonn, E., Yusuf, S., Dzavik, V., *et al.* (2001). Effects of ramipril and vitamin E on atherosclerosis: the study to evaluate carotid ultrasound changes in patients treated with ramipril and vitamin E (SECURE). *Circulation*, **103**, 919–25.

Lynch, J., Krause, N., Kaplan, G., Salonen, R. and Salonen, J. T (1997). Workplace demands, economic reward and progression of carotid atherosclerosis. *Circulation*, **96**, 302–7.

Lynch, J., Krause, N., Kaplan, G. A., Salonen, R. and Salonen, J. T. (1997). Workplace demands, economic reward, and progression of carotid atherosclerosis. *Circulation*, **96**, 302–7.

Mackinnon, A. D., Jerrard-Dunne, P., Sitzer, M., *et al.* (2004). Rates and determinants of site-specific progres-sion of carotid artery intima-media thickness: the carotid atherosclerosis progression study. *Stroke*, **35**, 2150–4.

Mackinnon, A. D., Jerrard-Dunne, P., Sitzer, M., *et al.* (2004). Rates and determinants of site-specific progres-sion of carotid artery intima-media thickness: the carotid atherosclerosis progression study. *Stroke*, **35**, 2150–4.

MacMahon, S., Sharpe, N., Gamble, G., *et al.* (1998). Effects of lowering average or below-average cholesterol levels on the progression of carotid athero-sclerosis. Results of the LIPID atherosclerosis substudy. *Circulation*, **98**, 1784–90.

MacMahon, S., Sharpe, N., Gamble, G., *et al.* (2000). Randomized, placebo-controlled trial of the angiotensin-converting enzyme inhibitor, ramipril, in patients with coronary or other occlusive arterial disease. PART-2 Collaborative Research Group. Prevention of Atherosclerosis with Ramipril. *Journal of the American College of Cardiology*, **36**, 438–43.

Manolio, T. A., Kronmal, R. A., Burke, G. L., *et al.* (1994). Magnetic resonance abnormalities and cardiovascular disease in older adults. *Stroke*, **25**, 318–27.

Manolio, T. A., Kronmal, R. A., Burke, G. L., O'Leary, D. H. and Price, T. R. (1996). Short-term predictors of incident stroke in older adults. The Cardiovascular Health Study. *Stroke*, **27**, 1479–86.

Manolio, T. A., Boerwinkle, E., O'Donnell, C. J. and Wilson, A. F. (2004). Genetics of ultrasonographic carotid atherosclerosis. *Arteriosclerosis, Thrombosis and Vascular Biology*, **24**, 1567–77.

Marcucci, R., Zanazzi, M., Bertoni, E., *et al.* (2003). Vitamin supplementation reduces the progression of atherosclerosis in hyperhomocysteinemic renal-transplant recipients. *Transplantation*, **75**, 1551–5.

Markussis, V., Beshyah, S. A., Fisher, C., *et al.* (1992). Detection of premature atherosclerosis by high-resolution ultrasonography in symptom-free hypopituitary adults. *Lancet*, **340**, 1188–92.

Matsumoto, K., Sera, Y., Abe, Y., *et al.* (2004). Metformin attenuates progression of carotid arterial wall thickness in patients with type 2 diabetes. *Diabetes Research and Clinical Practice*, **64**, 225–8.

McNeill, A. M., Rosamond, W. D., Girman, C. J., *et al.* (2004). Prevalence of coronary heart disease and carotid arterial thickening in patients with the metabolic syndrome (The ARIC Study). *American Journal of Cardiology*, **94**, 1249–54.

Melnick, S. L., Shahar, E., Folsom, A. R., *et al.* (1993). Past infection by chlamydia pneumoniae strain TWAR and asymptomatic carotid atherosclerosis. *American Journal of Medicine*, **95**, 499–504.

Mercuri, M., Bond, M. G., Sirtori, C. R., *et al.* (1996). Pravastatin reduces carotid intima-media thickness progression in an asymptomatic hypercholesterolemic Mediterranean population: the Carotid Atherosclerosis Italian Ultrasound Study. *American Journal of Medicine*, **101**, 627–34.

Miyazaki, H., Matsuoka, H., Cooke, J. P., *et al.* (1999). Endogenous nitric oxide synthase inhibitor: a novel marker of atherosclerosis. *Circulation*, **99**, 1141–6.

Nagata-Sakurai, M., Inaba, M., Goto, H., *et al.* (2003). Inflammation and bone resorption as independent factors of accelerated arterial wall thickening in patients with rheumatoid arthritis. *Arthritis and Rheumatism*, **48**, 3061–7.

Nathan, D. M., Lachin, J., Cleary, P., *et al.* (2003). Diabetes Control and Complications Trial; Epidemiology of Diabetes Interventions and Complications Research Group. Intensive diabetes therapy and carotid intima-media thickness in type 1 diabetes mellitus. *New England Journal of Medicine*, **348**, 2294–303.

Nordstrom, C. K., Dwyer, K. M., Merz, C. N., Shircore, A. and Dwyer, J. H. (2003). Leisure time physical activity and early atherosclerosis: the Los Angeles Atherosclerosis Study. *American Journal of Medicine*, **115**, 19–25.

North, K. E., MacCluer, J. W., Devereux, R. B., *et al.* (2002). Heritability of carotid artery structure and function: the Strong Heart Family Study. *Arteriosclerosis, Thrombosis and Vascular Biology*, **22**, 1698–703.

O'Leary, D. H., Polak, J. F., Kronmal, R. A., *et al.* (1992). Distribution and correlates of sonographically detected carotid artery disease in the Cardiovascular Health Study. *Stroke*, **23**, 1752–60.

O'Leary, D. H., Polak, J. F., Kronmal, R. A., *et al.* (1999). Carotid artery intima and media thickness as a risk factor for myocardial infarction and stroke in older adults. Cardiovascular Health Study Collaborative Research Group. *New England Journal of Medicine*, **340**, 14–22.

Pignoli, P., Tremoli, E., Poli, A., Oreste, P. and Paoletti, R. (1986). Intimal plus medial thickness of the arterial wall: a direct measurement with ultrasound imaging. *Circulation*, **74**, 1399–406.

Pitt, B., Byington, R. P., Furberg, C. D., *et al.* (2000). Effect of amlodipine on the progression of atherosclerosis and the occurrence of clinical events. PREVENT Investigators. *Circulation*, **102**, 1503–10.

Polak, J. F., Kronmal, R. A., Tell, G. S., *et al.* (1996). Compensatory increase in common carotid artery diameter. *Stroke*, **27**, 2012–15.

Polak, J. R., Shemanski, L., O'Leary, D. H., *et al.* (1998). Hypoechoic plaque at US of the carotid artery: an independent risk factor for incident stroke in adults aged 65 years or older. *Radiology*, **208**, 649–54.

Postiglione, A., Rubba, P., De Simone, B., *et al.* (1985). Carotid atherosclerosis in familial hypercholesterolemia. *Stroke*, **16**, 658–61.

Price, T. R., Manolio, T. A., Kronmal, R. A., *et al.* (1997). Silent brain infarction on magnetic resonance imaging and neurological abnormalities in community-dwelling older adults. *Stroke*, **28**, 1158–64.

Psaty, B. M., Furberg, C. D., Kuller, L. H., *et al.* (1999). Traditional risk factors and subclinical disease measures as predictors of first myocardial infarction in older adults. The Cardiovascular Health Study. *Archives of Internal Medicine*, **159**, 1339–47.

Raitakari, O. T., Juonala, M., Kahonen, M., *et al.* (2003). Cardiovascular risk factors in childhood and carotid artery intima-media thickness in adulthood: the Cardiovascular Risk in Young Finns Study. *Journal of the American Medical Association*, **290**, 2277–83.

Ranke, C., Hecker, H., Creutzig, A. and Alexander, K. (1993). Dose-dependent effect of aspirin on carotid atherosclerosis. *Circulation*, **87**, 1873–9.

Roman, M. J., Shanker, B. A., Davis, A., *et al.* (2003). Prevalence and correlates of accelerated atherosclerosis in systemic lupus erythematosus. *New England Journal of Medicine*, **349**, 2399–406.

Sabeti, S., Exner, M., Mlekusch, W., *et al.* (2005). Prognostic impact of fibrinogen in carotid atherosclerosis: nonspecific indicator of inflammation or independent predictor of disease progression? *Stroke*, **36**, 1400–4.

Salomaa V., Stinson V., Kark, J. D., *et al.* (1995). Association of fibrinolytic parameters with early atherosclerosis. The ARIC Study. *Circulation*, **15**, 1269–79.

Salonen, R. and Salonen, J. T. (1990). Progression of carotid atherosclerosis and its determinants: a population-based ultrasonography study. *Atherosclerosis*, **81**, 33–40.

Salonen, J. T. and Salonen, R. (1993). Ultrasound B-mode imaging in observational studies of atherosclerotic progression. *Circulation*, **87** (Suppl. II), II-56–II.

Salonen, R., Seppanen, K., Rauramaa, R. and Salonen, J. T. (1988). Prevalence of carotid atherosclerosis and serum cholesterol levels in eastern Finland. *Arteriosclerosis*, **8**, 788–92.

Salonen, R., Tervahauta, M., Salonen, J. T., *et al.* (1994). Ultrasonographic manifestations of common carotid atherosclerosis in elderly Eastern Finnish men. *Arteriosclerosis and Thrombosis*, **14**, 1631–40.

Salonen, R., Nyyssonen, K., Porkkala, E., *et al.* (1995). Kuopio Atherosclerosis Prevention Study (KAPS). *Circulation*, **92**, 1758–64.

Salonen, R. M., Nyyssonen, K., Kaikkonen, J., *et al.* (2003). Antioxidant Supplementation in Atherosclerosis Prevention Study. Six-year effect of combined vitamin C and E supplementation on atherosclerotic progression: the Antioxidant Supplementation in Atherosclerosis Prevention (ASAP) Study. *Circulation*, **107**, 947–53.

Sawayama, Y., Shimizu, C., Maeda, N., *et al.* (2002). Effects of probucol and pravastatin on common carotid atherosclerosis in patients with asymptomatic hypercholesterolemia. Fukuoka Atherosclerosis Trial (FAST). *Journal of the American College of Cardiology*, **39**, 610–16.

Schillinger, M., Exner, M., Mlekusch, W., *et al.* (2005). Inflammation and Carotid Artery – Risk for Atherosclerosis Study (ICARAS). *Circulation*, **111**, 2203–9.

Schott, L. L., Wildman, R. P., Brockwell, S., *et al.* (2004). Segment-specific effects of cardiovascular risk factors on carotid artery intima-medial thickness in women at midlife. *Arteriosclerosis, Thrombosis and Vascular Biology*, **24**, 1951–6.

Selhub, J., Jacques, P. F., Bostom, A. G., *et al.* (1995). Association between plasma homocysteine concentrations and extracranial carotid-artery stenosis. *New England Journal of Medicine*, **332**, 286–91.

Sharrett, A. R., Sorlie, P. D., Chambless, L. E., *et al.* (1999). Relative importance of various risk factors for asymptomatic carotid atherosclerosis versus coronary heart disease incidence. *American Journal of Epidemiology*, **149**, 843–52.

Sidhu, J. S., Kaposzta, Z., Markus, H. S. and Kaski, J. C. (2004). Effect of rosiglitazone on common carotid intima-media thickness progression in coronary artery disease patients without diabetes mellitus. *Arteriosclerosis, Thrombosis and Vascular Biology*, **24**, 930–4.

Simon, A., Gariepy, J., Moyse, D. and Levenson, J. (2001). Differential effects of nifedipine and co-amilozide on the progression of early carotid wall changes. *Circulation*, **103**, 2949–54.

Smilde, T. J., van Wissen, S., Wollersheim, H., *et al.* (2001). Effect of aggressive versus conventional lipid lowering on atherosclerosis progression in familial hypercholesterolaemia (ASAP): a prospective, randomized, double-blind trial. *Lancet*, **357**, 577–81.

Swan, L., Birnie, D. H., Inglis, G., Connell, J. M. and Hillis, W. S. (2003). The determination of carotid intima medial thickness in adults – a population-based twin study. *Atherosclerosis*, **166**, 137–41.

Sztajzel, R., Momjian, S., Momjian-Mayor, I., *et al.* (2005). Stratified gray-scale median analysis and color mapping of the carotid plaque: correlation with endarterectomy specimen histology of 28 patients. *Stroke*, **36**, 741–5.

Tang, R., Hennig, M., Thomasson, B., *et al.* (2000). Baseline reproducibility of B-mode ultrasonic measurement of carotid artery intima-media thickness: the European Lacidipine Study on Atherosclerosis (ELSA). *Journal of Hypertension*, **18**, 197–201.

Taylor, A. J., Kent, S. M., Flaherty, P. J., *et al.* (2002). ARBITER: Arterial Biology for the Investigation of the Treatment Effects of Reducing Cholesterol: a randomized trial comparing the effects of atorvastatin and pravastatin on carotid intima medial thickness. *Circulation*, **106**, 2055–60.

Taylor, A. J., Sullenberger, L. E., Lee, H. J., Lee, J. K. and Grace, K. A. (2004). Arterial Biology for the Investigation of the Treatment Effects of Reducing Cholesterol (ARBITER) 2: a double-blind, placebo-controlled study of extended-release niacin on atherosclerosis progression in secondary prevention patients treated with statins. *Circulation*, **110**, 3512–17.

Tell, G. S., Evans, G. W., Folsom, A. R., *et al.* (1994). Dietary fat intake and carotid artery wall thickness: The Atherosclerosis Risk in Communities (ARIC) Study. *American Journal of Epidemiology*, **139**, 979–89.

Terry, J. G., Tang, R., Espeland, M. A., *et al.* (2003). Carotid arterial structure in patients with documented coronary artery disease and disease-free control subjects. *Circulation*, **107**, 1146–51.

Tracy, R. P., Bovill, E. G., Yanez, D., *et al.* (1995). Fibrinogen and factor VIII, but not factor VII, are associated with measures of subclinical cardiovascular disease in the elderly. Results from the Cardiovascular Health Study. *Arteriosclerosis, Thrombosis and Vascular Biology*, **15**, 1269–79.

Van der Meer, I. M., de Maat, M. P., Bots, M. L., *et al.* (2002). Inflammatory mediators and cell adhesion molecules as indicators of severity of atherosclerosis: the Rotterdam Study. *Arteriosclerosis, Thrombosis and Vascular Biology*, **22**, 838–42.

Van der Meer, I. M., de Maat, M. P., Hak, A. E., *et al.* (2002). C-reactive protein predicts progression of atherosclerosis measured at various sites in the arterial tree: the Rotterdam Study. *Stroke*, **33**, 2750–5.

Van der Meer, I. M., Iglesias del Sol, A., Hak, A. E., *et al.* (2003). Risk factors for progression of atherosclerosis measured at multiple sites in the arterial tree: the Rotterdam Study. *Stroke*, **34**, 2374–9.

Van der Meer, I. M., Iglesias del Sol, A., Hak, A. E., *et al.* (2003). Risk factors for progression of atherosclerosis measured at multiple sites in the arterial tree: the Rotterdam Study. *Stroke*, **34**, 2374–9.

Vermeer, S. E., Den Heijer, T., Koudstaal, P. J., *et al.* (2003). Rotterdam Scan Study. Incidence and risk factors of silent brain infarcts in the population-based Rotterdam Scan Study. *Stroke*, **34**, 392–6.

Vermeulen, E. G., Stehouwer, C. D., Twisk, J. W., *et al.* (2000). Effect of homocysteine-lowering treatment with folic acid plus vitamin B6 on progression of subclinical atherosclerosis: a randomised, placebo-controlled trial. *Lancet*, **355**, 517–22.

Wallenfeldt, K., Bokemark, L., Wikstrand, J., Hulthe, J. and Fagerberg, B. (2004). Apolipoprotein B/apolipoprotein A-I in relation to the metabolic syndrome and change in carotid artery intima-media thickness during 3 years in middle-aged men. *Stroke*, **35**, 2248–52.

Wallenfeldt, K., Hulthe, J. and Fagerberg, B. (2005). The metabolic syndrome in middle-aged men according to different definitions and related changes in carotid artery intima-media thickness (IMT) during 3 years of follow-up. *Journal of Internal Medicine*, **258**, 28–37.

Wang, T. J., Nam, B. H., Wilson, P. W., *et al.* (2002). Association of C-reactive protein with carotid atherosclerosis in men and women: the Framingham Heart Study. *Arteriosclerosis, Thrombosis and Vascular Biology*, **22**, 1662–7.

Wiklund, O., Hulthe, J., Wikstrand, J., *et al.* (2002). Effect of controlled release/extended release metoprolol on carotid intima-media thickness in patients with hypercholesterolemia: a 3-year randomized study. *Stroke*, **33**, 572–7.

Wildman, R. P., Schott, L. L., Brockwell, S., Kuller, L. H. and Sutton-Tyrrell, K. (2004). A dietary and exercise intervention slows menopause-associated progression of subclinical atherosclerosis as measured by intima-media thickness of the carotid arteries. *Journal of the American College of Cardiology*, **44**, 579–85.

Willeit, J., Kiechl, S., Oberhollenzer, F., *et al.* (2000). Distinct risk profiles of early and advanced atherosclerosis: prospective results from the Bruneck Study. *Arteriosclerosis, Thrombosis and Vascular Biology*, **20**, 529–37.

Willeit, J., Kiechl, S., Oberhollenzer, F., *et al.* (2000). Distinct risk profiles of early and advanced atherosclerosis: prospective results from the Bruneck Study. *Arteriosclerosis, Thrombosis and Vascular Biology*, **20**, 529–37.

Wilson, P. W. F., Hoeg, J. M., D'Agostino, R. B., *et al.* (1997). Cumulative effects of high cholesterol levels, high blood pressure, and cigarette smoking on carotid stenosis. *New England Journal of Medicine*, **337**, 516–22.

Wong, M., Edelstein, J., Wollman, J. and Bond, M. G. (1993). Ultrasonic-pathological comparison of the human arterial wall. *Arteriosclerosis and Thrombosis*, **13**, 482–6.

Wu, H., Dwyer, K. M., Fan, Z., *et al.* (2003). Dietary fiber and progression of atherosclerosis: the Los Angeles Atherosclerosis Study. *American Journal of Clinical Nutrition*, **78**, 1085–91.

Xiang, A. H., Azen, S. P., Buchanan, T. A., *et al.* (2002). Heritability of subclinical atherosclerosis in Latino families ascertained through a hypertensive parent. *Arteriosclerosis, Thrombosis and Vascular Biology*, **22**, 843–8.

Zanchetti, A., Rosei, E. A., Dal Palu, C., *et al.* (1998). The Verapamil in Hypertension and Atherosclerosis Study (VHAS): results of long-term randomized treatment with either verapamil or chlorthalidone on carotid intima-media thickness. *Journal of Hypertension*, **16**, 1667–76.

Zanchetti, A., Bond, M. G., Hennig, M., *et al.* (2002). European Lacidipine Study on Atherosclerosis investigators. Calcium antagonist lacidipine slows down progression of asymptomatic carotid atherosclerosis: principal results of the European Lacidipine Study on

Atherosclerosis (ELSA), a randomized, double-blind, long-term trial. *Circulation*, **106**, 2422–7.

Zanchetti, A., Bond, M. G., Hennig, M., *et al.* (2004). Absolute and relative changes in carotid intima-media thickness and atherosclerotic plaques during long-term antihypertensive treatment: further results of the European Lacidipine Study on Atherosclerosis (ELSA). *Journal of Hypertension*, **22**, 1201–12.

Zanchetti, A., Crepaldi, G., Bond, M. G., *et al.* (2004). Different Effects of Antihypertensive Regimens Based on Fosinopril or Hydrochlorothiazide With or Without Lipid Lowering by Pravastatin on Progression of Asymptomatic Carotid Atherosclerosis: Principal Results of PHYLLIS – A Randomized Double-Blind Trial. *Stroke*, **35**, 2807–12.

Zannad, F., Visvikis, S., Gueguen, R., *et al.* (1998). Genetics strongly determines the wall thickness of the left and right carotid arteries. *Human Genetics*, **103**, 183–8.

Zannad, F. and Benetos, A. (2003). Genetics of intima-media thickness. *Current Opinion in Lipidology*, **14**, 191–200.

Zureik, M., Touboul, P. J., Bonithon-Kopp, C., *et al.* (1991). Cross-sectional and 4-year longitudinal associations between brachial pulse pressure and common carotid intima-media thickness in a general population. The EVA study. *Stroke*, **30**, 550–5.

Zureik, M., Touboul, P. J., Bonithon-Kopp, C., *et al.* (1999). Cross-sectional and 4-year longitudinal associations between brachial pulse pressure and common carotid intima-media thickness in a general population. The EVA study. *Stroke*, **30**, 550–5.

32

Monitoring pharmaceutical interventions with IVUS

Stephen J. Nicholls, Steven E. Nissen and E. Murat Tuzcu

The Cleveland Clinic Foundation, Cleveland OH, USA

Introduction

A number of therapeutic strategies have been demonstrated to have a profound impact on coronary artery disease. Accordingly, these agents have become an integral component of cardiovascular prevention regimens. In many cases, however, initiation of therapy after a clinical event is often too late, whether that is myocardial ischemia, transient ischemic attack or more focal infarction. In addition, the majority of clinical events are not prevented by the use of these therapies. As atherosclerotic cardiovascular disease remains the scourge of Western societies and is becoming increasingly prevalent within developing nations, there is an ongoing need to develop interventions that effectively reduce vascular risk.

While the final determinant of proof of efficacy of these agents resides in their ability to prevent clinical events, any assessment of an agent must be performed on the background of a combination of agents with proven efficacy. The background use of multiple efficacious agents has resulted in progressively lower event rates in patients assigned to placebo arms in clinical trials. As a result, an increasingly larger number of patients need to be followed for longer time periods in clinical trials to observe event rates that allow for an evaluation of the efficacy of these agents. As development of experimental agents is a long and costly process,

it has become increasingly attractive to assess the effect of agents on a number of surrogate endpoints, in order to provide preliminary information in the design of large-scale clinical event trials. The evolution of imaging modalities that visualize the arterial wall provide an opportunity to evaluate the effect of experimental strategies on the size and composition of atherosclerotic plaque.

Atherosclerosis imaging modalities

Despite its widespread use to guide the provision of revascularization strategies, coronary angiography has a limited ability to predict the likelihood of ischemic events. The majority of patients who experience a myocardial infarction, do so in a vascular territory supplied by a culprit lesion that is only mildly stenotic on angiography (Ambrose et al., 1988; Little et al., 1988; Giroud et al., 1992). This finding has supported the concept that the propensity to undergo plaque rupture and develop cardiac ischemia is a function of plaque activity, rather than its extent (Falk et al., 1995; Ross, 1999). However, it has become increasingly recognized that angiography, which provides a silhouette of the lumen, underestimates the extent of atherosclerosis (Topol and Nissen, 1995). Immense interest has therefore been stimulated to develop imaging modalities that visualize the arterial

Carotid Disease: The Role of Imaging in Diagnosis and Management, ed. Jonathan Gillard, Martin Graves, Thomas Hatsukami and Chun Yuan. Published by Cambridge University Press. © Cambridge University Press 2007.

wall and are more able to accurately quantify plaque burden. The application of intravascular ultrasound (IVUS) within the coronary arteries has allowed for an enhanced characterization of the size and distribution of atheroma and the natural history of the arterial wall's response to its accumulation.

IVUS

IVUS is performed safely at the time of diagnostic coronary angiography and involves the placement of a high frequency ultrasound transducer on the tip of a catheter within the major epicardial coronary arteries (Nissen and Yock, 2001) as described in Chapter 17. The high resolution tomographic cross-sectional images of the arterial wall, plaque and lumen that are generated can be employed by interventional cardiologists to guide the management of specific lesions (Fuessl *et al.*, 1999; Serruys *et al.*, 2004). IVUS has also been used to estimate the extent of atheroma throughout segments of coronary arteries (Mintz *et al.*, 2001). This is accomplished by continuous imaging while the catheter is withdrawn at a rate of 0.5 mm/s by connecting the catheter to a motorized pullback device.

The images that are generated can be used to estimate plaque burden. The leading edges of the external elastic membrane (EEM) and the lumen in a tomographic image can be traced by manual planimetry. The plaque area in that image is then determined as the difference between the areas occupied by the EEM and lumen (Mintz *et al.*, 2001) (Figure 32.1). As catheter withdrawal generates a series of consecutive images, summation of plaque areas from each of these images provides a volumetric estimate of the extent of atheroma within the arterial segment that was studied (Figure 32.2). In addition to quantification of plaque burden, IVUS also provides a broad characterization of plaque morphology, including the presence and extent of calcification. As the same arterial segment can be imaged at different

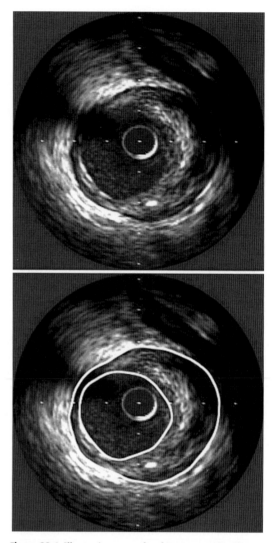

Figure 32.1 Illustrative example of a cross-sectional tomographic image of a coronary artery generated by intravascular ultrasound (top panel) with tracings of the leading edges of the external elastic membrane (outer circle) and lumen (inner circle) in the lower panel.

moments in time, it is now possible to investigate the natural history of plaque progression and to define how it is influenced by a multitude of antiatherosclerotic therapies (Figure 32.3).

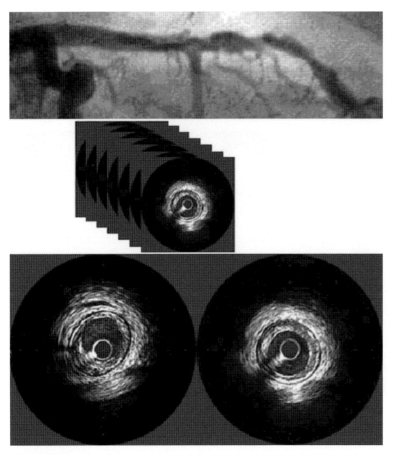

Figure 32.2 Representative images of withdrawl of the IVUS transducer through an arterial segment (top panel) generates a series of stacked tomographic images (middle panel). As the transducer is withdrawn at a constant rate of 0.5 mm/s, every sixtieth image represents images spaced precisely 1 mm apart and is selected for measurement.

Lessons from IVUS

The ability to visualize the entire arterial wall in vivo has allowed IVUS to be employed to characterize the accumulation of atherosclerotic plaque within the arterial wall. These IVUS studies revealed the diffuse nature of atherosclerosis, which exceeds the angiographically evident extent of the disease (Mintz *et al.*, 1995). IVUS has also confirmed the findings of necropsy studies (PDAY Research Group, 1990; Berenson *et al.*, 1992) and carotid intimal media thickness in population

studies (Urbina *et al.*, 2002; Knoflach *et al.*, 2003) that report the appearance of macroscopic atheroma early in life. Performing IVUS in donor coronary arteries shortly following cardiac transplantation in a cohort of 262 patients revealed that one in six hearts from teenage donors harbored significant atheroma, defined as a mean maximal plaque thickness greater than 0.5 mm. The prevalence of significant atheroma contained within the epicardial arteries of these apparently healthy hearts increased dramatically with age (Tuzcu *et al.*, 2001).

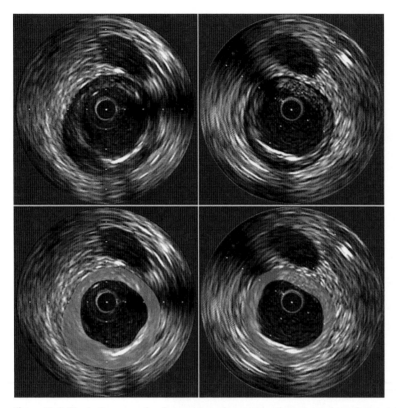

Figure 32.3 Illustrative example of regression of coronary atheroma evaluated at matched sites by IVUS pullbacks performed at baseline (left panels) and follow-up (right panels). Shading of the corresponding plaque area is depicted in the lower panels.

IVUS has also played a pivotal role in defining the remodeling response of the arterial wall in relation to accumulation of atherosclerotic plaque. Glagov and colleagues initially proposed that the arterial wall undergoes expansion, or remodeling, of the internal elastic lamina in response to the accumulation of atheroma (Glagov *et al.*, 1987). This process was initially described in necropsy studies and has subsequently been confirmed in vivo by IVUS studies (Losordo *et al.*, 1994; Pasterkamp *et al.*, 1995). In association with the early stages of arterial remodeling, luminal dimensions are preserved, making it possible that a substantial amount of atheroma might accumulate within the arterial wall before it is detected by angiography. A number of reports have

subsequently demonstrated that the arterial wall remodels in opposing directions in different clinical syndromes (Schoenhagen *et al.*, 2000). Culprit lesions are associated with expansive remodeling in the setting of acute coronary syndromes. In contrast, lesions are more likely to undergo constrictive remodeling in the setting of stable ischemia. The demonstration that the arterial wall undergoes changes in size and structure supports the concept that the vessel wall is not simply a passive player in atherosclerosis.

In addition to the characterization of the development and progression of atherosclerotic plaque, reports of IVUS studies have highlighted the multifocal nature of plaque rupture in the setting of acute coronary syndromes (Rioufol *et al.*, 2002;

Schoenhagen *et al.*, 2003). The finding of multiple ruptured plaques throughout the coronary arterial tree, rather than just the culprit vessel provides further evidence for the notion that the ischemic complications of atherosclerosis are triggered by systemic, rather than focal, factors (Ross, 1999; Lutgens *et al.*, 2003). It is therefore likely that as the majority of episodes of plaque rupture are clinically quiescent, factors that regulate thrombus formation are of critical importance in determining the likelihood of progression to ischemia (Naghavi *et al.*, 2003).

The application of IVUS has been employed to describe the natural history of vascular pathologies that extend beyond atherosclerosis. Serial IVUS studies have defined the factors that contribute to the development of restenosis following percutaneous intervention (Yeung *et al.*, 1995; Tuzcu *et al.*, 1996). As a result of its ability to detect early neointimal thickening, IVUS has also become the gold standard for the detection and monitoring of transplant vasculopathy (Kapadia *et al.*, 1999).

Impact of therapeutic strategies assessed by serial IVUS

As a result of the ability to repeat IVUS assessments of the same arterial segment at different points in time, it has now become possible to determine the impact that a large range of interventions exert on the development of atherosclerosis and neointimal hyperplasia. A number of reports have recently emerged that investigate the role of aggressive modification of both traditional and emerging risk factors.

Impact of infusing high density lipoproteins on plaque burden

A large body of evidence from population (Gordon *et al.*, 1977) and animal (Badimon *et al.*, 1989, 1990; Plump *et al.*, 1994; Rong *et al.*, 2001) studies suggest that high density lipoproteins (HDLs) exert a protective influence on the arterial wall.

While a number of strategies have been developed which promote both the quality and quantity of HDL, it remains uncertain whether these interventions are beneficial in humans. In an exciting proof of concept, serial IVUS was recently employed to demonstrate rapid regression of coronary atheroma in humans who received infusions of reconstituted HDL particles containing apolipoprotein A-I Milano (Nissen *et al.*, 2003). This extended the findings of preclinical reports which demonstrated carriers of the apoA-I Milano variant, with low HDL levels, are protected from cardiovascular disease (Franceschini *et al.*, 1980), and that infusions were beneficial in animal models of atherosclerosis (Shah *et al.*, 1998, 2001; Chiesa *et al.*, 2002).

In the IVUS study, 47 patients within 2 weeks of an acute coronary syndrome received weekly infusions of placebo or complexes of apoA-I Milano and phospholipid (ETC-216) for 5 weeks. IVUS studies were performed within the same coronary artery segment at baseline and within 2 weeks of the final infusion. Atheroma volume decreased by 4.2% in patients who received infusions of ETC-216, containing either 15 mg/kg or 45 mg/kg protein. The most dramatic effect was seen in those 10-mm subsegments that contained the greatest amount of atheroma. This study is supportive of the previous reports that demonstrated that combination therapy with niacin and a statin promoted plaque regression in angiographic studies (Brown *et al.*, 2001) and halted progression of carotid intimal medial thickness, presumably through their favorable effects on low density lipoprotein (LDL) and HDL (Taylor *et al.*, 2004). These profound findings have stimulated the need to perform large-scale studies to assess the potential clinical impact of interventions that promote HDL.

Impact of lipid lowering on atherosclerotic plaque

While a large body of evidence has demonstrated that clinical events are prevented by LDL lowering with statins (4S Investigators, 1994; Shepherd *et al.*, 1995; Sacks *et al.*, 1996; Downs *et al.*, 1998; LIPID Study Group, 1998; HPS Investigators, 2002), a number of important issues remain unresolved with regard to their clinical use. In particular, it remains to be unequivocally established whether a greater clinical benefit is derived from use of higher statin doses or their early administration following an acute ischemic syndrome. Considerable debate has focused on the target LDL levels. In addition, while a number of angiographic studies have reported that statin therapy can, at best halt progression of luminal stenoses (MAAS Investigators, 1990; Blankenhorn *et al.*, 1993; Jukema *et al.*, 1995; Pitt *et al.*, 1995; Arntz *et al.*, 2000), the benefit found in these studies appears to be less profound than their effect on clinical event rates. Extending on early reports of plaque regression following LDL apheresis in patients with drug refractory familial hypercholesterolemia (Koga *et al.*, 1992; Matsuzaki *et al.*, 2002), a number of studies using serial IVUS imaging have recently been reported demonstrating the impact of statin therapy on the volume of coronary atherosclerosis. For example, serial IVUS demonstrated plaque regression with a 6.3% reduction in plaque volume following 12 months of therapy with simvastatin 40 mg daily combined with a lipid-lowering diet (Jensen *et al.*, 2004).

IVUS assessment of the impact of aggressive lipid lowering

The lack of consensus regarding a possible LDL threshold, below which no further clinical benefit is derived, has stimulated ongoing debate with regard to what is an appropriate LDL target for patients with atherosclerotic cardiovascular disease. Serial IVUS recently reported the impact on coronary atheroma burden of moderate and intensive lipid-lowering strategies. In the Reversal of Atherosclerosis with Aggressive Lipid Lowering

(REVERSAL) study (Nissen *et al.*, 2004) 502 patients with coronary artery disease and an LDL-C level between 125 mg/dL and 210 mg/dL received either pravastatin 40 mg daily or atorvastatin 80 mg daily for 18 months. This resulted in reductions of LDL-C to 79 mg/dL and 110 mg/dL, with atorvastatin and pravastatin, respectively. The therapies differed in their ability to lower C-reactive protein (CRP), by 36.4% with atorvastatin and 5.2% with pravastatin. While atheroma volume increased by 2.7% with pravastatin, serial IVUS revealed that there was no change in patients treated with atorvastatin compared with baseline. A continuous relationship was demonstrated between changes in LDL cholesterol and atheroma volume. Consistent with the effect of infusing apoA-I Milano, the impact of lipid lowering was greatest in those 10-mm subsegments that harbored the greatest amount of plaque at baseline. In fact, it was demonstrated that both statins promoted atheroma regression in these regions. The demonstration that intensive lipid lowering alters the natural history of plaque progression parallels the recent finding of a 22% reduction in clinical endpoints that resulted from high dose compared with low-dose atorvastatin in the Treating to New Targets (TNT) study (LaRosa *et al.*, 2005).

IVUS assessment of the antiinflammatory properties of statins

It was apparent that LDL lowering did not account for all of the benefit that was derived from use of the intensive lipid-lowering strategy in REVERSAL. Examination of the regression lines demonstrating the relationship between changes in LDL cholesterol and plaque volume revealed that the lines for the different treatment strategies never met. In particular, it was noted that at any level of change of LDL cholesterol, the regression line favored a greater impact of atorvastatin on atheroma volume. This appeared to suggest that an additional 20% of lowering LDL cholesterol is required with pravastatin to achieve the same effect on plaque progression. This result provides further impetus for the suggestion that atorvastatin possesses beneficial properties that extend beyond their ability to lower LDL. One of these properties appears to be a reduction of vascular inflammation, as a continuous relationship was also demonstrated between CRP lowering and the rate of plaque progression (Nissen *et al.*, 2005). These results paralleled the findings of an incremental benefit of high-dose atorvastatin over pravastatin on clinical event rates and CRP in patients who participated in the Pravastatin or Atorvastatin Evaluation and Infection Therapy (PROVE-IT) study (Cannon *et al.*, 2004; Ridker *et al.*, 2005).

IVUS assessment of early statin administration

A number of studies have reported that initiation of statin therapy in the setting of an acute coronary syndrome results in an early beneficial reduction in clinical events (Schwartz *et al.*, 2001; Stenestrand and Wallentin, 2001). Serial IVUS was recently employed to demonstrate the beneficial impact of this strategy on coronary atheroma. Forty eight patients who received atorvastatin 20 mg daily or a placebo for 6 months following percutaneous intervention for an ST elevation myocardial infarction in the ESTABLISH study were assessed by serial IVUS (Okazaki *et al.*, 2004). A strong correlation was observed between the percentage change in atheroma volume and both LDL cholesterol at follow-up and the percent reduction in LDL cholesterol. A 13.1% reduction in plaque volume accompanied the 41.7% reduction in LDL cholesterol with atorvastatin therapy. In contrast, treatment with diet alone had no effect on levels of LDL cholesterol and was associated with an 8.7% increase in plaque volume.

Impact of intensive blood pressure lowering on plaque burden

In a novel experimental design, serial IVUS was employed as an endpoint, embedded within a large clinical event trial that assessed the impact of initiating antihypertensive therapy to patients with coronary artery disease with apparently normal blood pressure. The Comparison of Amlodipine vs. Enalapril to Limit Occurrences of Thrombosis (CAMELOT) study (Nissen *et al.*, 2004) randomized 1991 patients with coronary artery disease (CAD) and a diastolic blood pressure less than 100 mmHg to receive amlodipine 10 mg daily, enalapril 20 mg daily or placebo for 24 months. The use of concomitant therapies for secondary prevention was high, suggesting that these patients were extremely well treated. The 31% reduction in major adverse clinical events that resulted from amlodipine therapy was due to a 27% reduction in the need for coronary revascularization and 42% reduction in hospitalization for angina. The embedded IVUS substudy was performed in 274 of these subjects and found that while there was an increase in plaque volume in placebo-treated patients, there was no change in atheroma burden in patients treated with amlodipine. The difference between treatment groups was not statistically significant. The most profound impact was seen in those patients with baseline blood pressure greater than the mean. The assessment of clinical events and IVUS in these patients demonstrated complementary effects on events and plaque burden. These findings extended those seen with aggressive lipid lowering and suggested that current blood pressure treatment goals in patients with CAD may be suboptimal.

Monitoring vascular pathologies beyond atherosclerosis

In addition to the characterization of the natural history of atherosclerosis and its response to a range of antiatherosclerotic agents, IVUS has been employed to investigate the formation of neointimal hyperplasia in a range of clinical settings. In response to percutaneous angioplasty, IVUS characterized that the restenosis that ensues results from a combination of recoil and remodeling of the arterial wall, followed by neointima formation (Mintz *et al.*, 1997). Serial IVUS has therefore assumed a pivotal role in the assessment of novel strategies to prevent restenosis including intracoronary radiation (Morino *et al.*, 2001); bare metal and drug-eluting stents (Fuessl *et al.*, 1999; Serruys *et al.*, 2004) and emerging antiinflammatory and antiproliferative agents (Cote *et al.*, 1999; Tardif *et al.*, 2001, 2003).

Neointimal hyperplasia is also a well-recognized complication of solid organ transplantation which predicts a poor clinical outcome and has become the leading indication for repeat cardiac transplantation (Keck *et al.*, 1999; Kobashigawa *et al.*, 2005; Tuzcu *et al.*, 2005). IVUS has become the imaging modality of choice for the detection and monitoring of the rate of progression of transplant vasculopathy (Kapadia *et al.*, 1999). In search of therapeutic strategies that have a beneficial impact on this process, the search has focused on the inflammatory and proliferative events that promote neointima formation as potential targets for intervention (Pinney and Mancini, 2004).

Serial IVUS demonstrated that everolimus, an agent with antiproliferative and antiinflammatory properties, prevented the development of vasculopathy in 634 primary heart transplant recipients who received either 1.5 mg of everolimus, 3 mg of everolimus or 1–3 mg of azathioprine in combination with standard medical therapy for 12 months (Eisen *et al.*, 2003). The low and high doses of everolimus reduced the incidence of vasculopathy after 1 year by 33% and 42%, respectively. Everolimus also reduced the increase in average maximal intimal thickness by 60–70% and the combination of death, graft loss or retransplantation, loss to follow-up, acute rejection grade 3A or rejection with hemodynamic compromise by 22–42%. Further findings that experimental agents have complementary effects on vascular pathologies and clinical events supports the concept that serial IVUS can be used as a reliable indicator of clinical effect in the early stages of drug development.

Characterization of plaque composition

The importance of plaque composition as a determinant of its propensity to provoke ischemic events has become increasingly recognized (Falk *et al.*, 1995; Ross, 1999). This has resulted from the findings of a number of angiographic studies that the culprit lesion in the setting of myocardial infarction is only mild to moderately stenotic in the majority of cases (Ambrose *et al.*, 1988; Little *et al.*, 1988; Giroud *et al.*, 1992). Further, pathologic studies have established that atheroma containing large amounts of macrophages are more likely to be complicated by breakdown of fibrous cap integrity, the typical precipitant of clinical ischemia (Falk *et al.*, 1995; Ross, 1999). This concept that vascular inflammation is an important factor in the provocation of acute ischemia is supported by the finding that systemic levels of inflammatory markers, such as CRP, predict the likelihood of future clinical ischemic events (Lindahl *et al.*, 2000; Ridker *et al.*, 2002).

As a result, the search to identify imaging techniques that accurately characterize the composition of atherosclerotic plaque is potentially important in risk stratification and triage of preventive strategies. IVUS has a limited ability to characterize plaque composition. At best, IVUS is able to broadly distinguish the possibly lipidic (echolucent), fibrotic (echodense) and calcific components of plaque, but these observations frequently result in a suboptimal correlation with histological characterization (Mintz *et al.*, 2001). Spectral analysis of the radiofrequency backscatter detected by an IVUS catheter has been reported to characterize the relative composition of human coronary atheroma with good histopathological correlation when studied in the ex vivo setting and is available for clinical use (Nair *et al.*, 2002). Measuring reflected light by optical coherence tomography (OCT) images atheroma macrophage activity with high resolution (Tearney *et al.*, 2003; MacNeill *et al.*, 2004). The temperature (Verheye *et al.*, 2002; MacNeill *et al.*, 2003) and compressibility (MacNeill *et al.*, 2003; Schaar *et al.*, 2003) are also tested for assessment of inflammatory and lipid-rich plaques. However, the clinical utility of these approaches is questionable. Multiple plaque ruptures are typically present throughout the coronary arterial tree in acute coronary syndromes (Schoenhagen *et al.*, 2003). In addition, the marked clinical benefit from systemic therapies in secondary prevention suggests that it is identification of the vulnerable patient, rather than a single plaque, that is most important.

These approaches are also limited by the requirement for invasive cardiac catheterisation. The ideal scenario would involve the integration of systemic biomarkers with robust predictive power and noninvasive imaging modalities that accurately quantify plaque burden and characterize its composition throughout the arterial tree. Magnetic resonance has been reported to assess quantity and composition of aortic atheroma (Choudhury *et al.*, 2002; Saam *et al.*, 2005). Its resolution is limited for the coronary arterial tree and has not yet become available for clinical use. In contrast, the resolution of computed tomography (CT) allows for visualization of the coronary arteries in much shorter time spans and allows for detection of luminal stenoses (Achenbach and Daniel, 2004; Schoenhagen *et al.*, 2004; Schoepf *et al.*, 2004). Its ability to characterize plaque composition is limited at this point in time to a broad distinction of soft from calcific plaque. The emergence of hybrid systems that combine CT and positron emission tomography (PET), which has been reported to quantify plaque macrophage activity, may provide another option for noninvasive characterization of plaque (Rudd *et al.*, 2002). It remains to be seen whether further developments of any of these imaging modalities will result in the degree of precision required for accurate plaque characterization. In the case that these modalities reach clinical utility, the potential exists to assess the serial response of burden and composition of atherosclerotic plaque in response to a wide range of experimental anti-atherosclerotic agents.

Conclusion

The ability to image the entire arterial wall by placement of an IVUS catheter within the coronary artery has made a substantial contribution to our understanding of factors that influence the natural history of atherogenesis. In particular, the ability to image the same arterial segment in vivo and in a serial fashion has provided a novel and powerful research tool to assess the impact of experimental interventions on atherosclerotic plaque. Its use has provided important evidence to support the need for aggressive modification of risk factors in patients with established atherosclerotic disease. IVUS has also reignited the concept that regression of atheroma, in addition to modification of its composition, should be a major goal in the development of agents that influence atherogenesis. Accordingly, the use of imaging modalities that accurately assess plaque burden and composition will become an integral component in the design of clinical trials that assess the impact of emerging pharmacological strategies for the prevention of atherosclerotic cardiovascular disease.

REFERENCES

4S Investigators. (1994). Randomised trial of cholesterol lowering in 4444 patients with coronary heart disease: the Scandinavian Simvastatin Survival Study (4S). *Lancet*, **344**, 1383–9.

Achenbach, S. and Daniel, W. G. (2004). Imaging of coronary atherosclerosis using computed tomography: current status and future directions. *Current Atherosclerosis Reports*, **6**, 213–18.

Ambrose, J. A., Tannenbaum, M. A., Alexopoulos, D., *et al.* (1988). Angiographic progression of coronary artery disease and the development of myocardial infarction. *Journal of the American College of Cardiology*, **12**, 56–62.

Arntz, H. R., Agrawal, R., Wunderlich, W., *et al.* (2000). Beneficial effects of pravastatin (+/-colestyramine/niacin) initiated immediately after a coronary event (the randomized Lipid-Coronary Artery Disease L-CAD Study). *American Journal of Cardiology*, **86**, 1293–8.

Badimon, J. J., Badimon, L. and Fuster, V. (1990). Regression of atherosclerotic lesions by high density lipoprotein plasma fraction in the cholesterol-fed rabbit. *Journal of Clinical Investigation*, **85**, 1234–41.

Badimon, J. J., Badimon, L., Galvez, A., *et al.* (1989). High density lipoprotein plasma fractions inhibit aortic fatty streaks in cholesterol-fed rabbits. *Laboratory Investigation*, **60**, 455–61.

Berenson, G. S., Wattigney, W. A., Tracy, R. E., *et al.* (1992). Atherosclerosis of the aorta and coronary arteries and cardiovascular risk factors in persons aged 6 to 30 years and studied at necropsy (The Bogalusa Heart Study). *American Journal of Cardiology*, **70**, 851–8.

Blankenhorn, D. H., Azen, S. P., Kramsch, D. M., *et al.* (1993). Coronary angiographic changes with lovastatin therapy. The Monitored Atherosclerosis Regression Study (MARS). The MARS Research Group. *Annals of Internal Medicine*, **119**, 969–76.

Brown, B. G., Zhao, X.-Q., Chait, A., *et al.* (2001). Simvastatin and niacin, antioxidant vitamins, or the combination for the prevention of coronary disease. *New England Journal of Medicine*, **345**, 1583–92.

Cannon, C. P., Braunwald, E., McCabe, C. H., *et al.* (2004). Intensive versus moderate lipid lowering with statins after acute coronary syndromes. *New England Journal of Medicine*, **350**, 1495–504.

Chiesa, G., Monteggia, E., Marchesi, M., *et al.* (2002). Recombinant Apolipoprotein A-IMilano infusion into rabbit carotid artery rapidly removes lipid from fatty streaks. *Circulation Research*, **90**, 974–80.

Choudhury, R. P., Fuster, V., Badimon, J. J., *et al.* (2002). MRI and characterization of atherosclerotic plaque: emerging applications and molecular imaging. *Arteriosclerosis, Thrombosis and Vascular Biology*, **22**, 1065–74.

Cote, G., Tardif, J. C., Lesperance, J., *et al.* (1999). Effects of probucol on vascular remodeling after coronary angioplasty. Multivitamins and Protocol Study Group. *Circulation*, **99**, 30–5.

Downs, J. R., Clearfield, M., Weis, S., *et al.* (1998). Primary prevention of acute coronary events with lovastatin in men and women with average cholesterol levels: results of AFcaps/Texcaps. AirForce/Texas Coronary Atherosclerosis Prevention Study. *Journal of the American Medical Association*, **279**, 1615–22.

Eisen, H. J., Tuzcu, E. M., Dorent, R., *et al.* (2003). Everolimus for the prevention of allograft rejection and vasculopathy in cardiac-transplant recipients. *New England Journal of Medicine*, **349**, 847–58.

Falk, E., Shah, P. K. and Fuster, V. (1995). Coronary plaque disruption. *Circulation*, **92**, 657–71.

Franceschini, G., Sirtori, C. R., Capurso, A., 2nd, *et al.* (1980). A-IMilano apoprotein. Decreased high density lipoprotein cholesterol levels with significant lipoprotein modifications and without clinical atherosclerosis in an Italian family. *Journal of Clinical Investigation*, **66**, 892–900.

Fuessl, R. T., Hoepp, H. W. and Sechtem, U. (1999). Intravascular ultrasonography in the evaluation of results of coronary angioplasty and stenting. *Current Opinion in Cardiology*, **14**, 471–9.

Giroud, D., Li, J. M., Urban, P., *et al.* (1992). Relation of the site of acute myocardial infarction to the most severe coronary arterial stenosis at prior angiography. *American Journal of Cardiology*, **69**, 729–32.

Glagov, S., Weisenberg, E., Zarins, C. K., *et al.* (1987). Compensatory enlargement of human atherosclerotic coronary arteries. *New England Journal of Medicine*, **316**, 1371–5.

Gordon, T., Castelli, W. P., Hjortland, M. C., *et al.* (1977). High density lipoprotein as a protective factor against coronary heart disease. The Framingham Study. *American Journal of Medicine*, **62**, 707–14.

HPS Investigators. (2002) MRC/BHF Heart Protection Study of cholesterol lowering with simvastatin in 20,536 high-risk individuals: a randomised placebo-controlled trial. Investigators. *Lancet*, **360**, 7–22.

Jensen, L. O., Thayssen, P., Pedersen, K. E., *et al.* (2004). Regression of coronary atherosclerosis by simvastatin: a serial intravascular ultrasound study. *Circulation*, **110**, 265–70.

Jukema, J. W., Bruschke, A. V., van Boven, A. J., *et al.* (1995). Effects of lipid lowering by pravastatin on progression and regression of coronary artery disease in symptomatic men with normal to moderately elevated serum cholesterol levels. The Regression Growth Evaluation Statin Study (REGRESS). *Circulation*, **91**, 2528–40.

Kapadia, S. R., Nissen, S. E. and Tuzcu, E. M. (1999). Impact of intravascular ultrasound in understanding transplant coronary artery disease. *Current Opinion in Cardiology*, **14**, 140–50.

Keck, B. M., Bennett, L. E., Rosendale, J., *et al.* (1999). Worldwide thoracic organ transplantation: a report from the UNOS/ISHLT International Registry for Thoracic Organ Transplantation. *Clinical Transplants*, 35–49.

Knoflach, M., Kiechl, S., Kind, M., *et al.* (2003). Cardiovascular risk factors and atherosclerosis in young males: ARMY study (Atherosclerosis Risk-Factors in Male Youngsters). *Circulation*, **108**, 1064–9.

Kobashigawa, J. A., Tobis, J. M., Starling, R. C., *et al.* (2005). Intravascular ultrasound validation study among heart transplant recipients. Outcomes after 5 years. *Journal of the American College of Cardiology*, **45**, 1532–7.

Koga, N., Iwata, Y. and Yamamoto, A. (1992). Angiographic and pathological studies on regression of coronary atherosclerosis of FH patients who received LDL-apheresis treatment. *Artificial Organs*, **16**, 171–6.

LaRosa, J. C., Grundy, S. M., Waters, D. D., *et al.* (2005). Intensive lipid lowering with atorvastatin in patients with stable coronary disease. *New England Journal of Medicine*, **52**, 1425–35.

Lindahl, B., Toss, H., Siegbahn, A., *et al.* (2000). Markers of myocardial damage and inflammation in relation to long-term mortality in unstable coronary artery disease. FRISC Study Group. Fragmin during Instability in Coronary Artery Disease. *New England Journal of Medicine*, **343**, 1139–47.

LIPID Study Group. (1998). Prevention of cardiovascular events and death with pravastatin in patients with coronary heart disease and a broad range of initial cholesterol levels. The Long-Term Intervention with Pravastatin in Ischaemic Disease (LIPID) Study Group. *New England Journal of Medicine*, **339**, 1349–57.

Little, W. C., Constantinescu, M., Applegate, R. J., *et al.* (1988). Can coronary angiography predict the site of a subsequent myocardial infarction in patients with mild-to-moderate coronary artery disease? *Circulation*, **78**, 1157–66.

Losordo, D. W., Rosenfield, K., Kaufman, J., *et al.* (1994). Focal compensatory enlargement of human arteries in response to progressive atherosclerosis. In vivo documentation using intravascular ultrasound. *Circulation*, **89**, 2570–7.

Lutgens, E., van Suylen, R. J., Faber, B. C., *et al.* (2003). Atherosclerotic plaque rupture: local or systemic process? *Arteriosclerosis, Thrombosis and Vascular Biology*, **23**, 2123–30.

MAAS Effect of simvastatin on coronary atheroma: the Multicentre Anti-Atheroma Study (MAAS). Investigators (1990). *Lancet*, **344**, 633–8.

MacNeill, B. D., Lowe, H. C., Takano, M., *et al.* (2003). Intravascular modalities for detection of vulnerable plaque: current status. *Arteriosclerosis, Thrombosis and Vascular Biology*, **23**, 1333–42.

MacNeill, B. D., Jang, I. K., Bouma, B. E., *et al.* (2004). Focal and multi-focal plaque macrophage distributions in patients with acute and stable presentations of coronary artery disease. *Journal of American College of Cardiology*, **44**, 972–9.

Matsuzaki, M., Hiramori, K., Imaizumi, T., *et al.* (2002). Intravascular ultrasound evaluation of coronary plaque regression by low density lipoprotein-apheresis in familial hypercholesterolemia: the Low Density Lipoprotein-Apheresis Coronary Morphology and Reserve Trial (LACMART). *Journal of the American College of Cardiology*, **40**, 220–7.

Mintz, G. S., Kent, K. M., Pichard, A. D., *et al.* (1997). Intravascular ultrasound insights into mechanisms of stenosis formation and restenosis. *Cardiology Clinics*, **15**, 17–29.

Mintz, G. S., Nissen, S. E., Anderson, W. D., *et al.* (2001). American College of Cardiology Clinical Expert Consensus Document on Standards for Acquisition, Measurement and Reporting of Intravascular Ultrasound Studies (IVUS). A report of the American College of Cardiology Task Force on Clinical Expert Consensus Documents. *Journal of the American College of Cardiology*, **37**, 1478–92.

Mintz, G. S., Painter, J. A., Pichard, A. D., *et al.* (1995). Atherosclerosis in angiographically "normal" coronary artery reference segments: an intravascular ultrasound study with clinical correlations. *Journal of the American College of Cardiology*, **25**, 1479–85.

Morino, Y., Bonneau, H. N. and Fitzgerald, P. J. (2001). Vascular brachytherapy: what have we learned from intravascular ultrasound? *Journal of Invasive Cardiology*, **13**, 409–16.

Naghavi, M., Libby, P., Falk, E., *et al.* (2003). From vulnerable plaque to vulnerable patient: a call for new definitions and risk assessment strategies: Part I. *Circulation*, **108**, 1664–72.

Nair, A., Kuban, B. D., Tuzcu, E. M., *et al.* (2002). Coronary plaque classification with intravascular ultrasound radiofrequency data analysis. *Circulation*, **106**, 2200–6.

Nissen, S. E., Tuzcu, E. M., Libby, P., *et al.* (2004). Effect of antihypertensive agents on cardiovascular events in patients with coronary disease and normal blood pressure: the CAMELOT study: a randomized controlled trial. *Journal of the American Medical Association*, **292**, 2217–25.

Nissen, S. E., Tuzcu, E. M., Schoenhagen, P., *et al.* (2004). Effect of intensive compared with moderate lipid-lowering therapy on progression of coronary atherosclerosis: a randomized controlled trial. *Journal of the American Medical Association*, **291**, 1071–80.

Nissen, S. E., Tuzcu, E. M., Schoenhagen, P., *et al.* (2005). Statin therapy, LDL cholesterol, C-reactive protein, and coronary artery disease. *New England Journal of Medicine*, **352**, 29–38.

Nissen, S. E., Tsunoda, T., Tuzcu, E. M., *et al.* (2003). Effect of recombinant ApoA-I Milano on coronary atherosclerosis in patients with acute coronary syndromes: a randomized controlled trial. *Journal of the American Medical Association*, **290**, 2292–300.

Nissen, S. E. and Yock, P. (2001). Intravascular ultrasound: novel pathophysiological insights and current clinical applications. *Circulation*, **103**, 604–16.

Okazaki, S., Yokoyama, T., Miyauchi, K., *et al.* (2004). Early statin treatment in patients with acute coronary syndrome: demonstration of the beneficial effect on atherosclerotic lesions by serial volumetric intravascular ultrasound analysis during half a year after coronary event: the ESTABLISH Study. *Circulation*, **110**, 1061–8.

Pasterkamp, G., Wensing, P. J., Post, M. J., *et al.* (1995). Paradoxical arterial wall shrinkage may contribute to luminal narrowing of human atherosclerotic femoral arteries. *Circulation*, **91**, 1444–9.

PDAY Research Group (1990). Relationship of atherosclerosis in young men to serum lipoprotein cholesterol concentrations and smoking. A preliminary report from the Pathobiological Determinants of Atherosclerosis in Youth (PDAY) Research Group. *Journal of the American Medical Association*, **264**, 3018–24.

Pinney, S. P. and Mancini, D. (2004). Cardiac allograft vasculopathy: advances in understanding its pathophysiology, prevention, and treatment. *Current Opinion in Cardiology*, **19**, 170–6.

Pitt, B., Mancini, G. B., Ellis, S. G., *et al.* (1995). Pravastatin limitation of atherosclerosis in the coronary arteries (PLAC I): reduction in atherosclerosis progression and clinical events. PLAC I investigation. *Journal of the American College of Cardiology*, **26**, 1133–9.

Plump, A. S., Scott, C. J. and Breslow, J. L. (1994). Human apolipoprotein A-I gene expression increases high density lipoprotein and suppresses atherosclerosis in the apolipoprotein E-deficient mouse. *Proceedings of the National Academy of Science (USA)*, **91**, 9607–11.

Ridker, P. M., Cannon, C. P., Morrow, D., *et al.* (2005). C-reactive protein levels and outcomes after statin therapy. *New England Journal of Medicine*, **352**, 20–8.

Ridker, P. M., Rifai, N., Rose, L., *et al.* (2002). Comparison of C-reactive protein and low-density lipoprotein cholesterol levels in the prediction of first cardiovascular events. *New England Journal of Medicine*, **347**, 1557–65.

Rioufol, G., Finet, G., Ginon, I., *et al.* (2002). Multiple atherosclerotic plaque rupture in acute coronary syndrome: a three-vessel intravascular ultrasound study. *Circulation*, **106**, 804–8.

Rong, J. X., Li, J., Reis, E. D., *et al.* (2001). Elevating high-density lipoprotein cholesterol in apolipoprotein E-deficient mice remodels advanced atherosclerotic lesions by decreasing macrophage and increasing smooth muscle cell content. *Circulation*, **104**, 2447–52.

Ross, R. (1999). Atherosclerosis – an inflammatory disease. *New England Journal of Medicine*, **340**, 115–26.

Rudd, J. H., Warburton, E. A., Fryer, T. D., *et al.* (2002). Imaging atherosclerotic plaque inflammation with 18F-fluorodeoxyglucose positron emission tomography. *Circulation*, **105**, 2708–11.

Saam, T., Ferguson, M. S., Yarnykh, V. L., *et al.* (2005). Quantitative evaluation of carotid plaque composition by in vivo MRI. *Arteriosclerosis, Thrombosis and Vascular Biology*, **25**, 234–9.

Sacks, F. M., Pfeffer, M. A., Moye, L. A., *et al.* (1996). The effect of pravastatin on coronary events after myocardial infarction in patients with average cholesterol levels. Cholesterol and Recurrent Events Trial investigators. *New England Journal of Medicine*, **335**, 1001–9.

Schaar, J. A., De Korte, C. L., Mastik, F., *et al.* (2003). Characterizing vulnerable plaque features with intravascular elastography. *Circulation*, **108**, 2636–41.

Schoepf, U. J., Becker, C. R., Ohnesorge, B. M., *et al.* (2004). CT of coronary artery disease. *Radiology*, **232**, 18–37.

Schoenhagen, P., Halliburton, S. S., Stillman, A. E., *et al.* (2004). Noninvasive imaging of coronary arteries: current and future role of multi-detector row CT. *Radiology*, **232**, 7–17.

Schoenhagen, P., Stone, G. W., Nissen, S. E., *et al.* (2003). Coronary plaque morphology and frequency of ulceration distant from culprit lesions in patients with unstable and stable presentation. *Arteriosclerosis, Thrombosis and Vascular Biology*, **23**, 1895–900.

Schoenhagen, P., Ziada, K. M., Kapadia, S. R., *et al.* (2000). Extent and direction of arterial remodeling in stable versus unstable coronary syndromes: an intravascular ultrasound study. *Circulation*, **101**, 598–603.

Schwartz, G. G., Olsson, A. G., Ezekowitz, M. D., *et al.* (2001). Effects of atorvastatin on early recurrent ischemic events in acute coronary syndromes: the MIRACL study: a randomized controlled trial. *Journal of the American Medical Association*, **285**, 1711–18.

Serruys, P. W., Degertekin, M., Tanabe, K., *et al.* (2004). Vascular responses at proximal and distal edges of paclitaxel-eluting stents: serial intravascular ultrasound analysis from the TAXUS II trial. *Circulation*, **109**, 627–33.

Shah, P. K., Nilsson, J., Kaul, S., *et al.* (1998). Effects of recombinant apolipoprotein A-I(Milano) on aortic atherosclerosis in apolipoprotein E-deficient mice. *Circulation*, **97**, 780–5.

Shah, P. K., Yano, J., Reyes, O., *et al.* (2001). High-dose recombinant apolipoprotein A-IMilano mobilizes tissue cholesterol and rapidly reduces plaque lipid and macrophage content in apolipoprotein E-deficient mice. *Circulation*, **103**, 3047–50.

Shepherd, J., Cobbe, S. M., Ford, I., *et al.* (1995). Prevention of coronary heart disease with pravastatin in men with hypercholesterolemia. West of Scotland Coronary Prevention Study Group. *New England Journal of Medicine*, **333**, 1301–7.

Stenestrand, U. and Wallentin, L. (2001). Early statin treatment following acute myocardial infarction and 1-year survival. *Journal of the American Medical Association*, **285**, 430–6.

Tardif, J. C., Cote, G., Lesperance, J., *et al.* (2001). Impact of residual plaque burden after balloon angioplasty in the MultiVitamins and Probucol (MVP) trial. *Canadian Journal of Cardiology*, **17**, 49–55.

Tardif, J. C., Gregoire, J., Schwartz, L., *et al.* (2003). Effects of AGI-1067 and probucol after percutaneous coronary interventions. *Circulation*, **107**, 552–8.

Taylor, A. J., Sullenberger, L. E., Lee, H. J., *et al.* (2004). Arterial Biology for the Investigation of the Treatment Effects of Reducing Cholesterol (ARBITER) 2: a double-blind, placebo-controlled study of extended-release niacin on atherosclerosis progression in secondary prevention patients treated with statins. *Circulation*, **110**, 3512–17.

Tearney, G. J., Yabushita, H., Houser, S. L., *et al.* (2003). Quantification of macrophage content in atherosclerotic plaques by optical coherence tomography. *Circulation*, **107**, 113–19.

Topol, E. J. and Nissen, S. E. (1995). Our preoccupation with coronary luminology. The dissociation between clinical and angiographic findings in ischemic heart disease. *Circulation*, **92**, 2333–42.

Tuzcu, E. M., De Franco, A. C., Goormastic, M., *et al.* (1996). Dichotomous pattern of coronary atherosclerosis 1 to 9 years after transplantation: insights from systematic intravascular ultrasound imaging. *Journal of the American College of Cardiology*, **27**, 839–46.

Tuzcu, E. M., Kapadia, S. R., Sachar, R., *et al.* (2005). Intravascular ultrasound evidence of angiographically silent progression in coronary atherosclerosis predicts long-term morbidity and mortality after cardiac transplantation. *Journal of the American College of Cardiology*, **45**, 1538–42.

Tuzcu, E. M., Kapadia, S. R., Tutar, E., *et al.* (2001). High prevalence of coronary atherosclerosis in asymptomatic teenagers and young adults: evidence from intravascular ultrasound. *Circulation*, **103**, 2705–10.

Urbina, E. M., Srinivasan, S. R., Tang, R., *et al.* (2002). Impact of multiple coronary risk factors on the intima-media thickness of different segments of carotid artery in healthy young adults (The Bogalusa Heart Study). *American Journal of Cardiology*, **90**, 953–8.

Verheye, S., De Meyer, G. R., Van Langenhove, G., *et al.* (2002). In vivo temperature heterogeneity of atherosclerotic plaques is determined by plaque composition. *Circulation*, **105**, 1596–601.

Yeung, A. C., Davis, S. F., Hauptman, P. J., *et al.* (1995). Incidence and progression of transplant coronary artery disease over 1 year: results of a multicenter trial with use of intravascular ultrasound. Multicenter Intravascular Ultrasound Transplant Study Group. *Journal of Heart and Lung Transplantation*, **14**, S215–220.

33

Monitoring of pharmaceutical interventions: MR plaque imaging

Thomas Hatsukami

University of Washington, Seattle WA, USA

Cardiovascular disease is the leading cause of death worldwide (World Health Organization, 2004). The majority of cardiovascular disease complications are atherosclerosis related (Lusis, 2000), and the discovery of novel forms of treatment for atherosclerosis has been a top priority for the pharmaceutical and biotechnology industry. However, the process of assessing clinical efficacy is associated with extraordinary cost, in that trials utilizing clinical endpoints, such as myocardial infarction, stroke, or cardiovascular death, require large study populations followed for many years. Reliable imaging biomarkers of atherosclerosis would potentially yield significant benefits in terms of efficiency and cost-savings in the development of new compounds.

Background and definitions

In 2001, the National Institutes of Health convened an expert working group to provide standardized terminology with regard to biomarkers in clinical trials (2001). The panel defined *biological marker* (biomarker) as a characteristic that is objectively measured and evaluated as an indicator of normal biological processes, pathogenic processes, or pharmacologic responses to a therapeutic intervention. A *clinical endpoint* is a characteristic or variable that reflects how a patient feels, functions, or survives. A *surrogate endpoint* is a biomarker that is intended to substitute for a clinical endpoint. A surrogate endpoint is expected to predict clinical benefit (or harm or lack of benefit or harm) based on epidemiologic, therapeutic, pathophysiologic, or other scientific evidence. Therefore, surrogate endpoints are a subset of the biomarker class, and not all biomarkers fulfill the criteria to be considered a surrogate endpoint.

In order for a biomarker to achieve surrogate endpoint status for regulatory approval of new compounds, requirements include establishment of accuracy and reproducibility of the biomarker, documentation that the biomarker predicts clinical events, and evidence that improvement in the biomarker (in response to treatment) is associated with reduction in clinical events. To date, none of the modalities for atherosclerosis imaging have achieved surrogate endpoint status for regulatory approval of new compounds.

In order to use biomarkers in the initial assessment of new therapies, for example, to confirm pharmacologic activity and to evaluate dose-response relationships, the requirements are less stringent. For this purpose, the validity of the imaging biomarker to measure characteristics of the atherosclerotic lesion must be established. As reviewed in Chapter 14 (MR plaque imaging), the accuracy of magnetic resonance imaging (MRI) for quantitative characterization of carotid

Carotid Disease: The Role of Imaging in Diagnosis and Management, ed. Jonathan Gillard, Martin Graves, Thomas Hatsukami and Chun Yuan. Published by Cambridge University Press. © Cambridge University Press 2007.

atherosclerosis has been extensively evaluated using a histological gold standard (Toussaint et al., 1996; Yuan et al., 1998; Hatsukami et al., 2000; Cai et al., 2002; Kerwin et al., 2003; Trivedi et al., 2004; Cai et al., 2005; Kerwin et al., 2005; Saam et al., 2005; in press), and its precision has been documented in a number of reproducibility studies (Kang et al., 2000; Mitsumori et al., 2003; Saam et al., 2005). By providing a direct measure of atherosclerotic lesion size and composition, currently available MRI methodology can provide confirmation of the effect of new compounds on plaque in humans, as well as critical data to assist in the design of subsequent phase III trials, in terms of sample size calculation and dosing.

Feasibility of multicenter clinical trials and trial design parameters

For the performance of multicenter clinical trials, a natural question is whether a standardized imaging protocol can be used in a multicenter setting with comparable image quality and physical coverage in serial studies. In a recently published study (Chu et al., 2005), 39 subjects from five clinical sites (site 1: $n = 11$; site 2: $n = 16$; site 3: $n = 2$; site 4: $n = 3$; site 5: $n = 7$) were imaged on 1.5 T machines (from the same manufacturer) using a standardized carotid imaging protocol with five weightings (T_1, proton density (PD), T_2, time-of-flight (TOF), and contrast-enhanced T_1). MR technologists from the five sites received comprehensive protocol training. A maximum coverage of 24 mm (12 slices) was designed for each of four scans (baseline and at four, eight, and 13 weeks). The adequacy of coverage was calculated as the percentage of arteries with at least six slices matched across all four scans. Image quality (ImQ) was evaluated using an established five-point scale for each image, with a score of 1 representing poor image quality, and 5 being the best. An image quality score ≥3 was considered acceptable for image analysis. Across five sites, the mean ImQ was 3.4−4.2 for T_1 weighted, 3.6−4.4 for

contrast enhanced T_1 weighted, 3.4−4.2 for PD weighted, 3.3−4.2 for T_2 weighted, and 3.4−4.0 for TOF. The mean ImQ per site was 3.5−4.2. All sites generated at least six-slice coverage (mean = 8.0−9.1) for all index carotid arteries. The ImQ and coverage values were comparable among clinical sites. This study demonstrated that, with comprehensive protocol training, carotid MRI is technically feasible for use in multicenter studies.

In another study, images obtained from the placebo-control arm of a five-site carotid MRI study were analyzed to assess the variability of MRI for measuring lesion size and composition, and to provide sample size calculations for a variety of imaging endpoints. Twenty subjects from the placebo group underwent four scans in 13 weeks on GE 1.5 T scanners, using TOF, T_1 weighted/PD weighted/T_2 weighted and contrast-enhanced T_1-weighted images. Measurement variability was assessed by comparing quantitative data from the index carotid artery over the four time points. The normalized wall index (NWI) was calculated as wall volume divided by total vessel volume (NWI also referred to as the wall/outer wall ratio). The percent lipid-rich/necrotic core (%LR/NC) was measured as a proportion of the volume of the vessel wall. Measurement error was 5.8% for wall volume, 3.2% for NWI, and 11.1% for %LR/NC. Power analysis based on these values indicated that the following minimum numbers of subjects per arm would be required to demonstrate a 5% treatment effect with 80% power, $p < 0.05$: wall volume: $n = 43$; NWI: $n = 14$; %LR/NC: $n = 152$. Findings from this study demonstrated that in vivo MRI is capable of quantifying atherosclerotic lesion size and plaque composition in the setting of a multicenter trial with low interscan variability, and provided the basis for sample size calculation of future carotid MRI trials.

Clinical studies using carotid MRI

One of the earliest reports using MRI to investigate differences in plaque composition with intensive lipid-lowering therapy was a case-control study by Zhao *et al.* (2001). Eight patients with documented coronary artery disease, who had been receiving intensive lipid-lowering treatment (niacin 2.5 g/d, lovastatin 40 mg/d, and colestipol 20 g/d) for 10 years underwent MRI examination of their carotid arteries. MRI findings from this group were compared to those from eight coronary artery disease patients, matched for age (±3 years), baseline low-density lipoprotein cholesterol (LDL-C, ±5 mg/dL), and triglycerides (±50 mg/dL) but who had never been treated with lipid-lowering drugs. Patients treated with 10-year intensive lipid-lowering therapy, compared with control subjects, had significantly lower LDL-C levels (84 vs. 158 mg/dL, respectively; $p < 0.001$), higher high density lipoprotein cholesterol levels (51 vs. 37 mg/dL, respectively; $p < 0.001$), smaller

lipid core area (0.7 vs. 10.2 mm^2, respectively; $p = 0.01$) and percent lipid composition (1% vs. 17%, respectively; Figure 33.1). Findings from this study suggested that intensive lipid-lowering therapy was associated with less plaque lipid content, based on MRI criteria.

One of the first prospective studies using MRI to examine vessel wall area changes in response to lipid-lowering therapy was published by Corti and colleagues (Corti *et al.*, 2001, 2002, 2005). In this study, newly diagnosed hypercholesterolemic patients ($n = 51$) were randomized to 20 mg/day ($n = 29$) or 80 mg/day ($n = 22$) of simvastatin. Subjects underwent carotid and aortic MRI every 6 months, with a mean follow-up period of 18.1 months. The authors found that both doses of simvastatin were associated with significant reduction in vessel wall area (VWA) over time

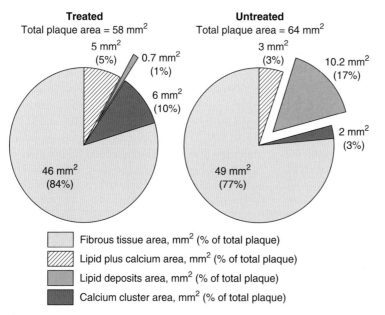

Figure 33.1 Carotid plaque tissue components as determined by magnetic resonance imaging (MRI) in patients who had received 10 years of intensive lipid-lowering therapy compared to untreated controls, matched for age and baseline low-density lipoprotein cholesterol and triglyceride levels. The treated plaques contained significantly less lipid than did the untreated plaques ($p = 0.01$). Fibrous tissue, calcium, and calcium plus lipid were not statistically different between the two groups. (Reproduced from Zhao *et al.* (2001). *Arteriosclerosis, Thrombosis and Vascular Biology*, **21**, 1623–9.)

in the carotid artery and aorta (analysis of variance $p < 0.001$). Aortic VWA decreased by 10% at 12 months and by 15% at 24 months. Carotid VWA decreased by 14% and 18% at 12 and 24 months, respectively. However, no change in lumen size was detected at 6 and 12 months. There was no significant difference between the two treatment arms for any of the vascular measurements. Post-hoc analysis demonstrated that patients achieving a mean LDL-C of ≤ 100 mg/dL had larger decreases in VWA, suggesting that the change in vessel size was more related to LDL-C reduction than dosage of simvastatin (Figure 33.2).

In another recently published study, Lima and colleagues reported evidence of significant regression in aortic atherosclerotic plaques by 6 months after initiation of therapy with simvastatin (Lima *et al.*, 2004). The thoracic aorta was imaged with MRI at baseline and 6 months in 27 patients who were treated with simvastatin 20–80 mg daily. The authors reported a reduction in aortic plaque (AP) volume from 3.3 ± 1.4 cm^3 at baseline to 2.9 ± 1.4 cm^3 at 6 months (12% reduction, $p < 0.02$). There was a slight trend toward luminal volume increase (from 12.0 ± 3.9 to 12.2 ± 3.7 cm^3,

$p < 0.06$). Consistent with the observation by Corti *et al.*, there was a significant correlation between plaque volume regression and changes in LDL-C levels (regression coefficient $= 7.07$ [95% CI 1.3–12.9] $p = 0.02$). The authors note that this study differs from the Corti study in that the former measured vessel wall changes in nonatherosclerotic arterial wall segments, whereas this study reports changes in atherosclerotic plaque. Furthermore, they were able to demonstrate changes as early as 6 months in this study. Despite the focus on atherosclerotic plaque, the authors noted that there were too few discrete plaques that had discernible components; therefore, characterization of plaque composition was not attempted.

Similar to the above studies that examined the effects of simvastatin, Yonemura and colleagues were able to show that regression of thoracic aortic plaques was demonstrated amongst patients treated with high-dose atorvastatin therapy (Yonemura *et al.*, 2005). In this study, 40 hypercholesterolemic patients were randomized to receive either 5 mg or 20 mg of atorvastatin. The thoracic and abdominal aorta was imaged with MRI at baseline

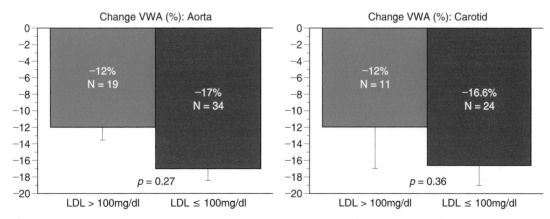

Figure 33.2 Effect of lipid lowering on aortic and carotid wall size measured by MRI. Subjects who achieved a low-density lipoprotein cholesterol (LDL) level ≤ 100 mg/dL demonstrated more regression in vessel wall area (VWA), compared to those levels greater than 100 mg/dL. Percent change in VWA was calculated based on last available MRI examination compared to baseline. (Reproduced from Corti *et al.* (2005). *Journal of the American College of Cardiology*, **46**, 105–22, with permission from American College of Cardiology Foundation.)

and 12 months after initiation of treatment. LDL-C was reduced by 34% and 47% in the low- and high-dose groups, respectively. Furthermore, C-reactive protein levels decreased by 28% and 47%, respectively, but the difference between the two dose groups was not significant. In the high-dose group, VWA in the thoracic aorta decreased by 18% ($p < 0.001$), whereas VWA increased by 4% in the low-dose group. In the abdominal aorta, there was no evidence of significant regression or progression in VWA (+3%) in the 20-mg group, but significant progression (+12%) in the 5-mg group ($p < 0.01$). Once again consistent with the other studies, the degree of plaque regression in thoracic aorta correlated with reduction in LDL-C ($r=0.64$; Figure 33.3). Notably, thoracic aortic regression

was also significantly associated with reduction in C-reactive protein levels ($r=0.49$).

Finally, initial results of the Outcome of Rosuvastatin treatment on carotid artery atheroma (ORION) trial were recently published comparing low- and high-dosages of rosuvastatin on carotid plaque morphology and composition with MRI (Hatsukami et al., 2005). Subjects ($n=43$) with fasting LDL-C levels ≥100 and <250 mg/dL and either 16−79% carotid stenosis by ultrasound or plaque with a lipid-rich necrotic core (LRNC) by MRI were randomized to low-dose (5 mg) or high-dose (40 or 80 mg) rosuvastatin therapy for 2 years. A standardized protocol was used to obtain four different contrast-weighted, cross-sectional images of bilateral carotid arteries

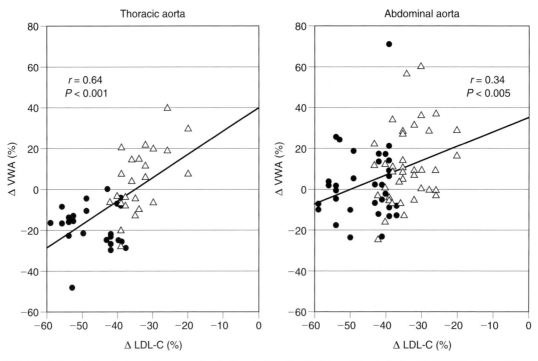

Figure 33.3 Correlations between the percent reduction in low-density lipoprotein-cholesterol (LDL-C) levels and the percent change in vessel wall area (VWA). The change in VWA in thoracic aortic plaques correlated well with the degree of LDL-C reduction ($r = 0.64$). A weak correlation was found in abdominal plaques ($r = 0.34$). Solid circles = 20-mg dose; open triangles = 5-mg dose. (Reproduced from Yonemura et al. (2005). *Journal of the American College of Cardiology*, **45**, 733−22, with permission from American College of Cardiology Foundation.)

(T_1 weighted, T_2 weighted, PD weighted, and 3D TOF images) at 1.5 T. Expert readers, blinded to dosage and time sequence, reviewed all imaging. As appropriate, data were analyzed by parametric or nonparametric tests. p-values represent within-group comparisons versus baseline. Thirty-five subjects (5 mg: $n = 15$; 40 mg: $n = 20$) had matched baseline and 2-year studies (63% men; mean age 65 years; mean baseline LDL-C 156 mg/dL). At 2 years, LDL-C was reduced from baseline by 39% and 58% in the low- and high-dose groups ($p < 0.001$). In the low- and high-dose groups, median % changes in carotid artery wall volume were 0.5% and −1.4%, respectively ($p = $ NS). Subjects whose wall volume regressed ($n = 16$) had an on-treatment mean LDL-C of 69 mg/dL (−56%), whereas subjects whose wall volume progressed ($n = 19$) had an LDL-C of 84 mg/dL (−45%). In plaques with a LRNC at baseline, the LRNC comprised 28.5% and 24.7% of the most diseased section (% LRNC) in the low- and high-dose groups. Low- and high-dose rosuvastatin reduced % LRNC at this location by 17.6% ($p = $ NS) and 35.5% ($p = 0.006$), with 75% and 90% of the plaques, respectively, showing regression from baseline. In patients without a LRNC lesion at baseline, none developed such a lesion after 2 years. In conclusion, both low and high doses of rosuvastatin were associated with significant reduction in LDL-C from baseline, and both groups did not show evidence of progression in wall volume over 2 years. This study was unique in that it is the first to note changes in composition in carotid plaque, with findings suggesting that aggressive LDL-C lowering was associated with regression of the lipid-rich necrotic core at the most diseased segments.

Summary

The accuracy and precision of MRI for quantitatively measuring atherosclerotic carotid morphology and composition have been extensively evaluated, as reviewed in Chapter 14. Sample-size calculations based on reproducibility data for carotid MRI indicate that clinical trials involving approximately 150 subjects per treatment arm would be sufficiently powered to detect a 5% difference in treatment effect. Although MRI has not yet fulfilled the rigorous criteria required for consideration as a surrogate endpoint for regulatory approval, it can currently serve an important function in terms of initial assessment of new compounds. Furthermore, MRI may provide valuable insight into pathophysiology and mechanisms of pharmacologic activity. Recently published studies document that MRI detects significant changes in the morphology of atherosclerotic plaque during the course of lipid-lowering therapy, and demonstrate the promise of this noninvasive imaging modality for use in clinical trials.

REFERENCES

Biomarkers Definitions Working Group. (2001). Biomarkers and surrogate endpoints: preferred definitions and conceptual framework. *Clinical Pharmacology and Therapeutics*, **69**, 89–95.

Cai, J. M., Hatsukami, T. S., Ferguson, M. S., *et al.* (2005). In vivo quantitative measurement of intact fibrous cap and lipid rich necrotic core size in atherosclerotic carotid plaque: a comparison of high resolution contrast enhanced MRI and histology. *Circulation*, **112**, 3437–44.

Cai, J. M., Hatsukami, T. S., Ferguson, M. S., *et al.* (2002). Classification of human carotid atherosclerotic lesions with in vivo multicontrast magnetic resonance imaging. *Circulation*, **106**, 1368–73.

Chu, B., Zhao, X. Q., Saam, T., *et al.* (2005). Feasibility of in vivo, multicontrast-weighted MR imaging of carotid atherosclerosis for multicenter studies. *Journal of Magnetic Resonance Imaging*, **21**, 809–17.

Corti, R., Fayad, Z. A., Fuster, V., *et al.* (2001). Effects of lipid-lowering by simvastatin on human atherosclerotic lesions: a longitudinal study by high-resolution, noninvasive magnetic resonance imaging. *Circulation*, **104**, 249–52.

Corti, R., Fuster, V., Fayad, Z. A., *et al.* (2005). Effects of aggressive versus conventional lipid-lowering therapy by simvastatin on human atherosclerotic lesions a prospective, randomized, double-blind trial with high-resolution magnetic resonance imaging. *Journal of American College of Cardiology*, **46**, 106–12.

Corti, R., Fuster, V., Fayad, Z. A., *et al.* (2002). Lipid lowering by simvastatin induces regression of human atherosclerotic lesions: two years' follow-up by high-resolution noninvasive magnetic resonance imaging. *Circulation*, **106**, 2884–7.

Hatsukami, T., Zhao, X. Q., Kraiss, L. W., *et al.* (2005). Assessment of rosuvastatin treatment on carotid atherosclerosis in moderately hypercholesterolemic subjects using high-resolution magnetic resonance imaging. *European Heart Journal*, **26** (abstract Suppl.), 626.

Hatsukami, T. S., Ross, R., Polissar, N. L. and Yuan, C. (2000). Visualization of fibrous cap thickness and rupture in human atherosclerotic carotid plaque in vivo with high-resolution magnetic resonance imaging. *Circulation*, **102**, 959–64.

Kang, X., Polissar, N. L., Han, C., Lin, E. and Yuan, C. (2000). Analysis of the measurement precision of arterial lumen and wall areas using high-resolution MRI in Process Citation. *Magnetic Resonance in Medicine*, **44**, 968–72.

Kerwin, W., Hooker, A., Spilker, M., *et al.* (2003). Quantitative magnetic resonance imaging analysis of neovasculature volume in carotid atherosclerotic plaque. *Circulation*, **107**, 851–6.

Kerwin, W., O'Brien, K. D., Ferguson, M. S., *et al.* (2005). Inflammation in carotid atherosclerotic plaque: A dynamic contrast-enhanced MR imaging study. *Radiology*, in press.

Lima, J. A., Desai, M. Y., Steen, H., *et al.* (2004). Statin-induced cholesterol lowering and plaque regression after 6 months of magnetic resonance imaging-monitored therapy. *Circulation*, **110**, 2336–41.

Lusis, A. J. (2000). Atherosclerosis. *Nature*, **407**, 233–41.

Mitsumori, L. M., Hatsukami, T. S., Ferguson, M. S., *et al.* (2003). In vivo accuracy of multisequence MR imaging for identifying unstable fibrous caps in advanced human carotid plaques. *Journal of Magnetic Resonance Imaging*, **17**, 410–20.

Saam, T., Ferguson, M. S., Yarnykh, V. L., *et al.* (2005). Quantitative evaluation of carotid plaque composition by in vivo MRI. *Arteriosclerosis, Thrombosis and Vascular Biology*, **25**, 234–9.

Toussaint, J. F., Lamuraglia, G. M., Southern, J. F., Fuster, V. and Kantor, H. L. (1996). Magnetic resonance images lipid, fibrous, calcified, hemorrhagic, and thrombotic components of human atherosclerosis in vivo. *Circulation*, **94**, 932–8.

Trivedi, R. A., U-King-Im, J M., Graves, M. J., Horsley, J., *et al.* (2004). Multi-sequence in vivo MRI can quantify fibrous cap and lipid core components in human carotid atherosclerotic plaques. *European Journal of Vascular and Endovascular Surgery*, **28**, 207–13.

World Health Organization. (2004). World Health Report 2004. Retrieved 2004, from http://www.who.int/whr/2004/en/index.html

Yonemura, A., Momiyama, Y., Fayad, Z. A., *et al.* (2005). Effect of lipid-lowering therapy with atorvastatin on atherosclerotic aortic plaques detected by noninvasive magnetic resonance imaging. *Journal of the American College of Cardiology*, **45**, 733–42.

Yuan, C., Beach, K. W., Smith, L. H. and Hatsukami, T. S. (1998). Measurement of atherosclerotic carotid plaque size in-vivo using high resolution magnetic resonance imaging. *Circulation*, **98**, 2666–71.

Zhao, X. Q., Yuan, C., Hatsukami, T. S., *et al.* (2001). Effects of prolonged intensive lipid-lowering therapy on the characteristics of carotid atherosclerotic plaques in vivo by MRI: a case-control study. *Arteriosclerosis, Thrombosis and Vascular Biology*, **21**, 1623–9.

34

Molecular imaging of carotid artery disease

James H. F. Rudd, Michael J. Lipinski, Fabien Hyafil and Zahi A. Fayad

The Zena and Michael A. Wiener Cardiovascular Institute, The Marie-Josée and Henry R. Kravis Cardiovascular Health Center,
Mount Sinai School of Medicine, New York NY, USA

Atherosclerosis and its complications are the scourge of Western civilization, and are becoming increasingly more frequent in the developing world (British Heart Foundation Health Promotion Research Group, 2005). Atherosclerosis affects medium- and large-sized arteries, with the carotid artery being the second most common site after the thoracic aorta (Svindland and Torvik, 1988).

Atherosclerosis is characterized by accumulation of lipid, inflammatory cells and connective tissue within the arterial wall. It is a chronic, progressive disease that has a long asymptomatic phase. The first pathological abnormality is the fatty streak, caused by an aggregation of lipid and macrophages in the subendothelial space. The fatty streak, often present within the aorta from the second decade of life (Ross, 1999), is thought to develop primarily in regions of endothelial dysfunction. Endothelial cells in regions of disrupted flow and low shear stress, often occurring in branch or bifurcation points of the arterial tree (Vander Laan et al., 2004), have decreased production of nitric oxide (Ku et al., 1985). The low shear stress also leads to increased expression of adhesion molecules and uptake of lipoproteins into the subendothelial space by means still unclear (Kinlay et al., 1998). Once oxidized, low density lipoproteins (LDL) are retained in the subendothelial space. Oxidized LDL (oxLDL) contains monocyte chemoattractant factors such as lysophosphatidylcholine and attracts further monocytes by triggering the release

of monocyte chemoattractant protein-1 (MCP-1) from endothelial cells and smooth muscle cells (Cushing et al., 1990). The newly expressed endothelial adhesion molecules, such as vascular cell adhesion molecule-1 (VCAM-1), intercellular adhesion molecule-1, E-selectin, and P-selectin, facilitate the internalization of monocytes into the subendothelium. Once there, monocytes transform into resident macrophages, bind oxLDL via scavenger receptors, and internalize the modified lipoprotein (Ross, 1999). The uptake of modified LDL is believed to be involved in the conversion of monocyte-derived macrophages into foam cells (Hamilton et al., 1999). The oxLDL induces the production of macrophage colony-stimulating factor (M-CSF) by vascular cells and macrophages, which can lead to macrophage proliferation. Eventually, the subendothelial accumulation of modified LDL and macrophage-derived foam cells leads to the formation of the atheromatous lipid core, which is hypocellular, avascular, and devoid of supporting collagen. The foam cells become necrotic, releasing their highly thrombogenic, enzymatically-modified lipids and tissue factor into the extracellular space of the core.

Fatty streaks may develop over time into mature atherosclerotic plaque. The central lipid core becomes bound on its luminal side by an endothelialized fibrous cap containing vascular smooth muscle cells and connective tissue, in particular collagen. This fibrous cap tends to be much thicker in the carotid arteries than in the coronary arteries due to the increased shear stress endured by the carotid arteries. Chronic exposure of endothelial cells to high levels of shear stress causes them to exhibit an atheroprotective phenotype (Traub and Berk, 1998) while low wall shear stress promotes arterial damage and plaque instability as described above. As the plaque grows, the affected artery expands outward so that the lumen diameter, and therefore blood flow, is preserved (a process known as positive remodeling [Glagov *et al.*, 1987]). Consequently, even large plaques can be accommodated without producing symptoms. Eventually the artery can expand no further, and the plaque begins to encroach into the lumen of the vessel, hindering blood flow during times of high demand.

Mature plaques may become calcified, especially the intimal portion. Carotid plaque calcification is commoner in asymptomatic plaques than symptomatic ones while symptomatic plaques contain more macrophages and inflammatory cells (Shaalan *et al.*, 2004; Spagnoli *et al.*, 2004). However, more than 35% of patients with calcified carotid plaques were found to have multiple coronary plaques, highlighting the widespread nature of atherosclerosis (Kato *et al.*, 2003). Additionally, patients with elevated blood C-reactive protein (CRP) levels, a marker of inflammation, were also found to have significantly more complex carotid plaques than those with normal levels (Lombardo *et al.*, 2004).

In the carotid artery, atherosclerotic plaques can remain quiescent for years (Svindland and Torvik, 1988). However, they can become symptomatic when they initiate clot formation in the vessel lumen, by either disturbing blood flow or allowing emboli to break off and lodge in the downstream cerebral circulation. This occurs either after fibrous cap rupture, with consequent exposure of the thrombogenic extracellular matrix of the cap and the tissue factor (TF)-rich lipid core to circulating blood, or less commonly, there can be erosion of the fibrous cap, again exposing TF and the thrombogenic subendothelial space. A recent histological analysis of 71 thrombosed plaques from stroke patients demonstrated that 90% of ischemic events were due to cap rupture with the remainder due to cap erosion (Spagnoli *et al.*, 2004). Both forms of plaque disruption invariably lead to local platelet accumulation and activation at the site of ulceration with subsequent thrombus formation. However, because of the brain's collateral circulation via the Circle of Willis, downstream embolism of thrombus plays a larger role in determining the severity of ischemia (transient ischemic attack [TIA] versus stroke) than hypoperfusion due to carotid artery occlusion (Yuan *et al.*, 2002a; Faxon *et al.*, 2004) – this is the opposite of the situation in the coronary arteries. Therefore, antiplatelet therapy is essential in patients at high risk of atherothrombotic cerebral events.

While symptomatic high-grade carotid lesions should be appropriately treated, screening high-risk patients with standard or molecular magnetic resonance imaging (MRI) may identify lesions prior to the development of symptoms. This could allow timely drug treatment aimed at either halting or even reversing the process of plaque progression and possibly prevent rupture (the statin drugs have proved efficacious in this regard [Cannon *et al.*, 2004]). Recently, developments in both MRI technology, computer software and a huge array of potential cellular and molecular targets are a step toward the identification of high-risk carotid disease and open the door toward using these targeted imaging agents as carriers for drug delivery specifically targeting atherosclerosis.

This chapter will cover these recent advances with particular respect to MRI. In order to grasp the concepts behind molecular MRI imaging, there will be a brief discussion of multicontrast MRI, highlighting its advantages and limitations where molecular MRI can be applied.

Multicontrast MRI

Multicontrast MRI of the plaque is based on successive T_1, T_2 and proton density-weighted sequences. Analysis of signal intensities detected by each of these sequences allows accurate differentiation of the atherosclerotic plaque components (lipid core, fibrous tissue, hemorrhage and calcification) by their different relaxation properties on MRI (Toussaint *et al.*, 1996; Fayad and Fuster, 2000). Development of dedicated software, which analyzes the signal intensities of multicontrast MRI on a pixel-by-pixel basis, has further improved the identification of atherosclerotic plaque components. An example of multicontrast MRI showing different plaque components and automatic segmentation of these plaques using a k-means cluster algorithm is shown in Figure 34.1 (Itskovich *et al.*, 2003).

The carotid artery plaque is ideally suited for imaging by multicontrast MRI. The superficial location of the carotid arteries without significant motion represents less of a technical challenge than imaging of the aorta or the coronary arteries. Recent advances in MR acquisition protocols have reduced scan times many-fold (Mani *et al.*, 2004). Carotid MR is robust and reproducible over time. For example, Yuan *et al.* demonstrated that in vivo multicontrast MR of human carotid arteries had sensitivity and specificity values of 85% and 92%, respectively, for the identification of a lipid core (Yuan *et al.*, 2001a, 2001b). Furthermore, in a case-controlled study, Zhao *et al.* studied the effect of statins on the composition of carotid plaques and demonstrated substantially reduced carotid plaque lipid content (with no substantial overall plaque area reduction) in patients treated for 10 years with an aggressive lipid-lowering regimen compared with untreated controls (Zhao *et al.*, 2001). This was further investigated recently,

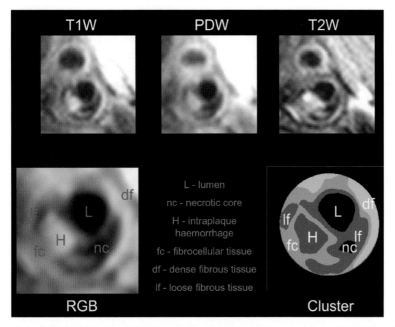

Figure 34.1 Multicontrast MRI images of a carotid artery. Top row shows T_1-weighted (T_1), proton density weighted (PD) and T_2-weighted (T_2) images of the same atherosclerotic plaque. The bottom left panel shows the (red-green-blue) RGB color composite image obtained by mapping the T_1-weighted image to the red, the PD-weighted image to the green and the T_2-weighted image to the blue channel, respectively. The bottom right panel shows the plaque segmented automatically into its various components using an automated k-means cluster analysis algorithm. Intraplaque hemorrhage (IH), necrotic core (nc), loose fibers (lf), dense fibers (df) and the fibrous cap (fc) can be clearly differentiated.

where a high-dose statin regimen was shown to be superior to low dose in terms of atheroma burden reduction (Corti *et al.*, 2005). Another important retrospective study imaged carotid arteries of patients with a history of recent transient ischemic attack or ischemic stroke compared with controls. Ruptured fibrous caps were detected with a much higher frequency by MRI (70%) in symptomatic patients than plaques with a thick fibrous cap (9%), confirming the ability of this technique to illustrate the underlying pathology (Yuan *et al.*, 2002b).

Recent histopathological studies (Burke *et al.*, 1999; Kolodgie *et al.*, 2003) suggest that intraplaque hemorrhage may play a role in plaque rupture. Therefore, particular efforts have been invested into its noninvasive detection with multicontrast MRI. A first study (Chu *et al.*, 2004) proved that multicontrast MRI can accurately image intraplaque hemorrhage in carotid atherosclerotic plaques using T_2^*-weighted sequences. Interestingly, a more recent prospective study (Takaya *et al.*, 2005) found that the detection of hemorrhage within carotid atherosclerotic plaques was associated with an accelerated increase of plaque volume over the following 18 months, supporting the hypothesis that intraplaque hemorrhage may be an atherogenic stimulus.

Molecular MR imaging of the carotid artery

Traditional plaque imaging modalities exploit anatomical variations between tissues to provide images. Molecular or target-specific imaging unites molecular and vascular biology with imaging modalities such as MRI. This allows the study of biological processes noninvasively, and with high-spatial resolution. Although standard MRI extracellular space contrast agents such as gadolinium (Gd)-DTPA may aid in the overall characterization of intermediate to advanced carotid lesions, the ability to deliver a large payload of paramagnetic particles that generate a high-signal intensity to a particular component of atherosclerosis may

greatly improve detection and determination of the composition of the plaque (Choudhury *et al.*, 2004; Lipinski *et al.*, 2004). The development of targeted imaging agents or molecular reporter systems, whether by specific antibodies or peptides, is extremely important as molecular targets are often present in very small levels (10^{-9}–10^{-13} M per gram of tissue) and pose a challenge to MRI imaging because of the inadequate signal intensity (i.e. sensitivity in the range of 10^{-3}–10^{-6} M) with standard untargeted contrast agents (Aime *et al.*, 2002).

Below we will discuss a variety of molecular targets that may provide improved imaging of carotid atherosclerotic plaque using MRI (Figure 34.2). Recent advances in contrast agent technology have enabled selection from a variety of contrast agents containing a high payload of paramagnetic and superparamagnetic particles that may be modified for targeting specific molecules in the plaque. It is important to remember that an animal model of spontaneous carotid plaque rupture does not exist. While novel contrast agents can be developed that target specific plaque components in different animal models of atherosclerosis, the ability to risk-stratify carotid atherosclerotic plaque with imaging cannot be determined until testing is performed prospectively in humans.

Endothelial dysfunction

Endothelial dysfunction is the earliest step in atherosclerosis, and the ability to image this stage of the disease might allow early lifestyle or therapeutic intervention to slow progression of disease. However, a great deal of the endothelium is dysfunctional in patients with atherosclerosis, especially in smokers and diabetics. While lesions prone to rupture in these patients may express adhesion molecules, those same adhesion molecules will be found throughout the vasculature and will therefore not be a specific marker for high-risk lesions.

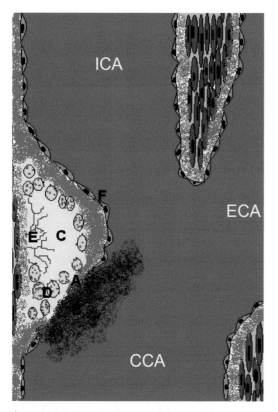

Figure 34.2 Schematic diagram of the carotid bifurcation to illustrate potential targets for molecular MRI imaging: (A) disrupted/thin fibrous cap; (B) thrombus; (C) lipid core; (D) macrophages (scavenger receptor in green); (E) neovascularisation; and (F) endothelial dysfunction.

The ability to image VCAM has been elegantly demonstrated by Kelly *et al*. They used a super-paramagnetic fluorescent nanoparticle coupled to a payload peptide that was internalized by endothelial cells expressing VCAM. This was tested in ApoE−/− mice fed a high cholesterol diet and was highly specific for VCAM-expressing cells, verified by immunohistochemistry (Kelly *et al.*, 2005).

MR imaging of the E-selectin molecule is also possible, at least in vitro. Kang *et al*. showed that a monoclonal antibody fragment tagged with iron oxide nanoparticles was specific for human endothelial cells expressing E-selectin in culture, with an increased binding of 200 times compared to control cells (Kang *et al.*, 2002). ICAM-1 receptors expressed on the cerebral vascular endothelium have been imaged with MR using antibody-conjugated paramagnetic liposomes (Sipkins *et al.*, 2000). MRI provided sufficient signal enhancement to determine areas of increased expression and binding was verified by fluorescent histopathology by looking at the fluorescently-tagged liposomes.

Angiogenesis

Recent investigations have focused on plaque neovascularization as an important factor contributing to atherosclerotic plaque vulnerability. The presence of neovessels is strongly associated with plaque inflammation and likelihood of rupture (Kumamoto *et al.*, 1995), presumably by allowing an alternative route for entry of monocytes and lymphocytes into the plaque. Gadolinium chelates represent the most commonly used MRI contrast agents for imaging new plaque vessels. These paramagnetic agents, i.e. they shorten the T_1 relaxation time of protons, increase the luminal signal on MRI after intravenous injection and are therefore good candidates for measuring plaque neovasculature. While Kerwin and colleagues demonstrated a correlation between the increase of signal intensity in carotid atherosclerotic plaques with gadolinium-enhanced MRI and the extent of neovessels in plaques measured histologically, this imaging modality is not specific for neovascularization and is limited since gadolinium chelates rapidly distribute into the extracellular space (Kerwin *et al.*, 2003). Further improvements in the quantification of plaque neovasculature with these agents will require the development of new kinetic models of the biodistribution of these contrast agents in atherosclerotic plaques (Lauffer *et al.*, 1998).

Alternatively, MRI contrast agents that remain within the blood, or diffuse more slowly into the extracellular space are currently being developed (Port *et al.*, 1999). For example, a novel agent targeting the integrin $\alpha_v\beta_3$ (specifically expressed on the endothelial surface of neovasculature) has been developed to identify regions in tissue or the vessel wall undergoing neovascularization. Winter *et al.* demonstrated in a rabbit model of atherosclerosis that regions of neovascularization in plaques had a 47% increase in signal intensity on MRI after the injection of $\alpha_v\beta_3$-targeted nanoparticles (Winter *et al.*, 2003b). Another epitope that has been successfully exploited for imaging angiogenesis within plaque (at least in ApoE−/− mice) is fibronectin. An antibody to an area of the fibronectin molecule that is conserved between species was raised (L19 against the ED-B epitope). The binding of antibody was confirmed both autoradiographically and by the use of a fluorescent probe, and was specific for the vaso vasorum of the atherosclerotic plaque (Matter *et al.*, 2004).

Thrombus

Intraluminal thrombosis represents the final step of the evolution of vulnerable atherosclerotic plaque and is an obvious target for new specific MRI contrast agents (see Chapter 22 also). Histological studies have demonstrated that superficial thrombus superimposed on a ruptured atherosclerotic plaque characterizes those plaques at high risk of ischemic events (Virmani *et al.*, 2000).

Several approaches have been taken to image the thrombus with MRI. Yu *et al.* used a gadolinium-loaded nanoparticle coupled to a fibrin antibody and tested this against an in vitro thrombus (Yu *et al.*, 2000). They were able to demonstrate significant signal enhancement using this approach, and confirmed tight binding of the antibody with scanning electron microscopy. A similar method, but using a different nanoparticle construct was employed by Winter *et al.* (2003a).

A recent paper analyzed the histology of intracoronary thrombi aspirated from 211 patients admitted with acute myocardial infarction. It was shown that over 50% of the culprit thrombi were at least days or weeks old (Rittersma *et al.*, 2005). Applying this work to the carotid circulation, a new fibrin-specific MR contrast agent has recently been designed. With this agent, thrombus resulting from plaque rupture has been identified using MR in a rabbit model. In the 25 arterial thrombi induced by carotid crush injury, Botnar *et al.* demonstrated a sensitivity and specificity of 100% for in vivo thrombus detection (Botnar *et al.*, 2004). Sirol *et al.* recently used the same fibrin-specific MR contrast agent (EP-1242, Epix Medical Inc, Cambridge MA) in 12 guinea pigs to demonstrate that the signal intensity of the thrombus was increased by over four-fold. The detection of thrombi was clearly improved from only a 42% pickup precontrast injection compared to 100% detection after injection (Sirol *et al.*, 2005a). The ability to identify different thrombus components with molecular MRI may allow the age of thrombus to be determined noninvasively. This has important clinical benefits because histological studies have shown that many microplaque rupture events with thrombus formation often predate the "catastrophic" rupture event that causes the clinical syndrome. The ability to detect these earlier warnings might allow intense therapy or device placement to avert symptoms. In this regard, our group has recently tested an experimental fibrin-targeted peptide (EP-2104R, Epix Medical Inc, Cambridge MA) for thrombus detection, and compared it to MRI without contrast and gadolinium-enhanced MRI (Sirol *et al.*, 2005b). Using this novel agent it was possible to discriminate between occlusive and nonocclusive thrombi, and also to track thrombus as it aged and became more organized by fibrous tissue infiltration. The new agent improved on the detection rate of both multi-contrast and gadolinium-enhanced MR (Figure 34.3).

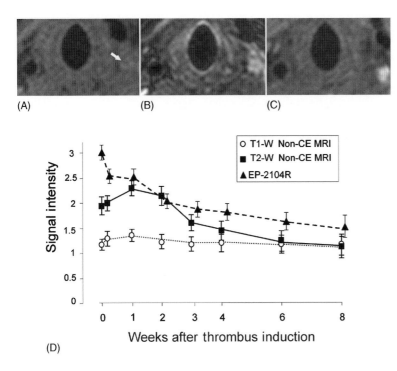

Figure 34.3 Transverse MRI images of a rabbit carotid artery 1 week after thrombus induction, imaged using a double inversion recovery turbo-spin echo sequence. T_1-weighted (A) and T_2-weighted (B) images were obtained without any injection of contrast agent. White arrow indicates location of the thrombus. Panel C displays the T_1-weighted images obtained 30 minutes after EP-2104R (Epix Medical Inc, Cambridge, MA) injection. Panel D displays the relative signal intensity changes (mean ± SD) over time for T_1-weighted (white circles), T_2-weighted (grey squares) and after EP-2104R injection (black triangles). This gadolinium based, fibrin-targeted MRI contrast agent demonstrates significant enhancement of the thrombus compared to T_1-weighted images ($p < 0.001$). Reproduced from Sirol *et al.* (2005b). *Circulation*, **112**, 1594–600.

Extracellular matrix

Other novel MRI contrast agents have been found to accumulate within atherosclerotic plaques. For example, gadofluorine (Schering AG, Berlin, Germany) is a lipophilic, macrocyclic, water-soluble, gadolinium chelate complex with a per-fluorinated side chain. Both Sirol and Barkhausen demonstrated that gadofluorine increased signal intensity by 207% in the aortic wall of athero-sclerotic rabbits but not in controls. A strong correlation was found between the intensity of MRI signal enhancement after the injection of gadofluorine and the presence of lipid-rich plaques on corresponding histological sections (Barkhausen *et al.*, 2003; Sirol *et al.*, 2004). This suggests a high affinity of gadofluorine for athero-sclerotic plaque (Figure 34.4). There is currently no evidence that gadofluorine binds to the lipid core, but rather ongoing work is suggesting that gado-fluorine may be confined to the extracellular space of atherosclerotic plaques and may interact with the abundant resident proteins in the extracellular matrix milieu.

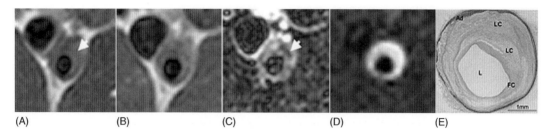

(A)   (B)   (C)   (D)   (E)

Figure 34.4 High-resolution in vivo MRI images of a rabbit aorta. T_1- (panel A), proton density- (panel B), T_2- (panel C)-weighted images were used to characterize the atherosclerotic plaque. The white arrows show the different areas of the atherosclerotic plaque (fibrous cap in T_1-weighted images (A) and a large lipid core in T_2-weighted images (C)). Panel D displays the same atherosclerotic lesion enhanced 24 hours after intravenous injection of gadofluorine (Schering AG, Berlin, Germany). Gadofluorine as previously reported by Sirol *et al.* (2004) improves in vivo atherosclerotic plaque detection. The corresponding histopathological section stained with combined Masson and Elastic Trichrom (CME) is shown in Panel E (magnification: 4×). Ad = adventitia, FC = fibrous cap; L = lumen; LC = lipid core.

Since the integrity of the fibrous cap is essential for separating the lumen from the thrombogenic core, identifying factors that lead to the disruption of the fibrous cap may aid in targeting patients prone to plaque rupture. Matrix metalloproteinases (MMPs) are responsible for the degradation of proteins in the extracellular matrix and the role of MMPs in plaque instability and matrix remodeling in atherosclerotic plaque has been well described (Rudd *et al.*, 2005). Therefore, the ability to detect MMP activity in the fibrous cap of carotid atherosclerosis with MRI may not only provide important information regarding risk of possible plaque rupture but may also allow tracking of MMP inhibition (Bremer *et al.*, 2001) and the effects of other therapies on MMP activity and thus plaque stability. While MMP detection with MRI is currently being pursued, MMP activity in the murine carotid arterial wall has been imaged in vivo using a novel radioligand specific to MMP and was able to determine regions with increased collagen breakdown (Schafers *et al.*, 2004).

Plaque inflammation

Resident plaque macrophages have been successfully imaged using ultrasmall superparamagnetic particles of iron oxide (USPIO) (see Chapter 20 also). These are are removed from the circulation by the reticuloendothelial system and accumulate in macrophages present in atherosclerotic plaques. Macrophages play a pivotal role in the destabilization of atherosclerosic plaques by secreting large quantities of fibrous cap-degrading MMPs, along with proinflammatory cytokines and tissue factor (Libby, 2001). Iron oxide contrast agents have superparamagnetic properties, i.e. they decrease T_2^* relaxation time by generating heterogeneities in the local magnetic field, and can be detected on MRI as signal voids on T_2^*-weighted sequences.

Kooi *et al.* studied 11 symptomatic patients scheduled for carotid endarterectomy with USPIO-enhanced MRI, and found a 24% decrease in signal intensity on corresponding T_2^*-weighted sequences, and histologically verified uptake of USPIO in 75% of ruptured or rupture-prone lesions (Kooi *et al.*, 2003). Trivedi *et al.* expanded on this work and demonstrated that the optimum time for imaging symptomatic carotid plaque was between 24 and 36 hours after injection of USPIO (Trivedi *et al.*, 2003, 2004). Recently, USPIO plaque imaging with MR has been validated against histopathology at timepoints out to 8 weeks in an animal model. Iron staining closely matched that of macrophage distribution within the plaque, but interestingly only a subset of smaller sized macrophages actively accumulated USPIO (Yancy *et al.*, 2005). New image acquisition methods that render the superparamagnetic signal loss as positive enhancement promises to improve the detection of plaques in vivo (Mani *et al.*, 2006). Finally, monocyte/macrophage recruitment into plaques after an inflammatory stimulus has been tracked by USPIO in a mouse model (Litovsky *et al.*, 2003), which might be useful in assessing the antiatherogenic potential of new drugs.

Macrophages within atherosclerotic plaques have also been targeted for imaging by the use of gadolinium-loaded immunomicelles. These agents, with diameters between 20 and 120 nm, are composed of phospholipids, a surfactant, and an aliphatic chain with Gd-DTPA attached at the polar head group. The polar head group of the aliphatic chain can be attached to antibodies directly or via a biotin-avidin bridge. Using this model, we have made micelles that have over 10 000 Gd ions on each micelle surface and the ability to specifically target the macrophage scavenger receptor (MSR). Promising work is currently underway and has demonstrated enhancement of murine atherosclerotic plaque on MRI using immunomicelles that target the MSR-A.

Our group recently developed another type of imaging agent based on a recombinant high-density lipoprotein (rHDL) molecule that incorporates gadolinium-DTPA phospholipids (Frias *et al.*, 2004). Natural HDL's role in the body is that of removing lipid from atherosclerotic plaque and returning it to the liver (reverse cholesterol transport). Elevated levels of HDL are associated with a reduction in plaque rupture events, presumably because of this protective effect (Wilson *et al.*, 2005). The rHDL imaging agent has a small diameter (7–12 nm) allowing it to diffuse into atherosclerotic plaques and, by using endogenous transport molecules, it does not trigger any immune reaction. Atherosclerotic plaques had a 35% increase of MRI signal intensity 24 hours after the injection of these rHDL particles in an ApoE knockout mouse model. Furthermore, fluorescent rHDL colocalized with macrophages present in atherosclerotic plaques with confocal microscopy. Figure 34.5 demonstrates the enhancement of atherosclerotic plaques after the injection of rHDL.

Conclusions and future directions

Thanks to the absence of ionizing radiation, molecular MRI represents the imaging technology of choice for the noninvasive high-spatial resolution detection and serial monitoring of atherosclerosis. High image quality and sensitivity to small changes in plaque size mean that there is little variance between measurements, permitting small sample sizes to be used in comparative studies. Thus, molecular MRI is ideally suited for use in evaluation of novel antiatheroma drugs.

The development of functional molecular imaging of atherosclerosis may also help to reveal the key pathological steps that lead from a stable atherosclerotic plaque to an acute ischemic event. However, recent clinical studies have underscored the multiple locations of vulnerable and ruptured atherosclerotic plaques and the diffuse inflammation of the arterial tree in patients with acute ischemic events compared to stable patients (Rioufol *et al.*, 2002). Therefore, the concept of detecting infrequent vulnerable atherosclerotic plaques with imaging and treating them individually has started to shift to a more global process of identifying vulnerable patients at high risk of acute clinical events, irrespective of the arterial location (Naghavi *et al.*, 2003).

In the future, molecular imaging with MRI of atherosclerosis may help to focus individual evaluation of cardiovascular risk and to optimize antiatherosclerotic therapies.

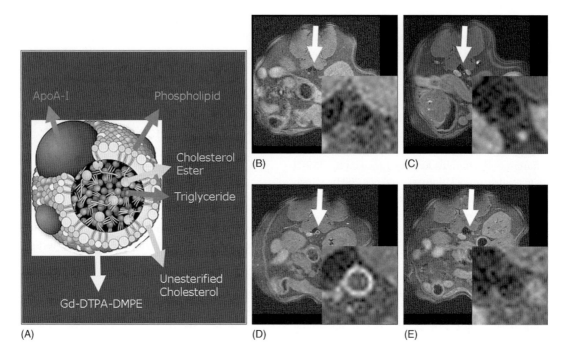

Figure 34.5 Panel A: this represents the recombinant HDL-like MRI contrast agent composed of an HDL-like particle and a phospholipid-based contrast agent (Gd-DTPA-DMPE). Transverse in vivo MR images of the abdominal aorta in an 8-week-old mouse at 9.4 Tesla before (B), 1 hour (C), 24 hours (D) and 48 hours (E) after the injection of recombinant HDL-like nanoparticles are displayed. The insets denote the magnification of the aortic region. Reproduced from Frias *et al.* (2004).

Acknowledgements

The authors of this work were supported by grants from the Fédération Française de Cardiologie, Paris, France (FH), the NIH/NHLBI (R01 HL071021 and R01 HL078667) (ZAF), the John E. Postley, Jr., M.D. Fund for the Imaging Science Laboratories (ZAF) and the British Heart Foundation (JR).

REFERENCES

Aime, S., Cabella, C., Colombatto, S., *et al.* (2002). Insights into the use of paramagnetic Gd(III) complexes in MR-molecular imaging investigations. *Journal of Magnetic Resonance Imaging*, **16**, 394–406.

Barkhausen, J., Ebert, W., Heyer, C., Debatin, J. F. and Weinmann, H. J. (2003). Detection of atherosclerotic plaque with gadofluorine-enhanced magnetic resonance imaging. *Circulation*, **108**, 605–9.

Botnar, R. M., Perez, A. S., Witte, S., *et al.* (2004). In vivo molecular imaging of acute and subacute thrombosis using a fibrin-binding magnetic resonance imaging contrast agent. *Circulation*, **109**, 2023–9.

Bremer, C., Tung, C. H. and Weissleder, R. (2001). In vivo molecular target assessment of matrix metalloproteinase inhibition., *Nature Medicine*, **7**, 743–8.

British Heart Foundation Health Promotion Research Group. (2005). *Coronary Heart Disease Statistics*. London, UK.

Burke, A. P., Farb, A., Malcom, G. T., *et al.* (1999). Plaque rupture and sudden death related to exertion in men with coronary artery disease. *Journal of the American Medical Association*, **281**, 921–6.

Cannon, C. P., Braunwald, E., McCabe, C. H., *et al.* (2004). Intensive versus moderate lipid lowering with statins after acute coronary syndromes. *New England Journal of Medicine*, **350**, 1495–504.

Choudhury, R. P., Fuster, V. and Fayad, Z. A. (2004). Molecular, cellular and functional imaging of atherothrombosis. *Nature Reviews. Drug Discovery*, **3**, 913–25.

Chu, B., Kampschulte, A., Ferguson, M. S., *et al.* (2004). Hemorrhage in the atherosclerotic carotid plaque: a high-resolution MRI study. *Stroke*, **35**, 1079–84.

Corti, R., Fuster, V., Fayad, Z. A., *et al.* (2005). Effects of aggressive versus conventional lipid-lowering therapy by simvastatin on human atherosclerotic lesions: a prospective, randomized, double-blind trial with high-resolution magnetic resonance imaging. *Journal of the American College of Cardiology*, **46**, 106–12.

Cushing, S. D., Berliner, J. A., Valente, A. J., *et al.* (1990). Minimally modified low density lipoprotein induces monocyte chemotactic protein 1 in human endothelial cells and smooth muscle cells. *Proceedings of the National Academy of Science USA*, **87**, 5134–8.

Faxon, D. P., Fuster, V., Libby, P., *et al.* (2004). Atherosclerotic vascular disease conference: writing group III: pathophysiology. *Circulation*, **109**, 2617–25.

Fayad, Z. A. and Fuster, V. (2000). Characterization of atherosclerotic plaques by magnetic resonance imaging. *Annals of the New York Academy of Science*, **902**, 173–86.

Frias, J. C., Williams, K. J., Fisher, E. A. and Fayad, Z. A. (2004). Recombinant HDL-like nanoparticles: a specific contrast agent for MRI of atherosclerotic plaques. *Journal of the American Chemical Society*, **126**, 16316–17.

Glagov, S., Weisenberg, E., Zarins, C. K., Stankunavicius, R. and Kolettis, G. J. (1987). Compensatory enlargement of human atherosclerotic coronary arteries. *New England Journal of Medicine*, **316**, 1371–5.

Hamilton, J. A., Myers, D., Jessup, W., *et al.* (1999). Oxidized LDL can induce macrophage survival, DNA synthesis, and enhanced proliferative response to CSF-1 and GM-CSF. *Arteriosclerosis, Thrombosis and Vascular Biology*, **19**, 98–105.

Itskovich, V. V., Choudhury, R. P., Aguinaldo, J. G., *et al.* (2003). Characterization of aortic root atherosclerosis in ApoE knockout mice: high-resolution in vivo and ex vivo MRM with histological correlation. *Magnetic Resonance in Medicine*, **49**, 381–5.

Kang, H. W., Josephson, L., Petrovsky, A., Weissleder, R. and Bogdanov, A., Jr. (2002). Magnetic resonance imaging of inducible E-selectin expression in human endothelial cell culture. *Bioconjugate Chemistry*, **13**, 122–7.

Kato, M., Dote, K., Habara, S., *et al.* (2003). Clinical implications of carotid artery remodeling in acute coronary syndrome: ultrasonographic assessment of positive remodeling. *Journal of the American College of Cardiology*, **42**, 1026–32.

Kelly, K. A., Allport, J. R., Tsourkas, A., *et al.* (2005). Detection of vascular adhesion molecule-1 expression using a novel multimodal nanoparticle. *Circulation Research*, **96**, 327–36.

Kerwin, W., Hooker, A. and Spilker, M. (2003). Quantitative magnetic resonance imaging analysis of neovasculature volume in carotid atherosclerotic plaque. *Circulation*, **107**, 851–6.

Kinlay, S., Selwyn, A. P., Libby, P. and Ganz, P. (1998). Inflammation, the endothelium, and the acute coronary syndromes. *Journal of Cardiovascular Pharmacology*, **32** (Suppl. 3), S62–6.

Kolodgie, F. D., Gold, H. K., Burke, A. P., *et al.* (2003). Intraplaque hemorrhage and progression of coronary atheroma. *New England Journal of Medicine*, **349**, 2316–25.

Kooi, M. E., Cappendijk, V. C., Cleutjens, K. B., *et al.* (2003). Accumulation of ultrasmall superparamagnetic particles of iron oxide in human atherosclerotic plaques can be detected by in vivo magnetic resonance imaging. *Circulation*, **107**, 2453–8.

Ku, D. N., Giddens, D. P., Zarins, C. K. and Glagov, S. (1985). Pulsatile flow and atherosclerosis in the human carotid bifurcation. Positive correlation between plaque location and low oscillating shear stress. *Arteriosclerosis*, **5**, 293–302.

Kumamoto, M., Nakashima, Y. and Sueishi, K. (1995). Intimal neovascularization in human coronary atherosclerosis: its origin and pathophysiological significance. *Human Pathology*, **26**, 450–6.

Lauffer, R. B., Parmelee, D. J., Dunham, S. U., *et al.* (1998). MS-325: albumin-targeted contrast agent for MR angiography. *Radiology*, **207**, 529–38.

Libby, P. (2001). Current concepts of the pathogenesis of the acute coronary syndromes. *Circulation*, **104**, 365–72.

Lipinski, M. J., Fuster, V., Fisher, E. A. and Fayad, Z. A. (2004). Technology insight: targeting of biological molecules for evaluation of high-risk atherosclerotic plaques with magnetic resonance imaging. *Nature Clinical Practice. Cardiovascular Medicine*, **1**, 48–55.

Litovsky, S., Madjid, M., Zarrabi, A., *et al.* (2003). Superparamagnetic iron oxide-based method for quantifying recruitment of monocytes to mouse atherosclerotic lesions in vivo: enhancement by tissue necrosis factor-alpha, interleukin-1beta, and interferon-gamma. *Circulation*, **107**, 1545–9.

Lombardo, A., Biasucci, L. M., Lanza, G. A., *et al.* (2004). Inflammation as a possible link between coronary and carotid plaque instability. *Circulation*, **109**, 3158–63.

Mani, V., Briley-Saebo, K. C., Itskovich, V. V., Samber, D. D. and Fayad, Z. A. (2006). Gradient echo acquisition for superparamagnetic particles with positive contrast (GRASP): Sequence characterization in membrane and glass superparamagnetic iron oxide phantoms at 1.5T and 3T. *Magnetic Resonance in Medicine*, **55**, 126–35.

Mani, V., Itskovich, V. V., Szimtenings, M., *et al.* (2004). Rapid extended coverage simultaneous multisection black-blood vessel wall MR imaging. *Radiology*, **232**, 281–8.

Matter, C. M., Schuler, P. K., Alessi, P., *et al.* (2004). Molecular imaging of atherosclerotic plaques using a human antibody against the extra-domain B of fibronectin. *Circulation Research*, **95**, 1225–33.

Naghavi, M., Libby, P., Falk, E., *et al.* (2003). From vulnerable plaque to vulnerable patient: a call for new definitions and risk assessment strategies: Part II. *Circulation*, **108**, 1772–8.

Port, M., Meyer, D., Bonnemain, B., *et al.* (1999). P760 and P775: MRI contrast agents characterized by new pharmacokinetic properties. *Magma*, **8**, 172–6.

Rioufol, G., Finet, G., Ginon, I., *et al.* (2002). Multiple atherosclerotic plaque rupture in acute coronary syndrome: a three-vessel intravascular ultrasound study. *Circulation*, **106**, 804–8.

Rittersma, S. Z., van der Wal, A. C., Koch, K. T., *et al.* (2005). Plaque instability frequently occurs days or weeks before occlusive coronary thrombosis: a pathological thrombectomy study in primary percutaneous coronary intervention. *Circulation*, **111**, 1160–5.

Ross, R. (1999). Atherosclerosis – an inflammatory disease. *New England Journal of Medicine*, **340**, 115–26.

Rudd, J. H., Davies, J. R. and Weissberg, P. L. (2005). Imaging of atherosclerosis – can we predict plaque rupture? *Trends in Cardiovascular Medicine*, **15**, 17–24.

Schafers, M., Riemann, B., Kopka, K., *et al.* (2004). Scintigraphic imaging of matrix metalloproteinase activity in the arterial wall in vivo. *Circulation*, **109**, 2554–9.

Shaalan, W. E., Cheng, H., Gewertz, B., *et al.* (2004). Degree of carotid plaque calcification in relation to symptomatic outcome and plaque inflammation. *Journal of Vascular Surgery*, **40**, 262–9.

Sipkins, D. A., Gijbels, K., Tropper, F. D., *et al.* (2000). ICAM-1 expression in autoimmune encephalitis visualized using magnetic resonance imaging. *Journal of Neuroimmunology*, **104**, 1–9.

Sirol, M., Aguinaldo, J. G., Graham, P. B., *et al.* (2005a). Fibrin-targeted contrast agent for improvement of in vivo acute thrombus detection with magnetic resonance imaging. *Atherosclerosis*, **182**, 79–85.

Sirol, M., Fuster, V., Badimon, J. J., *et al.* (2005b). Chronic thrombus detection with in vivo magnetic resonance imaging and a fibrin-targeted contrast agent. *Circulation*, **112**, 1594–600.

Sirol, M., Itskovich, V. V., Mani, V., *et al.* (2004). Lipid-rich atherosclerotic plaques detected by gadofluorine-enhanced in vivo magnetic resonance imaging. *Circulation*, **109**, 2890–6.

Spagnoli, L. G., Mauriello, A., Sangiorgi, G., *et al.* (2004). Extracranial thrombotically active carotid plaque as a risk factor for ischemic stroke. *Journal of the American Medical Association*, **292**, 1845–52.

Svindland, A. and Torvik, A. (1988). Atherosclerotic carotid disease in asymptomatic individuals: An histological study of 53 cases. *Acta Neurologica Scandinavica*, **78**, 506–17.

Takaya, N., Yuan, C., Chu, B., *et al.* (2005). Presence of intraplaque hemorrhage stimulates progression of carotid atherosclerotic plaques: a high-resolution magnetic resonance imaging study. *Circulation*, **111**, 2768–75.

Toussaint, J. F., LaMuraglia, G. M., Southern, J. F., *et al.* (1996). Magnetic resonance images lipid, fibrous, calcified, hemorrhagic, and thrombotic components of human atherosclerosis in vivo. *Circulation*, **94**, 932–8.

Traub, O. and Berk, B. C. (1998). Laminar shear stress: mechanisms by which endothelial cells transduce an atheroprotective force. *Arteriosclerosis, Thrombosis and Vascular Biology*, **18**, 677–85.

Trivedi, R., King-Im, J. and Gillard, J. (2003). Accumulation of ultrasmall superparamagnetic particles of iron oxide in human atherosclerotic plaque. *Circulation*, **108**, e140.

Trivedi, R. A., King-Im, J. M., Graves, M. J., *et al.* (2004). In vivo detection of macrophages in human carotid atheroma: temporal dependence of ultrasmall superparamagnetic particles of iron oxide-enhanced MRI. *Stroke*, **35**, 1631–5.

VanderLaan, P. A., Reardon, C. A. and Getz, G. S. (2004). Site specificity of atherosclerosis: site-selective responses to atherosclerotic modulators. *Arteriosclerosis, Thrombosis and Vascular Biology*, **24**, 12–22.

Virmani, R., Kolodgie, F. D., Burke, A. P., Farb, A. and Schwartz, S. M. (2000). Lessons from sudden coronary death: a comprehensive morphological classification scheme for atherosclerotic lesions. *Arteriosclerosis, Thrombosis and Vascular Biology*, **20**, 1262–75.

Wilson, P. W., D'Agostino, R. B., Parise, H., Sullivan, L. and Meigs, J. B. (2005). Metabolic syndrome as a precursor of cardiovascular disease and type 2 diabetes mellitus. *Circulation*, **112**, 3066–72.

Winter, P. M., Caruthers, S. D., Yu, X., *et al.* (2003a). Improved molecular imaging contrast agent for detection of human thrombus. *Magnetic Resonance in Medicine*, **50**, 411–16.

Winter, P. M., Morawski, A. M., Caruthers, S. D., *et al.* (2003b). Molecular imaging of angiogenesis in early-stage atherosclerosis with alpha(v)beta3-integrin-targeted nanoparticles. *Circulation*, **108**, 2270–4.

Yancy, A. D., Olzinski, A. R., Hu, T. C., *et al.* (2005). Differential uptake of ferumoxtran-10 and ferumoxytol, ultrasmall superparamagnetic iron oxide contrast agents in rabbit: critical determinants of atherosclerotic plaque labeling. *Journal of Magnetic Resonance Imaging*, **21**, 432–42.

Yu, X., Song, S. K., Chen, J., *et al.* (2000). High-resolution MRI characterization of human thrombus using a novel fibrin-targeted paramagnetic nanoparticle contrast agent. *Magnetic Resonance in Medicine*, **44**, 867–72.

Yuan, C., Kerwin, W. S., Ferguson, M. S., *et al.* (2002a). Contrast-enhanced high resolution MRI for atherosclerotic carotid artery tissue characterization. *Journal of Magnetic Resonance Imaging*, **15**, 62–7.

Yuan, C., Mitsumori, L. M Beach, K. W. and Maravilla, K. R. (2001a). Carotid atherosclerotic plaque: noninvasive MR characterization and identification of vulnerable lesions. *Radiology*, **221**, 285–99.

Yuan, C., Mitsumori, L. M., Ferguson, M. S, *et al.* (2001b). In vivo accuracy of multispectral magnetic resonance imaging for identifying lipid-rich necrotic cores and intraplaque hemorrhage in advanced human carotid plaques. *Circulation*, **104**, 2051–6.

Yuan, C., Zhang, S. X., Polissar, N. L., *et al.* (2002b). Identification of fibrous cap rupture with magnetic resonance imaging is highly associated with recent transient ischemic attack or stroke. *Circulation*, **105**, 181–5.

Zhao, X. Q., Yuan, C., Hatsukami, T. S., *et al.* (2001). Effects of prolonged intensive lipid-lowering therapy on the characteristics of carotid atherosclerotic plaques in vivo by MRI: a case-control study. *Arteriosclerosis, Thrombosis and Vascular Biology*, **21**, 1623–9.

35

Future technical developments

Brian K. Rutt and John A. Ronald

Robarts Research Institute, London ON, Canada

Introduction

In this chapter, we speculate on future developments that are expected to improve our ability to characterize carotid atherosclerotic plaque. To this end, we first introduce the term magnetic resonance (MR) "virtual histology" as a way of organizing our thoughts about these future developments. Then we discuss some technological advancements that should eventually allow MR "virtual histology" of atherosclerosis to become a reality, and the impact that these novel technologies will have on our ability to diagnose and treat atherosclerosis.

MR virtual histology and atherosclerosis

The "gold standard" of tissue identification used in pathology is the histological staining of sections of fixed tissue from the organ of interest. Histology utilizes specific stains to differentiate between tissues, thus separating tissue types with contrasting colors. For example, to identify collagen, we use a stain that is sensitive to the chemical structure of collagen. Histological analysis of atherosclerotic plaque often involves the comparison of normal or asymptomatic tissue to tissue from patients presenting with clinical symptoms, and the subsequent identification and interpretation of any structural or compositional differences between

these tissue types that may explain the clinical symptoms.

Of all the clinical imaging modalities used today, magnetic resonance imaging (MRI) is the most effective and flexible at providing contrast between different tissue types. It does this by probing the chemical environment (i.e. density, chemical and physical state of hydrogen nuclei) of different tissues. Hence adjacent tissues with different properties are contrasted against each other depending on the type of contrast mechanism chosen (e.g. T_1, T_2 and proton density [PD] weighted imaging). In general, the wide variety of contrast mechanisms, each with an associated pulse sequence to emphasize or "weight" that particular contrast mechanism, enable the acquisition of one region of anatomy with numerous contrast mechanisms. Historically, tissue classification by MRI was crude – allowing discrimination between water-based and fat-based tissues, for example, but not much beyond this. However, modern advances in the understanding of novel MRI contrast mechanisms and the development of associated pulse sequences to reveal these contrast mechanisms, as well as innovations in MR contrast agents and significant improvements in MR hardware, have now created the possibility of identifying or classifying many types of tissue using "multicontrast MRI". It is now thought that MRI has the potential to provide as much information about structural differences between pathological

Carotid Disease: The Role of Imaging in Diagnosis and Management, ed. Jonathan Gillard, Martin Graves, Thomas Hatsukami and Chun Yuan. Published by Cambridge University Press. © Cambridge University Press 2007.

tissue types as do histological staining techniques, and that MRI can even provide information about the cellular and molecular makeup of tissue, similar to immunohistochemical techniques. The use of MRI in this way can be considered a sort of "virtual histology", but has the enormous advantages over traditional histology in that it can be done noninvasively, longitudinally and in a living organism. In the future, this will allow better identification of pathological conditions, improved risk stratification of patients, and better tailoring of pharmaceutical or surgical interventions to a patient's needs.

Atherosclerotic lesion composition is now considered to be more important than lesion size for prediction of major cardiac or cerebrovascular events (Zaman *et al.*, 2000). Hence, noninvasive imaging modalities capable of examining lesion composition in a manner similar to histological methods are highly desirable. Development of MR virtual histology for the characterization of atherosclerotic plaque is, therefore, an important and ongoing research goal. MRI is also highly advantageous because it is capable of providing high-resolution images without requirement for invasive transducers or ionizing radiation, providing a desirable method for longitudinal studies of atherosclerosis. As shown in previous chapters, MRI has shown great potential for detailed analysis of plaque structure, cellular content, and even molecular content and activity, and together, these characteristics give MRI the most promising potential of all modalities for differentiating between stable and unstable plaque. For the above reasons, it is important to discuss current and future technical developments that will make MR virtual histology routine in both laboratory and clinic.

Pulse sequences

A variety of MR pulse sequences are available for carotid plaque imaging. The choice of pulse sequence(s) used for a given study should be considered carefully, as specific applications will benefit from certain pulse sequences. These include sequences used for determining lumen size, vessel wall boundaries, vessel wall composition, and contrast enhancement due to contrast agent administration.

Black-blood imaging

The sequence type used most often for vessel wall imaging is the "black-blood" sequence. Briefly, sequences of this type work by nulling signal normally obtained from blood flowing into the slice plane while maintaining signal from the surrounding tissue (i.e. the vessel wall). This increases the conspicuity of distinguishing the vessel wall from the lumen, allowing better identification of vessel wall/luminal boundaries for determining lumen and vessel wall size, and lesion composition. This has been found to be particularly advantageous when using semiautomated or automated algorithms designed to determine luminal and outer vessel wall boundaries (Steinman and Rutt, 1998). Typically, signal from flowing blood is nulled using either a double-inversion recovery (DIR) sequence (Edelman *et al.*, 1991) or by applying either one saturation band proximal to the image slice or saturation bands both proximal and distal to the image plane (Nayak *et al.*, 2001). Sequences employing fast imaging parameters, such as a fast-spin-echo (FSE)/rapid acquisition with relaxation enhancement (RARE) sequence, are then combined with either of the above nulling schema to acquire a single black-blood image (Simonetti *et al.*, 1996; Stemerman *et al.*, 1999). The major drawback of early black-blood techniques was the fact that they were single-slice noninterleaved techniques, resulting in long patient scan times. One resolution of this has been the use of a form of interleaving, in which during each imaging cycle multiple slices are read out in interleaved fashion, but the DIR inversion packet is applied to all slices prior to each readout (Parker *et al.*, 2002). In addition, sequences have been developed that allow sequential collection of multiple slices during each DIR prepulse, resulting in a further factor of 2 or more improvements in time efficiency (Song *et al.*, 2002), or repeating the entire DIR sequence for each slice, with adjustment of the inversion time in a slice-dependent fashion, to further increase efficiency (Yarnykh and Yuan, 2003). Combination and optimization of these various sequence modifications has resulted in the design of a newer sequence called rapid extended coverage (REX) DIR-RARE (Mani *et al.*, 2004). For aortic imaging, use of this sequence resulted in a dramatic 17-fold reduction in acquisition time, whilst maintaining image quality, versus single slice DIR-RARE imaging (Mani *et al.*, 2004).

Minimization of flow-artifacts in black-blood images is important to consider when developing new sequences, as these can influence the accuracy of lesion and luminal size measurements (Steinman and Rutt, 1998). Cardiac-gating of black-blood sequences has been shown to reduce these artifacts within images of the carotid bifurcation (Steinman and Rutt, 1998). However, recent evidence has shown that with the use of improved imaging techniques, such as REX-DIR-RARE, that gating may not be necessary for carotid imaging, allowing for reduction in scan time and improved patient comfort (Mani *et al.*, 2005). Further improvements in black-blood imaging sequences in terms of effective blood-suppression, reduction of acquisition times, and enhanced image quality are expected in the future. As a general rule, it is now felt that acquisition of 30–50 mm coverage in the superior-inferior direction, with 2–3 mm thickness per slice, in a total scan time of 5 minutes or less, is highly desirable for most clinical plaque characterization studies, and the above-mentioned sequence modifications are now reaching this target.

Further speed-up factors of 2 or 3 may be possible through the use of new parallel imaging techniques (such as SENSE, GRAPPA, etc.) in conjunction with large-scale coil arrays designed specifically for carotid bifurcation imaging (Itskovich *et al.*, 2004a; Leiner *et al.*, 2005).

However, such coil arrays are available for brain imaging and large field-of-view neurovascular imaging, but not in general for targeted carotid bifurcation imaging (for example six or more elements clustered tightly around the carotid bifurcation), and therefore, this form of sequence acceleration has only been applied in a very limited way to detailed carotid plaque characterization studies. Despite this limitation, the development of such coils, combined with the application of new parallel imaging techniques, is expected to lead to significant further gains in scan-time efficiency for black-blood carotid plaque imaging as well as other forms of carotid imaging.

Extension of the black-blood sequence concept to true three-dimensional acquisition would have importance in the push toward isotropically-resolved 3D voxels, which should improve plaque quantification. Some efforts have been successful here, mostly aimed at coronary vessel wall and plaque imaging (Botnar *et al.*, 2001; Kim *et al.*, 2002), but there has been limited application of such methods in carotid plaque imaging, likely due to the technical difficulties of motion artifact suppression and adequate blood-signal suppression over the entire 3D slab.

Considerations for multicontrast MRI

To be able to fully characterize a plaque using MRI it has become apparent that it is necessary to collect multiple images of the same plaque using different contrast mechanisms (i.e. different pulse sequence and timing parameters), so called multicontrast MRI. One of the major drawbacks of this technique is the length of time that is required to collect multiple images of different contrast weightings. To address this, one group has developed a DIR-FSE sequence capable of simultaneously collecting three conventional (T_1, T_2 and PD) contrast-weighted images during a single magnetization, which should dramatically reduce patient scan time and improve registration between contrasts (Kim *et al.*, 2004). On top of the challenge of long imaging times, it is also still the case that the optimal field strength, spatial resolution, choice and number of contrasts, and postprocessing tools required to achieve high accuracy and reliability in plaque characterization have not been firmly established. Clarke *et al.* (2003, 2006) has shown that one way to help define the number and type of contrast mechanisms necessary to identify plaque type in vivo is to perform high resolution ex vivo imaging of carotid endarterectomy specimens. This has the advantage of allowing acquisition of a large number of contrasts (this group used eight different contrasts), at high spatial resolution and signal-to-noise ratio, which would be impractical or impossible to achieve in vivo. An additional advantage of ex vivo specimen studies is the use of nontraditional contrast mechanisms, such as diffusion-weighted imaging (DWI), which are technically challenging to accomplish in vivo (and therefore not widely used) but may one day be feasible for in vivo imaging. Following ex vivo imaging of specimens, Clarke *et al.* co-registered MR images to digitized images of the corresponding histological section and a multispectral classification algorithm was trained to identify plaque components pixel-by-pixel based on their spectral signature over the given number of contrast mechanisms chosen. This work has shown that highly accurate classification of plaque can be accomplished using a combination of two conventional sequences (PD and T_1) plus DWI, the latter appearing to be the best at differentiating necrotic core from other plaque components. Figure 35.1 summarizes this work. This group showed that use of the optimal combination of contrast-weightings could accurately differentiate between necrotic material, fibrous tissue, calcification, hemorrhage, and loose connective tissue, and a high level of agreement between MR-based and histopathological American Heart Association classification of lesions was seen. The study also showed that the classification accuracy was significantly reduced when the most commonly used set of three contrast-weightings (PD, T_1, and T_2) was used in the classification process. Tables 35.1 and 35.2

summarize these findings. The understanding that DWI is extremely powerful at distinguishing between necrotic core and fibrous tissue, two of the most significant plaque components contributing to plaque vulnerability, provides incentive to develop new diffusion-weighted pulse sequences capable of high-resolution plaque imaging even in the presence of motion. Sequences based on noncartesian k-space coverage strategies, such as periodically overlapping parallel lines with enhanced reconstruction (PROPELLER) (Pipe *et al.*, 2002), and radial (Sarlls *et al.*, 2005) may have potential in this respect.

Additional postprocessing of the same ex vivo data performed by Ronen (Ronen, 2006) has investigated the influence of both signal-to-noise ratio (SNR) and spatial resolution on classification accuracy. Results show that within a realistic range of voxel size and SNR, SNR is more important than voxel size for achieving high classification accuracy when using three-contrast MRI. Studies such as these will continue to define the optimal pulse sequence types and parameters for accurate plaque compositional assessment, critical information that will enable standardization of protocols for future multicenter studies.

Quantitative mapping of plaques

Despite tremendous progress in the development and preliminary use of high-resolution multicontrast MRI for atherosclerotic plaque characterization, much remains to be done to develop and validate quantitative relaxometric methods for this application. Currently delineation of plaque constituents in vivo is most commonly performed manually, using relative intensity differences between structures in T_1, T_2, and PD images as the decision metric (Yuan and Kerwin, 2004). One reason that automatic classification of structures has not been more successful in vivo has been lack of an absolute image intensity scale, as well as inconsistent signal intensities due to inhomogeneous coil sensitivity profiles. Algorithms to approximately correct for radiofrequency coil

Table 35.1. Optimal subsets of MR contrast-weightings

Number of MR contrast-weightings	Optimal subset	Accuracy $\pm$ SD
1	T1w	57.2 $\pm$ 21.0
2	Dw, T1w	78.2 $\pm$ 7.9
3	Dw, T1w, PDw	82.9 $\pm$ 6.8
4	Dw, T1w, PDw, partial T2w	83.2 $\pm$ 6.3
5	Dw, T1w, PDw, partial T2w, T1w SPGR	83.6 $\pm$ 5.3
6	Dw, T1w, PDw, partial T2w, T1w SPGR, MT SPGR	84.7 $\pm$ 5.5
7	Dw, T1w, PDw, partial T2w, T1w SPGR, MT SPGR, T2w	84.3 $\pm$ 4.8
8	Dw, T1w, PDw, partial T2w, T1w SPGR, MT SPGR, T2w, FIESTA	84.3 $\pm$ 5.0

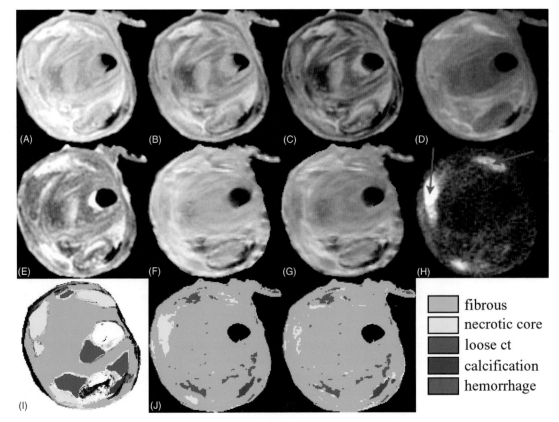

Figure 35.1 Severely stenotic plaque imaged with eight contrast-weightings: (A) PDw; (B) partial T2w; (C) T2w; (D) T1w; (E) FIESTA; (F) T1w SPGR; (G) T1w SPGR with MT; (H) Dw SE (arrows in [H] point to necrotic core, demonstrating Dw sensitivity and specificity for detecting necrotic core); (I) pathologist's segmentation; (J) classification using all eight contrast-weightings; (K) classification using seven contrast-weightings; diffusion excluded.

Table 35.2. Optimal subsets of MR contrast-weightings with Dw contrast excluded

Number of MR contrast-weightings	Optimal subset with diffusion-weighted contrast excluded	Accuracy $\pm$ SD
1	T1w	57.2 ± 21.0
2	T1w, PDw	68.9 ± 21.6
3	T1w, PDw, partial T2w	71.8 ± 20.7
4	T1w, PDw, partial T2w, FIESTA	72.7 ± 19.4
5	T1w, PDw, partial T2w, FIESTA, T2w	73.0 ± 18.5
6	T1w, PDw, partial T2w, FIESTA, T2w, MT SPGR	75.3 ± 16.3
7	T1w, PDw, partial T2w, FIESTA, T2w, MT SPGR, T1w SPGR	76.2 ± 14.5

inhomogeneity have been proposed (Murakami *et al.*, 1996; Han *et al.*, 2001). However, the use of quantitative T_1 and T_2 relaxation time and apparent diffusion coefficient mapping strategies would resolve these problems outright, and should in turn increase our ability to classify internal plaque components both manually and automatically. T_1 and T_2 values of atherosclerotic plaque components have been determined using MRI, although this literature is sparse and incomplete. Morrisett's study determined T_1 and T_2 values of micro-dissected sections of calcified regions, lipid-rich regions and thrombus, as well as T_2 values of calcified/solid lipid, cellular/extracellular matrix, fluid lipid and fibrous tissue, obtained from parametric images of plaque specimens (Morrisett *et al.*, 2003). Toussaint measured T_2 values both in vivo preendarterectomy and ex vivo postendarterectomy (Toussaint *et al.*, 1996). Newer quantitative mapping methods are becoming available that should permit the measurement of the important MR parameters at high resolution and in three dimensions, over the carotid plaque. For example, Deoni *et al.* have invented and implemented highly efficient, three-dimensional T_1 and T_2 mapping methodologies, termed driven equilibrium single pulse observation of T_1 (DESPOT1) and T_2 (DESPOT2), which are believed to be the most efficient combined T_1 and T_2 mapping methods developed to date (Deoni *et al.*, 2003, 2004a). An important extension of this method permits the derivation of quantitative diffusion coefficients

at high resolution in three dimensions (termed driven equilibrium single pulse observation in three dimensions [DESPOD]) (Deoni *et al.*, 2004b). The application of such mapping strategies may make highly reproducible quantitative plaque characterization a reality.

Contrast-enhanced imaging pulse sequences

Contrast-enhanced imaging of vessel wall has shown great potential for increasing our ability to identify the vulnerable plaque. These agents come in two flavors: gadolinium-based (Gd) agents and iron-based agents. To assess contrast enhancement using Gd-based positive contrast agents, typically black-blood sequences, such as T_1 DB-TSE, IR-D-FLASH (Koktzoglou, 2005) or IR-turbo FLASH (Barkhausen *et al.*, 2003), are employed. These sequences are adequate when the interval between pre- and post-contrast administration is long enough to allow for clearance of the agent from the blood. However, for agents that have a transient effect in the vessel wall, black-blood sequences require alterations in timing parameters (most notably inversion time, TI) to maintain a black-blood image due to T_1 shortening effects of the Gd agent in the blood. This change in T_1 has been shown to influence the ability to correctly assess contrast enhancement within the vessel wall, and therefore new sequences for contrast agents acting within a short time frame are being developed. One such sequence employing a quadruple set of preparative inversion recovery (QIR) pulses, called QIR-FSE, allows nulling of in-flowing blood with a range of T_1 values while maintaining the ability to accurately quantify tissue intensity values (Yarnykh and Yuan, 2002). In addition, Sirol *et al.* have developed a sequence, called IR-DIFF-TFL, using a combination of inversion-recovery (IR) and diffusion-based (DIFF) flow suppression prepulses and a segmented gradient echo sequence. This sequence has shown excellent results for nulling of blood signal when contrast agents with high R1 relaxivity values in blood (e.g. Gadofluorine, 17.4 L/mmol/s) are used (Sirol *et al.*, 2004).

Alternatively, iron-based contrast agents, typically ultra small superparamagnetic iron oxide (USPIO) nanoparticles, have been shown to be useful for imaging of macrophages in lesions in both animals and humans (Schmitz *et al.*, 2000, 2001; Ruehm *et al.*, 2001; Kooi *et al.*, 2003; Trivedi *et al.*, 2004). These agents are advantageous over Gd-based agents because of the increased detection sensitivity of MRI to iron-based agents versus Gd-based agents. The contentious disadvantage of USPIO use is that they are negative contrast agents and therefore the amount of agent, and therefore its target, within the tissue of interest is considered difficult to determine. However, some attempts at circumventing this problem have been made. In bright-blood sequences these agents cause a large susceptibility artifact due to T_2 and T_2^*-shortening effects that can extend into the lumen of the vessel. While this "blooming" artifact interferes with localization of agent, its size has recently been used as a surrogate for the amount of agent deposited in the lesion; positive correlations between area of luminal encroachment of the "blooming" artifact and both the area of macrophage-rich lesion and Prussian-blue iron staining within the corresponding histological sections were found (Hyafil *et al.*, 2006). In addition, some work has been done to develop pulse sequences that are iron-specific, creating a positive, rather than negative, contrast in the area where the iron-based agents have accumulated (Coristine *et al.*, 2004; Cunningham *et al.*, 2005; Pintaske *et al.*, 2005). This

would allow a more direct assessment of agent concentration within the vessel wall than methods such as the surrogates used above.

Both Gd- and iron-based contrast agent studies can also benefit from the application of quantitative mapping techniques such as DESPOT1 and DESPOT2 described above (Deoni *et al.*, 2003). Since Gd-based agents act by shortening T_1, while iron-based agents shorten T_2 and T_2^*, this means that measurement of these relaxation times should improve the sensitivity of MRI for characterizing those plaque pathophysiological features that govern contrast agent uptake.

It is expected that pulse sequence technology will continue to advance at a rapid pace, and will lead to novel contrast mechanisms as well as new capabilities to suppress motion artifacts and blood flow effects, and to highlight specific plaque components.

MR hardware

The three hardware subsystems that are important in the discussion of technical advancements are: (1) the MR machine; (2) the gradient coils; and (3) the radiofrequency (RF) coils. Here a brief introduction to each component and the novel innovations being developed will be discussed.

MR scanner and field strength

First high image quality can be thought of as the collection of images with a resolution and SNR sufficient to clearly identify the most important or relevant plaque constituents. Importantly, the signal-to-noise ratio in the resulting images is thought to scale linearly with the main magnetic field strength, reported in units of Tesla (T), of the MR machine used. Present-day clinical scanners work at 1.5 T (most commonly) or more recently 3 T, compared to the higher field strengths found in whole-body ultra-high-field scanners now available from the major vendors (e.g. 7 T) or animal machines (e.g. 11 T or higher). Despite the relative lack of published data on the value of field strengths higher than 1.5 T for carotid plaque imaging, it is beginning to be clear that imaging at 3 T will provide concrete benefits of higher SNR and possibly improved blood suppression and tissue contrast (especially in the presence of contrast agents). It is safe to assume that greater accuracy and/or more efficient scanning will be achievable when working at this higher field strength, and that the bulk of clinical research into human atherosclerotic plaque imaging will occur at 3 T in the future.

Gradient coils

Ex vivo plaque imaging has been an essential tool for the development of all forms of MR virtual histological techniques. This has been largely due to the ability to collect high quality images not easily obtainable in vivo. Most commonly, very high field scanners (e.g. 9.4 T) have been used for this purpose (Itskovich et al., 2003, 2004b). Alternatively, studies have shown that dedicated gradient coil inserts for low field strength clinical scanners are also capable of providing significant improvements in image quality (Martin et al., 1995; Clarke et al., 2003, 2006). Gradient hardware performance for conventional whole-body gradient coils is rapidly reaching the physiological limitation of peripheral nerve stimulation (Chronik and Rutt, 2001a,b; Zhang et al., 2003). Therefore, improvement of gradient performance for in vivo imaging will be dependent on the development of innovative concepts in local gradient hardware, such as insertable gradient coils for head/neck imaging (Chronik et al., 2000) or surface/open gradient coils (Green et al., 2005).

RF coils

In addition to gradient technology, the use of optimized RF coils continues to have a strong impact on image quality. The optimal RF coil design is dictated by its intended purpose. Examples include the use of small solenoid coils

for ex vivo imaging of specimens (Clarke et al., 2003, 2006), dedicated phased-array surface coils for superficial vessel imaging (Hayes et al., 1996; von Ingersleben et al., 1997; Hadley et al., 2000), and the design of intravascular coils for imaging of vascular beds not easily imaged with surface coils due to their depth within the body (Worthley et al., 2003; Larose et al., 2005). Finally, the advent of parallel imaging in the last 5–7 years is opening new doors and opportunities for generating high image quality in shorter scan times, utilizing large-scale arrays of RF coil elements (Itskovich et al., 2004a). It is expected that the use of 8-, 16- or 32-element arrays for carotid artery imaging will improve image quality or lead to considerably more time-efficient studies as these coils become available in the future. Figure 35.2 shows

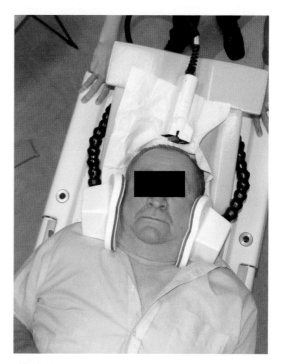

Figure 35.2 Bilateral 6-channel coil designed for high resolution carotid plaque imaging at 3T. Prototype designed by E. Boskamp, L. Blawat, A. Alejski and B. Rutt (GE Healthcare Technologies and Robarts Research Institute).

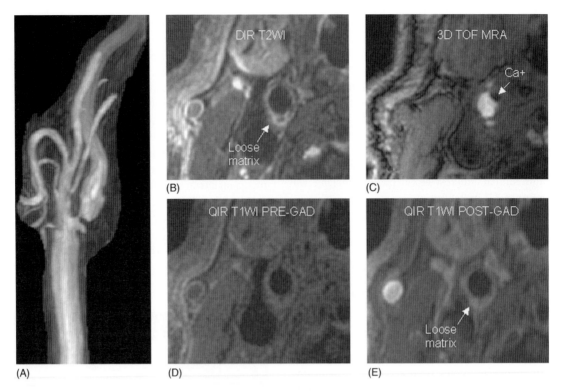

Figure 35.3 Contrast-enhanced MRA (A) and multicontrast imaging of carotid plaque (B–E), acquired using 6-channel carotid bifurcation coil (see Figure 35.2) at 3T. Images show excellent spatial resolution and signal-to-noise ratio, despite rapid scan time (less than 5 minutes per contrast-weighting) and large coverage (total of 18.2 mm slices in the superior-inferior direction). Images courtesy of K. DeMarco (Michigan State University).

a prototype 6-channel coil designed for carotid bifurcation imaging at 3 T, while Figure 35.3 shows high-resolution carotid plaque images produced with this coil in less than 5 minutes per contrast-weighting.

Images of atherosclerotic plaque have been obtained with in-plane voxel dimensions as low as 0.25 mm in the carotid, 0.8 mm in the aorta and 0.5 mm in the coronaries, and with slice thicknesses between 2 and 5 mm (Yuan *et al.*, 1996, 2001; Fayad and Fuster, 2000; Fayad *et al.*, 2000). Hardware advances, such as those described above, will permit the acquisition of such high resolution images in human studies within relatively short acquisition times, such as less than 5 minutes per MR contrast.

Future of contrast agents

In addition to the conventional and targeted contrast agents described in the previous chapters and sections, progress in the development of "activatable" agents for plaque imaging has also occurred. In one case, this has involved the development of a low molecular weight paramagnetic (Gd-based) enzyme pseudosubstrate that oligomerizes in the presence of myeloperoxidase (MPO) and hydrogen peroxide, resulting in signal amplification (Bogdanov *et al.*, 2002; Chen *et al.*, 2004). This amplification strategy makes this agent much more sensitive to its molecular target than the simpler targeted agents such as those described in previous chapters. MPO was chosen as an excellent molecular target for atherosclerotic plaque imaging for various reasons. Emerging evidence suggests that activated macrophages secrete various enzymes that mediate inflammation in atherosclerosis (Libby *et al.*, 2002). In particular, MPO appears to be a marker of active inflammation in high-risk ("vulnerable") atheromata (Sugiyama *et al.*, 2001; Heinecke, 2003). Furthermore, a recent clinical study has shown that elevated plasma MPO concentrations strongly predict adverse cardiovascular outcomes in patients with chest pain (Brennan and Hazen, 2003; Brennan *et al.*, 2003). Therefore, in vivo MRI of MPO activity may directly identify biologically vulnerable (active inflammatory) atherosclerotic lesions, thereby dramatically improving our capability to characterize atherosclerotic plaque. It is expected that considerable effort will be directed toward development of these types of "activatable" agents in the future using similar or novel amplification strategies. Clearly innovative advancements in the chemistry of contrast agents such as that described here will dramatically influence how MRI will be used to distinguish stable and unstable atherosclerotic lesions in future.

Summary

Recently, therapeutic strategies for treatment of atherosclerosis have changed focus from plaque reduction to plaque stabilization (Libby and Aikawa, 2002). This has largely occurred as a result of increasing experimental and clinical evidence showing that the mechanism whereby statin therapy lowers the risk of cardiovascular events is largely attributable to effects of these agents on lesion stability, related to altered plaque composition, rather than reduction in absolute plaque size (Brown *et al.*, 1993; Lee, 2000, Mitani *et al.*, 2003). However, current detection of arterial lesion burden is usually restricted to measures of luminal stenosis with angiography or lesion size using other modalities, neither of which necessarily

predict lesion stability. Overwhelming evidence supports the current concept that lesion stability is very closely linked with lesion composition and the underlying physiological processes occurring within the vessel wall (Ambrose *et al.*, 1985; Fuster *et al.*, 1992; Falk and Fernandez-Ortiz, 1995; Mann and Davies, 1996; Falk, 1999; Welt and Simon, 2001). Thus, the future of atherosclerotic plaque imaging will by definition be dominated by those modalities capable of characterizing lesion composition, ideally down to the cellular and molecular levels.

MRI is an excellent candidate method for this purpose because it can provide serial high-resolution images of the vessel wall without the requirement of invasive transducers or ionizing radiation. In addition, MRI is capable of identifying a large number of tissue types using both conventional and contrast-mediated techniques, making it possible to use such "MR virtual histology" to identify plaques in a way similar to histological identification of plaque type. To accurately distinguish between "unstable" and "stable" plaques, several MR techniques are available, including multicontrast MRI, cellular MR imaging and molecular MR imaging. In the future, convergence between these imaging techniques, all in the same patient, will most likely become a necessity in order to allow risk stratification of individual patients. This is for two reasons: atherosclerosis now being considered a multifactorial disease, and the identification of new imaging targets related to plaque stability. As we learn more about plaque biology and the underlying processes leading to plaque rupture and clinical events, more imaging targets will be recognized. The development of robust plaque characterization tools will also be important because novel therapeutic interventions may target stability in different ways and the outcome of those interventions will need to be assessed. Ultimately, it is expected that these techniques will lead to efficient titration and customization of therapeutic strategies for stabilization of vulnerable plaques throughout the body, leading to better patient care.

REFERENCES

Ambrose, J. A., Winters, S. L., Arora, R. R., *et al.* (1985). Coronary angiographic morphology in myocardial infarction: a link between the pathogenesis of unstable angina and myocardial infarction. *Journal of the American College of Cardiology*, **6**, 1233–8.

Barkhausen, J., Ebert, W., Heyer, C., Debatin, J. F. and Weinmann, H. J. (2003). Detection of atherosclerotic plaque with Gadofluorine-enhanced magnetic resonance imaging. *Circulation*, **108**, 605–9.

Bogdanov, A., Jr., Matuszewski, L., Bremer, C., Petrovsky, A. and Weissleder, R. (2002). Oligomerization of paramagnetic substrates result in signal amplification and can be used for MR imaging of molecular targets. *Molecular Imaging*, **1**, 16–23.

Botnar, R. M., Kim, W. Y., Bornert, P., *et al.* (2001). 3D coronary vessel wall imaging utilizing a local inversion technique with spiral image acquisition. *Magnetic Resonance in Medicine*, **46**, 848–54.

Brennan, M. L. and Hazen, S. L. (2003). Emerging role of myeloperoxidase and oxidant stress markers in cardiovascular risk assessment. *Current Opinion in Lipidology*, **14**, 353–9.

Brennan, M. L., Penn, M. S., Van Lente, F., *et al* (2003). Prognostic value of myeloperoxidase in patients with chest pain. *New England Journal of Medicine*, **349**, 1595–604.

Brown, B. G., Zhao, X. Q., Sacco, D. E. and Albers, J. J. (1993). Lipid lowering and plaque regression. New insights into prevention of plaque disruption and clinical events in coronary disease. *Circulation*, **87**, 1781–91.

Chen, J. W., Pham, W., Weissleder, R. and Bogdanov, A., Jr. (2004). Human myeloperoxidase: a potential target for molecular MR imaging in atherosclerosis. *Magnetic Resonance in Medicine*, **52**, 1021–8.

Chronik, B. A., Alejski, A. and Rutt, B. K. (2000). Design and fabrication of a three-axis edge ROU head and neck gradient coil. *Magnetic Resonance in Medicine*, **44**, 955–63.

Chronik, B. A. and Rutt, B. K. (2001a). A comparison between human magnetostimulation thresholds in whole-body and head/neck gradient coils. *Magnetic Resonance in Medicine*, **46**, 386–94.

Chronik, B. A. and Rutt, B. K. (2001b). Simple linear formulation for magnetostimulation specific to MRI gradient coils. *Magnetic Resonance in Medicine*, **45**, 916–19.

Clarke, S. E., Beletsky, V., Hammond, R. R., Hegele, R. A. and Rutt, B. K. (2006). Validation of automatically classified magnetic resonance images for carotid plaque compositional analysis. *Stroke*, **37**, 93–7.

Clarke, S. E., Hammond, R. R., Mitchell, J. R. and Rutt, B. K. (2003). Quantitative assessment of carotid plaque composition using multicontrast MRI and registered histology. *Magnetic Resonance in Medicine*, **50**, 1199–208.

Coristine, A. J. F. P., Deoni, S. C. L., Heyn C. and Rutt, B. K. (2004). Positive contrast labelling of spio loaded cells in cell samples and spinal chord injury. *International Society for Magnetic Resonance in Medicine 12th Annual Scientific Meeting and Exhibition*. Kyoto, Japan.

Cunningham, C. H., Arai, T., Yang, P. C., *et al.* (2005). Positive contrast magnetic resonance imaging of cells labeled with magnetic nanoparticles. *Magnetic Resonance in Medicine*, **53**, 999–1005.

Deoni, S. C., Peters, T. M. and Rutt, B. K. (2004a). Determination of optimal angles for variable nutation proton magnetic spin-lattice, T1, and spin-spin, T2, relaxation times measurement. *Magnetic Resonance in Medicine*, **51**, 194–9.

Deoni, S. C., Peters, T. M. and Rutt, B. K. (2004b). Quantitative diffusion imaging with steady-state free precession. *Magnetic Resonance in Medicine*, **51**, 428–33.

Deoni, S. C., Rutt, B. K. and Peters, T. M. (2003). Rapid combined T1 and T2 mapping using gradient recalled acquisition in the steady state. *Magnetic Resonance in Medicine*, **49**, 515–26.

Edelman, R. R., Chien, D. and Kim, D. (1991). Fast selective black blood MR imaging. *Radiology*, **181**, 655–60.

Falk, E. (1999). Stable versus unstable atherosclerosis: clinical aspects. *American Heart Journal*, **138**, S421–5.

Falk, E. and Fernandez-Ortiz, A. (1995). Role of thrombosis in atherosclerosis and its complications. *American Journal of Cardiology*, **75**, 3B-11B.

Fayad, Z. A. and Fuster, V. (2000). Characterization of atherosclerotic plaques by magnetic resonance imaging. *Annals of the New York Academy of Sciences*, **902**, 173–86.

Fayad, Z. A., Nahar, T., Fallon, J. T., *et al.* (2000). In vivo magnetic resonance evaluation of atherosclerotic plaques in the human thoracic aorta: a comparison with transesophageal echocardiography. *Circulation*, **101**, 2503–9.

Fuster, V., Badimon, L., Badimon, J. J. and Chesebro, J. H. (1992). The pathogenesis of coronary artery disease and the acute coronary syndromes (2). *New England Journal of Medicine*, **326**, 310–18.

Green, D., Leggett, J. and Bowtell, R. (2005). Hemispherical gradient coils for magnetic resonance imaging. *Magnetic Resonance in Medicine*, **54**, 656–68.

Hadley, J. R., Chapman, B. E., Roberts, J. A., et al. (2000). A three-coil comparison for MR angiography. *Journal of Magnetic Resonance Imaging*, **11**, 458–68.

Han, C., Hatsukami, T. S. and Yuan, C. (2001). A multi-scale method for automatic correction of intensity non-uniformity in MR images. *Journal of Magnetic Resonance Imaging*, **13**, 428–36.

Hayes, C. E., Mathis, C. M. and Yuan, C. (1996). Surface coil phased arrays for high-resolution imaging of the carotid arteries. *Journal of Magnetic Resonance Imaging*, **6**, 109–12.

Heinecke, J. W. (2003). Oxidative stress: new approaches to diagnosis and prognosis in atherosclerosis. *American Journal of Cardiology*, **91**, 12A–16A.

Hyafil, F., Laissy, J. P., Mazighi, M., et al. (2006). Ferumoxtran-10-enhanced MRI of the hypercholesterolemic rabbit aorta: relationship between signal loss and macrophage infiltration. *Arteriosclerosis, Thrombosis, and Vascular Biology*, **26**, 176–81.

Itskovich, V. V., Choudhury, R. P., Aguinaldo, J. G., et al. (2003). Characterization of aortic root atherosclerosis in ApoE knockout mice: high-resolution in vivo and ex vivo MRM with histological correlation. *Magnetic Resonance in Medicine*, **49**, 381–5.

Itskovich, V. V., Mani, V., Mizsei, G., et al. (2004a). Parallel and nonparallel simultaneous multislice black-blood double inversion recovery techniques for vessel wall imaging. *Journal of Magnetic Resonance Imaging*, **19**, 459–67.

Itskovich, V. V., Samber, D. D., Mani, V., et al. (2004b). Quantification of human atherosclerotic plaques using spatially enhanced cluster analysis of multicontrast-weighted magnetic resonance images. *Magnetic Resonance in Medicine*, **52**, 515–23.

Kim, S. E., Kholmovski, E. G., Jeong, E. K., et al. (2004). Triple contrast technique for black blood imaging with double inversion preparation. *Magnetic Resonance in Medicine*, **52**, 1379–87.

Kim, W. Y., Stuber, M., Bornert, P., et al. (2002). Three-dimensional black-blood cardiac magnetic resonance coronary vessel wall imaging detects positive arterial remodeling in patients with nonsignificant coronary artery disease. *Circulation*, **106**, 296–9.

Koktzoglou, I. H. K. R., Kane B. J., Tang, R., et al. (2005). Gadofluorine-enhanced magnetic resonance imaging of atherosclerotic plaque in swine. *International Society for Magnetic Resonance in Medicine 13th Scientific Meeting and Exhibition*. South Beach, Miami.

Kooi, M. E., Cappendijk, V. C., Cleutjens, K. B., et al. (2003). Accumulation of ultrasmall superparamagnetic particles of iron oxide in human atherosclerotic plaques can be detected by in vivo magnetic resonance imaging. *Circulation*, **107**, 2453–8.

Larose, E., Yeghiazarians, Y., Libby, P., et al. (2005). Characterization of human atherosclerotic plaques by intravascular magnetic resonance imaging. *Circulation*, **112**, 2324–31.

Lee, R. T. (2000). Plaque stabilization: the role of lipid lowering. *International Journal of Cardiology*, **74** (Suppl. 1), S11–15.

Leiner, T., Gerretsen, S., Botnar, R., et al. (2005). Magnetic resonance imaging of atherosclerosis. *European Radiology*, **15**, 1087–99.

Libby, P. and Aikawa, M. (2002). Stabilization of atherosclerotic plaques: new mechanisms and clinical targets. *Nature Medicine*, **8**, 1257–62.

Libby, P., Ridker, P. M. and Maseri, A. (2002). Inflammation and atherosclerosis. *Circulation*, **105**, 1135–43.

Mani, V., Itskovich, V. V., Aguiar, S. H., et al. (2005). Comparison of gated and non-gated fast multislice black-blood carotid imaging using rapid extended coverage and inflow/outflow saturation techniques. *Journal of Magnetic Resonance Imaging*, **22**, 628–33.

Mani, V., Itskovich, V. V., Szimtenings, M., et al. (2004). Rapid extended coverage simultaneous multisection black-blood vessel wall MR imaging. *Radiology*, **232**, 281–8.

Mann, J. M. and Davies, M. J. (1996). Vulnerable plaque. Relation of characteristics to degree of stenosis in human coronary arteries. *Circulation*, **94**, 928–31.

Martin, A. J., Gotlieb, A. I. and Henkelman, R. M. (1995). High-resolution MR imaging of human arteries. *Journal of Magnetic Resonance Imaging*, **5**, 93–100.

Mitani, H., Egashira, K. and Kimura, M. (2003). HMG-CoA reductase inhibitor, fluvastatin, has cholesterol-lowering independent "direct" effects on atherosclerotic vessels in high cholesterol diet-fed rabbits. *Pharmacology Research*, **48**, 417–27.

Morriset, J., Vick, W., Sharma, R., et al. (2003). Discrimination of components in atherosclerotic plaques from human carotid endarterectomy specimens by magnetic resonance imaging ex vivo. *Magnetic Resonance Imaging*, **21**, 465–74.

Murakami, J.W., Hayes, C.E. and Weinberger, E. (1996). Intensity correction of phased-array surface coil images. *Magnetic Resonance in Medicine*, **35**, 585–90.

Nayak, K.S., Rivas, P.A., Pauly, J.M., *et al.* (2001). Real-time black-blood MRI using spatial presaturation. *Journal of Magnetic Resonance Imaging*, **13**, 807–12.

Parker, D.L., Goodrich, K.C., Masiker, M., Tsuruda, J.S. and Katzman, G.L. (2002). Improved efficiency in double-inversion fast spin-echo imaging. *Magnetic Resonance in Medicine*, **47**, 1017–21.

Pintaske, J., Martirosian, P., Claussen, C.D. and Schick, F. (2005). Positive contrast in the detection of magnetically labeled cells by MRI – in vitro experiments. *Biomedical Technology (Berl)*, **50**, 271–6.

Pipe, J.G., Farthing, V.G. and Forbes, K.P. (2002). Multi-shot diffusion-weighted FSE using PROPELLER MRI. *Magnetic Resonance in Medicine*, **47**, 42–52.

Ronen, R.R., Clarke, S.E., Hammond, R.R. and Rutt, B.K. (2006). Resolution and SNR effects on carotid plaque classification. *Magnetic Resonance in Medicine*, **56**, 290–5.

Ruehm, S.G., Corot, C., Vogt, P., Cristina, H. and Debatin, J.F. (2002). Ultrasmall superparamagnetic iron oxide-enhanced MR imaging of atherosclerotic plaque in hyperlipidemic rabbits. *Academy of Radiology*, **9** (Suppl. 1), S143–4.

Ruehm, S.G., Corot, C., Vogt, P., Kolb, S. and Debatin, J.F. (2001). Magnetic resonance imaging of atherosclerotic plaque with ultrasmall superparamagnetic particles of iron oxide in hyperlipidemic rabbits. *Circulation*, **103**, 415–22.

Sarlls, J.E., Newbould, R.D., Altbach, M.I., *et al.* (2005). Isotropic diffusion weighting in radial fast spin-echo magnetic resonance imaging. *Magnetic Resonance in Medicine*, **53**, 1347–54.

Schmitz, S.A., Coupland, S.E., Gust, R., *et al.* (2000). Superparamagnetic iron oxide-enhanced MRI of atherosclerotic plaques in Watanabe hereditable hyperlipidemic rabbits. *Investigative Radiology*, **35**, 460–71.

Schmitz, S.A., Taupitz, M., Wagner, S., *et al.* (2001). Magnetic resonance imaging of atherosclerotic plaques using superparamagnetic iron oxide particles. *Journal of Magnetic Resonance Imaging*, **14**, 355–61.

Simonetti, O.P., Finn, J.P., White, R.D., Laub, G. and Henry, D.A. (1996). "Black blood" T2-weighted inversion-recovery MR imaging of the heart. *Radiology*, **199**, 49–57.

Sirol, M., Itskovich, V.V., Mani, V., *et al.* (2004). Lipid-rich atherosclerotic plaques detected by gadofluorine-enhanced in vivo magnetic resonance imaging. *Circulation*, **109**, 2890–6.

Song, H.K., Wright, A.C., Wolf, R.L. and Wehrli, F.W. (2002). Multislice double inversion pulse sequence for efficient black-blood MRI. *Magnetic Resonance in Medicine*, **47**, 616–20.

Steinman, D.A. and Rutt, B.K. (1998). On the nature and reduction of plaque-mimicking flow artifacts in black blood MRI of the carotid bifurcation. *Magnetic Resonance in Medicine*, **39**, 635–41.

Stemerman, D.H., Krinsky, G.A., Lee, V.S., *et al.* (1999). Thoracic aorta: rapid black-blood MR imaging with half-Fourier rapid acquisition with relaxation enhancement with or without electrocardiographic triggering. *Radiology*, **213**, 185–91.

Sugiyama, S., Okada, Y., Sukhova, G.K., *et al.* (2001). Macrophage myeloperoxidase regulation by granulocyte macrophage colony-stimulating factor in human atherosclerosis and implications in acute coronary syndromes. *American Journal of Pathology*, **158**, 879–91.

Toussaint, J.F., Lamuraglia, G.M., Southern, J.F., Fuster, V. and Kantor, H.L. (1996). Magnetic resonance images lipid, fibrous, calcified, hemorrhagic, and thrombotic components of human atherosclerosis in vivo. *Circulation*, **94**, 932–8.

Trivedi, R.A., U-King-Im, J.M., Graves, M.J., *et al.* (2004). In vivo detection of macrophages in human carotid atheroma: temporal dependence of ultrasmall superparamagnetic particles of iron oxide-enhanced MRI. *Stroke*, **35**, 1631–5.

Von Ingersleben, G., Schmiedl, U.P., Hatsukami, T.S., *et al.* (1997). Characterization of atherosclerotic plaques at the carotid bifurcation: correlation of high-resolution MR imaging with histologic analysis – preliminary study. *Radiographics*, **17**, 1417–23.

Welt, F.G. and Simon, D.I. (2001). Atherosclerosis and plaque rupture. *Catheterization and Cardiovascular Intervention*, **53**, 56–63.

Worthley, S.G., Helft, G., Fuster, V., *et al.* (2003). A novel nonobstructive intravascular MRI coil: in vivo imaging of experimental atherosclerosis. *Arteriosclerosis, Thrombosis, and Vascular Biology*, **23**, 346–50.

Yarnykh, V.L. and Yuan, C. (2002). T1-insensitive flow suppression using quadruple inversion-recovery. *Magnetic Resonance in Medicine*, **48**, 899–905.

Yarnykh, V. L. and Yuan, C. (2003). Multislice double inversion-recovery black-blood imaging with simultaneous slice reinversion. *Journal of Magnetic Resonance Imaging*, **17**, 478–83.

Yuan, C. and Kerwin, W. S. (2004). MRI of atherosclerosis. *Journal of Magnetic Resonance Imaging*, **19**, 710–19.

Yuan, C., Mitsumori, L. M., Beach, K. W. and Maravilla, K. R. (2001). Carotid atherosclerotic plaque: noninvasive MR characterization and identification of vulnerable lesions. *Radiology*, **221**, 285–99.

Yuan, C., Skinner, M. P., Kaneko, E., *et al.* (1996). Magnetic resonance imaging to study lesions of atherosclerosis in the hyperlipidemic rabbit aorta. *Magnetic Resonance Imaging*, **14**, 93–102.

Zaman, A. G., Helft, G., Worthley, S. G. and Badimon, J. J. (2000). The role of plaque rupture and thrombosis in coronary artery disease. *Atherosclerosis*, **149**, 251–66.

Zhang, B., Yen, Y. F., Chronik, B. A., *et al.* (2003). Peripheral nerve stimulation properties of head and body gradient coils of various sizes. *Magnetic Resonance in Medicine*, **50**, 50–8.

Index